T0320653

NEUROBIOLOGICAL ISSUES IN AUTISM

CURRENT ISSUES IN AUTISM

Series Editors: Eric Schopler and Gary B. Mesibov

University of North Carolina School of Medicine
Chapel Hill, North Carolina

AUTISM IN ADOLESCENTS AND ADULTS
Edited by Eric Schopler and Gary B. Mesibov

COMMUNICATION PROBLEMS IN AUTISM
Edited by Eric Schopler and Gary B. Mesibov

THE EFFECTS OF AUTISM ON THE FAMILY
Edited by Eric Schopler and Gary B. Mesibov

NEUROBIOLOGICAL ISSUES IN AUTISM
Edited by Eric Schopler and Gary B. Mesibov

SOCIAL BEHAVIOR IN AUTISM
Edited by Eric Schopler and Gary B. Mesibov

NEUROBIOLOGICAL ISSUES IN AUTISM

Edited by
Eric Schopler
and
Gary B. Mesibov

University of North Carolina School of Medicine
Chapel Hill, North Carolina

PLENUM PRESS • NEW YORK AND LONDON

Library of Congress Cataloging in Publication Data

Neurobiological issues in autism.

(Current issues in autism)
Based on the 6th Annual TEACCH Conference held in Chapel Hill in 1985.
Includes bibliographies and index.
1. Autism—Congresses. 2. Neurobiology—Congresses. I. Schopler, Eric. II. Mesibov,
Gary B. III. TEACCH Conference (6th: 1985: Chapel Hill, N.C.) IV. Series. [DNLM: 1.
Autism—congresses. 2. Neurobiology—congresses. WM 203.5 N494 1985]
RC553.A88N48   1987   616.89′82   87-2441
ISBN 0-306-42451-7

10 9 8 7 6 5 4 3 2

© 1987 Plenum Press, New York
A Division of Plenum Publishing Corporation
233 Spring Street, New York, N.Y. 10013

Printed in the United States of America

To the North Carolina children and adults with autism and their families in the hope that the exciting new developments in this book will lead to new ways to assist in their struggle

Contributors

MARGARET L. BAUMAN, Pediatric Neurology Unit, Massachusetts General Hospital, Boston, Massachusetts 02114

GEORGE R. BREESE, Departments of Psychiatry and Pharmacology, Child Development Institute and Mental Health Clinical Research Center, University of North Carolina, Chapel Hill, North Carolina 27514

MAGDA CAMPBELL, Department of Psychiatry, New York University Medical Center, New York, New York 10016

LARRY R. CHURCHILL, Departments of Social and Administrative Medicine and Religious Studies, University of North Carolina, Chapel Hill, North Carolina 27514

ROLAND D. CIARANELLO, Division of Child Psychiatry and Child Development, Department of Psychiatry and Behavioral Sciences, Stanford University School of Medicine, Stanford, California 94305

MARY COLEMAN, Children's Brain Research Clinic, Washington, DC 20008; and Georgetown University School of Medicine, Washington, DC 20007

ERIC COURCHESNE, Neurosciences Department, School of Medicine, University of California at San Diego, La Jolla, California 92093; and Neuropsychology Research Laboratory, Children's Hospital Research Center, San Diego, California 92123

ALAN W. CROSS, Departments of Social and Administrative Medicine and Pediatrics, University of North Carolina, Chapel Hill, North Carolina 27514

GERALDINE DAWSON, Department of Psychology, University of Washington, Seattle, Washington 98195

G. ROBERT DeLONG, Pediatric Neurology Unit, Massachusetts General Hospital, Boston, Massachusetts 02114

MARTHA B. DENCKLA, Developmental Neurology Branch, National Institute of Neurological and Communicative Disorders and Stroke, Bethesda, Maryland 20205

GLEN R. ELLIOTT, Division of Child Psychiatry and Child Development, Department of Psychiatry and Behavioral Sciences, Stanford University School of Medicine, Stanford, California 94305

RANDALL W. EVANS, Biological Sciences Research Center, University of North Carolina, Chapel Hill, North Carolina 27514

DEBORAH FEIN, Laboratory of Neuropsychology, Boston University Medical Center, Boston, Massachusetts 02118

SUSAN E. FOLSTEIN, Division of Psychiatric Genetics, Department of Psychiatry, Johns Hopkins University, Baltimore, Maryland 21205

DANIEL X. FREEDMAN, Department of Psychiatry, University of California at Los Angeles, Los Angeles, California 90024

WAYNE H. GREEN, Department of Psychiatry, New York University Medical Center, New York, New York 10016

THOMAS GUALTIERI, Department of Psychiatry, University of North Carolina, Chapel Hill, North Carolina 27514

NANCY M. P. KING, Department of Social and Administrative Medicine, University of North Carolina, Chapel Hill, North Carolina 27514

MARCEL KINSBOURNE, Eunice Kennedy Shriver Center for Mental Retardation, Waltham, Massachusetts 02254; and Harvard Medical School, Boston, Massachusetts 02115

EUGENE M. C. LEE, Child at Risk Project, Department of Psychiatry and Behavioral Sciences, University of Washington School of Medicine, Harborview Medical Center, Seattle, Washington 98104

CATHERINE LORD, Department of Pediatrics, University of Alberta, and Department of Psychology, Glenrose Hospital, Edmonton, Alberta T5G 0B7, Canada

GARY B. MESIBOV, Division TEACCH, University of North Carolina, Chapel Hill, North Carolina 27514

ROBERT A. MUELLER, Departments of Anesthesiology and Pharmacology, University of North Carolina, Chapel Hill, North Carolina 27514

JAAK PANKSEPP, Department of Psychology, Bowling Green State University, Bowling Green, Ohio 43403

DEBRA R. PATTERSON, Biological Sciences Research Center, University of North Carolina, Chapel Hill, North Carolina 27514

BRUCE PENNINGTON, University of Colorado Health Sciences Center, Denver, Colorado 80262

RICHARD PERRY, Department of Psychiatry, New York University Medical Center, New York, New York 10016

DANIEL J. RAITEN, Department of Behavioral Medicine, Children's Hospital, National Medical Center, Washington, DC 20010

ROBERT JAY REICHLER, Child at Risk Project, Department of Psychiatry and Behavioral Sciences, University of Washington School of Medicine, Harborview Medical Center, Seattle, Washington 98104

BERNARD RIMLAND, Institute for Child Behavior Research, San Diego, California 92116

JUDITH M. RUMSEY, Child Psychiatry Branch, National Institute of Mental Health, Bethesda, Maryland 20892

MICHAEL L. RUTTER, M. R. C. Child Psychiatry Unit, Department of Child and Adolescent Psychiatry, Institute of Psychiatry, University of London, De Crespigny Park, Denmark Hill, London SE5 8AF, England

TONY L. SAHLEY, Coleman Memorial Laboratory, Department of Otolaryngology, University of California, San Francisco, California 94143

ERIC SCHOPLER, Division TEACCH, University of North Carolina, Chapel Hill, North Carolina 27514

STEPHEN R. SCHROEDER, Department of Psychiatry, Child Development Institute, University of North Carolina, Chapel Hill, North Carolina 27514

MICHAEL C. SHARP, Department of Pediatrics, University of North Carolina, Chapel Hill, North Carolina 27514

ARTHUR M. SMALL, Department of Psychiatry, New York University Medical Center, New York, New York 10016

LUKE Y. TSAI, Department of Psychiatry, University of Kansas, Kansas City, Kansas 66103

LYNN WATERHOUSE, Child Behavior Study, Trenton State College, Trenton, New Jersey 08625

ARTHUR YUWILER, Neurobiochemistry Research, Veterans Administration, Los Angeles, California 90073; and Department of Psychiatry, University of California at Los Angeles, Los Angeles, California 90024

Preface

As a division of the School of Medicine at the University of North Carolina at Chapel Hill, TEACCH has always been involved in the latest biological research on autism and related developmental disabilities. However, until now there has not been sufficient information to justify a separate volume on this most important topic. Recent advances both in our understanding of the brain and in the technology to facilitate the measurement of neurological functioning have stimulated significant growth, which is reflected in this volume.

As with the preceding books in this series, Current Issues in Autism, this volume is based on one of the annual TEACCH conferences held in Chapel Hill each May. The books are not simply published proceedings of the conference papers, however. Instead, conference participants are asked to develop chapters around their presentations, and other international experts whose work is beyond the scope of the conference, but related to the major theme, are asked to contribute as well. These volumes are intended to provide the most current knowledge and professional practice available to us concerning major issues in autism.

In this volume, recent advances in our understanding of causes and neurological mechanisms are described by the leading scientists and clinicians in the field. The latest genetic and pharmacological research is also cited, along with speculations about future advances in the field. We believe that the information in this volume is the most current report of the state of the art in this rapidly expanding area and will be most useful to professionals and parents concerned with understanding and helping people with autism.

ERIC SCHOPLER
GARY B. MESIBOV

Acknowledgments

We are, of course, indebted to many people for their cooperation and assistance, and it is our great pleasure to acknowledge each of them. First, our thanks to Helen Garrison, who organized the conference that was the starting point for this book. Her thoroughness, attention to detail, and organizational ability have been impressive throughout this project. John Swetnam provided valuable editorial assistance in strengthening individual chapters and managing the overall product. Our secretarial staff, including Judy Carter, Deana Betterton, and Vickie Weaver, provided competent typing and secretarial assistance. We also thank our TEACCH colleagues for their thoughtful and stimulating suggestions.

As with all of the efforts in the TEACCH program, this book would not have been possible without the assistance of the families of autistic people in North Carolina, the state legislature, and the University of North Carolina School of Medicine. The ability of these three groups to cooperate in their ongoing efforts gives us all hope and optimism as we struggle to help those with this most difficult handicap.

E.S.
G.B.M.

Contents

Part I: Introduction and Overview

Chapter 1

INTRODUCTION TO NEUROBIOLOGICAL ISSUES IN AUTISM

Eric Schopler and Gary B. Mesibov

Tensions between Basic and Applied Research	3
Overview of the Book	5
Summary	11
References	11

Chapter 2

OVERVIEW OF BIOMEDICAL ISSUES IN AUTISM

Robert Jay Reichler and Eugene M. C. Lee

Specificity Model	14
Etiological Specificity	15
Biological Mechanisms and Models	16
Neurological/Anatomical Approach	16
Brain Anatomy and Autistic Symptoms	21
Neurochemistry	29
Genetics	32
Critique of Localization Approaches and Models	33
Developmental Approach	34
Summary and Conclusions	36
References	38

Chapter 3

NEUROBIOLOGICAL RESEARCH PRIORITIES IN AUTISM

Judith M. Rumsey and Martha B. Denckla

    Characterization and Classification of Behavioral Pathology   44
    Localization Research   47
    Neurochemistry   52
    Conclusion   53
    Glossary   54
    References   57

Chapter 4

ETHICAL ISSUES IN THE HEALTH CARE OF CHILDREN WITH DEVELOPMENTAL
HANDICAPS

Alan W. Cross, Larry R. Churchill, Michael C. Sharp, and Nancy M. P. King

    The Role of Ethical Reflection in Medicine   63
    The Case Approach to Ethical Analysis   65
    Case 1: Leonard   66
    Case 2: Monica   68
    Case 3: Charlie   70
    Case 4: Robert   72
    Case 5: Susan   74
    Case 6: Samantha   75
    Summary   78
    References   79

Part II: Neurological and Genetic Issues: Theory Based

Chapter 5

AUTISM: FAMILIAL AGGREGATION AND GENETIC IMPLICATIONS

Susan E. Folstein and Michael L. Rutter

    Introduction   83
    Characteristics of Autism   84

Evidence for Genetic Factors in Autism Derived from Family and
  Twin Studies of Cases of Unknown Etiology   86
Single Gene Disorders Associated with Autism   91
Genetic Evaluation and Counseling for Families with an Autistic
  Child   96
Conclusions   99
References   100

Chapter 6

CEREBRAL–BRAINSTEM RELATIONS IN INFANTILE AUTISM

Marcel Kinsbourne

Overactivation in Autism: Behavioral Observations   107
Overactivation in Autism: Psychopathological Observations   109
The Varieties of Hemispheric Dysfunction   110
Activational Pathology   111
Neurological Findings in Autism   111
Peripheral Laterality   112
Evidence on Peripheral Laterality in Infantile Autism   113
Hemisphere Dysfunction: Less Is More?   114
Evidence on Central Laterality in Infantile Autism   115
Ascending Activation and Laterality   117
Overactivation and Autistic Symptomatology   117
Approach versus Withdrawal and the Balance of Hemispheric
  Activation   119
References   120

Chapter 7

IMPLICATIONS OF SOCIAL DEFICITS IN AUTISM FOR NEUROLOGICAL
DYSFUNCTION

Deborah Fein, Bruce Pennington, and Lynn Waterhouse

Introduction   127
Social Deficits in Autism   127
Neurological Basis of Social Behavior   131
Neurological Involvement in Autism   136

Conclusions   139
References   140

Chapter 8

THE NEUROCHEMICAL BASIS OF SYMPTOMS IN THE LESCH–NYHAN
SYNDROME: RELATIONSHIP TO CENTRAL SYMPTOMS IN OTHER
DEVELOPMENTAL DISORDERS

George R. Breese, Robert A. Mueller, and Stephen R. Schroeder

Introduction   145
Neurological Symptoms   146
Neurochemical Assessment   146
Comparison with Parkinsonism and Huntington Chorea   148
Modeling the Neurochemical Deficit   149
Age-Dependent Responses: Neurobiological Considerations   150
Investigation of Dopamine Receptor Supersensitivity   152
Purinergic Mechanisms Associated with Self-Biting   153
Possible Treatment Strategies   153
Relevance of Neurochemical Findings to Other Developmental Disorders   155
Summary   155
References   156

Part III: Neurological and Genetic Issues: Empirical Basis

Chapter 9

THE SEARCH FOR NEUROLOGICAL SUBGROUPS IN AUTISM

Mary Coleman

Introduction   163
Genetic Disorders   164
Infectious Disorders   166
Birth Injury   167
Metabolic Diseases   167
Structural Changes in the Brain Associated with Autistic Symptoms   170
Other Disease Entities   171
Blindness and Deafness   173

Conclusion 173
References 174

Chapter 10

PRE-, PERI-, AND NEONATAL FACTORS IN AUTISM

Luke Y. Tsai

Prenatal Factors 180
Perinatal Factors 184
Neonatal Factors 186
Conclusions 187
References 187

Chapter 11

NEUROBIOLOGICAL IMPLICATIONS OF SEX DIFFERENCES IN AUTISM

Catherine Lord and Eric Schopler

Sex Differences in Incidence 192
Sex Ratios, Autism, and Mental Retardation 194
Genetic Implications of Differences in Sex Ratios 196
Relevance of Sex Differences in Normal Development to Autism 202
Sex Differences in Identification, Diagnosis, and Referral 206
Conclusion 207
References 207

Chapter 12

THE ROLE OF ABNORMAL HEMISPHERIC SPECIALIZATION IN AUTISM

Geraldine Dawson

Introduction 213
Review of the Evidence 213
Theories Regarding the Role of Abnormal Hemispheric Specialization
    in Autism 215
A Test of Some Predictions 219
The Possible Role of Abnormal Hemispheric Specialization in the Affective
    and Social Deficits of Autistic Children 221
Conclusion 223
References 224

Chapter 13

BRAIN LESIONS IN AUTISM

G. Robert DeLong and Margaret L. Bauman

Introduction 229
The Significance of Brain Lesions: Neurological versus Nonneurological
    Autism 229
Clinical Studies 230
Epidemiological Factors Associated with Encephalopathy 231
Neuroradiological Studies 231
Cases with Discrete Medial Temporal Lobe Lesions 235
Neuroanatomic Studies 237
Discussion 238
References 240

Part IV: Neurochemical, Biochemical, and Nutritional Issues

Chapter 14

NEUROCHEMICAL HYPOTHESES OF CHILDHOOD PSYCHOSES

Glen R. Elliott and Roland D. Ciaranello

Introduction 245
Evidence of Central Nervous System Abnormalities 246
Evidence of Abnormalities in Brain Neuroregulators 249
Future Directions for Research 254
References 256

Chapter 15

NEUROTRANSMITTER RESEARCH IN AUTISM

Arthur Yuwiler and Daniel X. Freedman

General Introduction 263
Transmitters 264

Conclusion 276
References 277

Chapter 16

A NEUROPHYSIOLOGICAL VIEW OF AUTISM

Eric Courchesne

Introduction 285
An Introduction to ERPs 287
ERP Research Requirements and Studies of Autism 292
ERP Studies in Autism 293
ERP Findings: Summary and Concluding Remarks 310
A Conjecture about the Pathophysiology of Autism 312
References 319

Chapter 17

NUTRITION AND DEVELOPMENTAL DISABILITIES: ISSUES IN CHRONIC CARE

Daniel J. Raiten

Introduction 325
Dietary Adequacy 327
Nutrition and Behavior 327
Pharmacology and Nutrition 330
References 334

Part V: Medication Issues

Chapter 18

OVERVIEW OF DRUG TREATMENT IN AUTISM

Magda Campbell, Richard Perry, Arthur M. Small, and Wayne H. Green

Introduction 341
Historical Background 346
Recent Studies 348
Conclusion 352
References 352

Chapter 19

POSSIBLE BRAIN OPIOID INVOLVEMENT IN DISRUPTED SOCIAL INTENT AND LANGUAGE DEVELOPMENT OF AUTISM

Jaak Panksepp and Tony L. Sahley

Background Information 357
Possible Neurochemical Dysfunctions in Autism 361
Concluding Remarks 366
References 367

Chapter 20

THE MEDICAL TREATMENT OF AUTISTIC PEOPLE: PROBLEMS AND SIDE EFFECTS

Thomas Gualtieri, Randall W. Evans, and Debra R. Patterson

Neuroleptic Drugs 374
Fenfluramine 377
"Megavitamin" Therapy 378
Anticonvulsant Drugs 384
References 385

Chapter 21

MEGAVITAMIN B6 AND MAGNESIUM IN THE TREATMENT OF AUTISTIC CHILDREN AND ADULTS

Bernard Rimland

The First Institute for Child Behavior Research Vitamin Study 390
The Institute for Child Behavior Research/University of California
    Medical School Vitamin B6 Study 394
Additional Studies in the United States of Vitamin B6 with Autistic
    Individuals 395
The French Studies of Vitamin B6 and Magnesium 396
Criticisms of Vitamin B6 Therapy with Autism 399
Discussion 402
References 404

INDEX 407

Introduction and Overview

Introduction to Neurobiological Issues in Autism

ERIC SCHOPLER and GARY B. MESIBOV

In one respect this book has been more difficult to edit than the previous four volumes in this series. These difficulties have been generated by the communication obstacles raised by technical terms and jargon. One voice from our editorial muse advises that we cannot expect to read about new scientific methods and procedures without learning the new terminology born of scientific progress. Another voice insists that it is the authors' responsibility to translate technical terms into understandable vocabulary, especially if they wish to have their work known to the general readers from various professional disciplines for whom this series is intended.

Editors usually have much better rapport with the second voice than the first. They know very well that if technical jargon prevents them from clearly understanding a chapter, the majority of general readers most certainly will not be able to follow the authors either. Our authors have worked diligently with us to reduce the obscuring effect of jargon. We believe that in this volume we have been most successful in our joint efforts, at least in part.

TENSIONS BETWEEN BASIC AND APPLIED RESEARCH

The debate about whose responsibility is the understanding of scientific terminology cannot be resolved simply by referring to our editorial roles. It is part of a broader set of tensions stacked behind the terms *basic* versus *applied* science. The traditional gap between these two enterprises is supposed to be bridged by the concept of "relevance." However, relevance is sometimes easier said than achieved. It is often prevented by some differences in assumptions, procedures, results, and implications of basic versus applied science.

We wish to review some of these differences because they encompass two conceptual priorities basic to our TEACCH program, priorities that also coincide with our purposes for producing this series of *Current Issues in Autism*. The first of these conceptual priorities is

ERIC SCHOPLER and GARY B. MESIBOV • Division TEACCH, University of North Carolina, Chapel Hill, North Carolina 27514.

to identify, develop, and disseminate the most current understanding of autism and related developmental disorders based on empirical research evidence. Conversely, we seek to replace fads, myths, and unscrupulous promises for cures with such research findings. The second is to make this information available to professionals and parents and to help them evaluate the implications of such knowledge for prevention and amelioration of the difficulties and suffering generated by such developmental disorders.

Thus, these volumes represent two types of relevance. One is the minimal relevance usually associated with the basic sciences that includes research theories and understanding of these disorders. This volume aims at understanding biological systems and processes associated with autism. The second, and for us the most important, type of relevance associated with clinical or applied research is the effective application of such knowledge to the treatment, amelioration, prevention, and cure of the disorder and its effects.

Historically, the concept of basic was applied to any of the sciences, e.g., anatomy, bacteriology, and biochemistry, considered fundamental to the science of medicine. More recently, it was also used to distinguish physics and chemistry, the "hard sciences," from the behavioral or "soft sciences."

There are many who believe that basic or hard sciences have a better purchase on the "truth" than do the applied or soft sciences. The latter were often compared pejoratively to literary criticism based on personal preference and untestable theory. This view of scientific knowledge had at least two unfortunate effects. The first was that basic scientists saw themselves mandated to pursue knowledge and truth regardless of its applied consequences. Such application, they reasoned, often represented only transitory interests dependent on the whims and wishes of politicians. Politicians, not scientists, would decide whether nuclear power would be used to generate power for war or for electric energy. This position enabled scientists to develop an array of nuclear and chemical technologies without having to investigate or even consider all the possible negative consequences or side effects of these techniques.

A second disadvantage of oversubscription to the basic science methods has been the inappropriate application of the basic science methods to the "soft" social sciences. The methods of the basic sciences have been aimed at discovering laws that regulate either living or inanimate matter through laboratory control over relevant variables. The soft sciences, on the other hand, involve the study of multiple, complex variables with subtle qualitative differences defined by social values or aspirations. Questions about, and problems with, these parameters do not lend themselves to the experimental methods of the basic sciences. Yet, after World War II, university graduate studies in the social science methods were primarily taught as extensions of the hard science methods. Moreover, it became public policy in the United States that scientific research be conducted and evaluated along the designs and experimental methods of the hard sciences. Grant applications and funding priorities were often set by the extent to which research proposals were cast in the trappings of experimental science. Such misdirected research designs often led to the development of new methodology or technical procedures. However, it also led to findings that were misleading or trivial.

Our infatuation with, and faith in, technical procedures has led to a profound confusion between medical technology and knowledge, a confusion increasingly recognized in recent years. However, it is not a new phenomenon. The grisly history of psychosurgery thoroughly documented by Valenstein (1986) illustrates the problem. Egres Moniz, an eminent neurologist, developed a technique for immobilizing psychiatric patients by destroying their frontal lobes with an instrument indistinguishable from an ice pick. This crude and ineffective technique, or "leucotomy," shunned even in the Soviet Union, probably represents one of the darkest chapters in modern medicine. For developing and implementing this procedure, especially in this country, Moniz was awarded the Nobel Prize in 1950. Moreover, the momentum of our technique worship maintained the use of this incredible procedure for over a decade before it was recognized that lobotomies were an inhumane and ineffective method of treating the mentally ill and the practice was discontinued.

Nevertheless, the emphasis on developing new technology continues to mushroom, and new technical procedures proliferate with increasing momentum. Not only are some of these excessively costly, but too often they promote neither the patient's welfare nor accurate diagnosis. Excessive diagnostic procedures often are rationalized by the need for defensive medicine, practiced against the threat of extravagant malpractice litigation. Ironically, the use of costly and irrelevant diagnostic technology may turn out to generate more litigation than it prevents.

The past tendency of separating grant applications for basic sciences from applied relevance is gradually being reversed. The growing recognition that basic science can lead to serious errors when relevance is ignored has prodded the NIH into placing increasing priority on the relevance of proposed research. This trend is reflected in the chapters of this book.

Today virtually all investigators in the field accept the overwhelming evidence that autism is biologically determined. As a result, research into the precise biological mechanisms has proliferated. In spite of recent concentrated efforts and the enormous expansion of our understanding, the autism syndrome remains somewhat elusive. It seems that the more we learn, the more we recognize the complexity of this syndrome. The problem appears to be that autism has multiple causes and multiple biological mechanisms. The purpose of this book is to provide the best current information on what we have learned about such mechanisms and the direction of the work still to be done.

OVERVIEW OF THE BOOK

The book is divided into five parts. Part I includes a general overview of the major issues involved in the neurobiological work. Part II includes the major neurological and genetic issues from a theoretical perspective. Part III encompasses these same issues with emphasis on empirical work. Part IV includes neurochemical, biochemical, and nutritional issues. The last section, Part V, deals with issues involving medication in autism.

The first section offers an overview of the major issues in the neurobiological area. Reichler and Lee's chapter on biological issues presents a developmental model, combining what is known about the autism syndrome with the most current information available about several aspects of brain functioning. They provide a most thoughtful and provocative reminder that the symptoms characterizing the autism syndrome have been reported as resulting from diverse parts of brain anatomy. Moreover, some of these behavioral functions do not appear at the same time and are developmentally determined. The authors raise the distinct possibility that research focused on specific sites with specific methods may not be able to unravel the biological mechanisms underlying autism. Moreover, studies designed across diagnostic categories, with a developmental perspective, may be the best hope for progress in understanding this disorder.

Rumsey and Denckla also outline some neurobiological research priorities for autism. They highlight some of the most important issues in the field for investigators to pursue. Overall, they have identified the need for more "hypothesis-driven" research. They also call for more work on identifying biological subgroups within autism, a thrust also identified by Schopler and Rutter (1978). They describe a need for ethological studies to clarify specific behavioral patterns, the interactions of these patterns with organic and environmental variables, and how they relate to nonhuman primates. Ethological studies should especially focus on social interactions.

Rumsey and Denckla also argue for more meaningful neuropsychological tests. Instruments for measuring social and/or affective responses are needed along with a better understanding of brain systems mediating social interaction. Although much work has been done in examining the communication problems in autism, we still need work with larger samples, more appropriate control groups, developmental norms, and better definitions of communicative intent.

Studies of motor difficulties in autism have suggested some interesting possibilities. Because this work involves minimal risk and is highly reliable, much can be gained from neuromotor assessment. Other priorities described by these authors derive from neuroanatomical, neurochemical, and physiological research. This chapter presents a rich discussion of where we are and some productive areas worth pursuing.

The final chapter in Part I is on ethical issues. With recent major advances in medical sciences, concern about ethical implications has grown. These concerns are very relevant to those working in the areas of autism and developmental disabilities.

In their chapter, Cross, Churchill, Sharp, and King present a system for analyzing ethical issues. Although these questions do not have right or wrong answers, the suggested analysis allows one to examine the ethical implications and possible courses of action for many situations. Their case study approach is effective in highlighting some of the major issues. Case studies dealing with patient–physician interactions, cultural differences, and abuses of dependency, among others, will give the reader an overview of some major ethical issues facing the field today and how they might be analyzed.

Part II describes some of the most important theoretical work in the neurobiological area. Folstein and Rutter begin this section with a most comprehensive analysis of the complex and important genetic work. They begin with a review of the family studies, tying in the autism research with the relationship between autism and other cognitive deficits. They also provide an excellent overview of segregation and linkage analysis, explaining the importance and potential benefits of each.

Following this review they specify the single gene disorders that are associated with autism, including PKU, tuberous sclerosis, and fragile X. This section includes some provocative ideas about the fragile X syndrome as well as the relationship between biochemical abnormalities and single gene disorders. They also suggest that our understanding of genetic factors is sufficient at this time to justify recommending comprehensive genetic counseling for families with autism. Finally, Folstein and Rutter describe how autism accompanied by severe mental retardation may differ more from autism without mental retardation than had been generally thought.

Marcel Kinsbourne introduces his theory of arousal as accounting for the behavioral characteristics observed in autistic individuals. He attributes these characteristics to excessive neurological arousal, a hypersensitivity of the right hemisphere to arousal and arousing events, and a possible left hemispheric impairment causing the right hemisphere to be disinhibited. In support of his theory, Kinsbourne presents evidence from animal and human studies of how overarousal can cause the avoidance of stimulation. He also traces alternative theories of hemispheric dysfunction and explanations of the laterality data in autistic individuals, arguing that overarousal obstructs the establishment of a consistent relationship between hand preferences and specific activities. Kinsbourne's hypotheses are intriguing and present an interpretation that is complementary to, though somewhat different from, that of the other chapters related to these issues (Chapters 7, 12).

Fein, Pennington, and Waterhouse argue in their chapter for the primacy of social deficits in autism. They suggest that the social problems we observe are not merely the outgrowth of cognitive deficits. They demonstrate the lack of correlation between social and cognitive deficits plus the implausibility of a totally cognitive explanation as evidence for this assertion.

Fein *et al.* then proceed with an analysis of the neurological bases of social behavior. Their discussion of the relationship between neurological functions and social behavior has important implications for research in autism. Their review on neurological testing is also important and informative.

Although the final chapter in this section by Breese, Mueller, and Schroeder does not focus on autism directly, their work could have profound implications for children with autism or other developmental problems. Their use of animal analogues with the Lesch–Nyhan syndrome could be a model for future work in autism and related developmental disabilities.

Lesch–Nyhan is an inborn error of purine metabolism expressed exclusively in males. It has some characteristics similar to other neurological problems such as Parkinson disease and Huntington chorea. As with autism, children with Lesch–Nyhan disease have elevated levels of serotonin.

In their chapter, Breese *et al.* present a biomedical approach to modeling the neurochemical deficits in Lesch–Nyhan disease. They show how the symptoms can be induced in laboratory animals, providing investigators with important information on neurological causes and possible treatments. The authors also discuss the mechanisms for other developmentally disabled children.

Part III reviews neurological and genetic issues from an empirical perspective. The chapters in this part represent the most up-to-date empirical work available. Mary Coleman opens this section with a discussion of neurological subgroups in autism. Although many have written about the need for defining such groups, Coleman's work has extended the concept. In her review she describes four basic subgroups: genetic disorders, infectious disorders, birth injuries, and metabolic diseases. The genetic work is reviewed quite thoroughly by Folstein and Rutter in this book so Coleman does not describe this group in much detail. There is some evidence that both pre- and postnatal infectious disorders can cause autism and form a second subgroup. However, except for rubella, the relationship between the infectious disorders and autism has not been conclusively demonstrated. Another subgroup that needs further documentation is birth injuries. Although such injury does not produce a homogeneous cause, further study may have important implications for prevention. There are strong indications of birth injuries in numerous case histories. Finally, there is some evidence that a fourth group might be those with metabolic disorders. These include problems with amino acid metabolism (PKU), purine synthesizing pathways, and carbohydrate metabolism.

In addition to her discussion of these major subgroups, Coleman describes structural changes in the brain associated with autistic symptoms, other disease entities (e.g., tuberous sclerosis), and blindness and deafness. Her work is in the forefront of a most promising area of inquiry.

Luke Tsai carefully reviews the pre-, peri-, and neonatal factors that relate to autism. His review of this important literature resonates with Reichler's perspective that no single factor is directly related to the autism syndrome. However, there are a number of pre- and perinatal factors that have a higher frequency in autistic children. These include older mothers, first-, fourth-, or later-born children, bleeding after the first trimester, use of medication, meconium in the amniotic fluid, and low Apgar scores. According to Tsai, the data do not suggest a unifying pathological process in autism but rather that various types of physical damage can produce the syndrome. Possibly there are other, as yet unidentified, factors involved. This review also suggests that neither a single postnatal factor nor a combination of these factors is associated with the autism syndrome.

Another important area of empirical research, sex differences in autism, is described in the chapter by Lord and Schopler. Despite the inadequacy of available data, the authors do an excellent job of reviewing what is known, its implications, and directions for future investigations. Although all studies find a higher incidence of autism in males as compared with females, the size of this difference varies, depending on the study. The authors describe some reasons for these differences, providing the reader with a greater understanding of these sex differences in the process.

Lord and Schopler then discuss the genetic implications of the sex ratios. This discussion nicely complements the genetic review of the Folstein and Rutter chapter. After reviewing evidence for X-linked, sex-linked, and autosomal patterns of genetic transmission, they argue that polygenic multifactorial models are more consistent with the present state of knowledge. They conclude with a discussion of what might be done and a call for more work in this important area. The potential for increasing our understanding of the autism syndrome through a better understanding of sex differences is quite compelling. The genetic reviews offered by this and the Folstein and Rutter chapter include the most thoughtful and up-to-date evaluation of genetic factors in autism.

Geraldine Dawson reviews another important area of empirical research in autism, hemispheric specialization. She reviews major findings with autistic people, including greater variability in their patterns of hemispheric specialization compared with normals, a greater tendency for right hemisphere dominance for functions typically associated with the left hemisphere, and a greater likelihood for older and higher-functioning autistic people to show more normal patterns of hemispheric specialization than younger, more impaired autistic children.

Following these major findings, Dawson reviews the existing theories of hemispheric specialization. These include the hypothesis of right hemispheric compensation for inadequate left hemispheric functioning, reduced hemispheric specialization, subcortical dysfunction, and the abnormal functional use of the hemispheres.

After her careful analysis of the shortcomings of each theory, Dawson develops her own model, based on the latest empirical research and understanding of the autism syndrome. Her model represents an exciting synthesis of current information and is an important addition to the autism literature.

In the final chapter of this section, DeLong and Bauman review the neurological evidence concerning brain lesions in autism. However, the reader should be cautioned that there is as yet no evidence of behavioral differences between autistic children showing specific brain lesions and those with no evidence of neurological damage.

The main conclusions that form the work of DeLong and Bauman are that anatomic abnormalities are relatively common in autistic brains, although they have little specificity (i.e., there is not generally a direct connection between a particular lesion and a specific behavior). Lesions are more prominent in the left than in the right hemisphere, with the most common abnormalities being enlargements of the ventricles, especially the lateral ventricles. The findings suggest central rather than cortical atrophy. The work on brain lesions in autism will probably increase in the years ahead as techniques for examining the brain become more sophisticated.

Part IV includes neurochemical, biochemical, and nutritional issues. Elliott and Ciaranello begin with a clear, concise, and most comprehensive review of various neurochemical hypotheses in autism. They carefully review studies on prevalence, risk factors, neuropathology, and the evidence of abnormalities in brain neuroregulators. Their chapter helps to explain possible relationships between neurobiological studies in these diverse areas.

In their discussion of future research directions they expect a wedding of computers and EEG systems to greatly enhance our ability to extract information on brain functioning. PET scans will soon enable us to look at many more key elements of brain functioning in children and adults. Another important technological advance is magnetic resonance (MR). MR imaging is rapidly replacing CT scans as the method of choice for obtaining anatomical information about the brain. Among other possibilities, this will allow for clearer discrimination among quite similar brain tissues. As our understanding of immunological mechanisms increases, we may learn more about mechanisms underlying autism. Advances in modern molecular biology will be of great help as well, especially when considered within the limits of specific technology suggested in Reichler and Lee's introductory chapter.

Yuwiler and Freedman present a thorough analysis of the neurotransmitter research. They accomplish this with a thorough review of the work on serotonin, catecholamines, and neuropeptides. Under each discussion they explore the research on tissue levels and pharmacology.

Their discussion of serotonin is especially important because of the large accumulation of related research. They describe some of the complexities of measuring and understanding the role of serotonin as well as the major implications of this research. Those interested in the latest evidence on fenfluramine will find a thorough review of this research here, and in chapters 18 and 20.

Although the current data do not allow for definitive conclusions on the relationship between brain transmitter systems and autism, a number of provocative hypotheses are advanced. Moreover, there is some convincing evidence that autistic people differ from the nonhandicapped population in their platelet serotonin uptake, free blood tryptophan, urinary HVA–creatinine ratios, circulating antibodies to 5HT 1A receptors or myelin basic protein, and in CSF endorphin H concentration. Better understanding of these differences and their implications could bring exciting advances to our understanding of the autism syndrome.

Eric Courchesne discusses autism from a neurophysiological perspective. In his chapter, he describes the attentional and conceptual problems associated with this disability, and also the neurophysiological mechanisms related to each. He discusses event-related potential (ERP) findings in autism that represent the major source of data on neurophysiological functioning.

The description of ERP findings begins with an informative description of how ERP data are collected and what they represent. Courchesne argues that ERP data gathered by him and his colleagues support the association of autism with cognitive dysfunction in at least three aspects of information processing: auditory and visual attention mechanisms, auditory autonomic orienting functioning, and auditory mechanisms using contextual information to modify memories or concepts. Along with the evidence for these hypotheses, Courchesne includes clear statements of what each of these deficits represents.

The final chapter in this section presents a comprehensive review of nutritional issues in developmental disabilities by Daniel Raiten. Although there are many discussions of dietary and nutritional issues, this chapter represents one of the few balanced, integrated, and comprehensive reviews of this complex area.

Following a nice historical overview, Raiten describes three major approaches to this area: dietary assessment, biochemical indices, and nutritional supplements. He critically reviews work along all of these lines, with special attention to megavitamin studies. The need for combining these three approaches is highlighted throughout.

Raiten then describes a study characterizing samples of developmentally disabled children in terms of their ability to obtain and assimilate dietary components. His discussion of factors influencing dietary practices is interesting and informative. This chapter also contains a useful discussion of methodological and design problems in this important area.

Part V includes chapters on an issue of great practical concern, drug treatments in autism. Magda Campbell has been in the forefront of this research for over a decade, and her chapter with Perry, Small, and Green reflects her experience and understanding.

The chapter begins with a historical review and then proceeds to discuss the use of haloperidol (Haldol), fenfluramine, and naltrexone. Since Campbell and her colleagues are responsible for much of the research on Haldol, her discussion of this drug is especially important.

Campbell explains how Haldol has been found to decrease behavioral symptoms and facilitate learning. Her data suggest that about 22% of the children placed on this medication develop the side effects known as dyskinesias. This percentage was not affected by brief "drug holidays." A period of 3 months of total cumulative exposure to this medication is required for tardive dyskinesias to develop.

Campbell includes important discussions of fenfluramine and naltrexone. Her discussion of fenfluramine will be of special interest because of the attention this drug has received recently. Naltrexone is one of the opiate antagonists described by Panksepp and Sahley (Chapter 19), and Campbell's discussion of that medication provides an interesting second perspective.

Panksepp and Sahley present a specific biochemical theory in their chapter, arguing that autism could result from excessive brain opioid activity in brain areas organizing sensory and social experience. They argue that this could also result in the delayed development that so frequently accompanies the autism syndrome.

Panksepp and Sahley present several sources of evidence for their hypothesis. First they describe the symptom similarities between autistic children and young animals tested with low doses of opioids. A second form of evidence relates to the research demonstrating that sterotypic and self-abusive behaviors may be mediated and maintained by high levels of B-endorphin.

This chapter concludes with a discussion of two major opiate receptor blocking agents, Norcan and Trexan. Naloxone (Norcan) is described as a relatively safe medication with no side effects like increased tolerance or addiction. A problem is that it cannot be administered orally and has a very brief period of effectiveness. Naltrexone (Trexan) can be orally administered and lasts for a few days. Future work might demonstrate these to have ameliorative effects for the symptoms of autism.

The chapter by Gualtieri, Evans, and Patterson provides an important discussion of the side effects of medication. They provide a comprehensive look at neuroleptic drugs, fenfluramine, megavitamins, and anticonvulsants. Their discussion of the latter two groups is especially interesting because most people do not think about possible side effects with megavitamins and anticonvulsants.

In addition to their discussion of specific drug groups, they make some excellent general points of significance to physicians and those working with them. They emphasize that drugs only treat symptoms and therefore must be integrated into an ongoing treatment program. They also argue for the need to train physicians working with developmentally disabled people to be more interested and knowledgeable about this population. These authors denounce the common practice of automatically raising dosages when there is no indication of a positive drug response to a lower dose. They argue that this practice is dangerous and lacks empirical verification. Those concerned about drug use with developmentally handicapped people will find this chapter most useful and important.

The final chapter in this book is by one of the pioneers of autism research, Bernard Rimland. Over the years Rimland has advocated the use of various megavitamin regimes as less intrusive than psychoactive drugs and equally effective for treating the symptoms of autism. His long-term advocacy for megavitamins is reflected in his anecdotal and autobiographical chapter organization. However, a significant number of empirical research studies are also reviewed, thus reminding us that, presentation style notwithstanding, megavitamin treatment merits the same consideration given to psychoactive drugs.

SUMMARY

In sum, it is our belief that this volume nicely accomplishes our two main objectives of identifying the most current understanding of autism based on biological research and then making this information available to parents and professionals. The volume represents a comprehensive treatment of what is known, what it might mean, and what one can expect in the near future. As we learn more about autism, we continually rediscover the complexity of this disability and the need to constantly update and reexamine our knowledge, theory, and practice in this field. It is our hope that this volume will be a major step in that direction.

REFERENCES

Schopler, E., & Rutter, M. (1978). Subgroups vary with selection purpose. In M. Rutter & E. Schopler (Eds.), *Autism: A reappraisal of concepts and treatment* (pp. 507–517). New York: Plenum Press.
Valendstein, E. S. (1986). *Great and desperate cures: The rise and decline of psychosurgery and other radical treatments for mental illness.* New York: Basic Books.

Overview of Biomedical Issues in Autism

ROBERT JAY REICHLER and EUGENE M. C. LEE

It has become a tradition, in papers attempting an overview or integrative analysis of issues in autism, to start out with a few protective remarks concerning the extreme difficulty of the task, and the problems of the current state of affairs that prevent a successful effort. The authors are then set free to roam and forage as they will, relatively protected from criticism. We shall not deviate from such a formidable and effective tradition. It is one of the advantages of a maintenance of sameness (which has a better adaptive connotation than the corollary resistance to change, which implies rigidity; Ciaranello, Vandenberg, & Anders, 1982).

Problems in clinical assessment of autistic patients is a ubiquitously recognized impediment to establishing behavioral–biological correlations. These, as partially iterated by Young, Kavanagh, Anderson, Shaywitz, and Cohen (1982) include inconsistent profiles across individuals who fulfill diagnostic criteria for autism (Fish & Ritvo, 1979; Ritvo & Freeman 1978); difficulty in obtaining cooperation from autistic patients; difficulty in finding measures for which levels of attention and motivation can be accurately measured or controlled; the lack of uniformly used and accepted, discreet, and operationally defined measures, which can be used across populations, including appropriate comparison and control subjects; the uncertain and inconsistent use of appropriate comparison and control populations; and changes in symptom and functional profiles, secondary to biological and behavioral interventions, as well as the developmental-maturational processes.

Furthermore, any effort to develop an integrated analysis or model is thwarted by the absence of any clearly demonstrated anatomical, physiological, or neurochemical basis for this syndrome. That is not to suggest that no abnormalities in these domains have been identified. Rather, it is the plethora of such abnormalities, found in multiple systems and functions, associated with a diversity of potential etiological agents and processes, that is confounding. As yet, no single measure of abnormality is consistently found in all or even most cases of autism, and none has been consistently shown to be unique or pathognomonic of autism. That is, all measures so far lack both specificity and selectivity.

ROBERT JAY REICHLER and EUGENE M. C. LEE • Child at Risk Project, Department of Psychiatry and Behavioral Sciences, University of Washington School of Medicine, Harborview Medical Center, Seattle, Washington 98104.

In this chapter we will discuss the limits of models focused on localized sites and on specific methodology. We will review the relevance of various biological mechanisms for autism in the area of neurology, biochemistry, and genetics. Within the limits of this chapter, we will not be able to treat each of these areas in equal detail. Instead, discussion is intended to provide a heuristic basis for replacing the localization model with a developmental multiple-systems model.

SPECIFICITY MODEL

DeMyer, Hingtgen, and Jackson (1981) have systematically reviewed the problem of varying rating scales with varying types, ranges, and numbers of items, and significant problems of reliability across scales and across investigators. The situation is further complicated by the relationship of various symptoms to chronological and mental age. One study compared autistic, normal, and retarded children between ages 2 and 5½ years of age using 67 objectively defined behaviors under controlled observation conditions, with abnormal subjects matched for mental and chronological age (Freeman, Ritvo, Guthrie, Schroth, & Ball, 1978). A discriminant analysis revealed only two behaviors ("repeats sound" and "communicates speech") that define the discriminant function and produce only 63% overall correct classification. It was not possible to separate the autistic from the retarded subjects in the presence of a normal sample, and there was evidence that many of the items were strongly related to both chronological and mental age. Autistic symptoms occur in an almost continuous pattern across various diagnostic groups, such as blindness, deafness, mental retardation, learning disorders (Wing 1969), and disintegrative psychosis (Corbett, Harris, Taylor, & Trimble, 1977). Capute, Derivan, Chauvel, and Rodriguez (1975) have demonstrated how frequently autistic symptoms are found in other developmentally disabled children.

It is often argued that while no symptoms or signs are pathognomonic or specific for autism, it is the syndromal occurrence that defines and delineates autism from other disorders. In one study DeMyer, Bryson, and Churchill (1973) found that the psychiatric diagnostic groups lay on a severity continuum. A cluster analysis showed much symptom overlap precluding any definition of cluster groups.

In addition, it is recognized that even with syndromal definition, autism is not a unitary entity and shows considerable heterogeneity (Coleman, 1979). Schopler and Reichler, with others (Schopler, Reichler, DeVillis, & Daly, 1980), using the Childhood Autism Rating Scale (CARS; Schopler, Reichler, & Renner, 1986), compared the CARS definition of autism with that of Ritvo and Freeman (1978) and Rutter (1978). While there is significant overlap there are also important differences. Of 266 children identified as autistic on the CARS, only 20.6% met Rutter's criteria for autism and 46.6% met the Ritvo and Freeman criteria. Ornitz (Ornitz, Guthrie, & Farley, 1978) reported on parental responses to a large behavioral inventory covering items considered symptomatic of autism. While 90% of autistic children were described as being "very hard to reach or in a shell more than rarely" and 85% ignored people as if they "did not exist" more than rarely, what is most striking are the percentages of autistic children who *do not* show many of these significant symptoms. For instance, 24% did not "avoid looking at people in the eye more than rarely," and over 50% "*did not* respond to affection by active withdrawal more than rarely." Indeed, most of the children did not become agitated or frightened by unfamiliar persons, and most did play interactive social games with mother. Similarly, 40% did not ignore toys, and 30% did not perform repetitive activities. Also, 25% did not show echolalia, 40% did not show delayed echolalia, and 30% did not ignore or fail to respond to sounds or excessively watch motions of their hands or fingers. Only a little more than 50% seemed preoccupied with spinning objects. In addition, a very large percentage of the children, from 70 to 90%, more than rarely showed normal modes of relating as well. This is a phenomenon that is regularly ignored. This striking inconstancy and heterogeneity of the syndrome leads to inconstant and inconsistent findings across studies. It has led at least one investigator, Mary Coleman, to suggest that we refer to autism as the "autistic syndromes" and attempt to define more homogeneous subgroups of autism, a matter discussed more by Coleman in Chapter 9 (Coleman, 1979).

There is also the persistent problem of identifying which symptoms are primary—that is, directly related to a putative biological dysfunction, and pathognomonic of the syndrome (DeMyer, 1979; Hingtgen & Bryson, 1972)—and which may be secondary, as a consequence of primary symptoms and variably associated with autism. For instance, Rutter, Bartak, and Newman (1971) conceptualized autism as a primary disorder of linguistic competence, Ornitz (1974) as a function of faulty sensory input, and Kanner (1943) as an inborn error of relating. This may be more of a conceptual or semantic problem than a biological one, with each perceiving a particular aspect of the whole. For example, Reichler and Schopler (1971) have shown that measures of sensory perception predict most of the variance associated with measures of relating to people. However, such conceptual biases may influence the diagnostic process and selection of patients studied (Schopler et al., 1986). Reichler and Schopler (1976) have previously reviewed nosological issues as a function of the purpose or question being posed and have suggested the need for different nosological systems for treatment and etiological purposes. Confounding of these functions often adds unnecessarily to confusion in research.

From a research point of view, this situation may be made worse by the current criteria in DSM-III. These criteria consist of five primary, unequal domains: the first, onset before 30 months of age (currently under reconsideration); the second, pervasive lack of responsiveness to other people; the third, gross deficits in language development; the fourth, peculiar speech patterns when speech is present; and the fifth, bizarre responses to various aspects of the environment. This system has collapsed many specific and not so clearly related items into a few more global areas. The effect of this may be to somewhat improve clinical diagnostic reliability at the cost of increasing heterogeneity in the population defined. Without further belaboring the point, there is general consensus that autism has significant heterogeneity in its presentation or definition that raises some question about whether it is reasonable to consider it a coherent syndrome.

ETIOLOGICAL SPECIFICITY

Despite the diversity and heterogeneity of the syndrome, it is almost universally accepted at this time that autism represents the expression of some underlying brain dysfunction (DeMyer et al., 1981; Rutter & Lockyer, 1967; Rutter, Bartak, & Newman, 1971). It cannot, however, be considered a disease in the sense that it is a variable expression associated with one primary or even several major etiological factors. In fact, it is generally recognized that autism is associated with multiple etiologies, any of which could potentially cause central nervous system dysfunction (Knobloch & Pasamanick, 1975; Damasio & Maurer, 1978; Ciaranello et al., 1982; Folstein & Rutter, 1978; Ornitz, 1978). Ornitz (1983) tabulated selected pathological conditions associated with autism showing 26 different conditions. Most striking is not only the diversity of agencies, ranging from genetic conditions such as Down syndrome to metabolic conditions such as phenylketonuria and infectious processes such as congenital rubella (Chess, 1977), but also the considerable temporal diversity ranging from prenatal conditions (see Chapter 10) such as mid-trimester bleeding, perinatal conditions such as high bilirubin, early postnatal developmental conditions such as infantile spasms and celiac disease, and late-occurring conditions such as herpes simplex encephalitides and tuberous sclerosis. Any conceptual model that endeavors to explain autism must therefore not only deal with the heterogeneity of expression but also account for the effects of diverse agents acting at presumably different stages of central nervous system maturation and development.

BIOLOGICAL MECHANISMS AND MODELS

There have been several approaches to the investigation of the underlying physiological mechanisms of autism. A number of investigators have dealt with these complex and diverse syndromes by postulating that the various etiological agents act through a unique biological or neurophysiological "final common pathway" (Ornitz, 1983, 1985; Maurer & Damasio, 1982). This conceptual framework reflects a rational and established scientific approach to problem solving, based on the principle of parsimony. But hypothesizing a single or unique mechanism does not necessarily correspond with reality. The verification of this conceptual model through empirical testing should also include parameters to demonstrate that (1) all cases that meet criteria for diagnosis show dysfunction in the putative mechanism, and (2) dysfunction in this mechanism does not occur in "noncases." If it does not occur in all cases, then either another mechanism must also be allowed (i.e., it is not unique) or a more encompassing single mechanism must be postulated. If the dysfunction can be demonstrated in noncases, then it is nonspecific, or the diagnostic definition must be broadened to allow for a broader spectrum of expression of symptomatology (Ornitz, 1978). This is the issue of selectivity and specificity for a dysfunctional mechanism leading to specific disorders. Further, it should be recognized that the conceptual effort to define a "final common pathway" is likely to confound research attempts to relate specific etiological factors to their sites or mechanisms of action.

Under this framework there are several models, including neuroanatomical, chemical, genetic, and developmental mechanisms, that have been identified as a basis for the dysfunctions and symptoms of autism. Rumsey reviews some of these models, and related research strategies and data, in greater detail in Chapter 3.

NEUROLOGICAL/ANATOMICAL APPROACH

Neuroanatomical emphasis is on the localization of brain regions responsible for behavioral manifestations or dysfunctions. As elaborated by Maurer and Damasio (1982), this involves identification of signs and symptoms, and correlating these with similar signs and symptoms occurring in better understood neurological disorders; and by reasoning from knowledge about the structure and functional connections of various brain regions, interpreting the signs and symptoms in terms of disturbed anatomy and physiology, and estimating the *localization* that could account for the data most parsimoniously. This approach, which has worked well in clinical neurology, takes advantage of the fact that most major systems (e.g., sensory, motor, and visual systems) have a stable organization—an isomorphism— throughout the course of the system from peripheral sites to cortical mapping. That is, the specific functions and organization of the system maintain a regular and constant relationship; for instance, in the sensory system, the representation of specific touch stimuli from the hand and the foot are in a fixed relationship throughout the course of the system. Secondly, the localization logic rests on the fact that different systems representing different functions approximate or cross only at certain known locations in the central nervous system. Therefore, for any combination of signs, and symptoms, there is a relatively unique location where all of the particular systems whose functions are disturbed are in geographical proximity. If these systems were either diffusely distributed or if they were uniformly represented through-out most or all of the course of the CNS, such an approach would be futile.

The functional components of the central nervous system (CNS) are constructed of cells called neurons, which have the ability to transmit information between them. Part of the neuron (Figure 1C) can be elongated to form a channel of transmission, called the axon, which in the brain and spinal cord generally travels in bundles called tracts. These tracts serve as communication pathways in the CNS. The neuron cell bodies cluster into groups, called nuclei, which are the structures we often refer to as brain areas. The spinal cord is located in our vertebrae and serves as a transmission link between the body and the brain and houses the mechanisms for reflexive behavior.

The brain can be discussed in three basic subdivisions: the forebrain, the midbrain, and the hindbrain (Figure 1B). There are several approaches used to describe and discuss the structures in the brain, and often neuroscientists refer to the region they are talking about in the context of, or relative to, other structures.

The hindbrain is further divided into the medulla, which is continuous with the spinal cord; the pons, which lies above the medulla; and the cerebellum, which hangs off the pons. The nuclei in these various regions network with each other to coordinate, maintain, and transmit sensory information upward to the brain and motor information downward to the body. The cerebellum and underlying nuclei (including the vestibular nuclei discussed later) chiefly function to maintain body balance and muscle coordination.

The midbrain nuclei serve to modulate and maintain sensory and motor processes, such as the control of eye movement in the visual system or the startle reactions to sound via the auditory system.

The forebrain lies above the midbrain and is divided into two cerebral hemispheres. Each hemisphere can be distinguished primarily by the functions it modulates. Both, however, have extensive connections between their components, and there are corresponding structures in both hemispheres. The most prominent structures are the cortex, hypothalamus, thalamus, basal ganglia, and limbic system (Figure 1B).

The cerebral cortex makes up the outer covering of the brain. It is the most recent in evolutionary development of the vertebrate nervous system. The peaks and valleys that create the grooves on the surface are known as sulci and fissures. The grooves provide artificial delineations on the cortex that are identified as lobes (Figures 1A). Four lobes are identified and studied in relation to the major functions they serve. In autism the frontal lobes have been of interest owing to their contribution to the modulation of emotion and higher-order mental processes such as thinking and memory, and the temporal lobes have been of interest because of their importance in the development of language ability and influence on social and emotional behavior.

The hypothalamus is a collection of several areas that controls several essential func-tions, including the control of the autonomic nervous system, regulation of several hormonal systems, and probable control of motivational behaviors, such as eating, drinking, and sex.

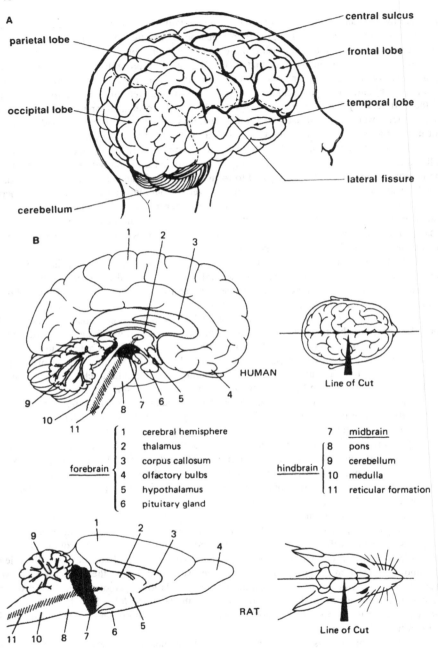

Figure 1. (A) Surface of the cortex. (B) Comparison of major subdivisions of the brain in humans and rats. (C) Golgi type I neuron. (B) and (C) are reprinted by permission of the publisher, from Schneider and Tarsis, 1980.

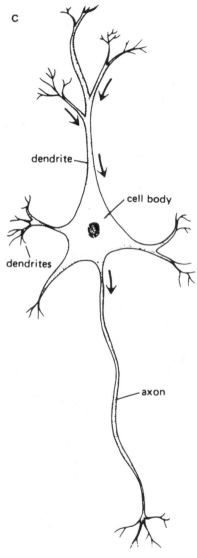

Figure 1 (*cont.*)

The thalamus is also a collection of several areas that function primarily to relay sensory information from the peripheral nervous system to the cortex.

The basal ganglia, which consist of three areas: the putamen, the globus pallidus, and the caudate, collectively coordinate muscle movement. Each area receives motor information from the cortex and relays it to lower structures and the spinal cord.

The limbic system (Figure 2) is a network of several structures. They include the amygdala, the hippocampus, the fornix, the mammillary bodies, and the septum. Each of these areas is believed to contribute to the control of emotional behavior and memory processing.

In this context you will see discussions of functions related to old brain and new brain. Old brain refers to the brain structures we share with lower animals, such as the hindbrain, which exist in reptiles and control some basic body functions such as breathing and heart rate. It also includes the deeper structures of the forebrain, such as the brainstem and the limbic system, which are also developed in higher vertebrates and control the expression of emotion and social behavior. New brain refers to the structures in mammals, such as the frontal lobes of the cortex, which reach their fullest development in the human brain and account for the abilities unique to man. The distinctions are relative to the regions discussed, and often different subcortical structures are referred to as old brain.

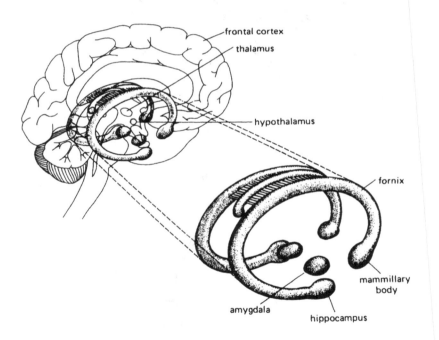

Figure 2. The limbic system. (Reprinted by permission of the publisher, from Schneider and Tarshis, 1980.)

The relationships between these structures and behavioral function are not uniform throughout the brain or throughout the animal kingdom. However, certain generalizations can be made: (1) The more primitive a behavior, such as reflexes, the more likely it is controlled or maintained by activity in lower brain regions (i.e., spinal cord, hindbrain, and midbrain). (2) The more complex the behavior, the more it could be influenced by activity in the forebrain. (3) The decision-making processes that characterize brain function generally take place in the forebrain but are influenced by events in the hindbrain and midbrain.

Before we leave this brief overview of the brain, a note may be made that the subdivisions of the brain mentioned are somewhat artificial and that it is impossible to attribute a single function to a single anatomical site (this issue will be presented in greater detail later in this chapter). Each area of the brain is related to almost every other area either directly or indirectly.

The spectrum of methods for determining structural neuropathophysiology includes gross differences as examined by imaging techniques, standard clinical neurological inference (Maurer & Damasio, 1982), neural localization studies as demonstrated by human and animal lesion and stimulation protocols, and neuropathological examination of brain differences at the gross and cellular level. There is a large degree of overlap between the various methods used in the neuroanatomical approach. In autism this approach has failed so far to uncover any definitive neurological mechanisms.

BRAIN ANATOMY AND AUTISTIC SYMPTOMS

Using this anatomical approach on a group of 17 autistic children, DeLong identified certain consistent changes in pneumoencephalographs (PEG: X rays with air injected into brain ventricles), apparently reflecting specific anatomical pathology (DeLong, 1978; Hauser, DeLong, & Rosman, 1975). These changes centered on the left temporal horn of the left lateral verticle. All of these cases clinically demonstrated a *primary language disorder*, characterized by a failure to develop expressive speech. Comprehension of spoken language, although delayed for age, was somewhat less deficient in 14 cases. These patients, with one exception, exhibited profound disturbances in relationship to people, with 12 of 17 identified as frankly autistic, and 5 considered somewhat symbiotic. Only 5 of 17 EEGs were considered normal. Five cases had normal nonverbal intelligence, 2 cases were mildly retarded, and 10 were significantly retarded. DeLong related these findings to syndromes associated with known lesions of the temporal lobes in adults, focusing on the Kluver–Bucy syndrome and Korsakoff psychosis. He demonstrated that the symptomatology is comparable, although varying, and thought to be dependent on whether lesions were unilateral or bilateral and the degree of involvement. Most striking in the Kluver–Bucy syndrome, which occurs after lesions to the medial anterior temporal lobes, are what has been described as an incapacity for adaptive social behavior, and loss of recognition of the significance of persons and events. Such patients show an "empty blandness," an absence of emotion or concern for others, and pursue no sustained purposeful activity. Korsakoff psychosis is considered an amnestic syndrome—a failure to register or recall recent experience beyond the immediate span of attention. DeLong argued that such impairments, occurring early in life, could lead to the gross dysfunctions and symptoms seen in autistic children.

However, another study reviewing pneumoencephalographs from children with a wide range of psychiatric syndromes reported cases of severe local dilatations in the temporal region with no specific clinical picture corresponding to these locations (Boesen & Aarkrog, 1967). Dalby (1975) presented pneumoencephalographic findings on a large group of children characterized by *developmental language retardation,* with 46% showing dilatation of the left temporal horn. Even DeLong presented control cases with abnormal PEG evidence of temporal lobe dilatation without autistic features. He also recognized that it is difficult to give an explanation for the deficit in social interaction directly from the temporal lobe lesions and attempted to derive these as secondary effects. Another investigator conducted a computerized tomographic (CT) brain scan study of 85 patients with childhood-onset pervasive neuropsychiatric disorders, including autism, pervasive developmental disorders, developmental language disorders, severe attentional deficit disorder with learning difficulties, and Tourette syndrome (Caparulo *et al.,* 1981). Twenty-four of the scans revealed clear abnormalities and 13% showed mild asymmetries in ventricular or hemispheral size. By diagnosis, abnormal scans were found in 59% of pervasive developmental disorders, 44% of language-impaired, and 38% of Tourette syndrome. No distinct abnormality was isolated by which diagnostic groups could be separated. A recent computer tomography comparison of 45 autistic and 19 control children demonstrated enlarged ventricles in less than 25% of the autistic subjects, and there were no significant correlations between ventricular measurements and the severity of autistic behavior (Campbell *et al.,* 1982).

While specific criticism can be made of these studies in terms of design and specific data, it is clear that they do not support the temporal lobe lesions as uniquely or uniformly associated with autism. Further, computerized tomography (CT) studies have not qualitatively (Caparulo *et al.,* 1981) or quantitatively (Damasio, Maurer, Damasio, & Chui, 1980) demonstrated any abnormalities related specifically to autism. Most imaging studies report no systematic correlation between abnormalities found upon imaging and functional abnormalities (Heir, LeMay, & Rosenberger, 1978; DeMyer *et al.,* 1981). A useful approach might be to examine a large number of patients with similar PEG or imaging lesions, and to attempt to identify discrete common factors, behaviors, or symptoms irrespective of clinical diagnosis.

A similar approach was taken by Ornitz (1983, 1985) though with a broadened concept of localization. He identified hyperactivity to auditory stimuli, visual ignoring, and a diminished response to tactile and painful stimuli as sensory disturbances very specific to the syndrome of autism. Ornitz noted, in contrast, the exaggerated reaction to similar stimuli that also occurs in autistic children. Motility disturbances were also identified as specific to the syndrome. He interpreted them as providing sensory input through stereotyped repetitive movement. These combined sensory and motility disturbances were described as faulty modulation of sensory input and motor output (Ornitz, 1974). He presented evidence that the vestibular system (the inner-ear orienting system and its associated brain centers) functions not only to maintain equilibrium and stabilize gaze "but also to modulate both input from other sensory modalities and also motor excitation" (Pomperano, 1967a, 1967b).

He argues that the dysfunction of central vestibular control mechanisms could account for a variety of physiological data in autistic children and for the disturbances of sensory modulation and motility. The spinning and rocking behaviors of autistic children were given as additional evidence of support for a vestibular dysfunction. Ornitz acknowledged that it is not possible to explain specific disturbances of language and communication, and relationships to objects and people, directly on the basis of central vestibular pathophysiology. However, he pointed out that the central nuclei of the vestibular system are embedded in the brainstem and are extensively interconnected through interacting neural loops to centers in the brainstem and diencephalon (Spyer, Ghelarducci, & Pompeiano, 1973). There is evidence that the brainstem plays a fundamental role in the elaboration of complex adaptation and individual behavior (Ornitz, 1983, 1985), a sense of continuity of self, and social reactivity to the environment. *By extrapolation,* brainstem dysfunction would be sufficient to explain the full gamut of autistic behaviors. Ornitz suggested that the mechanism underlying the autistic syndrome is likely to involve a *system dysfunction* rather than simple, local anatomical lesions. By combining these functions of the brainstem-vestibular system with rostrally directed (i.e., forward) connections to the thalamus, he postulated a brainstem-diencephalic theory that "takes the faulty modulation of sensory input into account by considering the multiple levels along the neuroaxis at which sensation is modulated." The basic assumption of the concept is that sensory input is insufficiently modulated so that normal sensory information is not available for processing by higher centers.

This approach to defining a broadened concept of an anatomically localized system has been extended to other areas of the brain. Damasio and Maurer (1978) have also focused systematically on disturbances of motility in autistic patients. By careful observations and measures, they define a pattern of motor defects, including abnormal control of movement such as akinesia (absence of or diminished movement); bradykinesia (delay in initiating, arresting, or changing motor patterns); or hyperkinesia (increased motor activity); abnormal involuntary motor movements, such as dykinesia (facial tics, limb movements, rhythmic flapping); alterations of muscle tone, such as hypertonia and hypotonia; and abnormal posture and gait, including inability to handle simultaneous motor tasks.

These disturbances most resemble neurological signs in analogous adult neurological disorders correlated with dysfunction of the basal ganglia and closely associated regions of older cortex located in the mesial aspects of the frontal and temporal lobes, also known as mesocortex, and the neostriatum. The amygdala is one structure located in the temporal lobes and is associated with the Kluver–Bucy syndrome when lesioned. A most striking phenomenon Damasio and Maurer (1978) describe is the asymmetry of the lower part of the face that was noticeable when the children smiled or spoke spontaneously, but not when they voluntarily moved their facial musculature on request. The phenomenon, an emotionally determined facial asymmetry, is known as emotional facial paralyses or reverse facial paralysis and has been interpreted as a sign of damage to the basal ganglia or the thalamus. Recent investigations indicate it is related to dysfunction of the older, sensorimotor cortex that integrates nonpyramidal (involuntary) motor systems located in the mesial frontal lobe. They also note the resemblance between the verbal defects of autism and the syndrome of mutism or relative speech inhibition that appears during the recovery from mesial frontal lobe lesions. They do not derive from impairment of primary linguistic processing but rather from a lack of initiative to communicate and from a lack of orientation toward stimuli, and they are suggestive evidence of an underlying impairment in "higher motor or perceptual control, or more generally in overall cognitive organization." Similar disturbances of attention and perception are associated with mesial frontal lobe regions. The authors explain ritualistic and compulsive behavior and disturbances in social relationship as secondary to the primary deficits described.

Direct neuropathological examination of tissue is one of the major approaches used to confirm the mechanisms proposed by neurological correlative approaches or to extend the list of neural regions that may play a role in the syndrome of autism. Bauman and Kemper (1985) report abnormalities in the cytoarchitecture of several limbic regions and the cerebellar system in the brain of a young autistic male, areas associated with both the Damasio–Maurer (limbic region) and Ornitz (cerebellar) models. Ritvo and colleagues found significantly decreased Purkinje cell densities in the cerebellar cortices and vermes of four autistic patients (Ritvo *et al.*, 1986).

The Damasio–Maurer model bears a striking resemblance to the approach taken by Ornitz. However, the location of the critical system is considerably forward of Ornitz's brainstem systems, in newer and higher level structures, although both systems interface in the thalamic-diencephalic region. The Damasio and Maurer model can be criticized for not addressing many of the physiological data reviewed by Ornitz. However, both conceptual models suffer from a lack of specific data to directly support them, and both use arguments from analogy to develop their models. In addition, each requires some extrapolation and assumptions that some essential features of the autistic syndrome are secondary to other primary dysfunctions. Lastly, neither explains the presence of some of these symptoms in nonautistic subjects or the lack of some symptoms in some autistic children, or provides an exclusive and unique model for explaining the syndrome. Indeed, a systematic review of animal and human lesion literature demonstrates that many of the features of autism can be provided by lesions at quite varying sites and levels of the central nervous system.

The following illustrates the diversity of functions and deficits associated with any specific brain structure and the considerable overlap of functions associated with different brain structures. The structures discussed are those implicated in several theories on the neurobiology of autism (Maurer & Damasio, 1982; Ornitz, 1983).

Each brain region is discussed in light of 12 primary functions in which autistic children show deficits. These functions fall into five major functional realms (modified from Ornitz *et al.*, 1978). This discussion is summarized in Table 1.

The table, and the following discussion, is based on both human and animal work examining the effects of lesions in these brain areas. We have indicated with a question mark (?) a functional area for which data are lacking or uncertain and which needs further research relative to the brain area discussed.

Frontal Lobes

The major functional roles of the frontal lobes are the formation of memory and the modulation of emotional expression. They possibly augment and/or parallel other systems that also play a role in memory formation and emotional expression.

1. Recognition: Frontal lobe lesions lead to a generalized decrease in recognition and memory task in adult humans (Milner, 1976). Monkeys with similar lesions demonstrate deficits in delayed response task and recent memory task (Fuster, 1980).

2. Affectionate and 3. Acknowledge: Affectionate bonding is difficult to identify in adult patients. However, frontal lobe lesions often result in patients with flat affect toward their environments and to others (Fuster, 1980; Maurer & Damasio, 1982). This deficit in social relating is also seen in other species with frontal damage (Fuster, 1980; Myers, Swett, & Miller, 1973).

4. Motivation: Decreased motivation to initiate activity with an object may also be attributed to a decrease in the ability to attend to an object, as found in monkeys with frontal lobe lesions (Fuster, 1980).

5. Modulate: Patients with frontal lobe damage also demonstrate a decreased ability to respond to stimuli in their environment (Fuster, 1980; Maurer & Damasio, 1982).

6. Orienting: Abnormal responses to sudden or orienting stimuli have not been reported in either patients or animals with frontal lobe lesions. However, if there is also involvement

Table 1. Brain Functions and Autistic Deficits

Brain function	Autistic features
I. Relating to people	
1. Recognition/responding to gaze	Children may be characterized by the avoidance of eye contact.
2. Affectionate bonding/socializing	The deficit here is characteristic of emotional remoteness and ignoring people as if they were not there.
II. Response to inanimate objects	
3. Acknowledges objects	Children often ignore toys as if they did not exist.
4. Motivation for change	Children often show a decreased motivation for change which includes repetitive behaviors or not wanting to attempt a task. This also is indicated by increased resistance to change in activities or environment.
III. Perception	
5. Modulatory response to stimulation	Children show a decreased modulatory response to stimulation and signs of neophobia. This is characterized by either hyperactivity, preoccupation, or hypersensitivity to stimuli or environment.
6. Orienting response	Children show a decreased or hyperreactivity and/or attention to sudden changes in stimuli or environment.
IV. Motor activity	
7. Stereotyped/repetitive	Children demonstrate a lack of control of stereotyped or repetitive behaviors such as hand flapping, whirling, and head or body rocking.
8. Posturing	Children may maintain a fixed uncomfortable position for extended periods of time.
9. Activity level	Children show episodic fluctuations in activity.
V. Language	
10. Communicative intent	Children show a decreased level of communicative intent.
11. Reception of language	There is echolalia and repeated verbalization of questions rather than answering, and poor comprehension.
12. Production of language	Children use speech with poor tone or rhythm (prosody), there is a misuse of pronouns.

of anterior septal regions, there is an increased response to all environmental stimuli (Isaacson, 1974; see septal section).

     ' 7. Stereotyped: Reports of motor stereotypy have been indicated in patients with limited frontal lobe damage (Fuster, 1980; Damasio & Maurer, 1978).

     8. Posturing: Posturing has not been reported in patients or animals with frontal lobe lesions.

     9. Activity: In patients with frontal lobe lesions there is a general decrease in activity (Crosby, Humphrey, & Lauer, 1962; Fuster, 1980). Activity levels in other species seem to present mixed results, such as monkeys in which frontal lobe lesions show an increased nonspecific level of activity.

     10. Communicative intent: Patients with frontal lobe damage present with a decrease in all social interactions, including communications (Fuster, 1980). There is a generalized decrease of expression and affect in these patients.

     11. Language reception and 12. Production: The reception and capacity to produce language in frontal patients seems to be intact. The frontal lobes seem to be more involved in the overlay of expression in one's language (Fuster, 1980).

Temporal Lobes

     Temporal lobe functions have been classified into the modulation of language, hearing, vestibular function, and motor activity. This discussion of functional deficits will focus on those lesions that affect only the temporal lobes and do not include underlying limbic structures. Amygdaloid and hippocampal lesion effects will be discussed separately below.

     1. Recognition: The temporal lobes may play a part in the integration of experiences into memories that are developed for the recognition of others. This function of the temporal lobes needs to be further examined in controlled studies.

     2. Affectionate: DeLong (1978) and Ornitz (1983) both postulate the involvement of the temporal lobes in affectionate bonding and in the presentation of decreased social interaction.

     3. Acknowledge: Damage to just the temporal lobes seems to show a deficit in attending to objects in one's environment. This may be attributed to dysfunctions in sensory modulation (Ornitz, 1983).

     4. Motivation: Despite the implications that the temporal lobes are involved in the modulation of sensory information, it is unclear how this may influence the motivational drive of an organism to initiate activity with an object.

     5. Modulate: Temporal lobe-lesioned individuals demonstrate a decrease in response to environmental stimuli (Ornitz, 1983).

     6. Orienting: Orienting response changes following temporal lobe lesions are not consistent within or between species studied.

     7. Stereotyped: The temporal lobes seem to play a part in the initiation of motor acts with interactions through the hippocampal system.

     8. Posturing: Currently it is unknown how the temporal lobe cortex may affect the functions leading to posturing.

     9. Activity: The motor effects of temporal lobe-lesioned animals have been attributed to the effects seen with hippocampal lesions—that is, the inability to maintain any particular behavior for a period of time. This has been interpreted as an increase in activity in animals with temporal lobe lesions.

10. Communicative intent: Ornitz (1983) has reported that damage to the temporal lobes may contribute to the decrease in communicative intent.

11. Reception and 12. Reproduction: The temporal lobes are noted to play a major role in the reception and initiation of language activity through both the sensory and motor components of speech (Crosby et al., 1962; Damasio & Maurer, 1978; Ojemann, 1976).

Amygdala

The amygdala is a highly heterogenous structure made up of several anatomical regions; when they are lesioned or stimulated, the result is a broad spectrum of modulated emotional reactions.

1. Recognition: Bilateral lesions to the amygdala produce a marked decrease in ability to interact socially with people or other animals (Isaacson, 1974; Ornitz, 1983).

2. Affectionate: Patients and monkeys with amygdaloid lesions also demonstrate a decrease in affective expression and bonding (DeLong, 1978; Isaacson, 1974).

3. Acknowledge: Rats with amygdaloid lesions will respond to novel or new objects placed in their environments and will demonstrate "normal" levels of exploratory behavior (Isaacson, 1974).

4. Motivation: Motivational levels in interacting with objects seems to be unchanged following amygdaloid lesions (Isaacson, 1974).

5. Modulate: There seems to be a decrease in response to novel objects in the patient's or animal's environment (DeLong, 1978; Isaacson, 1974).

6. Orienting: Amygdala-lesioned animals demonstrate a decrease in their responding to orienting stimuli (Isaacson, 1974).

7. Stereotyped and 8. Posturing: ?

9. Activity: The Kluver–Bucy syndrome following amygdaloid lesions results in a marked decrease in activity or the absence of sustained, purposive activity (Isaacson, 1974; Ornitz, 1983).

10. Communicative intent, 11. Reception, and 12. Production: ?

Hippocampus

The hippocampus is also a heterogenous structure that modulates motor behavior and the formation of types of memory or cognitions.

1. Recognition and 2. Affectionate: The Korsakoff syndrome following hippocampal lesions in man and animals results in impairments in the ability to recognize and interact socially with others (DeLong, 1978; Isaacson, 1974; O'Keefe & Nadel, 1978).

3. Acknowledge: There is a general tendency to ignore objects in one's environment and often carry out activity as if the object were not present (Crosby et al., 1962; Isaacson, 1974).

4. Motivation: In most species there is a general decrease in "motivational" intent to interact with objects (O'Keefe & Nadel, 1978).

5. Modulate: There is a decrease in responding to stimuli and changes in one's environment following extensive hippocampal lesions (Crosby et al., 1962; Isaacson, 1974).

6. Orienting: The orienting response in animals with hippocampal lesions has been noted to be markedly decreased. However, this may be secondary to the inability to hippocampal animals to maintain any response, and they may have "normal" orienting response without the ability to maintain those responses (Blanchard, Blanchard, Lee, & Fukunaga, 1977; Isaacson, 1974).

7. Stereotyped: Rats with hippocampal lesions demonstrate some stereotyped behaviors in an open field (Blanchard et al., 1977).

8. Posturing: With a generalized increase in activity there is a consequent decrease in the ability to posture or maintain any pose (Isaacson, 1974).

9. Activity: Hippocampal patients and animals generally demonstrate an increase in the levels of activity and have impairment in maintaining a particular behavior or pose (Blanchard et al., 1977, Isaacson, 1974).

10. Communicative intent: Hippocampal involvement in communications may be related to the impairments either in memory formation or in behavioral modulation.

11. Reception and 12. Production: ?

Other Brain Structures

A similar analysis could be made on other brain structures about which less is known. Four examples will be given. For the septal nuclei modulation of emotional responses and ideation have been associated with septal function. The general role of the septum in reactivity may account for the changes in emotional behavior following septal lesion or stimulation. Isaacson (1974) reported that most animals with septal lesions demonstrate increased responsiveness to social interaction and to other environmental stimuli.

The corpus striatum is a diverse collection of structures that need further study. Current functions attributed to the striatum range from cortical translation of descending commands, cognition, and the modulation of sensory information and arousal. When the caudate and globus palladus are included, Chozick (1983) noted the occurrence of amnesia associated with striatal damage that may effect recognition and interactions with others. Blanchard, Williams, Lee, and Blanchard (1981a) reported that specific striatal lesions result in decreased response to orienting stimuli, while Chozick (1983) and Isaacson (1974) found that injections of amphetamine into the corpus striatum often result in dose-dependent circling or posturing. Lesions to these regions will decrease the stereotyped behaviors, but often not the posturing induced by central amphetamine stimulation. Chozick (1983) reported increased activity levels in patients and animals with striatal damage, and Ojemann (1976) reported that stimulation of posterior regions of the striatum resulted in decreased ability to initiate speech.

Traditionally the thalamus has been noted as the major relay station of the brain which directs, integrates, and modulates information through the brain (Maurer & Damasio, 1982). These authors reported that damage of the dorsal thalamus resulted in a decreased ability to recognize others. Crosby et al. (1962) reported that lesions to this region resulted in decreased sensation of tactual stimulation.

A major role of the vestibular region is the integration of information from the vestibular system and the skin, joint, and tension receptors for maintaining posture and balance. Ornitz has implicated the vestibular nuclei and adjacent structures in the modulation of sensory information, and has hypothesized that the interaction of these structures may account for autistic symptoms. Ornitz (1983) has reported that lesions to the general vestibular region can result in impaired response to stimuli and orienting information. He noted that stereotypic behavior may be secondary to dysfunction of vestibular feedback positional and motion information. Crosby *et al* (1962) and Ornitz (1983) noted increased activity levels in patients and animals with lesions to the vestibular region.

The literature suggests that central gray (periaqueductal gray) plays a role in the modulation of pain stimuli and motor responses to pain or threat of attack. This region is dorsal and medial to the vestibular regions discussed above. Blanchard, Williams, Lee, and Blanchard (1981b) reported that rats with central gray lesions show increase in social responses to other rats in the colonies. He also reported a generalized decrease in response to environmental and orienting stimuli (Blanchard, Williams, Lee, & Blanchard, 1981b). In a parallel vein, Hasobuchi, Adams, and Linchitz (1977) induced catatonic posturing in rats by injecting naloxone into this region.

Table 2 represents a summary of the evidence for localized neural involvement for function deficit found in autism. The localization of specific functions is not as direct as researchers had hoped. Table 2 demonstrates the complexity and distributed nature of functions in the brain. Other areas of functional localization research, such as language, has demonstrated similar conclusions in which there is a lack of localization of functions or even subfunctions (Ojemann, 1976).

Functional localization models similar to anatomical models can be derived and supported from a neurochemical system basis (see Young *et al.*, 1982), and these overlap the anatomical systems already delineated.

NEUROCHEMISTRY

Neurochemistry is the study of the chemical and metabolic processes in the nervous system. A major emphasis has been on the investigation of the behavior and action of chemical substances which act as transmitters between neurons (i.e., neurotransmitters; see Chapter 15 for a more detailed discussion). The level of activity of neurotransmitters has been correlated with the level found in various body fluids. The most direct method for measuring the activity of a neurotransmitter in humans is by assaying levels found in the cerebrospinal fluid (CSF). While this assays only neurotransmitters produced by the CNS, the primary areas or systems of interest, even if over- or underactive, may contribute only a portion of total CNS output, and correlation with specific sites or subsystems may be obscured. In addition, since chemical substances in the CSF are picked up by the venous blood drainage of the CNS and eventually excreted through the kidneys, neurotransmitters and their metabolites have also been assayed in blood and urine as an estimate of neurotransmitter activity in the CNS. However, these two sources often provide confounded results since other systems in the body also utilize neurotransmitters and contribute to blood and urine levels. Another source for the study of the metabolic activity of the neurochemicals and a model of the brain's metabolism has been the platelets containing an enzyme that helps regulate the level of neurochemicals by metabolizing them to an inactive state (i.e., monoamine oxidase—MAO). Assays have measured neurotransmitters, their metabolites, and enzyme activity directly.

Strategies in neurochemical research on autism have recently been reviewed by Young and associates (1982) and in this volume by Rumsey and Denckla, Chapter 3, and by Yuwiler and Freedman, Chapter 15. The three major sources of material for the measurement discussed above have dominated the studies of neurochemical correlates of autism in the literature. An alternative strategy has been to correlate the dysfunctional features of autism with animal models of altered neurochemical states. Several of the neurotransmitters have

Table 2. Regional Neural Involvement in the 12 Functions/Deficits Found in Autism[a]

Neural region	Functions/deficits											
	Recognition	Affectionate	Acknowledge	Motivation	Modulate	Orienting	Stereotyped	Posturing	Activity	Communicative intent	Reception	Production
	1	2	3	4	5	6	7	8	9	10	11	12
Neocortex												
Frontal lobes	+	+	+	+	+	?	+	o	−	+	p+	p+
Temporal lobes	p?	+	+	p+	+	p+	+	?	+	+	o	o
Mesocortex												
Amygdala	+	+	o	o	+	+	?	?	+	?	?	?
Hippocampus	+	+	+	+	+	+	+	−	+	p+	?	?
Septum	?	+	?	?	+	+	?	?	p+	?	?	p+
Corpus striatum	p+	?	?	?	+	+	+	+	+	?	?	p+
Thalamus	+	?	−	?	+	?	?	+	+	?	?	?
Brainstem												
Vestibular region	?	?	?	?	+	+	+	?	p+	?	?	?
Central gray	?	?	−	?	+	+	?	+	?	?	?	?

[a](+) = lesion study shows possible contribution to function; (−) = lesion study shows possible countereffects to function; (o) = no effect relative to function; (p) = postulated to have effect on function; (?) = unknown.

been mapped onto anatomical systems in the brain. These systems have additional functional features that act independently and interact with other neurochemical or anatomical systems to modulate and control brain activities. Metabolic and neurochemical mapping may link the neuroanatomical theories of autism to the chemical systems.

Serotonergic activity in the brain is believed to primarily modulate several neural systems and to affect several physiological functions and behaviors, such as sleep, body temperature, and sensory perception. Repeated studies have found increased blood levels of serotonin in about one-third of autistic subjects examined (Young *et al.*, 1982). Young and associates (1982) identify five major sources of variance in the measurement of blood serotonin and report that the pathophysiology relating hyperserotonemia with autism is not clear. Cohen's group (Cohen, Caparulo, Shaywitz, & Bowers, 1977) reports no differences in levels of 5-hydroxyindoleacetic acid (5-HIAA, the principal metabolite of serotonin) when contrasting autistic patients with other diagnostic groups. When examined in relation to functional features, greater attentional dysfunction and impaired social relating correlated with lower CSF 5-HIAA levels. Ritvo (personal communication, 1983) has attempted to treat autistic children with fenfluramine, which reportedly lowers brain serotonin, with mixed results. This is discussed further in Chapter 20.

Dopamine is thought to affect several functions and behaviors, including motor control, cognitive activity, motivation, and attention. Measures of blood levels of dopamine, however, have consistently shown no relationship to CNS activity (Young *et al.*, 1982). CSF levels of homovanillic acid (HVA, the principal metabolite of dopamine) are not significantly different between autistic and other impaired children. HVA levels seem to be more related to the level of motor disturbance. That is, higher HVA levels are correlated with greater motor disturbance. Studies examining HVA levels and motor behaviors may need to also investigate covariates such as age, sex, and serotonin levels (Cohen, Caparulo, Shaywitz, & Bowers, 1977).

Two catecholamines often discussed concurrently, owing to their similar effects on behavior, are norepinephrine and epinephrine. Norepinephrine is associated with cardiovascular-respiratory function, appetite, activity level, arousal, anxiety, and response to stress. Measures of blood levels of norepinephrine seem to be elevated in autistic subjects relative to controls. Studies of serum dopamine-beta-hydroxylase (DBH, the enzyme that converts dopamine to norepinephrine) activity in autistic and psychotic children (Johnston & Singer, 1982; Young *et al.*, 1982) have produced mixed results. In light of the question of continuity between adult and childhood psychoses, DBH was of interest because of reports that schizophrenic adults show abnormal DBH activity. Studies of 24-hour urinary 3-methoxy-4-hydroxyphenethylene glycol (MHPG, the main CNS metabolite of norepinephrine) have reported decreased levels associated with increased arousal, anxiety, or stress observed in autistic children (Young, Cohen, Caparulo, Brown, & Mass, 1979).

Monoamine oxidase (MAO) activity is thought to be of importance for the modulation and control over the levels of serotonin, dopamine, and norepinephrine. Platelet MAO activity is studied because it is thought to represent a reasonable model of MAO activity in the brain and because of the ease of accessibility compared to either brain tissue or CSF. Cohen, Young, and Roth (1977) reported no significant differences in platelet MAO activity between individuals with childhood autism, normal children, and normal adults.

A relatively new technology that allows researchers to image the metabolic processes in intact living brains has been the development of the positron emission tomography (PET) scanners. PET studies have focused on the distribution and relative rates of glucose utilization in the brain that allows for the dynamic mapping of localized brain metabolism. Rumsey and associates (1985) reported normal rates in resting brain glucose utilization in 15 autistic male patients. A few patients showed one or more areas with "extreme" relative metabolic rates, but no group of areas was consistently abnormal across all patients. This approach could provide an anatomical focus for neurochemical research based on the metabolic aberrations found.

Advances in the mapping of neurochemical systems in the brain has only added another level of complexity to the anatomical localization of functional mechanisms. An example of this is the delineation of the types of motor behavior elicited by stimulating or lesioning different dopamine systems. For example, stimulation of the mesolimbic dopamine system induces locomotor activity in animals, but stimulation of the nigrostriatal dopamine system produces stereotypy and circling behavior (Iversen, 1977).

GENETICS

The genetic approach focuses on the identification of inheritable factors for aspects of a syndrome or condition. Support is established using strategies such as family history research, twin studies, and other sibling studies, as well as fragile X and other chromosomal studies.

In a review of possible genetic components of autism, Spence (1976) concluded that twin studies indicate that a possible polygenic or multifactorial genetic mechanism exists only for *some* aspects or symptoms of autism. These conclusions are complicated by the lack of family data, the variable clustering of symptoms in autism, and lack of evidence identifying specific genetic mechanisms.

Early twin studies have provided suggestive support for genetic transmission of autism, mainly for language-cognitive components (DeMyer et al., 1981; Folstein & Rutter, 1977). Recent studies based on a population identified in the UCLA registry for genetic studies in autism have analyzed both twin and family data to test several genetic hypotheses (Ritvo, Freeman, Mason-Brothers, Mo, & Ritvo, 1985, Ritvo, Spence, et al., 1985).

Ritvo, Freeman, et al., (1985) utilized the UCLA registry to identify 61 pairs of twins. They found 95.7% concordance for monozygotic twins and only 23.5% for dizygotic twins. The major dysfunctions found were with the *language* and *cognitive* features of autism. Also, 46 families were identified with multiple incidences of autism. Using classical segregation analyses, they report some evidence for possible autosomal recessive inheritance (Ritvo, Spence, et al., 1985). Some criticism has been raised of these studies because of possible selection biases, diagnostic imprecision, and unreliability of family data. A more detailed discussion is provided in Chapter 5.

A collaborative study between UCLA and the University of Oregon Health Sciences examined the hypothesis that parents of autistic children may share more human leukocyte antigens (HLA or histocompatibility antigens) than parents of normals (Stubbs, Ritvo, & Mason-Brothers, 1985). Increased similarity between the parents may decrease the protection of the fetus from the mother's immune system and be related to findings that mothers of autistic children tend to share some of the symptoms of preeclampsia and have an increased incidence of spontaneous abortions. The study found that 75% of the pairs of parents of autistic children shared at least one antigen while only 22% of the comparison groups shared an antigen.

As with other investigative approaches, the genetic studies provide additional evidence of the diversity of etiological factors and mechanisms which may relate to autism. Increased concordance rates and segregation analyses suggest direct genetic effects, but the increased relationship to language disorders suggests a more nonspecific genetic factor. The studies of HLA antigens points to yet a quite different effect, that of the mother's immune system.

CRITIQUE OF LOCALIZATION APPROACHES AND MODELS

Our examination of various approaches such as the neuroanatomical, neurochemical, and genetic models might suggest that any or all of these approaches may lead to discovery of mechanisms to explain the syndromes of autism. At face value, it would seem that the only hurdle may be that of current technical ability to adequately localize specific lesions or dysfunctional systems.

Lieblich (1982) presents a comprehensive critique of the current approaches and conceptualizations in neuroscience. He points out that behavioral effects, altered as a result of lesions or stimulation (electrical or chemical), or correlated with cellular and surface recording, may not be an accurate measure of activity or function of the brain region under study. The several issues include the distinction between acute and long-term changes, effects due to local activity or to the activity of distant related structures, the differentiation between methodological paradigms, variance due to individual differences, and the distinction between the mechanism underlying normal function and the mode of action of agents causing abnormal function.

The distinction between acute and long-term effects is illustrated by the behavioral effects following septal lesions, where animals demonstrated hyperreactivity and emotional changes. These changes do not last, and they raise the question of the septum's true role in the modulation of the behaviors exhibited after lesioning it—primarily whether the changes are due to other systems compensating for the loss of the septum and its "true" functions (Albert & Chew, 1980).

The septal example could also illustrate the issue of attributing function to a region without knowing if that region is directly involved with that function under normal conditions, or if the effect or behavioral change is due to related regions that may be connected or have "fibers of passage" coursing through that region.

The differentiation between methodological paradigms can be illustrated by the differences found between recording techniques and lesioning techniques. For example, certain neurons were found to be related to the spatial ability through cellular recording techniques. When, however, these same neurons were lesioned there were no behavioral deficits for spatial ability found (O'Keefe & Nadel, 1978).

An example that addresses all three issues is in the differences found following serotonin depletion. Electrolytic lesions of the raphe nuclei in the midbrain result in severe depletion of serotonin and a marked increase in motor behavior (Lorens, Goldberg, Hole, Kohler, & Srebro, 1976). In contrast, neurotoxic depletion of serotonin, in the same system, does not result in any increase in motor behavior (Hole, Fuxe, & Jonsson, 1976).

Individual differences refer to the tremendous genetic effects that may account for species, strain, sex, and other organism-specific differences found in response to various manipulations. For example, the considerable variability in the degree and nature of behavioral changes following pharmacological treatment has been correlated highly with genetic differences and stimulated the development of psychopharmacogenetics (Broadhurst, 1978).

Addressing the erroneous logic in ascribing a role in normal function to mechanisms used to create dysfunction, Lieblich (1982) states:

. . . measures of coherence and reproducibility cannot be sufficient to dispel suspicions that a phenomenon discovered by experimental manipulation of the brain is artifact. Arbib (1972) has presented the argument that taking out a resistor from a television set, inducing a loud howl, does not mean that the resistor is the howl center, or for that matter, that the resistor has anything to do with the control of sound in the set. . . . Why is it so difficult for anybody lesioning resistors to convince us that his resistors are somehow involved in the control of sound in an electronic device, while it is relatively easy to convince readers of brain research publications that the stimulation, lesion, or recording of brain tissue is somehow involved in the control of behavior.

This is akin to the old medical adage that cure of pneumonia with penicillin does not indicate the pneumonia is caused by the lack of penicillin.

Lastly, Lieblich raises the question as to whether passively measured activities (chemical or electrical) have a certain relationship to functions of the "current" brain. That is, although any measure discovered to characterize the brain or parts of it may have great potential significance, one cannot be logically assured that the measure is relevant to the capability of the brain at its current developmental stage. He provides, as an example, the presumed role of the neocortex in higher complex functions, such as maternal and play behaviors. When the neocortex was removed in hamsters the animals developed the usual hamster-typical behavior patterns. He points out that while the interaction of the development of the neocortex and limbic elements could have been necessary for the appearance of hamster-typical behaviors, it is not necessary for cortex to be present for the expression of these behaviors at a later period.

The problems of identifying an anatomical or neurochemical locus as the explanatory mechanism for autism is further complicated when developmental data are taken into account and effects take place interactively, not only anatomically across systems, but across time as well.

DEVELOPMENTAL APPROACH

Developmental effects interact with functional neuroanatomy or neurochemistry and can manifest behavioral alterations in several ways. These effects also present alternatives to the "final common pathway" emphasis for research and clinical approaches. This framework has generated several possible models to explain how developmental mechanisms could contribute to the understanding of autism and related disorders.

Ciaranello et al. (1982) review several possible neurodevelopmental factors that could be affected and lead to an autistic syndrome (see also Chapter 14). They note several extrinsic and intrinsic factors that alter the late phases of neuronal development, which in turn affect the anatomical connectivity between brain sites, hence modifying the development of receptors, biochemical capacity, and overall functionality of the CNS.

On the basis that dysfunctions occurring in earliest phases of CNS formation are often fatal and at least lead to gross lesions, and the general lack of features implicating early dysmorphogenesis of fetal development, they reason that most of the known or suggested etiological agents associated with autism tend to occur late in gestation. The authors conclude that these effects most likely occur in the end stages of neuronal development during a period of neuronal elaboration and synapse formation.

During this period, there is elongation of the axon and elaboration of complex dendritic trees that determine the functional connections and interneuronal communications that are established. These processes are affected not only by intrinsic cell factors, like genes, but also by extrinsic factors, such as contact with other nerve fiber inputs. These extrinsic effects are not exclusively in the presynaptic neuron but are also in the development and elaboration of the postsynaptic neuron. The postsynaptic neuron also has retrograde effects on the presynaptic neuron through its contact and development. Much of this elaborative process continues postnatally and is dependent on environmental stimuli acting on the CNS. For example, continuous illumination of rats from birth to 80 days of age leads to an increased number of dendritic spines in specific groups of pyramidal neurons in the visual cortex (Parnavelas, 1978). This functional activity may be a critical factor in modifying insufficient or partially abnormal dendritic architecture occurring with developmental failures. This is particularly intriguing in light of the prodigious amount of research on the effects of isolation on primates. Many aspects of the autistic syndrome have been produced in monkeys using a social isolation paradigm (Harlow & Harlow, 1965; Holson & Sackett, 1984; Sackett, 1972).

Tanguay and Edwards (1982) present a model that examines the possible effects of abnormalities occurring during critical phases in development that may act as neuropathological agents to "higher" or later developed neural regions and functions.

Goldman-Rakic, Isseroff, Schwartz, and Bugbee (1983) review the neurobiology of cognitive development and closely examine the role and correlates of prefrontal cortex development and cognitive development. They conclude that there are functional shifts in the organization of the prefrontal cortex that occur during development. This is illustrated by the findings that behavioral capacities of an animal suffering brain damage early in life may appear normal at first but fail to develop at the same rate or show deficits later when compared to intact animals.

Developmental timing of different mechanisms could be disrupted and lead to structural and functional deficits. The controller gene illustration is that of the biosynthesis of thyroid hormone and its role in the retraction of the tail of a developing frog. In the frog, the gland that generates the hormone develops to a point at which it produces an increased level of hormone. Parallel to this, the tail develops the receptors for the hormone (Miranda, Botti, Ragnelli, & diCola, 1982). This is analogous to the runners in a relay race in which one runner passing off the baton needs to maintain his rate and not slow down too soon and the receiving runner has to be prepared to increase his rate and grab the baton: If either runner is off, they may drop the baton; hence, there is a small "window" in which the actions of both runners need to be timed just right.

Behavioral patterns may also affect neural development and structure. As Gottlieb (1983) points out, "normal development is brought about by the meshing of a number of separate though interrelated time schedules. The probable bidirectionality between the activity of genes and neural structure and function can be highly significant for behavior well beyond the early period of development in which the formative reciprocal interactions took place." Forty years ago, the developmental psychologist McGraw (1946) indicated that structure and function likely have a mutual and interactive influence. She said: "It seems fairly evident that certain structural changes take place prior to the onset of overt function; it seems equally evident that cessation of neurostructural development does not coincide with the onset of function. There is every reason to believe that when conditions are favorable, function makes some contribution to further advancement in structural development of the nervous system." The effects of behavior and experience probably go beyond simple maintenance of existing structure and include facilitation of structure (i.e., possible acceleration or extension) and induction of new structure (Gottlieb, 1984). Visual, auditory, and tactile inputs may influence the infant's capacity to modulate state and motor responses (Parmelee & Sigman, 1976). It is not known how long this sensitive period for fine tuning of the CNS lasts in normal infants, but it is presumed to extend for at least the first several months of life. There is also likely to be some variation of this "plasticity" between different structures and different functions. Even less is known concerning the specific effects of disruptions to these processes in humans, how fixed they are, and to what extent they can be overcome by later structural reorganization under the influence of stimuli, training, and other behavior.

SUMMARY AND CONCLUSIONS

Many of the approaches discussed above attempt to deal with an important inference issue—that is, that the phenomenon they are studying is specific and distinguishable from other factors that may be acting on a patient with the autism syndrome. We have attempted to illustrate the limitations of these approaches to resolving the issue of understanding the etiology of autism and its underlying biological mechanisms. The heterogeneity of the signs, symptoms, and behaviors associated with the autism syndrome raises significant question about the appropriateness of studying autism as a specific or discrete disorder. Further, the complexity of functional anatomical overlap presented suggests that a simple association between any structure or system and the complex behavioral syndrome of autism is unlikely. The developmental perspective suggests that effects of structural and developmental alterations may occur at considerably different times than their behavioral manifestations, and further, that these alterations may interactively influence the development of other systems. This indicates that alterations in the system may be far-reaching in both location and time from the site of original effects. These factors suggest significant changes in the investigative approach to understanding autism.

1. While the nosological conceptualizations of autism as a syndrome may have clinical and even political utility (i.e., funding, programming), it is not likely to be conducive to productive biological research. Instead it is important to study the full range of developmentally disordered populations, as well as normal individuals, in order to identify the regularity of association between any particular functions, symptoms, and signs that may share common biological dysfunctions (Lieblich, 1982). This will also facilitate the collections of more coherent groups of subjects who share specific functional problems, in order to improve the potential for identifying such common biological factors.

2. As a corollary, since autism lacks relative specificity as a fixed syndrome in that it is so variable, it shares so many symptoms and signs with other disorders, and the symptoms and signs occur on a continuum of function, research efforts should focus on specific functions rather than on specific clinically derived groups (see also Schopler & Rutter, 1978). Studies should elucidate the relationship of specific functions and their related dysfunctions to biological structure and functions, and agents that may have etiological import. This will require quantitatively more precise measurement of a function than has been common in such research and, often, the redefinition of functions in terms of more atomic or basic elements. This implies the development of new instruments, tests, techniques, and strategies.

3. The overlap of functional and behavioral expression associated with diverse biological (CNS) structures should direct efforts at a more integrative approach to understanding of the nervous system and away from focusing on isolated structures or systems. Much more needs to be learned about the interactive effects of alterations in one system on the function of other systems. This suggests that investigators with interest in manipulating or studying

the function of a particular structure or system (e.g., stimulation, lesions) are obliged to measure *simultaneously* the alterations these interventions produce in other interrelated structures and functions.

4. Since we are focusing on developmental disorders, there needs to be an overlying developmental perspective in this research. Clearly, identifying a particular dysfunctional system in a 3-year-old autistic child may tell us little about the specific etiological agent or its actual site of action. This implies that we need to learn a great deal more about the pre-, peri-, and postnatal experiences of developmentally disordered children, including those with autism. We also need to investigate more thoroughly the effects of various agents and alterations at specific sites, at various stages of pre- and postnatal development, and the resultant consequences for later development in a wide range of sites and systems of the brain.

5. Finally, we must recognize that behavioral development and experiential factors may have substantial effects on the postnatal central nervous system. This does not support the previously drawn false conclusion that improper or inappropriate child rearing may cause autism. There is no evidence for this and much against it. This does suggest, however, that efforts at early identification of children with, or at risk, for developmental disorders (including, but not exclusively, autism) are essential for evaluating the effects of environmental interventions. The influence of such environmental effects may be relatively limited to specific periods of high plasticity in the CNS, and may consequently limit the impact of interventions that take place at ages 3, 4, or older, as is typical for autism and other developmental disabilities.

It should be recognized that many of the investigators whose work was reviewed in this chapter have in fact tended to focus on relatively specific functions rather than examine the syndrome of autism per se; that many have in fact used other developmentally disordered groups as comparisons in their studies, and some have even specifically investigated certain functions (e.g., language) across developmental disorders; and that there has been an increasing recognition of the need to explore more complex systems rather than identify selective specific foci.

We would argue, however, that our current level of knowledge, as reviewed in this chapter, calls for a more comprehensive refocusing of research efforts in the direction of a functional approach where multimethods and multimeasures are applied to the study of identified functions, such as language, perception, and motor activity. Then complex models, incorporating interactions between different CNS systems, may be developed to account for deficits to a function, how it differentiates or shows similarities to other functions, and their individual roles in autism and other disorders. From this approach, more complex models could be derived from the models of functions, understanding of the interactions between functions, and interactions between CNS systems.

Given a theoretical, logical, and data-based model of functions, clinical models can then be developed and used to verify or modify the model of functions involved. These models should include research strategies that can be implemented to control for or measure identified developmental, genetic, and environmental factors. For example, controlled natural history studies of autism and other developmental disorders could quantify some developmental and environmental factors leading to the risk of developing an autistic or other syndrome. Individual differences found in those developing these syndromes could then be identified.

This approach will result in an empirically developed, theoretically coherent, and hierarchically organized taxonomy of discrete functions, their interactions in the expression of complex behaviors, and the organization of their dysfunctions in rationally and systematically defined disorders.

ACKNOWLEDGMENTS

The work discussed here is supported in part by NIMH Grant No. 1R01 MH37997-01, Children at Risk for Anxiety Disorders, and NIMH Grant No. 1R01 MH40078-01A1, Children at Risk for Depression.

REFERENCES

Albert, D. J., & Chew, G. L. (1980). The septal forebrain and the inhibitory modulation in attack and defense in the rat: A review. *Behavioral Neurology and Biology, 30,* 357–388.

Arbib, M. A. (1972). *The metaphorical brain.* New York: Wiley.

Bauman, M., & Kemper, T. L. (1985). Histoanatomic observations of the brain in early infantile autism. *Neurology, 35,* 866–874.

Blanchard, D. C., Blanchard, R. J., Lee, E. M. C., & Fukunaga, K. K. (1977). Movement arrest and the hippocampus. *Physiological Psychology, 5,* 331–335.

Blanchard, D. C., Williams, G., Lee, E. M. C., & Blanchard, R. J. (1981a). Taming in the wild Norway rat following lesions in the basal ganglia. *Physiology and Behavior, 27,* 995–1000.

Blanchard, D. C., Williams, G., Lee, E. M. C., & Blanchard, R. J. (1981b). Taming of wild rattus Norvegicus by lesions of the mesencephalic central gray. *Physiological Psychology, 9,* 157–163.

Boesen, V., & Aarkrog, T. (1967). Pneumoencephalography of patients in a child psychiatric department. *Danish Medical Bulletin, 14,* 210–218.

Broadhurst, P. L. (1978). *Drugs and the inheritance of behavior: A survey of comparative psychopharmacogenetics.* New York: Plenum Press.

Campbell, M., Rosebloom, S., Perry, R., George, A. E., Richeff, I. T., Anderson, L., Small, A. A., & Jennings, S. J. (1982). Computerized oxial tomography in young autistic children. *American Journal of Psychiatry, 139,* 510–512.

Caparulo, B. K., Cohen, D. J., Rothman, S. L., Young, J. G., Katz, J. D., Shaywitz, S. E., & Shaywitz, B. A. (1981). Computed tomographic brain scanning in children with developmental neuropsychiatric disorders. *Journal of the American Academy of Child Psychiatry, 20,* 338–357.

Capute, A. J., Derivan, A. T., Chauvel, P. J., & Rodriguez, A. (1975). Infantile autism: I. A prospective study of the diagnosis. *Developmental Medicine and Child Neurology, 17,* 58–62.

Chess, S. (1977). Follow-up report on autism in congenital rubella. *Journal of Autism and Childhood Schizophrenia, 7,* 68–81.

Chozick, B. S. (1983). The behavioral effects of lesions of the corpus striatum: A review. *International Journal of Neuroscience, 19,* 143–160.

Ciaranello, R. D., Vandenberg, S. R., & Anders, T. F. (1982). Intrinsic and extrinsic determinants of neural development: Relation to infantile autism. *Journal of Autism and Developmental Disorders, 12,* 115–145.

Cohen, D. J., Caparulo, B. K., Shaywitz, B. A., & Bowers, M. B. (1977). Dopamine and serotonin metabolism in neuropsychiatrically disturbed children. *Archives of General Psychiatry, 34,* 545–550.

Cohen, D. J., Young, J. G., & Roth, J. A. (1977). Platelet monoamine oxidase in early childhood autism. *Archives of General Psychiatry, 34,* 534–537.

Coleman, M. (1979). Studies of the autistic syndromes. In R. Katzman (Ed.), *Congenital and acquired cognitive disorders. Research Publications, Association for Research in Nervous and Mental Disease, 57,* 265–275.

Corbett, J., Harris, R., Taylor, R., & Trimble, M. (1977). Progressive distintegrative psychoses of childhood. *Journal of Child Psychology and Psychiatry, 18,* 211–219.

Crosby, E. C., Humphrey, T., & Lauer, W. (1962). *Correlative neuroanatomy of the nervous system.* New York: Macmillan.

Dalby, M. (1975). *Air studies of speech-retarded children: Evidence of early lateralization of language function.* Abstract, First International Congress of Child Neurology, Toronto.

Damasio, A. R., & Maurer, R. G. (1978). A neurological model for childhood autism. *Archives of Neurology, 35,* 777–786.

Damasio, H., Maurer, R. G., Damasio, A. R., & Chui, H. C. (1980). Computerized tomographic scan findings in patients with autistic behavior. *Archives of Neurology, 37,* 504–510.

DeLong, G. R. (1978). A neuropsychologic interpretation of infantile autism. In M. Rutter & E. Schopler (Eds.), *A reappraisal of concepts and treatment.* New York: Plenum Press.

DeMyer, M. K. (1979). *Parents and children in autism.* Washington, D.C.: V. H. Winston.

DeMyer, M. K., Bryson, C. Q., & Churchill, D. W. (1973). The earliest indicators of pathological development: Comparison of symptoms during infancy and early childhood in normal, subnormal, schizophrenic and autistic children. In *Biological and environmental determinants of early development. Research Publications, Association for Research in Nervous and Mental Disease, 51,* 298–332.

DeMyer, M. K., Hingtgen, J. N., & Jackson, R. K. (1981). Infantile autism reviewed: A decade of research. *Schizophrenia Bulletin, 7*(3), 388–451.

Fish, B., & Ritvo, E. R. (1978). Psychoses of childhood. In J. D. Noshpitz & I. Berlin (Eds.), *Basic handbook of child psychiatry.* New York: Basic Books.

Fish, B., & Ritvo, E. R. (1979). Psychoses of childhood. In J. D. Noshpitz (Ed.), *Basic handbook of child psychiatry (Vol. 2). Disturbances in development* (pp. 249–304). New York: Basic Books.

Folstein, S., & Rutter, M. (1977). Genetic influences and infantile autism. *Nature, 265,* 726–728.

Folstein, S., & Rutter, M. (1978). A twin study of individuals with infantile autism. In M. Rutter & E. Schopler (Eds.), *A reappraisal of concepts and treatment.* New York: Plenum Press.

Freeman, B. J., Ritvo, E., Guthrie, D., Schroth, P., & Ball, J. (1978). The behavior observation scale for autism. Initial methodology, data analysis, and preliminary findings on 89 children. *Journal of the American Academy of Child Psychiatry, 17,* 576–588.

Fuster, J. M. (1980). *The prefrontal cortex: Anatomy, physiology, and neuropsychology of the frontal lobe.* New York: Raven Press.

Goldman-Rakic, P. S., Isseroff, A., Schwartz, M. L., & Bugbee, N. M. (1983). The neurobiology of cognitive development. In P. H. Mussen (Ed.), M. M. Haith & J. J. Campos (Vol. Eds.), *Handbook of child psychology* (Vol. 2). New York: Wiley.

Gottlieb, G. (1983). The psychobiological approach to developmental issues. In P. H. Mussen (Eds.), M. M. Haith & J. J. Campos (Vol. Ed.), *Handbook of child psychology* (Vol. 2). New York: Wiley.

Harlow, H. F., & Harlow, M. K. (1965). The affectional systems. In A. M. Schrier, H. F. Harlow, & F. Stollnitz (Eds.), *Behavior of nonhuman primates* (Vol. 2). New York: Academic Press.

Hasobuchi, Y., Adams, J. E., & Linchitz, R. (1977). Pain relief by electrical stimulation of the central gray matter in humans and its reversal by naloxone. *Science, 197,* 183–186.

Hauser, S. L., DeLong, G. R., & Rosman, N. P. (1975). Pneumographic findings in the infantile autism syndrome: A correlation with temporal lobe disease. *Brain, 98,* 667–668.

Heir, D. E., LeMay, M., & Rosenberger, P. B. (1978). Autism: Association with reversed cerebral asymmetry. *Neurology, 28,* 348–349.

Hingtgen, J. N., & Bryson, C. Q. (1972). Recent developments in the study of early childhood psychoses: Infantile autism, childhood schizophrenia, and related disorders. *Schizophrenia Bulletin, 5,* 8–54.

Hole, K., Fuxe, K., & Jonsson, G. (1976). Behavioral effects of 5,7-dihydroxy tryptamine lesions of ascending 5-hydroxytryptamine pathways. *Brain Research, 107,* 385–389.

Holson, R., & Sackett, G. P. (1984). Effects of isolation rearing on learning by mammals. *Psychology of Learning and Motivation, 18.*

Isaacson, R. (1974). *The limbic system*. New York: Plenum Press.

Iversen, S. D. (1977). Brain dopamine systems and behavior. In L. L. Iversen, S. D. Iversen, & S. H. Snyder (Eds.), *Handbook of psychopharmacology* (Vol. 8, pp. 333–384). New York: Plenum Press.

Johnston, M. V., & Singer, H. S. (1982). Brain neurotransmitters and neuromodulators in pediatrics. *Pediatrics, 70,* 57–68.

Kanner, L. (1943). Autistic disturbances of affective contact. *Nervous Child, 2,* 217–250.

Knobloch, H., & Pasamanick, B. (1975). Some etiologic and prognostic factors in early infantile autism and psychosis. *Pediatrics, 55,* 182–191.

Lieblich, I. (1982). Implication of the use of the genetic paradigm for brain research. In I. Lieblich (Ed.), *Genetics of the Brain*. New York: Elsevier.

Lorens, S. A., Goldberg, H. C., Hole, K., Kohler, C., & Srebro, B. (1976). Activity, avoidance learning and regional 5-hydroxytryptamine following intrabrain stem 5,7-dihydroxytryptamine and electrolytic midbrain raphe lesions in the rat. *Brain Research, 108,* 97–113.

Maurer, R. G., & Damasio, A. R. (1982). Childhood autism from the point of view of behavioral neurology. *Journal of Autism and Developmental Disorders, 12,* 195–205.

McGraw, M. B. (1946). Maturation of behavior. In L. Carmichael (Ed.), *Manual of child psychology*. New York: Wiley.

Milner, B. (1976). CNS maturation and language acquisition. In H. Whitaker & H. A. Whitaker (Eds.), *Studies in neurolinguistics*. New York: Academic Press.

Miranda, M., Botti, D., Ragnelli, A. M., & diCola, M. (1982). A study on melanogenesis and catecholamine biosynthesis during *Bufo bufo* development. *J. Exp. Zool., 224(2),* 217–222.

Myers, R. E., Swett, C., & Miller, M. (1973). Loss of social group affinity following prefrontal lesions in free-ranging macaques. *Brain Research, 64,* 257–269.

Ojemann, G. A. (1976). Subcortical language mechanisms. In H. Whitaker & H. A. Whitaker (Eds.), *Studies in Neurolinguistics*. New York: Academic Press.

O'Keefe, J., & Nadel, L. (1978). *The hippocampus as a cognitive map*. New York: Oxford University Press.

Ornitz, E. M. (1974). The modulation of sensory input and motor output in autistic children. *Journal of Autism and Childhood Schizophrenia, 4,* 197–215.

Ornitz, E. M. (1978). Biological homogeneity or heterogeneity? In M. Rutter & E. Schopler (Eds.), *A reappraisal of concepts and treatment*. New York: Plenum Press.

Ornitz, E. M. (1983). The functional neuroanatomy of infantile autism. *International Journal of Neuroscience, 19,* 85–124.

Ornitz, E. M. (1985). Neurophysiology of infantile autism. *Journal of the American Academy of Child Psychiatry, 24,* 251–262.

Ornitz, E. M., Guthrie, D., & Farley, A. J. (1978). The early symptoms of childhood autism. In G. Serban (Eds.), *Cognitive defects in the development of mental illness*. New York: Brunner/Mazel.

Parmelee, A. H., & Sigman, M. (1976). Development of visual behavior & neurological organization on pre-term and full-term infants. In A. D. Pick (Ed.), *Minnesota Symposia on Child Psychology* (Vol. 10). Minneapolis: University of Minnesota Press.

Parnavelas, J. G. (1978). Influence of stimulation of cortical development. In M. A. Corner, R. E. Baker, N. E. van de Poll, D. F. Swaab, & H. B. M. Uylings (Eds.), Maturation of the nervous system, *Progress in Brain Research, 48,* 247–259.

Pomperano, O. (1967a). The neurophysiologic mechanisms of the postural and motor events during desynchronized sleep. *Research Publications, Association for Research in Nervous and Mental Disease, 45,* 351–423.

Pomperano, O. (1967b). Sensory inhibition during motor activity in sleep. In M. D. Yahr & D. P. Purpura (Eds.), *Neurophysiological basis of normal and abnormal motor activities*. New York: Hewlett, Raven Press.

Reichler, R. J., & Schopler, E. (1971). Observations on the nature of human relatedness. *Journal of Autism and Childhood Schizophrenia, 1,* 283–296.

Reichler, R. J., & Schopler, E. (1976). Developmental therapy: A program model. In E. Schopler & R. J. Reichler (Eds.), *Psychopathology and child development*. New York: Plenum Press.

Ritvo, E. R., & Freeman, B. J. (1978). National Society for Autistic Children definition of the syndrome of autism. *Journal of the American Academy of Child Psychiatry, 17*, 565–576.

Ritvo, E. R., Freeman, B. J., Mason-Brothers, A., Mo, A., & Ritvo, A. M. (1985). Concordance for the syndrome of autism in 40 pairs of afflicted twins. *American Journal of Psychiatry, 142*, 74–77.

Ritvo, E. R., Freeman, B. J., Scheibel, A. B., Duong, P. T., Robinson, H., & Guthrie, D. (1986). Decreased Purkinje cell density in four autistic patients: Initial findings of the UCLA-NSAC Autopsy Research Project. *American Journal of Psychiatry, 43(7)*, 862–866.

Ritvo, E. R., Spence, M. A., Freeman, B. J., Mason-Brothers, A., Mo, A., & Marazita, M. L. (1985). Evidence for autosomal recessive inheritance in 46 families with multiple incidence of autism. *American Journal of Psychiatry, 142*, 187–192.

Rumsey, J. M., Duara, R., Grady, C., Rapoport, J. L., Margolin, R. A., Rapoport, S. I., & Cutler, N. R. (1985). Brain metabolism in autism. *Archives of General Psychiatry, 42*, 448–455.

Rutter, M. (1978). Diagnosis and definition of childhood autism. *Journal of Autism and Childhood Schizophrenia, 8*, 139–161.

Rutter, M., Bartak, L., & Newman, S. (1971). Autism—A central disorder of cognition and language? In M. Rutter (Ed.), *Infantile autism: Concepts, characteristics and treatment*. London: Churchill-Livingstone.

Rutter, M., & Lockyer, L. (1967). A five to fifteen year follow-up study of infantile psychosis. I. Description of the sample. *British Journal of Psychiatry, 113*, 1169–1182.

Sackett, G. P. (1972). *Isolation rearing in monkeys: Diffuse and specific effects on later behavior*. Colloques Internationaux du C.N.R.S., No. 198, Modèles animaux du comportement humain.

Schneider, A. M., & Tarshis, B. (1980). *An introduction to physiological psychology* (2nd ed.). New York: Random House.

Schopler, E., Reichler, R. J., DeVillis, R. F., & Daly, K. (1980). Toward objective classification of childhood autism: Childhood Autism Rating Scale (CARS). *Journal of Autism and Developmental Disorders, 10*, 91–103.

Schopler, E., Reichler, R. J., & Renner, B. R. (1986). The Childhood Autism Rating Scale (CARS): For diagnostic screening and classification of autism. New York: Irvington.

Schopler, E., & Rutter, M. (1978). Subgroups vary with selection purpose. In M. Rutter & E. Schopler (Eds.), *Autism: A reappraisal of concepts and treatment* (pp. 507–517). New York: Plenum Press.

Shaywitz, B. A., Cohen, D. J., Leckman, J. F., Young, J. G., & Bowers, M. B. (1980). Ontogeny of dopamine and serotonin metabolities in the cerebrospinal fluid of children with neurological disorders. *Developmental Medicine and Child Neurology, 22*, 748–754.

Spence, M. A. (1976). Genetic studies. In E. Ritvo (Ed.), *Autism: Diagnosis, current research and management* (pp. 169–174). New York: Halstead/Wiley.

Spyer, K. M., Ghelarducci, B., & Pompeiano, O. (1973). Responses of brain stem reticular neurons to tilting. *Brain Research, 56*, 321–326.

Stubbs, E. G., Ritvo, E. R., & Mason-Brothers, A. (1985). Autism and shared parental HLA antigens. *Journal of the American Academy of Child Psychiatry, 24*, 182–185.

Tanguay, P. E., & Edwards, R. M. (1982). Electrophysiological studies of autism: The whisper of the bang. *Journal of Autism and Developmental Disorders, 12*, 172–184.

Young, J. G., Cohen, D. J., Caparulo, B. K., Brown, S., & Maas, J. W. (1979). Decreased 24-hour urinary MHPG in childhood autism. *American Journal of Psychiatry, 136*, 1055–1057.

Young, J. G., Kavanagh, M. E., Anderson, G. M., Shaywitz, B. A., & Cohen, D. J. (1982). Clinical neurochemistry of autism and associated disorders. *Journal of Autism and Developmental Disorders, 12*, 147–165.

Neurobiological Research Priorities in Autism

JUDITH M. RUMSEY and MARTHA B. DENCKLA

Views regarding the etiology of infantile autism have shifted from early psychogenic hypotheses to today's neurobiologic hypotheses as a result of scientific research. Both careful biological and careful behavioral studies have contributed to this dramatic shift. Behavioral studies have shown that cognitive deficits in autism are present in infancy, are primary rather than secondary to social withdrawal, are strongly prognostic, and place children at greater risk for seizures (Rutter, 1983). Biological studies of autism have identified a high incidence of minor physical anomalies, dermatoglyphic abnormalities, perinatal complications, and seizures, as well as subtle anatomical abnormalities on CT scans and associations with established medical disease (e.g., phenylketonuria, rubella) (DeMyer, Hingtgen, & Jackson, 1981). Yet no specific biological markers have been identified, and our knowledge of autism's neurobiology remains quite limited.

This chapter attempts to identify research priorities that hold promise for advancing our understanding of the neurobiology of infantile autism. These priorities fall into three major categories, which correspond to the major subdivisions of this chapter. The first centers around the need to characterize more clearly the behavioral pathology that defines autism and to develop a classification system for subtyping the heterogeneity seen within this syndrome. The second category consists of research directed toward localizing dysfunction within the central nervous system. This includes indirect methods of examining brain anatomy and functioning, as well as direct postmortem studies of brain. Third and last is the need to further study and explore possible neurochemical abnormalities.

While this chapter considers each of these priority areas separately, in reality they overlap. For example, clarification of behavioral pathology (e.g., social impairments and communication deficits) may well suggest hypotheses concerning the localization of dysfunction within the central nervous system. Similarly, localization studies may suggest hypotheses concerning disordered neurochemistry. Thus, these divisions serve an organizational

JUDITH M. RUMSEY • Child Psychiatry Branch, National Institute of Mental Health, Bethesda, Maryland 20892.   MARTHA B. DENCKLA • Developmental Neurology Branch, National Institute of Neurological and Communicative Disorders and Stroke, Bethesda, Maryland 20205.

purpose and the lines of demarcation among them are somewhat arbitrary. Subdivisions within these categories reflect various research disciplines.

CHARACTERIZATION AND CLASSIFICATION OF BEHAVIORAL PATHOLOGY

Clearly operationalized research definitions of infantile autism are needed to advance our understanding of this syndrome. Ambiguity and variations in research definitions now complicate attempts to compare findings across studies. Clinical diagnosis continues to serve as the sole definition of autism in most research. This contrasts with the widespread reliance on standardized scales and other research instruments used to diagnose, subtype, and quantify other behaviorally defined disorders.

A clinical diagnosis of autism encompasses extreme heterogeneity with respect to intellectual and language functioning, behavioral pathology, and medical status. Autism is seen in association with identifiable neurological, infectious, and metabolic disease (or a history of such) and seizures, as well as in physically healthy individuals ("idiopathic autism"). Failures to adequately describe research samples with respect to concomitant developmental disorders and medical disease often make it difficult to interpret research findings. Thus, there remains a need to better characterize research samples and to classify the range of behavioral pathology associated with autism in a manner that may be meaningfully related to neurobiological abnormality.

This need can be addressed through the development of more adequate classification systems ("clinical nosology"), ethological studies, neuropsychological studies of social-affective functioning, and studies of communication in autism. Ethological studies can help elucidate the nature of autistic behavior and facilitate the development of animal models for studying this disorder. Neuropsychological studies can help define in brain-related terms the processing deficits that accompany the core social-affective symptoms of autism. Studies of language and communication can help refine our behavioral descriptions and research definitions, as well as provide information relevant to localization of dysfunction.

Clinical Nosology

Clearly operationalized classification schemes with demonstrated reliability and validity (discriminant, concurrent, and predictive) are still needed for diagnosing young children, particularly preschool-age children, (1) as autistic versus nonautistic mentally retarded or developmentally language-disordered and (2) as subtypes within the autistic spectrum.

There is an emerging consensus that social impairment—deviant and not merely delayed social responsiveness and social interaction—constitutes the core characteristic of autism and that communicative, particularly nonverbal, impairment constitutes an essential characteristic. In addition, repetitive behavior (stereotyped, compulsive, or ritualistic) is so often seen in conjunction with these impairments that it acts as a confirmatory diagnostic criterion. While this triad of symptoms provides a conceptual basis for differential diagnosis, operational definitions of these constructs require further development. An evaluation of available diagnostic scales is provided by Parks (1983), who notes a need for additional studies to establish discriminant validity.

High- and low-IQ autistic children differ significantly in their behavioral repertoires and symptomatology (Bartak & Rutter, 1976; Freeman et al., 1981), making developmental status paramount in evaluating the clinical significance of individual behavioral patterns. Changes in symptomatology with age further complicate matters (Rutter, 1970). Thus, developmental norms on autistic, normal, retarded, and dysphasic children are needed for relevant behavioral measures.

Clinical ratings on higher-order constructs (like social aloofness) might well be operationalized in direct examinations of more specific social, communicative, cognitive, play, and neuromotor skills in young preschool children. Differentiation of subtypes with differing neurobehavioral profiles might substantially decrease the heterogeneity apparent within autism and enhance opportunities for identifying biological correlates. Course and prognosis and a variety of biological measures should be studied in relationship to early differences in developmental and behavioral patterns.

Ethology

Ethological studies are needed to clarify behavioral patterns specific to autism, their interaction with other organismic variables (e.g., intelligence, linguistic competence, age) and environmental variables, and their counterparts in nonhuman primates. Observational studies should increasingly center on social interactions, e.g., parent–child, peer–child. Disordered early attachment and later disordered social reciprocity require operationalization. Studies in naturalistic settings (Donnellan, Anderson, & Mesaros, 1984; Mirenda, Donnellan, & Yoder, 1983; Richer & Coss, 1976; Sigman & Ungerer, 1983) have begun to appear in the literature and should identify qualitative behaviors of critical interest for further controlled study in laboratory settings.

Environmental influences on social approach and withdrawal behaviors should be determined through experimental studies. While some ethologists postulate that autistic children are motivated to avoid social encounters and that social approach behaviors on the part of others increase "flight" behaviors (Richer, 1978; Tinbergen & Tinbergen, 1976), others (e.g., Clark & Rutter, 1981; McHale, Simeonsson, Marcus, & Olley, 1980) find that social approaches and demands increase social interaction. The quality of social interaction, however, remains quite deviant and requires further description and specification.

A clear, specific behavioral profile for autism (which includes responses to environmental variables) mapped onto an appropriate developmental chart will permit the construction of equivalent profiles in nonhuman primates, paving the way for valid animal models of autism. The shift from an emphasis on linguistic (Churchill, 1972) to social/communicative dysfunction, involving nonverbal and prelinguistic behavior as well (Rutter, 1983), increases opportunities for identifying autistic behaviors (e.g., failures of social attachment, generalized communicative impairments) that can be measured in nonhuman primates. Effects of circumscribed lesions on communicative and social competence have been studied in monkeys (primarily adults) to some extent. However, attempts to model infantile autism are a very recent development and require the establishment of specific behavioral equivalencies.

Clinical Neuropsychology

Neuropsychological tests meaningfully related to understanding the autistic spectrum are also needed. Constructs such as sociability and the perception and expression of affect need to be operationalized. Standardized instruments relevant to social or affective issues are either nonexistent or inapplicable to young communicatively impaired children, so that their development constitutes a research priority. Such measures should bridge a wide developmental span, ranging from primitive social drive to subtle expressive capacities and empathy. Again, multiple contrast groups (e.g., dysphasic, retarded, and normal children matched for chronological age and for mental age) should advance our understanding of whatever social-affective characteristics emerge as autistic "signatures."

It remains difficult to conceptualize just what sort of learning or information-processing deficit in infancy could selectively impair social development, while sparing many aspects of sensory-motor-cognitive capacity, a dissociation that becomes more striking in adolescence and adulthood. Rutter (1983) has concluded that the social abnormalities of autistic patients probably stem from a special sort of cognitive deficit, one in the domain of social and emotional "give and take," rather than a cognitive deficit extrinsic to sociability (i.e., explicable by general language, attentional, sensory, or perceptual aspects of cognition as tapped by standard cognitive measures). Further documentation and exploration of the special difficulty autistic individuals demonstrate clinically with tasks involving social context or content are needed. To date, few experimental studies have systematically addressed this issue of selective social impairment.

Additional research issues are the relative contributions of motivational versus social skill deficits and the receptive versus expressive nature of social impairments in autistic persons of different ages. Some level of social motivation appears to develop in some proportion of autistic persons over time. While young autistic children either passively accept cuddling or stubbornly resist social contact, older autistic persons may initiate and persistently engage in social approaches characterized by a glaring lack of skill. Whether skill deficits preceded or followed the social isolation is unclear. Whether these deficits are based on poor social comprehension or whether they are primarily expressive in nature is also unknown.

Language and Communication

While severe language impairment is a universal feature of infantile autism in young children, the precise nature of the impairment and its developmental course vary. Language may be absent, deficient, or excessive and deviant. Comparative studies of autistic, retarded, and dysphasic children (Bartak, Rutter, & Cox, 1977; Cantwell, Baker, & Rutter, 1978; Cohen, Caparulo, & Shaywitz, 1976; Tager-Flusberg, 1981; Waterhouse & Fein, 1982) have taught us that some features of autistic language—most notably phonology and syntax— follow a normal developmental course and thus, when impaired, can be characterized as "delayed." Other features (e.g., delayed echolalia, repetitions of one's own utterances, thinking aloud/action accompaniments, metaphorical language, dysprosodies, paucity of spontaneous speech [Cantwell & Baker, 1978; Prior, 1977; Shapiro, Roberts, & Fish, 1970; Simmons & Baltaxe, 1975]) are specific to autism. Autistic speech has also been described as rigid and socially inappropriate, overly literal, and perseverative (Tager-Flusberg, 1981; Waterhouse & Fein, 1982). These deviant features include disturbances of the pragmatic aspects of speech and language, features that are intimately tied to social functioning.

While clinically described by several investigators, these pragmatic disturbances have largely eluded formal definition and description. Recent preliminary studies of pragmatic disturbances in small samples of autistic children and in individual cases suggest more communicative speech with a familiar caretaker than with a stranger (Bernard-Opitz, 1982), the use of echolalia to maintain interaction (Prizant & Duchan, 1981), and more qualitative than quantitative differences in interactive acts (Wetherby & Prutting, 1984). The latter hint at skill deficits in these limited samples.

Nonverbal communicative disturbances are now also recognized as specific features of autism. During infancy, deficiencies are seen in mime, gesture, imitation, and social attachment behaviors (Bartak, Rutter, & Cox, 1975; Cohen et al., 1976; Wing, 1971). During childhood, autistic children do not appear frustrated by their oral communication deficits and fail to compensate nonverbally, as do dysphasic, deaf, and nonautistic retarded children (Bartak et al., 1975; Boucher, 1976; Cohen et al., 1976).

Systematic studies of pragmatic and extralinguistic disturbances using adequate samples are needed to characterize communicative deviance in autism. Better definition of nonverbal impairments may permit their study in animal models. Both may carry researchers away from left perisylvian brain regions, known to underlie linguistic skills, in the search for localized brain abnormalities (Damasio & Maurer, 1978; Fein, Humes, Kaplan, Lucci, & Waterhouse, 1984).

LOCALIZATION RESEARCH

While there is little doubt that autism is a brain disorder, where in the brain the anatomical substrates of autistic symptoms lie remains a mystery. The history of clinical neurology teaches us that localization, the "where" of brain–behavior relationships, is a useful and time-saving step for uncovering pathophysiological mechanisms and, still further down the line, fundamental disease etiologies. Without the localization step, direct attacks upon biochemical or other pathophysiological mechanisms can be like random ad hoc searches for the proverbial needle in a haystack.

Anatomic localization research relevant to autism can proceed simultaneously in animal experiments and in patient populations with motor examinations, in vivo brain imaging (anatomical and physiological), and neuropathological studies, each of which is discussed below. Comparisons of clinical and animal studies testing similar hypotheses concerning brain circuits subserving equivalent behaviors may narrow the candidates for anatomic localization.

Hypothesis-driven anatomic research has been greatly facilitated by thoughtful neurological surveys such as that of Damasio and Maurer (1978). Briefly, this review suggested that neuroanatomic substrates for autism be sought through analogies between neurobehavioral symptoms in autism and those in adults with acquired focal brain lesions. The neurobehavioral symptoms of autism, as outlined by Damasio and Maurer, include (1) diminished emotional reactivity to aversive aspects of the environment or pain and reduced spontaneous exploration, (2) failure to structure visual exploration, (3) diminished capacity to inhibit strongly established responses, (4) memory dysfunction, with habit memory or learning preponderant over "conscious" associative learning, (5) akinesia, dyskinesia, choreoathetoid posturing, other involuntary or ticlike movements, and (6) impaired modulation of movements and imprecision of coordination. By analogy, these implicate the (1) anterior cingulate cortex, (2) orbitofrontal cortex, (3) amygdala, (4) hippocampus, (5) basal ganglia, and (6) cerebellum as possible lesion sites. Highlighted were the mesolimbic cortex and neostriatum, which constitute principal regions of termination of dopaminergic neurons.

Other localization hypotheses (DeMyer et al., 1981) have not been as fully elaborated. Several investigators (Baltaxe & Simmons, 1975; Prior, 1979) have hypothesized selective impairment of the left hemisphere in autism, primarily because of associated language deficits. This hypothesis is increasingly being challenged by findings of nonverbal and extralinguistic impairments (Fein *et al.*, 1984). DeLong (1976) and others (Hauser, DeLong, & Rosman, 1975; Hetzler & Griffin, 1981) have hypothesized that mesial temporal structures are dysfunctional in autism and that damage to these structures may be unilateral (left) in some patients and bilateral in others. Neuroanatomical, neuromotor, and neurophysiological studies can test these alternative hypotheses.

Much of our knowledge concerning brain–behavior relationships is based on studies of adults with acquired lesions. However, one must be cautious in drawing inferences about children or developmental disorders from data on localization of dysfunction in adults. Early cerebral insult may result in greater functional reorganization of the brain than is seen in the case of adult-acquired lesions. Notable in this regard is the fact that children with unilateral left hemisphere lesions resulting in acquired aphasias frequently show good spoken language recovery (Alajouanine & Lhermitte, 1965; Basser, 1962). In addition, neuronal connections may be deranged in developmental disorders (Galaburda, Sherman, Rosen, Aboitiz, & Geschwind, 1985), further complicating inferences about localization of dysfunction. Thus, an autistic child who eventually develops language may display abnormal cerebral organization of language functioning. Neurophysiological techniques can be used to test hypotheses about the organization, or possible reorganization, of cortical functions in autism.

Motor Studies

Relatively immune to cultural influences, motor examinations may provide localization clues when abnormalities are compared with those seen in neurological disorders with known focal pathology. Damasio and his colleagues (Damasio & Maurer, 1978; Vilensky, Damasio, & Maurer, 1981) have clinically described motility disturbances suggestive of extrapyramidal dysfunction in autism. These include akinesia, bradykinesia, abnormalities of postural fixation, abnormal righting reflexes, alterations of muscle tone, "reverse" facial movement dysfunction (mimetic/emotional facial weakness), gait disturbances, and involuntary movements. Kinesiologic analysis of gait in autism using high-speed motion picture techniques (Vilensky *et al.*, 1981) has shown similarities to gait disturbances measured in Parkinsonian adults. Additional controlled, quantitative studies of motility would be useful, particularly if done longitudinally, since clinical experience suggests that extrapyramidal motoric disturbances are more striking in older autistic populations.

Another motor measure likely to yield useful results is that of prosody—the stresses, inflections, and rhythm of speech. Autistic spectrum disorders are clinically characterized by prosodic disturbances that appear to encompass both syntactic and affective components of vocal contour (Baltaxe & Simmons, 1983). Such disturbances may implicate right anterior cortical or subcortical, extrapyramidal involvement (Kent & Rosenbek, 1982). Thus, acoustic spectral analysis of autistic speech, separately analyzed for informational (denotative) and affective (connotative) dysfunction, is of research interest. The receptive versus expressive nature of dysprosodies in autism could be clarified with tests of the ability to perceive and interpret affective and nonaffective aspects of prosody.

Neuroanatomical Imaging

Autism has been studied with *in vivo* neuroanatomical imaging techniques for approximately 10 years now. Computerized tomographic (CT) scan studies have identified gross abnormalities, such as lesions, only in a minority of patients, generally those with identified neurological disorders (Damasio, Maurer, Damasio, & Chui, 1980; Gillberg & Svendsen, 1983). Even then, no single abnormality has been discernible. Thus, most CT-scan studies have applied quantitative measures in a search for subtle abnormalities.

Quantitative studies show that, contrary to early report (Hier, LeMay, & Rosenberg, 1979), autistic patients do not, as a group, show abnormal anterior or posterior cerebral asymmetries (Damasio et al., 1980; Gillberg & Svendsen, 1983; Tsai, Jacoby, & Stewart, 1983; Tsai, Jacoby, Stewart, & Beisler, 1982). Ventricular asymmetries identified in patients with neurological disease (Damasio et al., 1980) have not been replicated with less biased measures in idiopathic cases of autism (Rosenbloom et al., 1984). Ventricular enlargement is seen in a minority of physically healthy autistic subjects across methods when retarded controls are not included (Campbell et al., 1982; Caparulo et al., 1981; Rosenbloom et al., 1984). The percentage of autistic patients showing abnormalities appears low relative to children with other developmental disorders, language impairments, and Tourette syndrome, and abnormalities seen across these groups appear to be nonspecific (Caparulo et al., 1981).

A more specific finding is that of increased fourth ventricular width and cerebellar atrophy recently reported in a CT study of autistic children (Bauman, LeMay, Bauman, & Rosenberger, 1985). This warrants additional investigation, because recent neuropathological studies (Bauman & Kemper, 1985; Ritvo et al., 1986) have found evidence of cerebellar abnormality.

Another discrete abnormality identified in an earlier pneumoencephalographic study (Hauser, DeLong, & Rosman, 1975) is the dilatation of the temporal horn of the left lateral ventricle, which suggested flattening and atrophy of the hippocampus. While discrete enlargement of the left temporal horn has not been reported in CT studies, this may be a function of differences in methods rather than an indication that such discrete enlargement does not exist (Muramoto, Kuru, & Sugishita, 1979). Thus, this finding warrants replication with noninvasive methods.

Magnetic resonance imaging (MRI) will permit better delineation of these posterior fossa structures (cerebellum, fourth ventricle) than does CT and scanning at planes other than the transverse plane used in CT. Coronal images should permit a better evaluation of temporal horn abnormalities than either CT, which is relatively insensitive to discrete temporal horn abnormalities, or pneumoencephalography, which may distort the ventricles. In addition to these advantages, the lack of ionizing radiation (X rays) in MRI makes the scanning of normal controls and developmental studies (repeated scans) feasible. However, because autistic children and young normal children may require sedation to remain still for scanning, risk factors may still limit child brain imaging.

Animal Models

The practical and ethical constraints inherent in human research necessitate the development of an animal model of autism. Such a model would permit more rigorous control over biological and behavioral variables and allow development to be studied within a compressed time frame. Behavioral and cognitive dysfunctions seen in autism can potentially be induced through discrete surgical ablations. Their developmental course, interactions with environmental and genetic variables, and responses to experimental treatments can then be examined. Nonhuman primates are, of course, the best candidates for an animal model of autism because of their genetic, anatomical, physiological, cognitive, social, and behavioral similarities to humans.

Our ability to evaluate the validity of a model of autism will, of course, be limited by our lack of knowledge concerning its biology and etiologies. Validity will have to be assessed initially on the basis of behavioral symptomatology, making good ethological studies and clear "diagnostic criteria" for the model imperative. Nevertheless, considerable success has been achieved in elucidating biological factors operative in human psychopathology (e.g., anxiety) using animal (monkey) models whose starting point is behavior (Suomi, 1982).

Behavioral and neuropsychological analogies between autism and better-understood neurological disorders, such as those outlined by Damasio and Maurer (1978), implicating bilateral mesial frontal and temporal, striatal, and limbic structures, provide starting points for developing an animal model of autism. These circuits, in addition to subserving social interaction, are entwined with those crucial to motor and memory functioning. The latter (motor, memory) may be easier to observe and measure and thus may serve as "markers" for more elusive social behaviors.

Prior research on the social-behavioral effects of lesions in monkeys supports the leads suggested by clinical research. For instance, limbic lesions have been shown to disrupt social behavior in adult monkeys (Aggleton & Passingham, 1981; Kling, 1972). Striatal lesions can result in the fragmentation of communication (i.e., conspecific signaling within the colony) (MacLean, 1978; Murphy, MacLean, & Hamilton, 1981). Infants with amygdalar lesions may initially appear normal but "grow into" their social abnormalities over time (Thompson, 1981). Thus, limbic and striatal lesions disrupt brain circuits that subserve social competence.

In addition to such social analogies, distinctive neuropsychological profiles can provide a basis for validating animal models. The strategy of replicating in monkeys distinctive neuropsychological profiles associated with autism will require clarification of such profiles, including memory profiles, and the establishment of equivalency of the tests applied (Squire & Zola-Morgan, 1983). Test batteries developed for evaluating memory dysfunction in monkeys can be applied to autistic children to help establish this equivalency (Merjanian *et al.*, 1984). While the variables controlling human performance may be more complex, tests developed for monkeys require little linguistic competence or cooperation, a distinct advantage when testing autistic children.

Bachevalier and Mishkin (personal communication) at the National Institute of Mental Health have begun studying both social-behavioral and cognitive development in rhesus monkeys with neonatal limbic lesions (combined bilateral hippocampal-amygdalar lesions, hippocampus only, amygdala only) and cortically lesioned (anterior temporal) and nonlesioned controls. Preliminary results suggest that monkeys with neonatal limbic lesions show striking deficits in social interaction, more stereotyped and self-directed activity (e.g., rocking, finger staring), and memory deficits when compared with their normal and cortically lesioned controls.

This sort of approach can help define what lesions are both necessary and sufficient to disrupt social development. It may be that the full autistic spectrum encompasses a range of lesions (anatomical or neurochemical) that impact upon social behavior and other behaviors (motor, cognitive). Any research that helps define and unravel the social circuitry of the brain should ultimately help us to understand autism.

Neurophysiology

Given the limited success of neuroanatomical imaging in identifying abnormalities in autism, physiological techniques may play a more vital role in identifying localized brain dysfunction in this disorder. In the area of neurophysiology, one useful tool is positron emission tomography, or PET, which provides three-dimensional images of a variety of biochemical processes. While most early PET studies have measured brain energy metabolism, regional blood volumes, blood flow, tissue drug levels, and receptor binding are now being measured as well. Findings of hypometabolic lesions not detectable *in vivo* by other methods in various neurological disorders, including tuberous sclerosis (Szelies *et al.*, 1983), epilepsy (Kuhl, 1984), early Alzheimer's disease (Foster *et al.*, 1984), and visual field defects (Reivich, Gur, & Alavi, 1983), attest to the sensitivity of metabolic studies with PET.

In contrast to findings of hypometabolism in such neurological disorders, normal to diffusely elevated rates of cerebral glucose utilization (but no convincing evidence of focal abnormalities) were found in 10 physically healthy, unmedicated autistic men, who were studied in a resting, sensory-restricted state. Future studies should employ behavioral tasks designed to activate particular brain circuits hypothesized to be dysfunctional in autism (e.g., limbic, frontal, left cortical) in order to enhance the sensitivity of this technique to localized abnormalities (Meyer, Sakai, Yamaguchi, Yamamoto, & Shaw, 1980) in developmental disorders.

Hypothesis testing employing such activation tasks can also proceed using Xenon 133 inhalation methods for determining regional cerebral blood flow. This technique provides an indirect measure of brain metabolism and reflects activity at the cortex but yields little information about subcortical physiology. Both the ability of autistic persons to activate various cortical regions and the organization of cortical functions (i.e., whether autistic patients show normal or unusual patterns of language lateralization) can be studied with this two-dimensional method.

PET studies of specific neurotransmitter receptor classes in autism represent a priority. Dopaminergic, opiate, and benzodiazepine receptors can now be studied selectively (Comar *et al.*, 1979; Frost, *et al.*, 1985; Wagner *et al.*, 1984). Hypotheses concerning dopaminergic (Damasio & Maurer, 1978) and opiate (Weizman *et al.*, 1984) abnormalities (see Neurochemistry section) await testing with these methods.

Neuropathology

Aside from postmortem brain changes characteristic of specific disease states sometimes associated with autistic behavior (e.g., tuberous sclerosis; Creak, 1963), neuropathology has been sparsely represented in research efforts relevant to autism. Initial studies of seven cases (Darby, 1976; Williams, Hauser, Purpura, DeLong, & Swisher, 1980) were negative.

A new era with respect to neuropathology now seems to have dawned with Bauman and Kemper's (1985) identification of microscopic abnormalities in limbic regions and the cerebellar system in the brain of a 29-year-old autistic man, who died by drowning. Preserved olivary neurones, increased cell packing densities, reduced size of neurones, and a lamina dissicans, or "clear zone," in entorhinal cortex, which normally disappears by 15 months of age, indicated failures of early brain development. Cerebral cortical cytoarchitectonics, thalamic nuclei, basal ganglia, basolateral amygdala, and dentate nycleus were normal.

Two additional new reports provide some support for these findings. Normal cell counts were found in the primary auditory cortex, auditory association cortex, and Broca's speech area in an adult female patient studied by Coleman, Romano, Lapham, and Simon (1985). Decreased Purkinje cell densities were found in the cerebella of four autistic patients studied by Ritvo and his colleagues (Ritvo et al., 1986). The specificity of these findings is not clear, however, since these studies examined only limited brain structures.

The examination of additional whole autistic brains with the detailed techniques used by Bauman and Kemper (1985) is a major research priority for the 1980s. More normal control brains need to be examined to address the issue of normal variability given the subtle nature of the findings. In addition, careful clinical data characterizing the patient's autism are essential, given that autism is both rare and heterogeneous. The case examined by Bauman and Kemper (1985) was in life a severely retarded, nearly mute, and later epileptic autistic man. That the cortex was so normal and the limbic system so specifically afflicted is startling and probably of great theoretical significance. It is important that these early findings not be overgeneralized, because they represent autism in its greatest severity, and the neuropathology represents but one possibility.

Cases of autism with established neuropathology should also be examined postmortem in order to localize known pathology and contrast this with localized lesions of the same type in nonautistic cases, e.g., mentally retarded, learning-disabled, or epileptic. The phakomatoses (neurofibromatosis of von Recklinghausen, tuberous sclerosis, incontinentia pigmentae) present with a good range of behavioral symptoms, not yet explored in terms of anatomic significance. Thus, the same disease process, pathologically, could be demonstrated in differing brain regions and correlated with different clinical syndromes.

NEUROCHEMISTRY

As is true of biological research on other psychiatric disorders, abnormalities of neurotransmitters and their metabolites have been pursued in autism for many years. Although elevations of serotonin ("hyperserotonemia") have been documented in autistic patients (Hanley, Stahl, & Freedman, 1977), neither specificity to autism nor pathophysiologic significance has been established. Thus, there remains a need to characterize patients with high versus low blood serotonin. There is also a need for study of the curious dissociation suggested by findings of hyperserotonemia in some studies (Campbell, Friedman, DeVito, Greenspan, & Collins, 1974; Campbell et al., 1975; Hanley et al., 1977), but decreased 5-hydroxyindoleacetic acid (5-HIAA), serotonin's principal metabolite, in others (Cohen, Caparulo, Shaywitz, & Bowers, 1977; Cohen, Shaywitz, Johnson, & Bowers, 1974). Simultaneous measurements (within the same patients) of serotonin and 5-HIAA are needed.

Young, Kavanagh, Anderson, Shaywitz, and Cohen (1982) have summarized possible new research directions in the study of dopamine and norepinephrine metabolism in autism. Further characterization of levels of plasma homovanillic acid (HVA), dopamine's major metabolite, examination of relationships between brain dopaminergic activity and abnormal movements, replication of reports of adrenergic abnormalities, the use of pharmacological challenges to adrenergic function, and attempts to relate adrenergic measures to clinical features such as arousal, anxiety, and memory functioning are recommended directions.

It must be noted, however, that neurochemical alterations often appear to be phenomena in need of explanation, rather than providing clear explanations of disease processes. Similarly, the approach of drawing inferences about disordered chemistry from medication effectiveness has not been particularly profitable. Most effective neuropsychiatric medications, including vitamins and other dietary supplements, have a multiplicity of neurochemical effects, limiting the inferences that can be drawn from drug-induced improvement.

An entirely new chemical approach, that of immunochemistry, has appeared this year in the literature on autism. Todd and Ciaranello (1985) found an antibody to serotonin receptors in the blood of 7 of 13 autistic children, as compared with 0 of 13 controls. This either could indicate an autoimmune disease or could be secondary to neuronal deterioration. Clearly, this type of research is a priority for the coming half decade, as are immunological tests of a broader nature, owing to the increased theoretical interest in the connection between developmental disabilities (ranging from dyslexia to autism) and familial autoimmune disease tendencies (Geschwind, personal communication; Geschwind & Behan, 1982). Antibody screening in autism and in relatives of autistic patients should be undertaken as a possible clue to genetics as well as a clue of possible direct pathogenetic significance in the individual.

Other exciting publications relating to autism bring to prominence the role of purines in subtypes of the disorder. The first patient with unusual autistic behavior and a purine disorder was described by Nyhan, James, Teberg, Sweetman, and Nelson in 1969. The enzyme in this case was an error in PRPP-synthetase (Becker, Raivio, Bakay, Adams, & Nyhan, 1980). A 1976 study by Coleman and her colleagues found that 22% of 69 patients had elevations of uric acid in the urine. Since then, Gruber, Jansen, Willis, and Seegmiller (1985) have found inosinate dehydrogenase deficiency in some of these patients. More recently, Jaeken and Van den Berghe (1984) described a third form of purine autism in which the error is in adenylosuccinase lyase. Since this initial finding, an additional four patients have been identified (Gruber & Coleman, personal communication). Gruber and Coleman have developed a "dipstick" for urine to detect this rare form of autism, which will make it possible to screen large autistic populations. A research drug is available for this particular inborn error of purine metabolism. Such reports require replication and then further investigation into pathophysiology, i.e., just how purine metabolism goes awry and interferes with brain functioning.

Coleman and Blass (1985) also report four patients with autism and lactic acidosis. They raise the possibility that inborn errors of carbohydrate metabolism are among the etiologies of autism. The enzymatic defects responsible for lactic acidosis should be investigated. Since lactate NMR spectroscopy is on the near horizon, this technique could be used in conjunction with studies of blood lactate and pyruvate to detect brain metabolic status before and after possible dietary interventions.

Another promising biochemical avenue involves the role of endogenous opioids in autism. Significantly reduced blood levels of endorphin have been reported in autistic children by Weizman and his colleagues (Weizman *et al.*, 1984). They hypothesize that deficient endorphin activity may underlie overresponsiveness to sensory stimuli (light, pain, or sounds), catastrophic reactions to change, lability, anxiety, and thought and perceptual disorders. In contrast to this, however, some animal work (Panksepp, Siviy, & Normansell, 1985) suggests a possible link between overactivity of the endogeneous opioids and autism. Since 1978, a body of basic research has suggested that there is an important relationship between social attachment in infant animals and brain opioid systems (Panksepp, 1979). Separation distress, as measured by distress vocalizations, appears to be inhibited by endorphins, so that overactivity in some brain opioid systems might suppress normal social attachment.

CONCLUSION

In conclusion, a variety of promising new leads and new technologies offer hope and direction. Both rigorous behavioral and rigorous biological investigations are needed to advance our understanding of autism's neurobiology. Careful descriptions of naturalistic behavior, elucidation of underlying deficits and processes through direct clinical examinations of social, cognitive, communicative, and motor behavior, and a clinically based, empirically validated classification system for this heterogeneous disorder should significantly advance the behavioral side of the brain–behavior equation we seek to define in autism. Hypothesis-driven anatomical examinations, *in vivo* and postmortem, as well as animal models, should provide needed localization clues. Additional clarification of serotonergic and catecholaminergic findings, exploration of new leads suggesting possible dysfunction of immunological, metabolic, and brain opioid systems, and physiological study of information processing and localized brain dysfunction will, one hopes, prove revealing of both the mechanisms and etiologies of this diverse and complex disorder of human behavior.

GLOSSARY

Acoustic spectral analysis   Analysis of acoustic information (e.g., speech sounds) into their component frequencies.

Adenylosuccinase lyase   An enzyme that promotes the formation of a double bond in adenylosuccinate, which is involved in the metabolism of inosine and adenosine, both purines. This step is preparatory to the transformation of adenylosuccinate into adenosine triphosphate (ATP).

Adrenergic   Activated by, characteristic of, or secreting epinephrine or substances with similar activity.

Akinesia   Absence or poverty of movement or delay in initiation of movement, not resulting from weakness or an inability to use a motor pattern (i.e., not apraxia).

Alzheimer disease   Progressive disease characterized by widespread cortical degeneration and the most common cause of dementia.

Amygdala   A set of nuclei in the base of the temporal lobe and part of the limbic system.

Anomalies, minor physical   Minor physical abnormalities, especially ones that result from imperfect fetal development.

Auditory cortex, primary   Area on the superior temporal gyrus which receives auditory input from subcortical structures (medial geniculate of the thalamus) and which is organized according to audible frequencies.

Auditory cortex, association   Cortex in the superior temporal lobe that integrates auditory information.

Autoimmune disease   Disease characterized by a specific immune response against constituents of the body's own tissues (autoantigens).

Basal ganglia   A group of subcortical nuclei which form part of each cerebral hemisphere and which include the corpus striatum (caudate and lenticular nuclei). Damage to these structures causes "extrapyramidal" disturbances.

Benzodiazepine receptors   Postsynaptic binding sites for benzodiazepines, a group of antianxiety drugs, which include Valium and Librium.

Bradykinesia   Slowness of movement, encompassing delay in initiating or arresting movement, delay in changing a motor pattern, and rapid fatigue on prolonged tasks.

Broca's area   A region located on the inferior frontal gyrus of the left hemisphere, which subserves the motor aspects of language production.

Cerebellum (plural, cerebella)   A semidetached mass of neural tissue that covers most of the posterior surface of the brainstem and whose integrity is necessary for equilibrium, muscle tone, postural control, and the coordination of voluntary movements.

Choreoathethoid posturing   Abnormal involuntary movements and body postures, generally implicating dysfunction of the extrapyramidal motor system (e.g., basal ganglia).

Cingulate cortex, anterior   The continuation of the superior frontal gyrus onto the medial surface of the hemispheres and part of the limbic system.

Coronal   A plane (at a right angle to the floor in the case of humans) that divides the head into anterior and posterior portions.

Cytoarchitectonics   The study of the organizing structure and distribution of cells in an organ or tissue, especially that in the cerebral cortex.

Dentate nucleus   One of the deep nuclei of the cerebellum.

Dermatoglyphic abnormalities   Abnormal patterns of ridges of the skin of the fingers, palms, toes, and soles, of medical interest clinically and as a genetic indicator, particularly of chromosomal abnormalities.

Dopamine   A neurotransmitter and immediate precursor of norepinephrine. High concentrations of dopamine (but not norepinephrine) are found in the caudate and putamen.

Dopaminergic neurons   Neurons that transmit the neurotransmitter dopamine.

Dopaminergic receptors   Receptors activated by the neurotransmitter dopamine.

Dyskinesia   Impairment of voluntary movement, resulting in fragmentary or incomplete movements.

Endorphin   An endogeneous and natural chemical that binds to opiate receptors in the brain.

Entorhinal cortex   An area which lies adjacent to the primary olfactory cortex at the base of the brain and which serves as olfactory association cortex with limbic functions.

Extrapyramidal   The anatomical motor system which excludes the pyramidal system and which includes the cerebellum and basal ganglia (caudate, amygdala, lentiform nucleus). Destruction of pyramidal fibers causes paralysis, while extrapyramidal damage does not, but rather results in various abnormalities of movement (e.g., tremor, poverty, or slowness of movement).

Frontal   Pertaining to the frontal lobes, which are involved in reasoning, planning, and emotional functioning.

Hippocampus   Structure in the anterior medial temporal lobe implicated in human memory and learning.

Hypometabolic lesions   Tissue showing lowered energy metabolism.

Hypometabolism   Abnormally lowered energy production or utilization.

Immunochemistry   That branch of biological science concerned with the physical chemical basis of immune phenomena and their interactions.

Incontinentia pigmentae   A hereditary condition occurring almost exclusively in females in which pigmented skin lesions are associated with developmental defects of the eyes, bones, and central nervous system.

Inosinate dehydrogenase   An enzyme involved in removing hydrogen from inosine, one of several purines.

Lactate   Any salt of lactic acid.

Lactic acidosis   Pathologic condition resulting from the accumulation of lactic acid.

Limbic   Pertaining to the limbic system, which includes the hippocampus, amygdala, septum, cingulate gyrus, and dentate gyrus.

Magnetic resonance imaging (MRI)   A new technique for visualizing brain anatomy in three dimensions through the manipulation of magnetic fields.

Mesial temporal   Pertaining to the portion of the temporal lobes adjacent to the midline of the brain.

Mesial   Near the midline.

Mesolimbic cortex   Horseshoe-shaped rim of cortex that lies on the mesial aspects of the frontal and temporal lobes and includes several limbic structures.

Metabolite   Any product of metabolism, the chemical processes involved in energy production and utilization.

Neostriatum   The striatum, which consists of the caudate and putamen, part of the basal ganglia.

Neurofibromatosis of von Recklinghausen   A congenital disorder characterized by development of multiple tumors of the spinal or cranial nerves, tumors of the skin, and cutaneous pigmentation.

Neurotransmitters   Chemicals that are released by neurons across synapses and taken up (postsynaptically) by other neurons, thus chemically transmitting information.

Norepinephrine   Noradrenalin, a hormone secreted by neurons that acts as a neurotransmitter.

NMR spectroscopy   A technique for measuring concentrations of certain chemicals or certain biological processes in tissue by manipulating magnetic fields.

Olivary neurons   Neurons of the inferior olivary nucleus, which provide afferents (inputs) to the cerebellum.

Opiate receptors   Structures on the postsynaptic membranes of neurons to which opiates (heroin, morphine) bind.

Opioids, endogeneous   Naturally occurring chemicals that act on the same receptors as do the opiates (heroin, morphine).

Orbitofrontal cortex   Cortex on the inferior portions of the frontal lobes.

Perisylvian   Around the Sylvian fissure, a region that in the left hemisphere subserves language.

Phakomatoses   A group of hereditary syndromes characterized by tumors of the eye, skin, and brain.

Pneumoencephalographic   Pertaining to pneumoencephalography.

Pneumoencephalography   A radiologic technique for visualizing the fluid-containing structures of the brain by replacing cerebrospinal fluid with air.

Positron emission tomography (PET)   A technique for three-dimensional imaging of biochemical processes in the brain, which makes use of tracers labeled with radioactive material, which are injected into the patient and detected with an external scanner.

Posterior fossa   The space containing the cerebullum, which is separated from the more anterior cerebrum by a membrane called the tentorium.

Purines   Building blocks of nucleic acids, such as DNA and RNA, that govern the cellular synthesis of proteins.

Purine disorder   Disorder characterized by abnormal levels of purines in cells, possibly due to defects in enzymes involved in purine synthesis or enzymes involved in DNA or RNA synthesis.

Purkinje cell   Large branching neuron in the cortex of the cerebellum and the only type of neuron whose axons leave the cortex.

Pyruvate   Chemical involved in the energy metabolism of cells.

PRPP-synthetase   5-phosphoribosyl-1-pyrophosphate synthetase, an enzyme involved in the biosynthesis of purines.

Receptor binding   The temporary attachment of neurotransmitters to structures on the postsynaptic membranes of neurons.

Reverse facial movement dysfunction   Asymmetry of the lower portion of the face apparent in spontaneous, but not in voluntary, facial expression, generally interpreted as a sign of damage to the basal ganglia or thalamus.

Righting reflexes   Involuntary activity resulting in the assumption of one's original position following a departure from it.

Serotonin   5-hydroxytryptamine (5-HT), a neurotransmitter present in high concentrations in the hypothalamus, midbrain, and caudate.

Striatal   Pertaining to the striatum, which consists of of the caudate and and the putamen, part of the basal ganglia.

Thalamic nuclei   Groups of nerve cell bodies in the thalamus with varying functions. Prominent among these functions is the receipt and processing of sensory information.

Tourette syndrome   A syndrome of facial and vocal tics with onset in childhood, progressing to generalized jerking movements in any part of the body.

Transverse plane   A plane which parallels or nearly parallels the floor in the case of humans and which is commonly used in CT scanning.

Tuberous sclerosis   A congenital, sometimes familial, disease that begins in early childhood and is characterized by progressive mental deterioration, convulsions, and the appearance of tumors of the skin and viscera.

Uric acid   An end product of purine metabolism.

Ventricle   A small cavity, such as one of the several cavities, or fluid-containing chambers of the brain.

Visual field defects   Loss of sight in one or more portions of one's field of vision, generally with preserved vision in other portions of the field.

Xenon 133 inhalation method   A method for measuring changes in cerebral blood flow that employs a mildly radioactive gas (xenon 133), which the patient inhales.

REFERENCES

Aggelton, J. P., & Passingham, R. E. (1981). Syndrome produced by lesions of the amygdala in monkeys. *Journal of Comparative and Physiological Psychology, 95*(6), 961–977.

Alajouanine, T. H., & Lhermitte, F. (1965). Acquired aphasia in children. *Brain, 88,* 653–662.

Baltaxe, C. A. M., & Simmons, J. Q. (1975). Language in childhood psychosis: A review. *Journal of Speech and Hearing Disorders, 40,* 439–458.

Baltaxe, C. A. M., & Simmons, J. Q. (1983). Communication deficits in the adolescent and adult autistic. *Seminars in Speech and Language, 4*(1), 27.

Bartak, L., & Rutter, M. (1976). Differences between mentally retarded and normally intelligent autistic children. *Journal of Autism and Childhood Schizophrenia, 6,* 109–120.

Bartak, L., Rutter, M., & Cox, A. (1975). A comparative study of infantile autism and specific developmental receptive language disorder. I. The children. *British Journal of Psychiatry, 126,* 127–145.

Bartak, L., Rutter, M., & Cox, A. (1977). A comparative study of infantile autism and specific developmental language disorders: III. Discriminant function analysis. *Journal of Autism and Childhood Schizophrenia, 7,* 383–396.

Basser, L. S. (1962). Hemiplegia of early onset and the faculty of speech with special reference to the effects of hemispherectomy. *Brain, 85,* 427–460.

Bauman, M., & Kemper, T. L. (1985). Histoanatomic observations of the brain in early infantile autism. *Neurology, 35,* 866–874.

Bauman, M. L., LeMay, M., Bauman, R. A., & Rosenberger, P. B. (1985). Computerized tomographic (CT) observations of the posterior fossa in early infantile autism. *Neurology, 35,* (Suppl. 1), 247.

Becker, M. A., Raivio, K. O., Bakay, B., Adams, W. B., & Nyhan, W. L. (1980). Variant human phosphoribosylpyrophosphate synthetase altered in regulatory and catalytic functions. *Journal of Clinical Investigation, 65,* 109–120.

Bernard-Opitz, V. (1982). Pragmatic analysis of the communicative behavior of an autistic child. *Journal of Speech and Hearing Disorders, 47,* 99–109.

Boucher, J. (1976). Is autism primarily a language disorder? *British Journal of Disorders of Communication, 11,* 135–143.

Campbell, M., Friedman, E., DeVito, E., Greenspan, L., & Collins, P. J. (1974). Blood serotonin in psychotic and brain-damaged children. *Journal of Autism and Childhood Schizophrenia, 4,* 33–41.

Campbell, M., Friedman, E., Green, W. H., Collins, P. J., Small, A. M., & Breuer, H. (1975). Blood serotonin in schizophrenic children. *International Journal of Pharmacopsychiatry, 10,* 213–221.

Campbell, M., Rosenbloom, S., Perry, R., George, A., Kricheff, I., Anderson, L., Small, A., & Jennings, S. (1982). Computerized axial tomography in young autistic children. *American Journal of Psychiatry, 139*, 510–512.

Cantwell, D., & Baker, L. (1978). Imitations and echoes in autistic and dysphasic children. *Journal of the American Academy of Child Psychiatry, 17*, 614–624.

Cantwell, D., Baker, L., & Rutter, M. (1978). A comparative study of infantile autism and specific developmental receptive language disorder: IV. Analysis of syntax and language function. *Journal of Child Psychology and Psychiatry, 19*, 351–362.

Caparulo, B., Cohen, D., Rothman, S., Young, J., Katz, J., Shaywitz, S., & Shaywitz, B. (1981). Computed tomographic brain scanning in children with developmental neuropsychiatric disorders. *Journal of the American Academy of Child Psychiatry, 20*, 338–357.

Churchill, D. (1972). The relation of infantile autism and early childhood schizophrenia to developmental language disorders of childhood. *Journal of Autism and Childhood Schizophrenia, 2*, 182–197.

Clark, P., & Rutter, M. (1981). Autistic children's responses to structure and to interpersonal demands. *Journal of Autism and Developmental Disorders, 11*, 201–217.

Cohen, D., Caparulo, B., & Shaywitz, B. (1976). Primary childhood aphasia and childhood autism. *Journal of the American Academy of Child Psychiatry, 15*, 604–645.

Cohen, D. J., Caparulo, B. K., Shaywitz, B. A., & Bowers, M. B., Jr. (1977). Dopamine and serotonin metabolism in neuropsychiatrically disturbed children: CSF homovanillic acid and 5-hydroxyindoleacetic acid. *Archives of General Psychiatry, 34*, 545–550.

Cohen, D. J., Shaywitz, B. A., Johnson, W. T., & Bowers, M. B., Jr. (1974). Biogenic amines in autistic and atypical children: Cerebrospinal fluid measures of homovanillic acid and 5-hydroxyindoleacetic acid. *Archives of General Psychiatry, 31*, 845–853.

Coleman, M. (1976). *The autistic syndromes.* New York: Elsevier/North-Holland.

Coleman, M., & Blass, J. P. (1985). Autism and lactic acidosis. *Journal of Autism and Developmental Disorders, 15*, 1–8.

Coleman, P. D., Romano, J., Lapham, L., & Simon, W. (1985). Cell counts in the cerebral cortex of an autistic patient. *Journal of Autism and Developmental Disorders, 15*, 245–255.

Comar, D., Zarifian, E., Verhas, M., Soussaline, F., Maziere, M., Berger, G., Loo, H., Cuche, C., Kellershohn, C., & Deniker, P. (1979). Brain distribution and kinetics of 11C-chloropromazine in schizophrenics. *Psychiatry Research, 1*, 23–29.

Creak, E. M. (1963). Schizophrenic syndrome in childhood. *Cerebral Palsy Bulletin, 3*, 501–503.

Damasio, A. R., & Maurer, R. G. (1978). A neurological model for childhood autism. *Archives of Neurology, 35*, 777–786.

Damasio, H., Maurer, R., Damasio, A., & Chui, H. (1980). Computerized tomographic scan findings in patients with autistic behavior. *Archives of Neurology, 37*, 504–510.

Darby, J. K. (1976). Neuropathologic aspects of psychosis in children. *Journal of Autism and Childhood Schizophrenia, 6*, 339–352.

DeLong, G. (1976). A neuropsychologic interpretation of infantile autism. In M. Rutter & E. Schopler (Eds.), *Autism: A reappraisal of concepts and treatment.* New York: Plenum Press.

DeMyer, M., Hingtgen, J., & Jackson, R. (1981). Infantile autism reviewed: A decade of research. *Schizophrenia Bulletin, 7*, 388–451.

Donnellan, A., Anderson, J., & Mesaros, R. (1984). An observational study of stereotypic behavior and proximity related to the occurrence of autistic child–family member interactions. *Journal of Autism and Developmental Disorders, 14*, 205–210.

Fein, D., Humes, M., Kaplan, E., Lucci, D., & Waterhouse, L. (1984). The question of left hemisphere dysfunction in infantile autism. *Psychological Bulletin, 95*, 258–281.

Foster, N., Chase, T., Mansi, L., Brooks, R., Fedio, P., Patronas, N., & Di Chiro, G. (1984). Cortical abnormalities in Alzheimer's disease. *Annals of Neurology, 16*, 649–654.

Freeman, B. J., Ritvo, E. R., Schroth, P. C., Tonick, I., Guthrie, D., & Wake, L. (1981). Behavioral characteristics of high- and low-IQ autistic children. *American Journal of Psychiatry, 138*, 25–29.

Frost, J. J., Wagner, H. N., Dannals, R. F., Ravert, H. T., Links, J. M., Wilson, A. A., Burns, D., Wong, D. F., McPherson, R. W., Rosenbaum, A. E., Kuhar, M. J., & Snyder, S. H. (1985). Imaging opiate receptors in the human brain by positron tomography. *Journal of Computer Assisted Tomography, 9*, 231–236.

Galaburda, A. M., Sherman, G. F., Rosen, G. D., Aboitiz, F., & Geschwind, N. (1985). Developmental dyslexia: Four consecutive patients with cortical anomalies. *Annals of Neurology, 18*, 222–233.

Geschwind, N., & Behan, P. (1982). Left-handedness: Association with immune disease, migraine, and developmental learning disorder. *Proceedings of the National Academy of Sciences, 79*, 5097–5100.

Gillberg, C., & Svendsen, P. (1983). Childhood psychosis and computed tomographic brain scan findings. *Journal of Autism and Developmental Disorders, 13*, 19–82.

Gruber, H. E., Jansen, I., Willis, R. C., & Seegmiller, J. E. (1985). Alterations of the inosinate branchpoint enzymes in cultured human lymphoblasts. *Biochimica et Biophysica Acta, 846*, 135–144.

Hanley, H. G., Stahl, S. M., & Freedman, D. X. (1977). Hyperserotonemia and amine metabolites in autistic and retarded children. *Archives of General Psychiatry, 34*, 521–531.

Hauser, S., DeLong, G., & Rosman, N. (1975). Pneumographic findings in the infantile autism syndrome. *Brain, 98*, 667–688.

Hetzler, B. E., & Griffin, J. L. (1981). Infantile autism and the temporal lobe of the brain. *Journal of Autism and Developmental Disorders, 11*, 317–330.

Hier, D., LeMay, M., & Rosenberg, P. (1979). Autism and unfavorable left-right asymmetries of the brain. *Journal of Autism and Developmental Disorders, 9*, 153–157.

Jaeken, J., & Van den Berghe, G. (1984). An infantile autistic syndrome characterised by the presence of succinylpurines in body fluids. *Lancet, 2*, 1058–1061.

Kent, R. D., & Rosenbek, J. C. (1982). Prosodic disturbance and neurologic lesion. *Brain and Language, 14*, 259–291.

Kling, A. (1972). Effects of amygdalectomy on social-affective behavior in non-human primates. In B. E. Eleftheriou (Ed.), *The neurobiology of the amygdala*. New York: Plenum Press.

Kuhl, D. (1984). Imaging local brain function with emission computed tomography. *Radiology, 150*, 625–631.

MacLean, P. D. (1978). Effects of lesions of globus pallidus on species-typical display behaviors of squirrel monkeys. *Brain Research, 149*, 175–196.

McHale, S. M., Simeonsson, R. J., Marcus, L. M., & Olley, J. G. (1980). The social and symbolic quality of autistic children's communication. *Journal of Autism and Developmental Disorders, 10*, 299–310.

Merjanian, P. M., Nadel, L., Jans, D. D., Granger, D. A., Lott, I. T., & Kean, M. L. (1984). Involvement of the hippocampus and amygdala in classical autism: A comparative neuropsychological study. *Society for Neuroscience Abstracts, 10*(1), #156.9, p. 524.

Meyer, J. S., Sakai, F., Yamaguchi, F., Yamamoto, M., & Shaw, T. (1980). Regional changes in cerebral blood flow during standard behavioral activation in patients with disorders of speech and mentation compared to normal volunteers. *Brain and Language, 9*, 61–77.

Mirenda, P., Donnellan, A., & Yoder, D. (1983). Gaze behavior: A new look at an old problem. *Journal of Autism and Developmental Disorders, 13*, 397–409.

Muramoto, O., Kuru, Y., & Sugishita, M. (1979). Pure memory loss with hippocampal lesions. *Archives of Neurology, 36*, 54–56.

Murphy, M. R., MacLean, P. D., & Hamilton, S. C. (1981). Species-typical behavior of hamsters deprived from birth of neocortex. *Science, 213*, 459–461.

Nyhan, W. L., James, J. A., Teberg, A. J., Sweetman, L., & Nelson, L. G. (1969). A new disorder of purine metabolism with behavioral manifestations. *Journal of Pediatrics, 74*, 20–27.

Panksepp, J. (1979). A neurochemical theory of autism. *Trends in Neuroscience, 2*, 174–177.

Panksepp, J., Siviy, S. M., & Normansell, L. A. (1985). Brain opioids and social emotions in the biology of attachment. In M. Reite & T. Fields (Eds.), *Psychobiology*. New York: Academic Press.

Parks, S. L., (1983). The assessment of autistic children: a selective review of available instruments. *Journal of Autism and Developmental Disorders, 13*, 255–267.

Prior, M. (1977). Psycholinguistic disabilities of autistic and retarded children. *Journal of Mental Deficiency Research, 21*, 37–45.

Prior, M. (1979). Cognitive abilities and disabilities in infantile autism: A review. *Journal of Abnormal Child Psychology, 7*, 357–380.

Prizant, B. M., & Duncan, J. F. (1981). The functions of immediate echolalia in autistic children. *Journal of Speech and Hearing Disorders, 46*(3), 241–249.

Reivich, M., Gur, R., & Alavi, A. (1983). Positron emission tomographic studies of sensory stimuli, cognitive processes and anxiety. *Human Neurobiology, 2*(1), 25–33.

Richer, J. (1978). The partial noncommunication of culture to autistic children—An application of human ethology. In M. Rutter & E. Schopler (Eds.), *Autism: A reappraisal of concepts and treatment*. New York: Plenum Press.

Richer, J., & Coss, R. (1976). Gaze aversion in autistic and normal children. *Acta Psychiatrica Scandinavica, 53*, 193–210.

Ritvo, E. R., Freeman, B. J., Scheibel, A. B., Duong, P. T., Robinson, H., Guthrie, D., and Ritvo, A. (1986). Lower Purkinje cell counts in the cerebella of four autistic subjects. Initial findings of the UCLA-NSAC autopsy research project. *American Journal of Psychiatry, 13*, 862–866.

Rosenbloom, S., Campbell, M., George, A., Kricheff, I., Taleporos, E., Anderson, L., Reuben, R., & Korein, J. (1984). High resolution CT scanning in infantile autism: A quantitative approach. *Journal of the American Academy of Child Psychiatry, 23*, 72–77.

Rutter, M. (1970). Autistic children: Infancy to adulthood. *Seminars in Psychiatry, 2*, 435–450.

Rutter, M. (1983). Cognitive deficits in the pathogenesis of autism. *Journal of Child Psychology and Psychiatry, 24*, 513–531.

Shapiro, T., Roberts, A., & Fish, B. (1970). Imitation and echoing in schizophrenic children. *Journal of the American Academy of Child Psychiatry, 9*, 548–567.

Sigman, M., & Ungerer, J. (1984). Cognitive and language skills in autistic, mentally retarded, and normal children. *Developmental Psychology, 20*, 293–302.

Simmons, J., & Baltaxe, C. (1975). Language patterns of adolescent autistics. *Journal of Autism and Childhood Schizophrenia, 5*, 331–351.

Squire, L., & Zola-Morgan, S. (1983). The neurology of memory: The case for correspondence between the findings for human and nonhuman primates. In J. Deutsch (Ed.), *The physiological basis of memory*. New York: Academic Press.

Suomi, S. J. (1982). Relevance of animal models for clinical psychology. In P. Kendall & J. Butcher (Eds.), *Handbook of research methods in clinical psychology*. New York: Wiley.

Szelies, B., Herholz, K., Heiss, W. D., Rackl, A., Pawlik, G., Wagner, R., Ilsen, H. W., & Wienhard, K. (1983). Hypometabolic cortical lesions in tuberous sclerosis with epilepsy: Demonstration by positron emission tomography. *Journal of Computer Assisted Tomography, 7*, 946–953.

Tager-Flusberg, H. B. (1981). On the nature of linguistic functioning in early infantile autism. *Journal of Autism and Developmental Disorders, 11*, 45–56.

Thompson, C. I. (1981). Long-term behavioral development of Rhesus monkeys after amygdalectomy in infancy. In Y. Ben-Ari (Ed.), *The amygdaloid complex* (INSERM Symposium No. 20). Amsterdam: Elsevier/North-Holland Biomedical Press.

Tinbergen, E. A., & Tinbergen, N. (1976). The aetiology of childhood autism: Criticism of the Tinbergens' theory: A rejoinder. *Psychological Medicine, 6*, 545–550.

Todd, R. D., & Ciaranello, R. D. (1985). Demonstration of inter- and intraspecies differences in serotonin binding sites by antibodies from an autistic child. *Proceedings of the National Academy of Sciences, 82*, 612–616.

Tsai, L. Y., Jacoby, C. G., & Stewart, M. A. (1983). Morphological cerebral asymmetries in autistic children. *Biological Psychiatry, 18*, 317–327.

Tsai, L., Jacoby, C. G., Stewart, M. A., & Beisler, J. M. (1982). Unfavourable left-right asymmetries of the brain and autism: A question of methodology. *British Journal of Psychiatry, 140*, 312–319.

Vilensky, J. A., Damasio, A. R., & Maurer, R. G. (1981). Gait disturbances in patients with autistic behavior. *Archives of Neurology, 38*, 646–649.

Wagner, H. N., Burns, D., Dannals, R. F., Wong, D. F., Langstrom, B., Duelfer, T., Frost, J. J., Ravert, H. T., Links, J. M., Rosenbloom, S. B., Lukas, S. E., Kramer, A. V., & Kuhar, M. J. (1984). Assessment of dopamine receptor densities in the human brain with carbon-11-labeled N-methylspiperone. *Annals of Neurology, 15*(Suppl.), S79–S84.

Waterhouse, L., & Fein, D. (1982). Language skills in developmentally disabled children. *Brain and Language, 15*, 307–333.

Weizman, R., Weizman, A., Tyano, S., Szekely, G., Weissman, B. A., & Sarne, Y. (1984). Humoral-endorphin blood levels in autistic, schizophrenic and healthy subjects. *Psychopharmacology, 82*, 368–370.

Wetherby, A. M., & Prutting, C. A. (1984). Profiles of communicative and cognitive-social abilities in autistic children. *Journal of Speech and Hearing Research, 27*, 364–377.

Williams, R. S., Hauser, S. L., Purpura, D. P., DeLong, G. R., & Swisher, C. N. (1980). Autism and mental retardation: Neuropathologic studies performed in four retarded persons with autistic behavior. *Archives of Neurology, 37*, 749–753.

Wing, L. (1971). *What is an autistic child?* London: National Society for Autistic Children.

Young, J. G., Kavanagh, M. E., Anderson, G. M., Shaywitz, B. A., & Cohen, D. J. (1982). Clinical neurochemistry of autism and associated disorders. *Journal of Autism and Developmental Disorders, 12*, 147–166.

Ethical Issues in the Health Care of Children with Developmental Handicaps

ALAN W. CROSS, LARRY R. CHURCHILL,
MICHAEL C. SHARP, and NANCY M. P. KING

THE ROLE OF ETHICAL REFLECTION IN MEDICINE

Over the last several decades medical care has become considerably more complex. As our understanding of medical problems and their treatment has expanded, we are faced with multiple diagnostic and therapeutic options that demand consideration and decision. Within this maze of technical choices are many issues that involve the personal values of both the patient and the health professional. The moral value systems of the patient and the health professional will come into conflict at times. Not infrequently, the values of society as expressed in laws and the policies of public agencies will also come into conflict with those of the patient and health professional. Medical ethics is the discipline that examines moral values and studies these value conflicts within the health care setting.

Like all disciplines, medical ethics uses words and concepts that must be defined to avoid misunderstanding. The term *moral values*, or morality, refers to standards for good behavior. Moral values may be expressed in absolute terms as *rules*, such as "Thou shalt not kill," or in more flexible terms as *principles*, such as "Patients' freedom to make their own choices should be protected." Sometimes rules and principles are expressed by using the language of *rights*. For example, the principle just stated may also appear as "the patient's right to decide." The existence of a right always implies that someone else owes, to the holder of the right, a specific *duty* to protect or uphold it. In our example, the physician would be said to have a duty to offer the patient the opportunity to decide. The example

ALAN W. CROSS • Departments of Social and Administrative Medicine and Pediatrics,   LARRY R. CHURCHILL • Departments of Social and Administrative Medicine and Religious Studies,   MICHAEL C. SHARP • Department of Pediatrics, and   NANCY M. P. KING • Department of Social and Administrative Medicine, University of North Carolina, Chapel Hill, North Carolina 27514.

shows that both the right and the corresponding duty actually derive from a single principle. Most rights language derives from principles of law, but rights can as readily spring from philosophical principles that may not be expressed in the law.

Personal values are those aspects of an individual's life and behavior that he or she deems important. They may be moral values, representing standards we accept as the "shoulds" and "musts" of our life, or they may be merely matters of taste, such as a standard of dress or deportment or a preference for chocolate. Ethics, which is often equated with morality, will be used here to refer only to the *discipline* that studies morals and values in conflict (Beauchamp & Childress, 1979).

The increasing complexity of medicine does not alone account for the greater prominence of medical ethics as a discipline. There are social forces that have contributed to this phenomenon. The consumer movement of the 1960s and 1970s was expressed in medicine as a need for greater attention to the rights of patients in determining their own medical care. The medical paternalism that had long been accepted was challenged. Health professionals were forced to pay greater attention to patients' values and their right to exercise those values in their own care. This right is now largely accepted in theory, although there is still much debate about its practical application. The traditions of medicine and the laws of society have not kept pace with the technology of medicine, leaving both the patient and the health professional uncertain as to the meaning and scope of the principle of autonomy (Moorkin, 1977). Reflection and debate on these issues will continue.

A recently emerging additional force that complicates and at times conflicts with the principle of patient autonomy is the "right to life" movement, frequently, but not exclusively, associated with moral and political conservatism. This philosophy has particularly affected discussion of the moral issues relating to children with handicaps and their families. Elevation of the principle of the sanctity of life above that of family privacy, and at times even above the patient's freedom to choose, has brought forward some of the most vexing issues we face. Parental rights to make choices on behalf of their children with handicaps have been called into question through the Baby Doe case and the legislation and federal regulations that emerged from that controversy (*Federal Register*, 1982, 1984). We are still in the midst of this debate and it is not yet clear how these issues can or will be sorted out.*

Prominent among the questions raised by both the patients' rights movement and the right to life movement is determining exactly who should speak for children with handicaps; the debate has ranged far beyond issues of life and death, into all treatment decisions in all treatment settings. Health care professionals no longer enjoy an absolute prerogative to make decisions for child patients, either directly or indirectly through influence upon parents. And although parents' right to decide has been challenged by these rights movements, in theory and in practice parents still represent the dominant decision-making force (Gaylin & Macklin, 1982). Attempts by society to regulate these decisions through state and federal legislation,

---

*Baby Doe was born in April 1982 with Down syndrome and esophageal atresia. His parents and doctors allowed him to die without the surgery that would have repaired his esophagus. The Reagan administration attempted to prevent recurrences of this withholding of care by appealing to laws that prohibit discrimination against the handicapped. When these regulations were invalidated by the courts, Congress passed a law that addressed these problems under the child abuse and neglect laws. Accompanying federal regulations, released in April 1985, essentially support parental decision making, so long as "medically indicated" treatment is given; treatment may not be withheld for reasons of quality of life or parental convenience (*Federal Register*, 1985; Murray, 1985; Pless, 1983).

hospital ethics committees, and local social service agencies have not yet established a clearly superior mechanism for decision making.

Many people have turned to ethics in hopes that it would provide simple answers to complex social and professional questions of rights and responsibilities in health care settings. Although ethics seeks to illuminate the many subtle issues in this set of problems, it does not represent a shortcut or a means of achieving simple solutions. In fact, it often makes the problems more complex, by identifying numerous issues that previously had gone unrecognized. In this chapter we will explore some ways in which ethics and medicine interrelate. Although our purpose is to clarify how ethics can serve medicine, we will also seek to illustrate its limitations.

THE CASE APPROACH TO ETHICAL ANALYSIS

Ethical discussions are at risk of becoming theoretical and removed from the realities of patients, families, health professionals, and the larger society of which they are all a part. In an effort to avoid this, we have chosen to build this chapter around the stories of six persons with handicaps. Through these narrative cases we illustrate some of the common problems that confront children with handicaps, their families, the health professionals that serve them, and the larger society. These cases deliberately proceed from infancy through adolescence, retracing the steps that families follow as their child with a handicap grows.

The systematic analysis of moral issues involves a several-step process. First, the significant moral problems need to be identified and distinguished from problems that are not moral. Next the origin and meaning of the values in conflict must be explored. Then rules, principles, and rights that pertain to the moral problem should be applied. Finally, the consequences of different actions need to be enumerated before a choice is ultimately made. Because of limitations of space it is impossible to work through each step in this process for each of the six cases. Instead each case has been chosen to particularly highlight one of the steps in the process. The first case (Leonard) shows some of the difficulties in distinguishing value conflicts from other problems. The second case (Monica) explores the social and cultural origins of value conflicts and the potential impact of the illness on patient behavior. The third case (Charlie) illustrates a subtle conflict and the application of a moral principle to explore the issues. The fourth case (Robert) examines the multiple dimensions of a principle and the various consequences of its application. The fifth case (Susan) expands the discussion to illustrate a value conflict between a family and a community demonstrating the social dimension of ethics and law. The final case (Samantha) explores multiple consequences of a complex social and legal problem.

Although the authors' views will inevitably be apparent, the purpose of the discussion is not to impose any single set of moral values on the reader. Plugging a single set of rules or principles into every case and deriving a simple answer is a very attractive approach to reducing the complexities of modern medicine. However, such oversimplification runs the risk of causing inflexibility and blind spots in our examination of moral problems, resulting too often in poor choices that overlook issues of critical importance to the individuals involved. The goal of ethical analysis is to reduce the incidence of poor choices by systematic exploration of moral conflicts, their origins, the principles at play and the many potential solutions. This requires an open-minded examination that usually results in even greater complexity. The possible solutions that emerge may all have merits and drawbacks, and a single "right" answer may remain elusive. Nonetheless, the premise of all ethical analysis is that examined and self-conscious choices will usually be superior to those which rely on moral habits, hunches, or convention. The cases are fictional. Although they may remind readers of actual dilemmas, they are only the creation of the authors in an attempt to illustrate realistic conflicts.

CASE 1: LEONARD

Distinguish Value Conflicts from Other Problems

Leonard is a 1-year-old white male firstborn child brought by his mother to the pediatrician for a routine well-child visit. In the course of the 10-min. encounter the busy pediatrician determines that the child is growing well, has had no recent illnesses, is sleeping and eating well, and appears quite happy. He is not yet walking. The physical exam is normal. As the pediatrician rises to leave the room, the mother blurts out her concern that her baby is not normal. He first rolled over at age 5 months and did not sit alone until 9 months of age. He has only just recently mastered crawling. The mother also notes that he does not interact with her nearly as much as her friend's child, who is only 10 months old. He will smile at her if she gets his attention, but he often seems to be in a world of his own. With some difficulty she asks if he might be deaf. The pediatrician reaches his hand around Leonard's head and rubs his fingers together next to Leonard's right ear. The child turns immediately to the sound. He does the same on the left. In a calm but authoritative manner, the physician reassures the mother that her baby's hearing is OK. He explains that many children do not follow the simple descriptions of development seen in the baby books. He also points out that the development of the motor milestones does not correlate very closely with ultimate intelligence. He indicates that this is very common in his experience and that the child will catch up soon. He suggests that she remind him of this concern if it is still there on the next visit in 3 months' time. As Leonard's pediatrician leaves the room, the mother feels confused. On the one hand, she feels as though her concerns are legitimate and have not been taken seriously. On the other hand, she wonders if she is not merely an overanxious mother fretting about inconsequential problems.

Identifying the Problems

The first step in ethical analysis is identifying the moral problems and distinguishing them from other aspects of the situation. This is particularly difficult in the outpatient setting, where life-and-death crises, with their clear and dramatic moral issues, rarely occur and instead value conflicts are embedded in the complex interaction between patient and health professional (Szasz & Hollander, 1956). This interaction can be described as having four dimensions, which are inevitably intertwined and often difficult to sort out. The first is the information dimension, which includes the information from the patient that describes aspects of the health problem and the information from the health professional that explains the nature of, and appropriate management for, the problem. The second dimension is sensitivity, which includes the capacity of the health professional to understand and empathize with the patient. At times the patient is also called upon to be sensitive to the health professional. The third is the moral dimension, which includes all of the personal and moral values brought to the encounter by both physician and patient. The fourth is the communication dimension, which involves the use of both verbal and nonverbal skills to communicate effectively.

Problems that cause dissatisfaction can arise in each of these dimensions. Problems in one dimension may initially be disguised as problems from a different dimension. What on the surface looks like a value conflict may turn out to be a breakdown in communication or a gap in information. Errors in one dimension may also cause problems in the others; for example, poor communication skills may lead to gaps in information. Similarly, attention to one dimension may avoid problems in another: Sensitivity to the cultural background of the patient might identify potential value conflicts that could be explored with effective communication skills.

Because these four dimensions are so intricately entwined it is at times very difficult to sort them out. A pure analysis of the moral problems might demand such a sorting, but in reality, success at ethical analysis is dependent on success in all four dimensions.

The interaction between Leonard's mother and his pediatrician illustrates the complexities of the relationship between the moral dimension and the other components of the provider–patient interaction, particularly in ambulatory care settings. A conflict has arisen that leaves the mother confused and dissatisfied. Despite the tendency to presume that the role of ethics is to eliminate from the health encounter all conflicts and dissatisfactions regardless of their cause, the problem sources here may be manifold and are not necessarily primarily morally based. If we examine this encounter in terms of the four dimensions discussed above, we see problems in each.

First, inadequate information has clearly contributed to the conflict here. Leonard's pediatrician may have been inadequately informed about the presentation of developmental delays or autism. He may also have been unaware of the inaccuracy of the method he used for testing the baby's hearing. Likewise, the mother may be unaware of the wide range of normal development. If both doctor and mother were better informed some of the conflict could have been avoided. In cases like this one, both parties have some responsibility to acquire and transmit necessary information, with the physician of course bearing the far greater responsibility with regard to medical knowledge.

Second, the doctor may have been insensitive to the magnitude of the mother's concerns and, thus, unaware that the minimal reassurance he offered was grossly inadequate. The mother, in turn, did not understand the pressure of the pediatrician's busy practice; thus, she delayed expressing her major concern until the time allotted for the appointment was nearly complete. If the physician had been more sensitive and the mother less hesitant, this additional portion of the conflict might also have been avoided.

Even the greatest sensitivity to another's concerns is unavailing unless it is accompanied by skill in communicating with the other. Felt concern and respect must be demonstrated and careful observation and listening must be reflected in both the tone and the content of the physician's responses if successful communication of information, understanding, and values is to take place and the conflict is to be successfully resolved. In situations like the one described in this case, the greater weight of responsibility falls to the physician to manage the encounter, to make the mother feel free to ask questions and to express concerns (Balint, 1964). The fears and anxieties that accompany illness often compromise the patient's ability to communicate effectively. The physician's skills can frequently overcome this problem.

Understanding the Value Conflicts

Finally, it is clear that this pediatrician's style of practice reflects certain personal and professional values. He has chosen, perhaps with too little consideration of the consequences, to have a high-volume, brief-encounter office practice that has little flexibility for accommodating the needs of a mother who brings a complex problem to the office. This choice may reflect a conscious effort to provide these services to a larger number of patients to avoid having to turn patients away. It may also reflect his personal discomfort with discussing emotionally charged issues over which he has little curative control. His inadequacy in meeting the mother's needs may further reflect his personal choice to give little priority to his own continuing education in the area of developmental delays. Again, this may reflect a deliberate choice to educate himself in other aspects of pediatrics at the expense of developmental delays. These are all personal and professional values that have a clear effect on the nature of the care that Leonard's pediatrician provides. They make it more likely that problems with information, sensitivity, and communication will arise with many of his patients.

Exploring Solutions and Their Consequences

Ethical reflection would provide this physician with an opportunity to consciously probe these values and their implications, and perhaps to explore alternative approaches, such as prompt referral to someone whose interests and practice are more suited to the needs of Leonard and his mother. No physician can be competent in all areas, and a knowledge of one's gaps in expertise and an awareness of when referral is appropriate—for whatever reason—are minimal requirements of good professional practice.

CASE 2: MONICA

Cultural Barriers and Adjusting to Chronic Illness

Monica is a 3-year-old black child referred to the medical center by the public health nurse at a local health department. Monica has a delay in language development and a vocabulary of only a few words. She keeps to herself most of the time, shunning interactions with either adults or children. She does not appear to understand even simple commands. Two previous appointments for this child's evaluation were not kept by the mother, who lives 30 miles from the medical center. The mother works in a hosiery mill and lives in a rural community with her three children and her own mother. The public health nurse contacted social services, and arrangements were finally made to bring the mother and child to this appointment. During the interaction with the evaluation team, the mother answers most questions monosyllabically. She rarely makes eye contact. Quiet hostility is apparent when she is asked questions about her marital status, living situation, employment, and alcohol consumption. The mother appears loving toward the child, although she admits to resorting to spanking on the occasions when the child does not cooperate.

On evaluation, Monica displays global developmental delays and communication problems consistent with autism. Members of the evaluation team are alarmed by the mother's failure to keep the first two appointments. They are concerned about the poor social circumstances of this family and the low education level of the mother, and they believe that she is unlikely to carry through with any of the therapeutic plans they believe essential for Monica's optimum development. In reviewing the findings and making recommendations, they suggest special classes five days per week at the medical center. They indicate the mother's need to participate in these sessions to learn the skills necessary to help Monica. The mother and child fail to appear at the first of these interventions.

Identifying the Problems

In this case, unlike the first, the health professionals involved have recognized the existence of a problem or conflict in their encounter with Monica and her mother and must move to identify its source and rectify it if possible. One means of alleviating or avoiding problems is to attempt to reach some agreements about the encounter. Disagreement in the outpatient setting often originates from one of three areas. Health professionals and patients need some agreement in each of these areas if they are to work effectively together. (1) There should be some common understanding of the *nature of the problem* that brings the two parties together, (2) there should be a common set of *goals* for the interaction, and (3) there should be some common understanding of the *roles* to be played by the patient and the health professional. Agreement is never complete in all of these areas, but efforts to identify and negotiate disagreements will reduce conflict and frustration.

Understanding the Value Conflicts

As in the first case, insensitivity and poor communication of important information play significant roles here. In this case, however, to communicate effectively with, and respond sensitively to Monica's mother requires a deeper understanding of cultural values and their influence on customs of parenting and on the interpretation of illness.

Health professionals are frequently faced with social and cultural gaps between themselves and their patients. Personal values are in part culturally determined. When we deal with individuals from diverse strata of our society, socially and culturally determined values may be at the heart of value conflicts. When doctor and patient speak from different cultures, words have different meanings and nonverbal cues have different significances. Verbal communication itself may be less valued in this mother's culture. These communication gaps will not be overcome without effort.

The failure to keep appointments may reflect, not a lack of concern on the mother's part for her child's welfare, but rather problems with the automobile that serves as her only means of transportation. Lack of a telephone and inability to pay for long-distance calls may be the root explanation of the mother's failure to cancel the appointment and schedule another. The loss of a day's wages to participate in the teaching sessions may represent an unreasonable sacrifice. Inattention to such important information and its implications might lead the health professional to make inappropriate assumptions about the mother's concern for her child or willingness to participate actively in her treatment.

Negotiating Solutions

Some of the value differences apparent between Monica's mother and these health professionals are probably embedded in culture; others reflect different personal values. The sorting of these two categories is often difficult. It is important to determine whether this mother has a different view of what her child needs from that held by the health professionals who would like to assist her. The health professionals perceive that an extensive educational intervention will bring the greatest benefit. The mother, on the other hand, may perceive Monica differently, believing her problem to be an act of God unlikely to be changed by any human interventions. As long as this basic value difference remains hidden, the health care team will be frustrated in its efforts on behalf of the child. If this value conflict comes to light, it may be possible for the health professionals to negotiate some form of compromise with the mother. But the initiation of any compromise whatever requires a willingness to learn each other's perspective. Initially an agreement might be reached on a very limited set of services offered within the community. If these services can be shown to benefit the child, the mother might be willing to proceed one step further. If, on the other hand, the expectations raised by the health professionals are not achieved, the mother may choose to retreat to her original inclination to do nothing.

Entangled in this maze of information, communication, and value problems is the ongoing process of a family coming to grips with a handicap in one of its children. This process creates barriers that may be misinterpreted as value conflicts. Denial, guilt, fear, depression, and hostility all represent common responses to this stressful situation. The choice of responses will be influenced by culture and personality and will often vary across individuals in the same family. In addition to distinguishing these reactions from value conflicts, the health professional should assist the family in understanding these reactions so as to diminish the family's interference with the best interests of the child.

CASE 3: CHARLIE

Subtle Abuses of Dependency

Charlie is a 4½-year-old child in the early phase of an intensive treatment program for autism. He is an only child. His father is a university professor, and his college-educated mother, Alice, has recently left her job as a research assistant to dedicate whatever energy is required to provide the very best care possible for Charlie. Alice is a delightful and pleasant woman who has been a model parent in her meticulous attention to every suggestion made by the teacher. Joan, the special education teacher, has had over 15 years of experience working with autistic children and their families. She is a very warm person who has spent hours working with Alice explaining the nature of Charlie's problem and the appropriate educational and behavioral interventions and patiently answering hundreds of questions that Alice has posed to her. Joan is delighted to work with this highly motivated mother and believes that Charlie can accomplish more than most children with his problem because of Alice's skills and efforts on Charlie's behalf. Likewise, Alice is appreciative of Joan's attention and looks to her for guidance on every aspect of Charlie's care. The researcher who was Alice's employer has recently won a large grant and calls her to offer her part-time employment and a significant role in the administration of this new research project. Alice, very interested in this new possibility for professional growth, consults Joan about the feasibility of accepting this professional challenge. Joan is quick to indicate her opinion that this would have a deleterious effect on Charlie, and without further discussion Alice nods her head in agreement and turns down the offer.

Exploring the Moral Conflicts

This case might appear to be an example of an ideal interaction. A motivated and bright mother is working with a caring and talented teacher. They share a common agenda of achieving the best possible results for Charlie. The aspect of this relationship that demands attention is the dependence that Alice has on the teacher and the power and influence that the teacher has over Alice.

Many patients become deeply indebted to health professionals who assist them. The sense of helplessness in the face of disease can lead some patients or their parents to become very dependent on their health care providers. This is particularly true when that health care provider is warm, caring, and willing to spend whatever time is needed with the patient or parent. Some measure of dependence is a natural part of the interaction and may serve a therapeutic purpose in helping a patient work through grief, change unhealthy life patterns, or accept an illness.

In most circumstances, health professionals should be seeking to give those they advise and care for greater independence in caring for their own needs. For most patients, this arises naturally from the desire to be independent. In some cases, however, both the patient and the health professional may derive rewards from a dependent relationship and may seek to enlarge the dependence rather than reduce it.

As a result of this dependence, the health professional can acquire considerable power over patients and their families. The exercise of this power, either purposefully or inadvertently, can compromise patient or family freedom. Joan is in a position to impose her own values on Alice, and because of her high regard for Joan, Alice is likely to accept those values without much question. Their relationship could be characterized by a subtle but powerful paternalism. In this regard, this situation is morally similar to cases in which physicians use threats of dire consequences to coerce patients into consenting to treatments. Although such physicians are faulted for blatant uses of power and callous attitudes, it is often overlooked that the power of a caring, dependent relationship can be abused as well. The power can be even more abusive if it is accepted without question by the patient. The consequences of this paternalism and loss of autonomy are just as great as in the more blatant examples.

Applying a Moral Principle

The health professional can never fully understand the patient and all of the forces in the patient's life. Therefore, the health care provider who makes decisions for patients and families runs the risk of inadvertently ignoring issues that would ultimately prove to be of critical significance to the patient. This is justified only if the patient's judgment is so clouded as to make him or her even more likely to overlook such critical issues. Even under such circumstances, however, the health professional must avoid the "golden rule" and strive instead to do *what the patient would choose for himself* if he were able (Cross & Churchill, 1982). This reduces the risk of the health professional's imposing values on the patient. This represents the principle of patient autonomy.

Abuse of dependency not only can lead to poor, restricted, or coerced choices but it may also breed greater dependency. The termination of such dependent relationships can be very traumatic. When the dependent patient attempts to escape the dependency, the therapeutic relationship may be destroyed by the resentment generated. In our case, Alice is fully competent to make her own decision and Joan's goal should be to help Alice accomplish this. Joan can offer some expert opinion on the impact of the decision on Charlie's progress, but beyond that Joan's opinion is personal—not expert—and needs to be labeled as such. Other issues that need to be weighed include the personal benefits to Alice, the financial benefits to the family, the potential for an increased role for the father in Charlie's care, and the prevention of Alice's "burnout." These issues are best considered by Alice, although Joan might assist Alice in considering them. However, in serving as a counselor Joan must be fully aware of the power she possesses and diligently avoid abusing it, even inadvertently.

CASE 4: ROBERT

Consent for Experimentation

Robert is an 11-year-old autistic child who has thrived in a special education program run in a large medical center near his home. Dr. Matthews is a psychologist who is in charge of the program and has worked closely with Robert and his family over the previous 8 years. Dr. Matthews has recently received a grant to study certain metabolic pathways in autistic children to determine whether this condition is an inborn error of metabolism. Dr. Matthews approaches Robert's parents to seek their permission to have Robert participate in his study. The study would require 5 days of hospitalization on a special research unit in the medical center. It would require several blood tests each day as well as the collection of all of his urine and stools over that time period. The parents would be free to visit and Robert's usual school and behavioral program would be continued during this time.

Dr. Matthews points out the importance of research on children with poorly understood problems like autism. He hopes and sincerely believes that his research will bring us closer to understanding the nature of this complex problem. The benefits of this research might not help Robert but may help autistic children of the future, Dr. Matthews explains to the parents.

The parents agree to allow Robert to participate, but when they return home they have some misgivings. They feel a great debt to Dr. Matthews and his program since it has provided an important service to their child at no cost to them. They also believe that further research in this condition is important. But they also realize that Robert will be upset by this 5-day experience. He inevitably becomes hard to control when he is in a strange environment. Drawing blood will require several people to hold him down because he is unlikely to be cooperative.

Robert's parents recognize that Robert could never adequately understand what is being asked of him and therefore could not consent for himself. But this realization only makes the task more difficult for them as they seek to consent fairly on their son's behalf. After much consideration, they call Dr. Matthews and rescind their consent. His obvious disappointment leads them to further worry whether this choice will influence the services they receive from his program hereafter.

Applying a Principle to the Moral Problem

This case illustrates multiple dimensions of informed consent. Because of their legal status as minors, all 11-year-olds would need to have parental consent to participate in such a research project (Holder, 1977). If their 11-year-old is of normal mental ability, most parents would discuss this consent with their child and take into account his or her feelings and opinions about the potential benefits of the experiment as well as the risks he or she would be subjected to by participation. Many researchers even demand a signed consent from a child of this age in addition to that of the parents. This is appropriate since most 11-year-olds are quite able to consent and participate with understanding.

However, with a developmentally handicapped child, or a normal child of a much younger age, the parents are forced to make the decision without the benefit of their child's meaningful input. One might interpret this as meaning that parents are free to do what they wish. To be legally and ethically sound, however, a proxy consent should include a careful consideration of all the issues that might be important to the handicapped child if he or she were able to make the choice for himself or herself. In other words, when you act on behalf of another you must be careful to act in the other's interests. It was after careful consideration of all of Robert's interests that the parents changed their decision.

Assessing the Consequences of Different Actions

Another issue raised by this case is the conflict of interest in Dr. Matthews's dual roles as therapist and researcher (Churchill, 1980). The parents' initial consent was probably based on their feeling of gratitude to Dr. Matthews for all he had done for their child. They therefore viewed participation in his research as a way to pay him back in part for his past help. Although Dr. Matthews did not expressly appeal to that sense of obligation, he made no effort to negate the impact that it might inappropriately have on their consent.

Although doing favors is appropriate between friends and peers, participating in research out of fear of offending the researcher is not an appropriate reason for consenting to take part in a research project. Dr. Matthews probably could never eliminate all feelings of obligation in Robert's parents even if he strongly stated that he did not wish them to consent simply to please him. It would have been more appropriate for the consent to be requested by someone in the research project who had no prior relationship with Robert or his parents.

Of course, because it would be deceptive to conceal Dr. Matthews's participation from Robert's parents, they might be affected by his involvement even though he himself does not seek their consent. Thus, although it can be minimized by careful and sensitive discussion, the dilemma cannot be eliminated so long as Robert is sought as a subject. Perceived obligation to physicians is a powerful, often subtle force that frequently contaminates consent for research. In our case, the disappointment registered in Dr. Matthews's voice when the parents rescinded their consent has at least temporarily altered their therapeutic relationship with Dr. Matthews in a potentially negative way. We are often lax in providing safeguards against such conflicts of interest and the potentially negative effects on the relationship of the health professional to the patient (Lebacqz & Levine, 1978).

Once these conflicts are dealt with, there is still the problem of achieving appropriate informed consent. Such consent must include a truthful rendition of all the information that would be needed for the parents to choose on behalf of their child. This would include a detailed description of what would be done as well as the potential risks involved. An accurate, nontechnical description of the purpose of the research project and its potential benefits is also needed. Complete freedom of choice must be guaranteed and no undue rewards or veiled threats should undermine this freedom. The consent must be reversible at any time and the family must have access to a higher authority within the research institution to deal with any grievances that might arise in the research setting. Even if these principles are adhered to, the actual process of achieving good informed consent is a difficult one, requiring careful attention to all of the dimensions of the physician–patient relationship discussed in these cases (Miller, 1980; President's Commission, 1982).

CASE 5: SUSAN

A Handicapped Child and Her Family versus Society

Susan is a 12-year-old mildly autistic child whose parents recently moved to a suburban community in the Midwest. Susan had been thriving in a special education setting designed for children with problems like hers. When her mother registered her for school in the new town, she brought extensive reports of Susan's educational program and progress. Although Susan's parents had received favorable reports about the new school system and its resources for autistic children, the school administrator coolly indicated that no such services existed in this community. When the parents discovered that Susan was to be placed in a Trainable Mentally Handicapped class with 11 other children and only one teacher, they were horrified. By chance they met the parents of another handicapped child who was placed in the same class. Through them they learned of the teacher's lack of special training and that the "education" was largely custodial care. At first confused, they quickly became angry and set about learning the education laws of this new state. They contacted the parents of the other children in this class along with several others in the school district and formed an advocacy group. When the group's requests for increased services were met by a lack of cooperation, a lawyer was hired. The legal action took 11 months, and another 6 months were needed to hire the appropriate special teachers. During this period, this family found itself greeted by hostility from others in the community who disagreed with spending the school's scarce resources for such a small group of children who were unlikely ever to contribute much to society.

Exploring Value Conflicts in Communities

On one level, this might be interpreted as a purely legal question, with parents using the courts to achieve the educational opportunities that the law intended for their child to receive. However, in this situation the law represents an expression of a set of values. The principle expressed in the law is that society accepts responsibility for the education of children with handicaps. This law, however, was not accompanied by adequate funding to be effectively implemented. Allocating adequate resources to the education of the handicapped child would require taking money from other programs likewise mandated by law. The citizens of the community have been unwilling to vote in the necessary tax increases to allow all educational mandates to be fulfilled adequately. In this community the decision appears to have been made, either deliberately or by default, that only minimal resources will be allocated for handicapped children in the schools. This is, therefore, a value conflict between the parents of these handicapped children and the citizens of the community in which they live (Kopelman & Moskop, 1984). The courts are merely the battleground for this value conflict.

Many families of children with handicaps are enmeshed in similar conflicts with the communities in which they live. They are often faced, as this family was, with choosing between the long-term interests of their child and the friendship of their neighbors. The frustrations of these battles and the loneliness which they often bring is a serious problem in the survival of these families. Although these battles do not always directly involve the health professional, he or she should remember that many such families may be choosing to devote substantial family resources to changing local, state, or federal policy on issues affecting their child. Such value decisions may end up influencing their relationship with the physician, because the parents' primary focus of attention is, at least temporarily, outside of the home. Thus, an understanding of these parents' public advocacy role is a necessary part of understanding them and their child. In addition, some physicians, upon ethical reflection, may decide that their own knowledge of the effects of handicapping conditions upon children puts them in a position to influence policy, as experts or advocates or both, and thus justifies time spent in such efforts.

CASE 6: SAMANTHA

The Young Adult, Sexual Abuse, and Reproductive Rights

Samantha is a 22-year-old mildly retarded female who has recently moved into a group home for retarded adults because the failing health of her elderly parents has made it difficult for them to care for her. Six months after Samantha's move to the group home, the house mother realizes that it has been at least 2 months since Samantha had a period. A pregnancy test confirms her fears and Samantha is gently questioned concerning her sexual behavior. With some difficulty she admits that she has had sex with the driver of the van that takes her to work each day. When she is told that she is pregnant, she smiles and says, "A baby in my tummy. Oh, I'm going to be a mommy." Samantha's parents are most distraught by the news since they are devout Catholics with strong convictions against abortion. They are, however, overwhelmed by the concept of raising a grandchild in the face of their realization that they are unable even now to care for Samantha. Samantha is no longer a minor and has not been adjudicated incompetent. By her own report she willingly participated in the sexual intercourse. No charges are pressed against the van driver, who has denied paternity. He quits his job and moves to another town.

Exploring the Interaction of Moral, Legal, and Social Dilemmas

Samantha's pregnancy is a potentially tragic circumstance that is likely to give rise to a number of complex legal, societal, and personal moral dilemmas. Many people are likely to be left feeling that the decision not to bring the van driver to trial is an injustice. However, a number of different concerns exist from the viewpoint of the legal system. Samantha, because she is chronologically adult, is presumed competent to make decisions on her own behalf until the contrary can be determined by a court. Three different legal determinations are at issue in this case. Two of these involve questions of Samantha's competence.

The first matter is whether the act of intercourse between Samantha and the driver ought to be treated as rape. Most crucial in this determination is Samantha's ability to give an effective consent to the act—whether she understood its implications and possible consequences and whether she is able to consent freely or might have been easily swayed by an exertion of apparent authority by the driver. Once presented with clear evidence of her handicap, a court would have to conduct a rather searching and particularized examination of her ability to make the decision in question under the circumstances described. The court will not view her competence as an all-or-nothing question but will examine it only for this decision. It is likely, however, that a court will be aided in this determination by hearing evidence about Samantha's competence in other areas.

If she is determined incapable of consenting to intercourse, a separate question remains: whether the driver knew or should have known that her mental limitations rendered her consent invalid. On the one hand, the driver occupied a position of special trust. Thus, he could be held to knowledge of Samantha's limited capacities even if he did not in fact know her limitations. On the other hand, Samantha was living relatively independently; she may have presented an appearance of considerable capability, and the driver may not have been given any job training to alert him to the nature of the handicaps of his passengers.

Despite our judgments about the morality of the van driver's actions, there is in addition a practical determination to be made here by the district attorney's office. To substantiate a charge of rape, much depends on Samantha's testimony. The judge and jury must determine both her competence and how she appeared to the van driver, as well as relying upon her description of the circumstances of the moment. If she is a good witness, the jury might believe a defense contention that she is, or appears, competent to consent to intercourse. If she is a poor witness, the jury might not be convinced that intercourse with the van driver even took place. A decision not to prosecute must be based on an evaluation of the likelihood that prosecution will be successful. In this case, a concerned physician might offer to assist the district attorney in preparing Samantha to testify, in assembling persuasive evidence regarding her competence, or in making the case that the van driver should have known—by virtue of job training, perhaps—of Samantha's limitations. Here a significant consideration is that without public examination of the circumstances of the incident, it is very difficult to evaluate fairly the blameworthiness of the van driver's action—unless the decision not to prosecute is also taken as a tacit determination by the district attorney that the facts as he found them did not warrant society's full opprobrium.

Once the decision not to prosecute has been made, two concerns remain. One is the legal question of paternity, which is at issue regardless of Samantha's competence and may be pursued because Samantha has named the driver as a possible father. The other is the problem of the van driver's future employment. Suppose he seeks a similar position in his new home and his prospective employer asks for references—should the physician relay these untested allegations? Suppose he seeks a different kind of job—is this behavior relevant as bearing on his general moral character even if comparable responsibility is not involved? Suppose further that there is no request for references but it is learned that he is employed in a similar position elsewhere—should the new employer be warned? These possibilities all raise questions of the law of defamation, but, more important, they raise questions, for the physician, of moral responsibility and fairness. These questions should not be answered entirely by legal concerns, but it must be remembered that the van driver's right to fair treatment, under these facts, is also morally based and not merely a matter of legal technicality. Thus, the physician who feels a strong moral responsibility to protect Samantha and others like her, and believes the driver to have shirked his moral responsibility as well, is nonetheless faced with a moral dilemma.

The third legal determination of potential significance in this case has to do with Samantha's capacity to bear and raise a child. In a strict sense, her expressed desire to become a mother cannot be treated as a refusal of medically indicated treatment unless abortion is medically indicated for her; thus, her choice to remain pregnant cannot legally be determined incompetent the way a refusal of surgery or medication could be. If abortion were medically indicated, someone else—a court-appointed guardian or the court itself—would have to choose for her. Her family's opposition to abortion would certainly figure into that decision (whether her parents were appointed guardians or not), unless continued pregnancy would endanger her life.

A difficult question is raised, however, when Samantha's ability to raise and care for a child is determined. The court could decide that Samantha's limitations and her parents' age and circumstances necessitate foster care placement for the baby. The court may also determine whether Samantha can consent to giving the child up for adoption once it is born. If her consent would be valid, she may agree to this course of action. If she refuses, in many states her parental rights may be terminated voluntarily, on the basis of her inability to care for the child. The legal proceeding in this instance is complicated and extensive because of the magnitude of the right at issue.

This tragedy might have been prevented by preparing Samantha to deal responsibly with her own sexuality. She needed an understanding of her own sexual desires and their proper expression, as well as warnings about the people who might take advantage of her. She needed lessons in birth control, and, most important, she needed someone she could comfortably talk with about these matters. Unfortunately, our society often prefers to deny the sexuality of people with handicaps.

All of the legal discussion of Samantha's competence so far has implied legal recogniton of the reality that people like Samantha are neither wholly competent nor wholly incompetent, and that each action and decision they make can be evaluated individually, taking account both of the individual circumstances and their own unique degree and kind of ability. The law in a number of states explicitly recognizes this variation in individual decision-making ability by means of the principle of limited guardianship. All states permit a court to determine that people like Samantha are incompetent and to appoint a guardian to act for them in all official capacities: financial, contractual, and the like. A number of states also permit the court to find such persons competent in some areas but incompetent in others, and to appoint a guardian whose powers are *limited* to making decisions the partially competent person cannot make (President's Commission for the Study of Ethical Problems, 1982).

Another approach to Samantha's problem initially might have been the utilization of this power of the legal system to declare her specifically incompetent in certain areas and to appoint a limited guardian to assist her. In reality, the social system does this by providing group homes and other means of support for the less competent, but this assistance may be given legal force by the formal naming of a guardian with control over a few specific dimensions of the life of a less competent adult. Such control would neither fully curtail Samantha's freedom nor erroneously assume her full competence. Although this approach might have been less useful in Samantha's case than better counseling, training, and supervision would have been, it can be very effective for financial matters and health care decisions. For example, it might have proved most advisable for Samantha that a limited guardian be appointed to make decisions for her regarding birth control. If sterilization had emerged as the choice in Samantha's best interests, that decision would probably have required court intervention, even if a guardian had already been appointed, because of its irreversibility (Macklin & Gaylin, 1981).

SUMMARY

Each of the six cases discussed in this chapter has emphasized a slightly different problem. In Leonard's case, some basic mechanics of the patient–provider relationship have gone awry; in Monica's, the basics are there but finding common ground requires further effort and insight on the part of the provider. Charlie's case emphasizes the subtlety with which a health professional may unwittingly exercise power to control a situation that is better controlled by the patient, while Robert's case illustrates the similar problems that arise when the clinician's research interests alter the balance in an ongoing relationship. Finally, the cases of Susan and Samantha demonstrate circumstances wherein the provider may feel the need or desire to step beyond the role of actor in individual interactions with patients and take cognizance of the larger framework of society and community. These two cases implicitly present the physician with two courses of action: (1) a continued focus of the individual patient–provider relationship, albeit with a new awareness and anticipation of potential problems and value choices from that larger framework which will affect the plan of care, and (2) an additional role as patient advocate in the public sector.

Ethical problems have many faces. Insensitivity, bad communication, and failure to reduce or minimize cultural and class barriers to health services present ethical problems just as serious as abuses of professional power or experimentation without proper consent. To probe any of these issues in depth would require more space than is available here. Our approach has been to display the wide range of encounters in which value conflicts may reside, hoping thereby to remind professionals and families of the delicacy and intricacy of our values in caring for autistic and handicapped children. More comprehensive discussions of the ethical problems we have introduced can be found in the references below.

Readers will have seen, as they proceeded through the chapter, that many of the issues emphasized in one case also appear in the other cases even though they are not specifically discussed. Common themes should naturally emerge. The four dimensions of the patient–physician relationship should be identifiable in every case, and lack of commonality of goals and roles may be found in more than just Monica's case. The problem of power, and the many ways in which the health professional's power may be misused, also may be seen in most of the cases. And it should be plain that those common themes are themselves intricately related. For example, the misuse of power and the lack of common ground in the encounter can either cause or result from failures of information, communication, and sensitivity. In addition, the problems identified may be interpreted and addressed either as matters of ethics or as matters of personal and professional skill and knowledge in effective interaction. What this shows is that both principled and practical inquiry are necessary to good patient care, and that many different ways of describing and rectifying ethical problems are available and workable so long as health professionals are able to identify and examine them.

REFERENCES

Balint, M. (1964). The apostolic function. In *The doctor, his patient and the illness*. New York: International Universities Press.

Beauchamp, T., & Childress, J. (1979). *Principles of biomedical ethics*. New York: Oxford Univeristy Press.

Churchill, L. R. (1980). Physician–patient/investigator–subject: Exploring the logic and tension. *Journal of Medicine and Philosophy, 5*, 215–224.

Cross, A., & Churchill, L. R. (1982). Ethical and cultural dimensions of informed consent, *Annals of Internal Medicine, 96*, 110.

Federal Register, May 18, 1982; January 12, 1984.

Federal Register, April 15, 1985.

Gaylin, W., & Macklin, R. (1982). *Who speaks for the child?* New York: Plenum Press.

Holder, A. R. (1977). *Legal issues in pediatric and adolescent medicine*. New York: Wiley.

Kopelman, L., & Moskop, J. (1984). *Ethics and mental retardation*. Dordrecht: Reidel.

Lebacqz, K. L., & Levine, R. J. (1978). Informed consent in human research: Ethical and legal aspects. In *Encyclopedia of Bioethics* (Vol. 2). New York: Free Press.

Macklin, R., & Gaylin, W. (Eds). (1981). *Mental retardation and sterilization: A problem of competency and paternalism*. New York: Plenum Press.

Miller, L. J. (1980). Informed consent. *Journal of the American Medical Association, 244*, 2100–03 (Part I); 2347–50 (Part II).

Moorkin, G. (1977). Paternalism. *Monist, p. 56*.

Murray, T. H. (1985). The final anticlimactic rule on Baby Doe. *Hastings Center Report, 15*, 5–9.

Pless, J. E. (1983). The story of Baby Doe. *New England Journal of Medicine, 309*, 664.

President's Commission for the Study of Ethical Problems. (1982). *Medical and biomedical and behavioral research* (Vol. 1). Report. *Making health care decisions: The ethical and legal implications of informed consent in the patient–practitioner relationship*. Washington, DC: U.S. Government Printing Office, 1982.

Szasz, T., & Hollander, M. (1956). The basic models of the doctor–patient relationship. *Archives of Internal Medicine, 97*, 585–592.

Neurological and Genetic Issues

Theory Based

Autism

Familial Aggregation and Genetic Implications

SUSAN E. FOLSTEIN and MICHAEL L. RUTTER

INTRODUCTION

Autism is a syndrome (Kanner, 1943) defined, not by etiology or pathology, but by particular behaviors and a characteristic natural history. The three clinical features essential for diagnosis are (1) deficits in the capacity to form relationships, associated with a poor appreciation of socioemotional cues, a lack of modulation of behavior according to social context, and a weak integration of social, emotional, and communicative behaviors; (2) deficits in the use of language for social communication, associated with poor synchrony and reciprocity in conversational interchange, impaired use of variations in cadence to reflect communicative modulation, together with abnormalities of language including stereotyped usages and delayed echolalia; and (3) restricted, repetitive, and stereotyped patterns of behavior, associated with abnormal preoccupations with part-objects or nonfunctional elements of play materials, and distress over changes in small details of the environment (Rutter & Schopler, 1986).

Although the majority of individuals with autism are also mentally retarded, the syndrome occurs in people with normal intelligence. The outcome, heavily influenced by IQ level and language development, is very poor when the IQ is below 50 or when there is no useful speech by the age of 5 years. However, even when intelligence is normal, social handicaps continue into adult life (Lotter, 1974, 1966; Rumsey et al., 1985; Rutter, 1970).

While a single pathology or pathophysiology may be discovered that will account for all cases of autism, it is clear that there is no single etiology. Although the etiology is still unknown in most cases, evidence from both biological and epidemiological studies demonstrates two principles about etiology of autism. First, there are many etiologies of autism, as would be expected in a syndrome defined only by its clinical features. At present, however, it is not known whether the majority of cases among those currently idiopathic will eventually be shown to have a single cause, or whether we will continue to "chip away" small numbers

SUSAN E. FOLSTEIN • Division of Psychiatric Genetics, Department of Psychiatry, Johns Hopkins University, Baltimore, Maryland 21205. MICHAEL L. RUTTER • M.R.C. Child Psychiatry Unit, Department of Child and Adolescent Psychiatry, Institute of Psychiatry, University of London, De Crespigny Park, Denmark Hill, London SE5 8AF, England.

of cases, with no single etiology accounting for the bulk of cases. The second principle is that the etiologies of autism are organic rather than psychosocial in nature. Among the rare cases of autism for which an etiology is apparent, there are examples of both physical-environmental (especially infections and perinatal trauma) and genetic causes. This chapter will present the evidence for the existence of one or more genetic factors in the etiology of the bulk of autism where the cause is unknown, and will review the evidence that autism can be associated with particular single gene disorders.

CHARACTERISTICS OF AUTISM

Before discussing the evidence for genetic factors in the etiology of autism, it is helpful to consider some characteristics of the syndrome that may enable us make reasonable hypotheses about etiology.

First, the age of onset is in infancy. Abnormalities may be evident from the first year and are almost always noticeable by 30 months. Unlike schizophrenia, with which autism has been commonly grouped, there is no prolonged period of relatively normal development before symptoms begin. Similarly, the distribution of the ages of onset of autism and schizophrenia do not overlap; with but few exceptions, there is at least a 5-year gap between the latest onset of autism and the earliest onset of adult-type schizophrenia (Kolvin, 1971; Rutter, 1974). These facts, along with the failure to find an excess of schizophrenia in the families of autistic children and the essential differences in the clinical features, make it unlikely that there is any etiological or pathophysiological connection between schizophrenia and autism. The age of onset also implies that some pathophysiological mechanism is operating at birth, if not before. Age at onset does not, however, help us predict the nature of etiology. Infections can have either immediate effects (as in congenital rubella) or delayed effects (as in postencephalitic Parkinsonism). Similarly, the manifestations of genetic conditions can begin at any time during life.

Second, although autism is strongly associated with mental retardation, the accompanying risks and neurological findings are different. Like mental retardation, autism is associated with an increased rate of pre- and perinatal abnormalities, but the increase is mainly in minor abnormalities, rather than the major abnormalities found in association with mental retardation (Deykin & MacMahon, 1980; Finegan & Quadrington, 1979; Gillberg & Gillberg, 1983). There is also a difference in the pattern of seizure development. While most children with severe mental retardation develop seizures in infancy or early childhood (Richardson, Koller, Katz, & McLaren, 1980), autistic children who develop seizures commonly do so around the time of puberty (Deykin & MacMahon, 1979). Also, while severe mental retardation is almost always associated with some kind of fairly obvious neuropathology (Crome & Stern, 1972), the few autopsy studies of autism either have revealed no detectable abnormalities or have shown rather subtle abnormalities that are not easily interpretable (Bauman & Kemper, 1985; Coleman, Romano, Lapham, & Simon, 1985; Darby, 1976; Harcherik et al., 1985; Williams, Hauser, Purpura, DeLong, & Swisher, 1980).

In addition, while autism is associated with disorders that also cause mental retardation, cases are not evenly distributed among those disorders; i.e., some disorders commonly cause both mental retardation and autism (e.g., infantile spasms, Riikonen & Amnell, 1981; and congenital rubella, Chess, Korn, & Fernandez, 1971; Chess, Fernandez, & Korn, 1978), while other conditions that are usually associated with intellectual impairment rarely give rise to autism (e.g., Down syndrome and cerebral palsy; Wing & Gould, 1979).

These different associations suggest that while there is some overlap in the specific disorders known to cause the two conditions, that overlap is quite small. It seems likely, therefore, that we must look for different etiologies of autism than those we have found for mental retardation. However, as will become clear below, we do not wish to suggest that the *types* of etiologies need be different. Single gene disorders may cause autism and single gene disorders may cause mental retardation, but the differences in the clinical features of these two syndromes lead us to hypothesize that the specific genes that are eventually found to explain autism will be different from the genes that, when abnormal, lead primarily to mental retardation.

Third, the cognitive deficits in autistic children, even in those who are not mentally retarded, tend to follow a distinctive and highly unusual pattern. Generally, they do poorly on tasks requiring sequential skills, conceptualization, and abstraction, and well on strictly nonverbal visual-spatial tasks (Rutter, 1979, 1983). In addition, they are impaired in their ability to discriminate social and emotional cues (Rutter, 1983). This distinctive pattern of cognitive deficits, present across IQ groups, suggests a common pathophysiology; whether it also implies a common etiology is less certain.

Finally, as suggested above, there is huge variation in the severity of the cognitive handicaps seen in autism. The IQ ranges from profoundly retarded to above average. Language development varies from virtually absent to nearly normal. The upper end of cognitive variability is extended even further if Asperger syndrome (Wing, 1981) and the possibly equivalent schizoid disorder of childhood (Chick, Waterhouse, & Wolff, 1979; Wolff & Barlow, 1979; Wolff & Chick, 1980) are included in the definition of autism. In these conditions, IQ is normal and there are no serious delays in language development. Deficits are virtually limited to social relationships that are strikingly similar to the social deficits in autism. Despite these deficits, persons with Asperger syndrome often attain a degree of social independence in adult life. There is the possibility, therefore, that lesser variants of autism may exist that have not been readily recognized. If these exist, the phenotype of autism used for genetic studies may need redefinition.

Such a wide variation in cognitive capacity usually implies etiologic diversity. Even when cases originally included in a phenotype with a wide IQ range all have genetic causes, multiple mutations have often been discovered (Laird & Schimke, 1979; McKusick, 1969). For example, the mucopolysaccharidoses were originally lumped together as "gargoylism" or "Hurler syndrome," on the basis of their similar physical characteristics. Within this original syndromic designation, intelligence ranged from normal to profoundly retarded. The IQ range within the current subgroups, defined by recessive mutations at particular loci, is quite narrow (McKusick, 1983). Similarly, the Marfan syndrome, caused by at least one autosomal dominant mutation, and homocystinuria, caused by autosomal recessive mutations at several loci (Valle, Pai, Thomas, & Pyeritz, 1980), were originally thought to be one disorder with a wide range in IQ. It was not until homocystine was found in the urine of a subset of the cases that the subtle differences in the physical features and IQ ranges of the two syndromes were appreciated.

On the other hand, a single etiology can result in a wide variation of handicap. Nongenetic examples are congenital rubella and cerebral palsy caused by perinatal trauma. Within genetic disorders there are examples among both recessive and dominant conditions. Patients with sickle cell anemia who also have persistent fetal hemoglobin have significantly less severe clinical manifestations of sickle cell anemia (Dover, Boyer, & Pembrey, 1981). Affected patients, within individual kindreds (all necessarily having the same mutation), of neurofibromatosis, tuberous sclerosis, or Joseph's disease (Rosenberg & Pettegrew, 1980) can show wide variations in the severity of symptoms. This phenomenon is called variable expressivity. In addition, some family members who "must" have the affected gene on the basis of family patterns of inheritance have no detectable symptoms. Disorders where this occurs are said to have incomplete penetrance. Milder manifestations of recessive conditions, both autosomal and X-linked, are sometimes seen in carriers. Mild mental retardation can be seen in the female carriers of fragile X and will be further discussed in that section. In some disorders that appear to be genetically determined, but appear not to transmit in a Mendelian fashion, (e.g., Tourette syndrome and stuttering; Kidd & Pauls, 1982), variable expressivity has been used as evidence for multifactorial etiology (i.e., the interaction of some unknown number of genes and environmental factors). However, it must be said that multifactorial inheritance has yet to be demonstrated for a human disorder at the molecular level. And evidence is mounting that some of the conditions consistent with multifactoral models, such as Tourette syndrome, could be inherited as Mendelizing traits with incomplete penetrance and variable expressivity.

Thus, on the basis of clinical features alone, it is hazardous at best to make specific predictions about whether there is one etiology or many. Similarly, it is impossible to predict, without additional data, whether a major etiology is more likely to be traumatic, infectious, or genetic. And finally, the symptoms alone do not allow us to confidently postulate a particular type of genetic transmission. Nevertheless, the data do suggest that it is necessary to search for etiologies that are not synonymous with those for schizophrenia or mental retardation, that organic causes are likely to predominate among the etiologies, and that the etiologies of autism associated with severe mental handicap may differ from that of autism in the presence of normal intelligence. With these considerations in mind, we will review the available evidence for genetic contributions to the etiology or etiologies of autism. As noted above, these data will be divided into two sections: first, the evidence for genetic factors in currently idiopathic autism, and second, a review of a few genetic disorders for which an association with autism has been reported.

EVIDENCE FOR GENETIC FACTORS IN AUTISM DERIVED FROM FAMILY AND TWIN STUDIES OF CASES OF UNKNOWN ETIOLOGY

The first step when investigating a syndrome for the possibility of genetic etiology is to look at familial aggregation of the disorder and patterns of disorder in twins. These studies include only cases where the etiology is unknown, i.e., in cases not associated with any etiologically defined disorder.

Interpretation of twin and family data is fraught with hazards, and several factors must be borne in mind when examining such data. First, family and twin data are prone to sampling biases. Unless sampling is systematic, "interesting families" with several affected members are more likely to be reported than those with just one affected child. Similarly, monozygotic twin pairs are more likely to be reported than dizygotic pairs and concordant pairs more than discordant ones. Second, whenever diagnostic methods and criteria are less than fully objective, there is wide scope for bias in diagnosing secondary cases in the family. Great caution is needed in the interpretation of studies where the diagnosis of family members (secondary cases) was not independent of, and blind to, the diagnosis of the proband (the case by which the family was identified). If the investigator making the diagnosis knows that the case is a member of a family with another affected member, he may be tempted to apply less stringent criteria. Similar cautions apply to studies where the diagnostic criteria are not fully specified.

However, cases with "similar" phenotypes are not to be overlooked or dismissed as irrelevant. As discussed earlier, genetic influences may apply to some deficit that is broader than the autism phenotype as strictly defined, so that investigation of familial aggregation of a range of disorders is warranted. The hazard here is in the interpretation of such familial aggregation: Learning disorders and developmental delays in speech and language are common (Silva, 1986; Yule & Rutter, 1985), so that such investigations must include systematic measurements and the use of a comparison group.

A final hazard in the interpretation of twin and family data concerns the methods of genetic analysis. As already noted, genetic heterogeneity must be presumed at this stage of our knowledge, and analyses that assume that any sample of autism represents an etiologically homogeneous population can be misleading.

Family Studies

Most epidemiological studies of autistic children have not included cases with known (or presumed) genetic etiologies, such as phenylketonuria or hypsarrhythmia. Even without the inclusion of these cases, some familial aggregation of autism has been noted. Very approximately, some 2% of families have two autistic children (August, Stewart, & Tsai, 1981, Folstein & Rutter, 1977; Rutter, 1967). While this number is small, it is 50 to 100 times what would be expected by chance according to the accepted prevalence rate of autism (2–4 per 10,000 school-age children) (Lotter, 1967; Treffert, 1970; Wing, O'Conner, & Lotter, 1967; Wing, Yeates, Brierley, & Gould, 1976). These estimates of rates in sibs are, however, in need of replication using standardized methods of assessment (Gottesman & Shields, 1982; Hanson & Gottesman, 1976). With the exception of August et al. (1981), none of the investigators systematically examined the secondary cases in the families in the same way as the probands. So it may be that these are mentally retarded children or perhaps mildly autistic children who would not meet the same criteria as those by which their proband autistic sibs were ascertained. While August et al. examined all the secondary cases, the authors do not state whether these diagnoses were blind to that of the proband.

It appeared in August's case series that familial cases were also mentally retarded, and other data to be described below suggest that it may not be autism so much as mental retardation that is familially aggregated. One exception is the report of Burgoine and Wing (1983) on triplets with Asperger syndrome. We have also observed familial aggregation of Asperger syndrome in a male proband, in his maternal uncle, and in his mother's male first cousin. As discussed earlier, Asperger syndrome is probably equivalent to autism without mental retardation (Wing, 1981). It may be that different kinds of questions must be asked when inquiring about the family history if familial aggregation of the milder variants of autism is to be detected.

Twin Studies

Even if the 1 to 3% rate of autism in sibs can be confirmed, familial aggregation does not necessarily imply genetic etiology. Infectious conditions can show familial aggregation, and there may be a tendency for mothers to have repeated complications of pregnancy and birth (Stanley & Alberman, 1984).

Better evidence for the importance of genetic factors has come from the study of twins. First came a number of reports of individual pairs of twins (reviewed by Folstein &

Rutter, 1977; Ritvo, Freeman, Mason-Brothers, Mo, & Ritvo, 1985; Rutter, 1967). The great majority of these pairs was reported to be concordant for autism. However, no definite genetic inferences could be made from these case reports for several reasons (discussed in detail by Gottesman & Shields, 1982). First, the number of reported monozygotic pairs far exceeded the number of reported dizygotic pairs, indicating a reporting bias. In the population, dizygotic pairs are twice as common as monozygotic pairs; when only same-sex pairs are considered, the proportions are about equal (Mittler, 1971). Second, for reasons described above, the proportion of concordant pairs in reports of individual pairs was probably over-estimated. Third, some publications failed to specify diagnostic methods and criteria. And finally, there was a failure in some cases to confirm the appearance of monozygosity by blood typing or dermatoglyphics and to describe the nature of the physical dissimilarities on which dizygosity was based. Twins who are similar in appearance are usually monozygotic, but like siblings, dizygotic pairs can look quite similar. The documentation of dizygosity is somewhat easier—if the pair differs in physical characteristics such as color and texture of hair, ear form, and eye color, dizygosity is virtually certain and need not be confirmed by other methods. However, dissimilarities in these characteristics must be marked in order to be sure of dizygosity. Twins who are actually monozygotic may be thought by friends and family to be dizygotic twins because they are easily distinguished by their demeanor and facial expression. This is particularly true if one of the twins is autistic.

For all these reasons, it was necessary to study a total population sample of twins before drawing any conclusions about possible genetic influences in the etiology of autism. In 1977 Folstein and Rutter reported a study of English autistic twins who were systematically ascertained through multiple sources. We specifically urged the reporting of dizygotic as well as monozygotic pairs and emphasized that we were equally interested in discordant and concordant pairs. According to our checks, our final sample of 21 pairs meeting diagnostic criteria appeared to be a reasonably complete sample within the school-age range (Folstein & Rutter, 1977). Zygosity was checked by multiple blood group analyses (or, as in one case, by dermatoglyphics) in all pairs who were not clearly dizygotic by a systematic inspection of physical features. The diagnostic criteria were consistent, and final diagnoses were made blind to zygosity and twin pair membership.

In this total population of 21 pairs of same-sex twin pairs, the concordance rate for autism was 36% in the monozygotic pairs and 0% in the dizygotic pairs. The concordance could not be explained by complications of pregnancy or delivery or by postnatal illness, and the results therefore supported the hypothesis that autism could be inherited. However, a twin study cannot indicate whether there is one genetic etiology or many, or whether one or more genetic mechanisms are operating. Nor is the absolute proportion of concordant monozygotic pairs related to the proportion of "genetic cases" in the population, because of the postconception environmental differences that occur in monozygotic twins.

The concordance rate for monozygotic pairs was considerably lower than would have been predicted from an analysis of the individual twin reports, and also lower than that recently reported by Ritvo, Freeman, et al. (1985), who claimed 95.7% concordance in MZ pairs and 23.5% in DZ pairs. Although the authors purported to use methods similar to those of Folstein and Rutter, in fact, they relied largely on voluntary replies from families to announcements of the study placed in the newsletter of the National Society for Autistic Children, along with a few local case referrals. The NSAAC announcements (The Advocate, 1980) did request discordant as well as concordant pairs, but this request was buried in the middle of several paragraphs requesting multiple case families by the same research group. As expected from the methods of case ascertainment, the sample contains a marked excess of monozygotic pairs. The report (Ritvo, Freeman, *et al.*, 1985) stated that the proportion of MZ to DZ pairs was equal, but because opposite-sex pairs are included, there should have been twice as many DZ as MZ pairs for the sample to be representative with respect to zygosity. The inclusion of opposite-sex pairs added to the difficulties in interpretation because of the very different rates of autism in males and females. Although the authors criticized other studies for failing to confirm dizygosity by blood groupings, most of their zygosities were based on parental report. Finally, no mention was made of any attempt to diagnose autism in the twins, blind to pair membership. In short, this study adds little to our knowledge about genetic factors in autism, and furthermore, it is misleading in its assertions and conclusions.

While the familial aggregation noted in case series, and the data from the twin studies, indicate that genetic factors are likely to be important in autism, these kinds of studies tell us little about the nature of the genetic defect, or whether there is one defect or many. All these investigations took place before the discovery of the association of autism with fragile X. How much of the familial aggregation of autism in sibs or how much of the twin concordance could be thus accounted for is unknown.

Other Disorders in Family Members

Even more striking than the familial aggregation of autism is the aggregation of disorders of general intelligence, and of reading and language in families of autistic children. This was first noticed by Bartak, Rutter, and Cox (1975), where a family history of reading or language disabilities was found in at least one first-degree relative of 5 of the 19 families (26%) studied. In these families, ascertained through an autistic child with an IQ above 70, no excess of mental retardation was noted, although this was not systematically studied. This familial aggregation of reading and language disorders in family members is not likely to be accounted for by fragile X because the autistic children had high IQs, an uncommon occurrence with fragile X.

Folstein and Rutter (1977) reported similar findings in their twin study. The concordance rate for disorders of cognition and language was considerably higher than the concordance rate for autism. Nine of the 11 monozygotic pairs (82%) were concordant for language or cognitive disorder, compared with only 1 of the 10 dizygotic pairs (10%). The severity of the disorders varied from rather mild, as evidenced by the need for tutoring in reading and grammar, to moderately disabling, exemplified by one co-twin with an IQ of 55 who needed special schooling.

The data on birth complications suggested an explanation for the findings. While the nonautistic but cognitively disabled monozygotic co-twins had normal or near normal birth histories, their autistic co-twins did not. Several had suffered significant perinatal problems. This suggested that while autism itself was sometimes inherited (as evidenced by the four monozygotic pairs who were concordant for autism), it appeared that more often a language or cognitive deficit was inherited, which, when combined with an environmental insult such as birth difficulties, resulted in autism. This conclusion does not necessarily apply to autism in general because twins are more prone than single births to birth injuries, and the injuries reported in case series of nontwin autistic children have been relatively mild. On the other hand, it is possible that a mild birth injury could have a greater impact in a child who was genetically predisposed to abnormal language or cognitive development.

Cognitive abnormalities among the siblings of autistic children were also reported by August *et al.* (1981). These investigators tested all the sibs of 41 autistic probands using standard IQ tests and tests of reading, spelling, and math. The age-matched siblings of children with Down syndrome served as the comparison group. The rate of cognitive abnormalities was 15% in the sibs of the autistic probands, compared with 3% among the sibs of the Down controls. All of the cognitively disabled children came from 8 of the 41 families, and all the probands in these 8 families were mentally retarded, suggesting that often it may not be autism but mental retardation that is familially aggregated. The familial aggregation of cognitive disabilities in this study could not all have been due to fragile X because 3 of the 8 families with cognitively disabled sibs were ascertained through female autistic probands. Baird and August (1985) have recently confirmed their earlier findings in another sample, and they did find 1 family where aggregation was accounted for by fragile X (August & Lockhart, 1984).

Another study of siblings using only IQ tests (Minton, Campbell, Green, Jennings, & Samit, 1982) also found a high rate of mental retardation among the siblings of autistic probands. In this study, the verbal scores of the siblings were significantly lower than performance scores, a pattern also seen in autistic children and in children with developmental language disorders.

Segregation Analysis

For several years, Ritvo and his group have been accumulating volunteer families with autism in two or more siblings. In collaboration with Spence (Ritvo, Spence, *et al.*, 1985), an attempt was made at segregation analysis, i.e., the investigation of possible genetic mechanisms for inheritance in autism using mathematical analysis of the case material. The authors reported that their data were consistent with autosomal recessive inheritance, and not consistent with multifactorial models. While they used analytic methods that controlled for the bias of sample ascertainment through multiple-case families, the methods presumed that the same segregation ratio was operating in the nonascertained families—that is, that the sample was homogeneous with respect to genetic mechanism. While this result is intriguing, it is somewhat confusing in light of the great excess of affected males and of male–male sib pairs in their sample. This is typical, of course, of autism samples, but it is not ordinarily expected in autosomal recessive inheritance where the sex ratio should be equal. Clearly, even if all of autism were inherited as single gene disorders, either some families would have to be X-linked to account for the excess of males or some powerful modifying factor must be postulated that somehow inhibits expression in females.

Autosomal recessive inheritance, or a mixture of autosomal and X-linked recessives, is by no means impossible in autism. One would expect somewhat more familial aggregation (McKusick, 1969), but that may be less than expected under certain circumstances. If family size is small, if the phenotype inhibits further reproduction, or if there is variable expressivity so that not all cases are detected, familial aggregation may be quite minimal.

Linkage Analysis

Using 34 families from this same sample, the same investigators (Spence *et al.*, 1985) undertook a limited linkage analysis. The purpose of genetic linkage analysis is to investigate whether a trait or disorder (e.g., autism) is systematically associated with some marker that is known to be the product of a single genetic locus. A positive result provides evidence for single gene transmission and for the association of a particular disorder with a particular genetic locus. The finding of a genetic linkage between a disorder and a marker does not imply that the marker, such as a blood group or HLA pattern, is related to the cause of the disorder, but simply that the gene for the trait or disorder under test and the gene for the marker are close neighbors on a particular chromosome.

On the assumption that there is a unique chromosomal location for some gene for autism, Spence *et al.* looked for linkage to HLA (chromosome 6) and 19 other autosomal markers in 34 families with two or more autistic children. One family with fragile X was omitted. No other markers located on the X chromosome were checked. No convincing linkages to the autosomal markers were found, and there was some suggestion of differences between families with only boys and families with one or more girls.

One should by no means conclude that Mendelian inheritance is thus ruled out. More complex analyses are needed to take into account the likely etiological and genetic heterogeneity even in autism samples chosen for having more than one affected case. Linkage studies need to be undertaken using the more numerous and more informative markers that are now available in the form of highly polymorphic anonymous DNA fragments. For a discussion of this method of genetic linkage analysis, see Gusella *et al.* (1984).

SINGLE GENE DISORDERS ASSOCIATED WITH AUTISM

Up to this point, we have been considering the evidence for genetic factors in the etiology of autism that is idiopathic in terms of current knowledge. Cases of autism are occasionally found that are not discernibly different from idiopathic autism, but for which an etiology is apparent. And there are a few etiologically defined conditions that may be associated with autism more often than expected by chance. Genetic etiologies include fragile X, and possibly tuberous sclerosis and phenylketonuria. The best documented association with an infectious disease is that between autism and congenital rubella (Chess *et al.*, 1978).

There are several difficulties in interpreting reports of such associations. First, reports are seldom based on systematically collected samples, so that the strength of the association with autism is not clear. That is to say, how many cases of autism are associated with the condition, and how many cases with the condition are also autistic? Second, many of the cases reported are not described well enough to be able to determine whether or not they meet currently accepted diagnostic criteria. (Some cases clearly do not meet criteria.) Third, it remains a puzzle what pathophysiological mechanism might unite these diverse etiologically defined conditions that are associated with autism. There is no obvious common pathophysiology among such diverse conditions as congenital rubella (an infection), hypsarrhythmia (a particular EEG pattern), recessively inherited phenylketonuria and the X-linked fragile X condition. However, investigations that might answer that question, such as PET scanning or postmortem neurochemical investigations of autistic children with known etiologies, have never been attempted.

With the possible exception of fragile X, such cases represent a tiny proportion of all cases of autism, but it is worthwhile reviewing these often cited associations to see just how much evidence there is for them, and because they may suggest clues about the etiology of idiopathic cases.

Phenylketonuria

Historically, the first genetic condition to be reported in association with autism was phenylketonuria. Phenylketonuria (PKU) is an inborn error of metabolism, inherited as an autosomal recessive disorder (Folling, 1934) and usually, but not universally, associated with mental retardation. All newborns are now screened for PKU, and a phenylalanine-free diet is instituted within the first weeks of life. The diet substantially diminishes the cognitive and behavioral handicap, although Stevenson and colleagues (Stevenson *et al.*, 1979) found a high rate of behavioral deviance in an unselected school-age sample with PKU that had been treated from infancy. None were autistic or had other behaviors common to autistic children.

From the few reports that describe the behavior of children with PKU prior to the availability of early treatment, it is clear that in addition to (and sometimes independent from) mental retardation, the children's behavior was severely deviant. In more than half the cases, the children were unfriendly, were often mute, and had repetitive behaviors. This literature is reviewed in an often quoted paper by Friedman (1969), who asserts that most children with untreated PKU are autistic. However, it is not entirely clear from his paper how autism was conceptualized. In most of the papers referred to by Friedman, the behavioral descriptions were not sufficiently detailed (Bjornson, 1964; Kratter, 1959; Leland, 1957; Sutherland, Berry, & Shirkey, 1960) to provide convincing evidence that the children actually met criteria for autism, although in most cases at least one autistic symptom was described.

It is of interest that not all socially unresponsive children with PKU were mentally retarded by IQ testing (Bjornson, 1964; Blainy & Gulliford, 1956; Cowie, 1951; Sutherland *et al.*, 1960), and reports from the 1950s and 1960s suggest that when dietary treatment was instituted after infancy, IQ showed no improvement, but that autistic symptoms frequently disappeared (Armstrong, Low, & Bosma, 1957; Armstrong & Tyler, 1955; Berry, Sutherland, Guest, & Umbarger, 1958; Bickel, Gerrard, & Hickmans, 1954; Blainy & Guilliford, 1956; Lewis, 1959; Woolf, Griffiths, & Moncrieff, 1955).

In his review, Friedman concluded that autism and mental retardation were separate manifestations of PKU, as evidenced by the presence of autistic symptoms in normally intelligent children with PKU and by the improvement of autistic symptoms, but not mental retardation, when a phenylalanine-free diet was begun after infancy.

Untreated PKU and PKU treated after infancy provide a useful illustration of the separability of autistic symptoms, if not autism, and mental retardation within a single condition and within a single case. This observation supports the hypothesis that on a pathophysiological level, autism and mental retardation have different mechanisms.

Tuberous Sclerosis and Neurofibromatosis

There may also be a specific association between autism and tuberous sclerosis, a neurocutaneous disorder inherited as an autosomal dominant trait. In severe cases the manifestations include mental retardation that is not present from birth but gradually worsens, facial nevi or adenoma sebaceum (also absent in younger children) commonly seen in a "butterfly" distribution over the cheeks, and epilepsy (Rosenberg & Pettegrew, 1980). The disease is transmitted by an affected parent who has milder manifestations. The most common type of EEG pattern in epileptic infants with tuberous sclerosis is hypsarrhythmia (Hunt, 1983a, 1983b, 1983c), and the reported association with autism is not with tuberous sclerosis itself but rather with hypsarrhythmia, which can have other etiologies (Riikonen & Amnell, 1981; Taft & Cohen, 1971). The cases reported both by Taft and Cohen and by Riikonen and Amnell were well described and typically autistic. The prevalence of autism in a case series of children with tuberous sclerosis has not been reported, so that the strength of the association with autism is unknown. In her series of 97 children with tuberous sclerosis, Hunt (1983c) alluded to a high prevalence of communication disorders, especially in those children with hypsarrhythmia, but she did not report specific psychiatric diagnoses.

Another neurocutaneous disorder, neurofibromatosis, also inherited as an autosomal dominant with variable severity of symptoms, was recently reported in association with autism. Neurofibromatosis, also called von Recklinghausen disease, is characterized by flat, pigmented nevi, tumors (neurofibromas) of the cranial and peripheral nerves and skin, and a predisposition to other tumors. Gillberg and Forsell (1984) reported neurofibromatosis in 6% of autistic children who were ascertained through a community survey. While it is only a single report and needs confirmation, it warrants follow-up because of the systematic nature of the sample. It is somewhat surprising that the association has not been noted previously, but without systematic family histories and physical examinations on each case, the diagnosis could easily be missed. The manifestations in parents are usually mild, and even in severe cases, signs accumulate only with age so that young children may have few stigmata.

Even if there is no specific association with autism, the neurocutaneous disorders may be useful in the investigation of the neuropathology or pathophysiology of autism. Both neurofibromatosis and tuberous sclerosis have brain lesions that are variable in location, so that neuropathological studies comparing cases with and without associated autism may suggest brain areas central to the pathophysiology of autism.

These single gene disorders reported in association with autism are autosomal disorders, and thus the sex ratio of affected persons would be expected to be equal, while the sex ratio in autism is about 4:1 males (see Chapter 11). It is not clear from the various case reports whether the children with autosomal disorders who are also autistic are for some reason more likely to be boys, but in the few reports where sex is mentioned, the ratio of boys to girls appears to be equal. For the most part, these disorders have not appeared in association with "pure" autism, but rather with autism accompanied by severe mental retardation, although exceptions are reported. It does appear that the sex ratio among severely retarded autistic children is somewhat less skewed to males (Lord, Schopler, & Revick, 1982), so that it is possible that among the severely retarded autistic population autosomal recessive conditions may have some numerical importance.

Fragile X

One single gene disorder, fragile X, has recently been discovered that is X-linked, is found predominantly in males, and appears to have a specific association with autism.

The clinical features are somewhat variable, but in its most severe form, the affected males are mentally retarded and, after puberty, have enlarged testicles. They tend to be hypotonic and to have somewhat long faces and large ears, but as children they do not appear particularly dysmorphic (Brondum-Nielsen, 1983). This syndrome of X-linked mental retardation was clinically recognized before the discovery of its association with fragile X and was known as the Martin–Bell syndrome (Martin & Bell, 1943).

Males with the genotype vary in IQ. Most are severely retarded but a few are normally intelligent and have offspring (Sherman, Morton, Jacobs, & Turner, 1984; Varley, Holm,

& Eren, 1985). Female carriers are occasionally mildly mentally retarded, possibly related to whether their normal or their fragile X is inactivated (Knoll, Chudley, & Gerrard, 1984; Turner, Brookwell, Daniel, Selikowitz, & Zilibowitz, 1980). In one report (Largo & Schinzel, 1985), IQ was reported to vary inversely with age, suggesting that damage to the brain is progressive. There are a few reports of prominent language impairment, but beyond the physical stigmata and mental retardation, the phenotype has yet to be characterized in a large sample.

The association of the Martin–Bell syndrome with a fragile site at the end of the long arm of the X chromosome was first reported by Lubs (1969), but the association was not confirmed until Sutherland (1977) discovered that demonstration of the fragile site required folate-poor tissue culture media. Even under optimal growing conditions, only a minority of the cells show the fragile site, and it cannot always be demonstrated in female carriers. The prevalence of fragile X is still uncertain, but it is probably the second (after Down syndrome) most common genetic cause of mental retardation. Estimates of incidence vary between 1 and 3 per 1000 live births (Blomquist, Gustavson, Holmgren, Nordenson, & Palsson-Strae, 1983; Blomquist, Gustavson, Holmgren, Nordenson, & Sweins, 1982; Herbst & Miller, 1980).

Fragile sites on chromosomes are areas that appear thinner than the rest of the chromosome when observed in metaphase preparations, as if that length of the chromosome were fragile and could easily break apart. Fragile sites have been observed on several chromosomes, but except for the site at Xq27 associated with the Martin–Bell syndrome, they have not been associated with any specific disorder (Sutherland, 1985).

Even though fragile X is transmitted in a Mendelian fashion, the genetics and the genetic counseling are complex (Fryns, 1984; Sherman *et al.*, 1985). For example, in families with fragile X, evidence suggests that the mothers of sporadic male cases are highly likely to be carriers, implying that new mutations occur most often in males (the maternal grandfather) at spermatogenesis. Recurrence rates of mental retardation in subsequent male offspring may be less than the theoretical 50% because not all males with fragile X are retarded; in addition, there is some risk for mild mental retardation to female offspring of carriers (Hagerman & McBogg, 1983; Sherman *et al.*, 1984).

The first case descriptions of autism in association with fragile X appeared simultaneously in 1982 (Brown *et al.*, 1982; Meryash, Szymanski, & Gerald, 1982). Meryash *et al.* described a 6-year-old boy with a long face, hypotonia, delayed motor development, severe mental retardation, and autistic features. Brown's cases were not described individually but were retarded and had large testes. The autistic children reported subsequently (August & Lockhart, 1984; Blomquist *et al.*, 1985; De Arce & Kearns, 1984; Fryns, 1984; Gillberg, 1983; Jorgensen, Nielsen, Isager, & Mouridsen, 1984; Kerbeshian, Burd, & Martsoff, 1984; Largo & Schinzel, 1985; Levitas *et al.*, 1983; McGillivray, Herbst, Dill, Sandercock, & Tischler, 1986; Watson *et al.*, 1984) have all been males, and most appear from the case descriptions to have considerable mental retardation, although few IQ scores have yet appeared. In Blomquist's series, two children had IQs above 70 (Blomquist *et al*, 1983).

While some reports include clinical descriptions of autistic children, others simply state that the children met either DSM-III (American Psychiatric Association, 1980) or Rutter's criteria (Rutter, 1967). Two authors provide some details. Among six fragile X autistic children reported by Levitas *et al.* (1983), one did not meet the criterion for language deviation and none had pronoun reversal, but all were socially deviant and had repetitive and stereotyped behaviors. Five of the six were self-abusive. Largo and Schinzel (1985) reported 13 boys from three fragile X families, with no apparent selection for autism. These cases are less well described, but most had some autistic symptoms, and several would meet criteria for autism. Five were self-abusive and an additional 4 were aggressive to others. From these limited clinical descriptions, it appears that some, and possibly most, fragile X males have some autistic symptoms and a portion are classically autistic. Although based on small numbers, they may tend to have less pronoun reversal and more self-abuse than average for autism.

It is not yet clear how many autistic boys have fragile X. Watson *et al.* (1984) reported a rate of 5%. The rate was 10% among their cases who were living in institutions. McGillivray *et al.* (1986) found fragile X in 12% of an institutionalized sample of autistic children, and Blomquist *et al.* (1985) found fragile X in 16% of autistic children ascertained through a variety of sources. In a sample ascertained because of severe language disability, Jorgensen *et al.* (1984) diagnosed autism in 11 of 23 children. One of the 11 autistic children had fragile X. At the other extreme, some investigators have found *no* fragile X among their autistic samples (Goldfine *et al.*, 1985; Pueschel, Herman, & Groden, 1985; Venter, Hof Coetzee, Van der Walt, & Retief, 1984). The reasons for this variation are not yet clear, but they may have to do with diagnostic criteria for autism and possibly with the methods used to detect fragile X. The procedure is by no means routine, and methods used to increase the expression of the fragile site may lead to false positives (De Arce & Kearns, 1984; Hagerman & McBogg, 1983).

Given the uncertain prevalence of fragile X and of autism, the latter of which varies widely depending on the diagnostic criteria (Gottesman & Shields, 1982; Wing & Gould, 1979), and given the uncertain rate of fragile X in autistic populations and the unknown rate of autism among boys with fragile X, it is impossible to say at the present time how strong the association is between autism and fragile X. Both are relatively common conditions and both are associated with mental retardation, so that some association would be expected by chance. Further studies are needed that address the rate of autism in an unselected fragile X population, and that compare the rate of fragile X in autistic samples according to their clinical features.

Nearly all the genetic studies of idiopathic autism described in earlier sections of the chapter were carried out before the reports of the association between autism and fragile X. Could the concordance of twins or familial aggregation in sibs be accounted for by the fragile X mutation? Most of the concordant twin pairs and sib pairs have been male (Folstein & Rutter, 1977; Ritvo, Freeman, *et al.*, 1985), so the possibility exists. However, among Ritvo's 34 families with autism in two or more sibs discussed above, only 1 fragile X family was found (Spence *et al.*, 1985). Also as mentioned above, Baird and August (1985) found fragile X in only one of their familial cases. Therefore, it is clear that fragile X will account for some but not all of the familial aggregation of autism. At the present, we can only conclude that some children with autism have fragile X, but how many have it, or whether their autistic features are always typical, is not clear. From a practical viewpoint, the diagnostic evaluation of an autistic boy should include a karyotype for fragile X, preferably carried out in a laboratory experienced with the procedure.

Biochemical Abnormalities: Their Relationship to Single Gene Disorders

Over the years many investigators have reported autism in association with abnormal levels of various metabolites (see Coleman, 1979; Young, Kavanagh, Anderson, Shaywitz, & Cohen, 1982; for reviews). Often it has not been possible to replicate the results (e.g., Boullin, Coleman, O'Brien, & Rimland, 1971; Boullin *et al.*, 1982; Gillberg, Trygstad, &

Foss, 1982; LeCouteur, Trygstad, Howlin, Robertson, & Rutter, 1986), and sometimes the reported cases are not clearly autistic (e.g., Jaeken & Van den Berghe, 1984).

Even when the findings have been replicated, as in the finding of elevated serotonin in about a third of autistic children (Young *et al.*, 1982), the meaning of the finding has not been clear. First similar elevations are often found in nonautistic retarded children (Rutter, 1978). While this is certainly reason for pause, it does not necessarily render the finding meaningless. Different metabolic abnormalities, associated with different phenotypes, can result in similar abnormalities in bodily fluids.

The second reason that the findings are confusing is that surprisingly few attempts have been made to study family patterns. Abnormal metabolites are most often due to some recessively inherited disorder, which can be confirmed by finding similar abnormalities in other affected family members, or finding intermediate levels in parents who would be obligate carriers in the case of autosomal recessive inheritance. In the only systematic study of serotonin levels in parents and sibs (Kuperman, Beeghly, Burns, & Tsai, 1985), there was a tendency for levels to aggregate in families, but there was no reported relationship of levels to clinical abnormalities in other family members.

Histidenemia has also been reported in a few autistic children. Studies of other family members have in this instance clearly documented that the association is by chance (Folstein & Rutter, 1977; Kotsopoulos & Kutty, 1979).

GENETIC EVALUATION AND COUNSELING FOR FAMILIES WITH AN AUTISTIC CHILD

The evaluation of every newly diagnosed autistic child should include a medical work-up for genetic disorders, beginning with a thorough family history, a history of perinatal injury and other illnesses, an examination looking for physical stigmata of genetic and neurological disorders, and some screening tests for the genetic disorders that may be associated with autism.

Taking a Family History

In taking the family history, it is important to ask not only about autism and mental retardation but also about problems with reading and language, and about social eccentricities. However, it must be cautioned that we are currently uncertain if and how these milder conditions contribute to the risk for recurrence of autism. The family history should be systematic, asking in turn about each first- and second-degree relative, and must be extensive enough to be able to detect X linkage or autosomal dominant patterns where not all heterozygotes are severely affected, as in fragile X, tuberous sclerosis, or neurofibromatosis. A family history that included only first-degree relatives (parents, sibs, and children of the proband) would not reveal the pattern of X-linked inheritance.

A family pattern is consistent with X-linkage if no male-to-male transmission is found. Affected cases should all be males, although carrier females may occasionally have mild symptoms, at least in the case of fragile X. This may also be true for other X-linked forms of cognitive disability. New mutations do occur in fragile X, and the failure to find other affected family members does not rule out the need for a karyotype. Figure 1 shows a pedigree for a fragile X family.

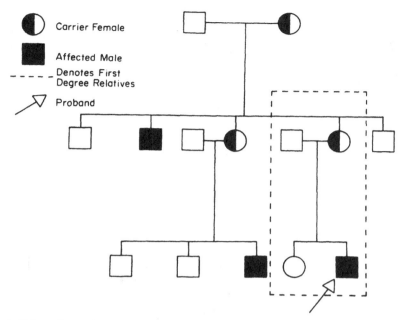

Figure 1. This pedigree demonstrates X-linked recessive inheritance, with only males affected and no male-to-male transmission. Note that no familial aggregation would be discovered if our information was limited to first-degree relatives (enclosed by box).

In autosomal recessive disorders, there are not usually any other affected family members, and any other cases will be found among siblings. Affected sib pairs are equally likely to be same-sexed or opposite-sexed, and the proband either male or female. Sometimes there is consanguinous mating, although this may have occurred several generations earlier. If the parents' families came from the same isolated community, investigation of the ancestors for consanguinity may be indicated. Figure 2 shows a family with phenylketonuria, an autosomal recessive condition, with only one affected child. In autosomal recessive disorders, the risk to subsequently conceived sibs of the proband is 25%. However, the risk to offspring of normal sibs is very small. Even if the sib is a carrier, the probability of marrying another carrier is small unless the family lives in an inbred, isolated community.

In autosomal dominant inheritance, one expects cases over several generations and in several collateral lines, but usually only in one parental line. However, not all affected persons will necessarily show the complete phenotype for the condition, so it is necessary to be familiar with the range of symptoms in order to take an accurate pedigree. The only autosomal dominant disorders that are known to be associated with autism are quite rare.

History of Early Injury and Illness

In a genetic evaluation for autism it is equally important to look for detectable non-genetic causes. At present, this endeavor is limited to history taking. A detailed history of complications of pregnancy and delivery, as well as serious illnesses or accidents within the

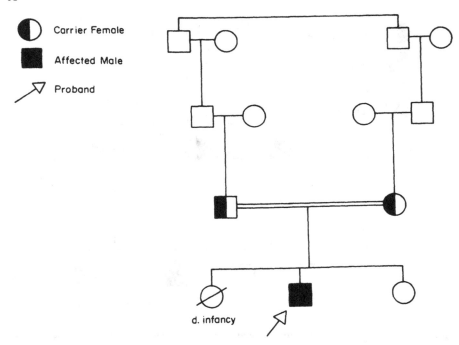

Figure 2. This pedigree demonstrates autosomal recessive inheritance with normal carrier parents and one affected child. The recurrence risk for subsequent children is 25%. The double line indicates consanguinity. The parents are related through their grandparents.

first 3 years of life, is needed. If there is any suggestion of trouble, the medical record should be carefully reviewed. Sometimes the situation in the delivery room is minimized to the mother but accurately documented in the record.

Because of the possible interaction between genetic predisposition and mild pre- and perinatal difficulties, it is not possible to discount a risk of recurrence of autism based on a mildly abnormal birth history or mild illness early in life. Also, parents often search their memories for possible explanations for their child's disorder and put undue emphasis on minor events in their attempt to find a cause. However, if there is a documented serious condition such as intracranial hemorrhage, perinatal hypoxia followed by seizures in the neonatal period, or some other severe insult, it is most likely an adequate explanation for the autism syndrome.

Physical Examination and Tests

The physical and neurological examination must be thorough, with the child undressed, so that abnormalities of pigmentation seen in the neurocutaneous disorders can be observed, and so that testicular size can be examined. Testicular size before puberty may be in the normal range in fragile X. Ear size, which may be large in children with fragile X, should be noted, and minor congenital anomalies (Waldrop & Halverson, 1971) systematically documented.

Blood should be sent for amino acid screening and karyotyping, specifically requesting fragile X testing for males, and if there is a history of gradual decline or suggestive findings on the physical examination, appropriate examinations for mucopolysaccharidoses and other storage diseases may be indicated. These more specialized examinations should be undertaken in consultation with a specialist in medical genetics.

Genetic Counseling

The purpose of genetic counseling as it applies to autism is to provide the parents, and occasionally the adult sibs, of an autistic child with information about the risk for recurrence of autism in subsequent pregnancies. As information about possible genetic contributions to autism are disseminated, we expect that more families will request genetic counseling.

At the present time, accurate predictions of risk are possible only in a small minority of cases with some detectable single gene disorder (such as the fragile X). In these cases, the risk is linked with that for the medical disorder with which the autism is associated. Referral to a medical geneticist is indicated in such instances in order both to carry out the investigations of other family members needed for an accurate appraisal of risk and to provide the knowledge needed for skilled genetic counseling.

In the cases where autism is associated with a clear history of severe perinatal or postnatal trauma giving rise to neurological complications at the time, and where there is no family history of autism or cognitive disabilities, it may be inferred that the risk of recurrence is probably very low.

The more usual circumstance, however, is of autism for which there is no known single gene disorder and no known nongenetic cause. In these cases the recurrence risk for autism has never been estimated. We estimate that about 1 to 3% of families have two autistic children and that 10 to 15% of the families have children with cognitive disabilities (including both persistent mental retardation and transient language handicaps). However, even if these figures are accurate, they cannot be translated into a risk for recurrence of autism in a subsequent pregnancy. In samples of families where the affected child is frequently an *only* or *lastborn* child (as is often the case for autism), observed familial aggregation will be unusual, even if the recurrence risk for a subsequent pregnancy is actually high.

CONCLUSIONS

Family and twin studies of idiopathic autism have shown that autism is occasionally aggregated in families and that disorders of cognition and language are found commonly among the family members of autistic probands. While there are no firm data about the aggregation of social eccentricities in the families of autistic probands, such as found in Asperger syndrome, clinical experience suggests that it may well occur. The actual prevalence of such disorders in first-degree relatives is not known. No studies have tested parents and few studies have tested sibs systematically for cognitive and language disorders. No studies of any kind have tested family members for social deficits similar to those seen in autism.

These limited data are open to numerous possible explanations and interpretations. It may be that many different etiologies will be found for autism, some of which will surely be genetic. It is equally possible that the bulk of classically diagnosed cases will share a single etiology, perhaps an inherited deficit in social and language processing that interacts with a variety of mild environmental insults that together result in the full autism syndrome. With respect to genetic mechanisms, there are also numerous possibilities that are not mutually exclusive, ranging from one or more single gene mutations to complex multifactorial determinations.

Several different kinds of studies are needed in order to sort out the various possibilities. A detailed family study based on a systematically ascertained sample is perhaps the most pressing need. In addition to a detailed clinical and laboratory examination of each autistic proband, all first-degree relatives should be examined and tested for social and cognitive deficits, and detailed pedigrees of the extended families should be collected. Such a family study population would provide a systematically ascertained, diagnosed, and examined sample, appropriate for use in a variety of genetic and biochemical analyses. Rates and patterns of family transmission and their relationship to the clinical features of the autistic proband could be studied. The sample could be tested for its compatibility with a variety of models of inheritance. Families could be screened for fragile X and other genetic disorders, and families appropriate for detailed molecular genetic study could be found. This could include both biochemical and state-of-the-art genetic linkage analyses that have become possible through advances in molecular genetics.

REFERENCES

Advocate, The. (1980). National Society for Autistic Children. *12* (March and July), Nos. 4 and 5.

American Psychiatric Association. (1980). *Diagnostic and statistical manual of mental disorders* (3rd ed.). Washington, DC, Author.

Armstrong, M. D., Low, N. L., & Bosma, J. F. (1957). Studies on phenylketonuria, IX. Further observations on the effect of phenylalanine-restricted diet on patients with phenylketonuria. *American Journal of Clinical Nutrition, 5*, 543–554.

Armstrong, M. D., & Tyler, F. H. (1955). Studies on phenylketonuria, I. Restricted phenylalanine intake and phenylketonuria. *Journal of Clinical Investigation, 34*, 565–580.

August, G. J., & Lockhart, L. H. (1984). Familial autism and the fragile X chromosome. *Journal of Autism and Developmental Disorders, 14*, 197–204.

August, G. J., Stewart, M. A., & Tsai, L. (1981). The incidence of cognitive disabilities in the siblings of autistic children. *British Journal of Psychiatry, 138*, 416–422.

Baird, T. D., & August, G. J. (1985). Familial heterogeneity in infantile autism. *Journal of Autism and Developmental Disorders, 15*, 315–321.

Bartak, L., Rutter, M., & Cox, A. (1975). A comparative study of infantile autism and specific developmental receptive language disorder. I. The children. *British Journal of Psychiatry, 126*, 127–145.

Bauman, M., & Kemper, T. L. (1985). Histoanatomic observations of the brain in early infantile autism. *Neurology, 35*, 866–874.

Berry, H. K., Sutherland, B. S., Guest, G. M., & Umbarger, B. (1958). Chemical and clinical observations during treatment of children with phenylketonuria. *Pediatrics, 21*, 929–940.

Bickel, H., Gerrard, J., & Hickmans, E. M. (1954). The influence of phenylalanine intake on the chemistry and behavior of a phenylketonuric child. *Acta Paediatrica, 43*, 64–77.

Bjornson, J. (1964). Behavior in phenylketonuria: Case with schizophrenia. *Archives of General Psychiatry, 10*, 65–70.

Blainy, J. D., & Gulliford, R. (1956). Phenylalanine-restricted diets in the treatment of phenylketonuria. *Archives of Disease in Childhood, 31*, 452–566.

Blomquist, H. K., Bohman, M., Edvinsson, S. O., Gillberg, C., Gustavon, K-H., Holmgren, C., and Wahlstrom, J. (1985). Frequency of the fragile X syndrome in infantile autism. A Swedish multicenter study. *Clinical Genetics, 27*, 113–117.

Blomquist, H. K., Gustavson, K-H., Holmgren, G., Nordenson, I., & Palsson-Strae, U. (1983). Fragile X syndrome in mildly mentally retarded children in a Northern Swedish county. A prevalence study. *Clinical Genetics, 24*, 393–398.

Blomquist, H. K., Gustavson, K-H., Holmgren, G., Nordenson, I., & Sweins, A. (1982). Fragile site X-chromosomes and X-linked mental retardation in severely retarded boys in a northern Swedish county. A prevalence study. *Clinical Genetics, 21*, 209–214.

Boullin, D. J., Coleman, M., O'Brien, R. A., & Rimland, B. (1971). Laboratory predictions of infantile autism, based on 5-hydroxy-tryptamine efflux from blood platelets and their correlation with the Rimland E2 scores. *Journal of Autism and Childhood Schizophrenia, 1*, 63–71.

Boullin, D. J., Freeman, B. J., Geller, E., Ritvo, E., Rutter, M., & Yuwiler, A. (1982). Toward the resolution of conflicting findings (Letter to the Editor). *Journal of Autism and Developmental Disorders, 12*, 97–98.

Brondum-Nielsen, K. (1983). Diagnosis of the fragile X syndrome (Martin-Bell syndrome). Clinical findings in 27 males with the fragile site at Xq^{28}. *Journal of Mental Deficiency Research, 27*, 211–226.

Brown, W. T., Jenkins, E. C., Friedman, E., Brooks, J., Wisniewski, K., Raguthu, S., & French, J. (1982). Autism is associated with the fragile X syndrome. *Journal of Autism and Developmental Disorders, 12*, 303–308.

Burgoine, E., & Wing, L. (1983). Identical triplets with Asperger's syndrome. *British Journal of Psychiatry, 143*, 261–265.

Chess, S., Fernandez, P. B., & Korn, S. J. (1978). Behavioral consequences of congenital rubella. *Journal of Pediatrics, 93*, 699–703.

Chess, S., Korn, S. J., & Fernandez, P. B. (1971). *Psychiatric disorders of children with congenital rubella.* New York: Brunner/Mazel.

Chick, J., Waterhouse, L., & Wolff, S. (1979). Psychological construing in schizoid children grown up. *British Journal of Psychiatry, 135*, 425–430.

Coleman, M. (1979). Studies of the autistic syndromes. In Robert Katzman (Ed.), *Congenital and acquired cognitive disorders.* New York: Raven Press.

Coleman, P. D., Romano, J., Lapham, L., & Simon, W. (1985). Cell counts in cerebral cortex of an autistic patient. *Journal of Autism and Developmental Disorders, 15*, 245–255.

Cowie, W. A. (1951). An atypical case of phenylketonuria. *Lancet, February*, 272–273.

Crome, L., & Stern, J. (1972). *Pathology of mental retardation* (2nd ed.). Edinburgh: Churchill-Livingstone.

Darby, J. K. (1976). Neuropathologic aspects of psychosis in children. *Journal of Autism and Childhood Schizophrenia, 6*, 339–352.

De Arce, M., & Kearns, A. (1984). The fragile X syndrome: The patients and their chromosomes. *Journal of Medical Genetics, 21*, 84–91.

Deykin, E. Y., & MacMahon, B. (1979). The incidence of seizures among children with autistic symptoms. *American Journal of Psychiatry, 136*, 1310–1312.

Deykin, E. Y., & MacMahon, B. (1980). Pregnancy, delivery and neonatal complications among autistic children. *American Journal of Diseases of Children, 134*, 860–864.

Dover, G. J., Boyer, S. H., & Pembrey, M. E. (1981). F-cell production in sickle cell anemia: Regulation of genes linked to beta-hemoglobin locus. *Science, 211*, 1441–1444.

Finegan, J., & Quadrington, B. (1979). Pre-, peri-, and neonatal factors and infantile autism. *Journal of Child Psychology and Psychiatry, 20*, 119–128.

Folling, A. (1934). Phenylpyruvic acid as a metabolic anomaly in connection with imbecility. *Zeitschrift für Physiologische Chemie, 224*, 169–176.

Folstein, S., & Rutter, M. (1977). Infantile autism: A genetic study of 21 twin pairs. *Journal of Child Psychology and Psychiatry, 18*, 297–231.

Friedman, E. (1969). The "autistic syndrome" and phenylketonuria. *Schizophrenia, 1*, 249–261.

Fryns, J. P. (1984). The fragile X syndrome: A study of 83 families. *Clinical Genetics, 26*, 497–528.

Gillberg, C. (1983). Identical triplets with infantile autism and the fragile X syndrome. *British Journal of Psychiatry, 143*, 256–260.

Gillberg, C., & Forsell, C. (1984). Childhood psychosis and neurofibromatosis—More than a coincidence? *Journal of Autism and Developmental Disorders, 14*, 1–8.

Gillberg, C., & Gillberg, I. C. (1983). Infantile autism: A total population study of nonoptimal, pre-, peri-, and neonatal conditions. *Journal of Autism and Developmental Disorders, 13*, 153–166.

Gillberg, C., Trygstad, O., & Foss, I. (1982). Childhood psychosis and urinary excretion of peptides and protein-associated peptide complexes. *Journal of Autism and Developmental Disorders, 12*, 229–241.

Goldfine, P. E., McPherson, P. M., Heath, G. A., Hardesty, V. A., Beauregard, L. J., & Gordon, S. (1985). Association of fragile X syndrome with autism. *American Journal of Psychiatry, 142*, 108–110.

Gottesman, I. I., & Shields, J. (1982). *Schizophrenia: The epigenetic puzzle*. Cambridge: Cambridge University Press.

Gusella, J. F., Tanzi, R. E., Anderson, M. A., Hobbs, W., Gibbons, K., Raschtchian, R., Gilliam, T. C., Wallace, M. R., Wexier, N. S., & Conneally, P. M. (1984). DNA markers for nervous system diseases. *Science, 225*, 1320–1326.

Hagerman, R. J., & McBogg, P. M. (1983). *The fragile X syndrome, diagnosis, biochemistry, and intervention*. Dillon, Colorado: Spectra Publishing.

Hanson, D. R., & Gottesman, I. I. (1976). The genetics, if any, of infantile autism and childhood schizophrenia. *Journal of Autism and Childhood Schizophrenia, 6*, 209–234.

Harcherik, D. F., Cohen, D. J., Ort, S., Paul, R., Shaywitz, B. A., Volkmar, F. R., Rothman, S. L. G., & Leckman, J. F. (1985). Computed tomographic brain scanning in four neuropsychiatric disorders of childhood. *American Journal of Psychiatry, 142*, 731–734.

Herbst, D. S., & Miller, J. R. (1980). Non-specific X-linked mental retardation. II. The frequency in British Columbia. *American Journal of Medical Genetics, 7*, 461–469.

Hunt, A. (1983a). Tuberous sclerosis: A survey of 97 cases. I: Seizures, pertussis immunization and handicap. *Developmental Medicine and Child Neurology, 25*, 346–347.

Hunt, A. (1983b). Tuberous sclerosis: A survey of 96 cases. II: Physical findings. *Developmental Medicine and Child Neurology, 25*, 350–352.

Hunt, A. (1983c). Tuberous sclerosis: A survey of 96 cases. III: Family aspects. *Developmental Medicine and Child Neurology, 25*, 353–357.

Jaeken, J., & Van den Berghe, G. V. (1984). An infantile autistic syndrome characterised by the presence of succinylpurines in body fluids. *Lancet, November*, 1058–1061.

Jorgensen, O. S., Nielsen, K. B., Isager, T., & Mouridsen, S. E. (1984). Fragile X chromosome among child psychiatric patients with disturbances of language and social relationships. *Acta Psychiatrica Scandinavica, 70*, 510–514.

Kanner, L. (1943). Autistic disturbances of affective contact. *Nervous Child, 2*, 217–250.

Kerbeshian, J., Burd, L., & Martsoff, J. (1984). A family with fragile X syndrome. *Journal of Nervous and Mental Disease, 172*, 549–551.

Kidd, K. K., & Pauls, D. L. (1982). Genetic hypotheses for Tourette syndrome. In T. N. Chase & A. J. Friedhoff (Eds.), Gilles de la Tourette syndrome, *Advances in Neurology, 35*, 243–249.

Knoll, J. H., Chudley, A. E., & Gerrard, J. W. (1984). Fragile (X) X-linked mental retardation. II. Frequency and replication pattern of fragile (X) (q28) in heterozygotes. *American Journal of Human Genetics, 36*, 640–645.

Kolvin, I. (1971). Psychoses in childhood—A comparative study. In M. Rutter (Ed.), *Infantile autism: Concepts, characteristics and treatment*. London: Churchill-Livingstone.

Kotsopoulos, S., & Kutty, K. M. (1979). Histidinemia and infantile autism. *Journal of Autism and Developmental Disorders, 9*, 55–60.

Kratter, F. E. (1959). The physiognomic, psychometric, behavioral and neurological aspects of phenylketonuria. *Journal of Mental Science, 105*, 421–427.

Kuperman, S., Beeghly, J. H. L., Burns, T. L., & Tsai, L. Y. (1985). Serotonin relationships of autistic probands and their first-degree relatives. *Journal of the American Academy of Child Psychiatry, 24*, 186–190.

Laird, G. J., & Schimke, R. N. (Eds.). (1979). *Clinical genetics: A source book for physicians.* New York: Wiley.

Largo, R. H., & Schinzel, A. (1985). Developmental and behavioural disturbances in 13 boys with fragile X syndrome. *European Journal of Pediatrics, 143*, 269–275.

LeCouteur, A., Trygstad, O., Howlin, P., Robertson, S., & Rutter, M. (1986). *Urinary peptide findings in autism: A non-replication.* Manuscript in preparation.

Leland, H. (1957). Some psychological characteristics of phenylketonuria. *Psychological Reports, 3*, 373–376.

Levitas, A., Hagerman, R. J., Braden, M., Rimland, B., McBogg, P., & Matteus, I. (1983). Autism and the fragile X syndrome. *Journal of Developmental and Behavioural Pediatrics, 3*, 151–158.

Lewis, E. (1959). The development of concepts in a girl after dietary treatment for phenylketonuria. *British Journal of Medical Psychology, 32*, 282–287.

Lord, C., Schopler, E., & Revick, D. (1982). Sex differences in sex ratios in autism. *Journal of Autism and Developmental Disorders, 12*, 317–330.

Lotter, V. (1966). Epidemiology of autistic conditions in young children. I. Prevalence. *Social Psychiatry, 1*, 124–137.

Lotter, V. (1967). Epidemiology of autistic conditions in young children. II. Some characteristics of the parents and children. *Social Psychiatry, 1*, 163–173.

Lotter, V. (1974). Factors related to outcome in autistic children. *Journal of Autism and Childhood Schizophrenia, 4*, 263–277.

Lubs, H. A. (1969). A marker X chromosome. *American Journal of Human Genetics, 21*, 231.

Martin, J. P., & Bell, J. (1943). A pedigree of mental defect showing sex-linkage. *Journal of Neurology and Psychiatry, 6*, 154–157.

McGillivray, B. C., Herbst, D. S., Dill, F. J., Sandercock, H. J., & Tischler, B. (1986). Infantile autism: An occasional manifestation of fragile (X) mental retardation. *American Journal of Medical Genetics, 23*, 353–358.

McKusick, V. A. (Ed.). (1969). *Human genetics.* Englewood Cliffs, New Jersey: Prentice-Hall.

McKusick, V. A. (1983). *Mendelian inheritance in man. Catalogs of autosomal dominant, autosomal recessive, and X-linked phenotypes* (6th ed.). Baltimore: Johns Hopkins University Press.

Meryash, D. L., Szymanski, L. S., & Gerald, P. S. (1982). Infantile autism associated with the fragile X syndrome. *Journal of Autism and Developmental Disorders, 12*, 295–301.

Minton, J., Campbell, M., Green, W., Jennings, S., & Samit, C. (1982). Cognitive assessment of siblings of autistic children. *Journal of the American Academy of Child Psychiatry, 213*, 256–261.

Mittler, P. (1971). *The study of twins.* Harmondsworth: Penguin.

Pueschel, S. F., Herman, R., & Groden, G. (1985). Brief report: Screening children with autism for fragile X syndrome and phenylketonuria. *Journal of Autism and Developmental Disorders, 15*, 335–343.

Richardson, S. A., Koller, H., Katz, M., & McLaren, J. (1980). Seizures and epilepsy in a mentally retarded population over the first 22 years of life. *Applied Research in Mental Retardation, 1*, 123–138.

Riikonen, R., & Amnell, G. (1981). Psychiatric disorders in children with early infantile spasms. *Developmental Medicine and Child Neurology, 23*, 747–760.

Ritvo, E. R., Freeman, B. J., Mason-Brothers, A., Mo, A., & Ritvo, A. M. (1985). Concordance for the syndrome of autism in 40 pairs of afflicted twins. *American Journal of Psychiatry, 142*, 74–77.

Ritvo, E. R., Spence, M. A., Freeman, B. J., Mason-Brothers, A., Mo, A., & Marazita, M. L. (1985). Evidence for autosomal recessive inheritance in 46 families with multiple incidences of autism. *American Journal of Psychiatry, 142*, 187–192.

Rosenberg, R. N., & Pettegrew, J. D. (1980). Genetic disease of the nervous system. In J. M. Dietschy (Ed.), R. N. Rosenberg (Vol. Ed.), *The science of clinical medicine:* Vol. 5. *Neurology* (pp. 165–242). New York: Gruen & Stratton.

Rumsey, J. M. Duara, R., Grady, C., Rapoport, J. L., Margolin, R. A., Rappoport, S. I., & Cutler, N. R. (1985). Brain metabolism in autism: Resting cerebral glucose utilization as measured with positron emission tomography (PET). *Archives of General Psychiatry, 15*, 448–457.

Rutter, M. (1967). Psychotic disorders in early childhood. In A. Coppen & A. Walk (Eds.), *British Journal of Psychiatry*, Special publication No. 1, Ashford Kent: Headley Bros.

Rutter, M. (1970). Autistic children: Infancy to adulthood. *Seminars in Psychiatry, 2*, 435–450.

Rutter, M. (1974). The development of infantile autism. *Psychological Medicine, 4*, 147–163.

Rutter, M. (1978). Serotonin, platelets and autism (Editorial). *British Medical Journal, 1*, 1651–1652.

Rutter, M. (1979). Language, cognition and autism. In R. Katzman (Ed.), *Congenital and acquired cognitive disorders*. New York: Raven Press.

Rutter, M. (1983). Cognitive deficits in the pathogenesis of autism. *Journal of Child Psychology and Psychiatry, 24*, 513–531.

Rutter, M., & Schopler, E. (1986). Autism and pervasive developmental disorders: Concepts and diagnostic issues. In M. Rutter, H. Tuma, & I. Lann (Eds.), *Assessment, diagnosis, and classification in child and adolescent psychiatry*. New York: Guilford Press.

Sherman, S. L., Jacobs, P. A., Morton, N. E., Froster-Iskenius, U., Howard-Peebles, P. N., Nielson, K. B., Partington, M. W., Sutherland, G. R., Turner, G., & Watson, M. (1985). Further segregation analysis of the fragile X syndrome with special reference to transmitting males. *Human Genetics, 69*, 289–299.

Sherman, S. L., Morton, N. E., Jacobs, P. A., & Turner, G. (1984). The marker (X) syndrome: A cytogenetic and genetic analysis. *Annals Human Genetics, 48*, 21–37.

Silva, P. A. (1986). Epidemiology, longitudinal course, and some associated factors: An update. In M. Rutter, W. Yule, & M. Bax (Eds.), *Language development and disorders* (Series in Clinics and Developmental Medicine). London: Spastics International/Blackwell Scientific.

Spence, M. A., Ritvo, E. R., Marazita, M. L., Funderburk, S. J., Sparkes, R. S., & Freeman, B. J. (1985). Gene mapping studies with the syndrome of autism. *Behavior Genetics, 15*, 1–13.

Stanley, F., & E. Alberman (Eds.). (1984). *The epidemiology of the cerebral palsies* (Clinics in Developmental Medicine, No. 87). London: Blackwell Scientific/Philadelphia: J. B. Lippincot.

Stevenson, J., Hawcroft, J., Lobascher, M., Smith, I., Wolff, O. H., & Graham, P. J. (1979). Behavioural deviance in children with early-treated phenylketonuria. *Archives of Disease in Childhood, 54*, 14–18.

Sutherland, B. S., Berry, H. K., & Shirkey, H. C. (1960). A syndrome of phenylketonuria with normal intelligence and behavior disturbances. *Journal of Pediatrics, 57*, 521–525.

Sutherland, G. R. (1977). Fragile sites on human chromosomes: Demonstration of their dependence on the type of tissue culture medium. *Science, 197*, 265–266.

Sutherland, G. R. (1985). Heritable fragile sites on human chromosomes. XII. Population cytogenetics. *Annals of Human Genetics, 49*, 153–162.

Taft, L. T., & Cohen, H. J. (1971). Hypsarrhythmia and infantile autism: A clinical report. *Journal of Autism and Childhood Schizophrenia, 1*, 327–336.

Treffert, D. A. (1970). Epidemiology of infantile autism. *Archives of General Psychiatry, 22*, 431–438.

Turner, G., Brookwell, R., Daniel, A., Selikowitz, M., & Zilibowitz, M. (1980). Heterozygous expression of X-linked mental retardation and X-chromosome marker fra(X)(q27). *New England Journal of Medicine, 303*, 662–664.

Valle, D., Pai, G. B., Thomas, G. H., & Pyeritz, R. E. (1980). Homocystinuria due to cystathionine beta-synthase deficiency: Clinical manifestations and therapy, *Johns Hopkins Medical Journal, 146,* 110–111.

Varley, C. K., Holm, V. A., & Eren, M. O. (1985). Cognitive and psychiatric variability in three brothers with fragile X syndrome. *Developmental and Behavioral Pediatrics, 6,* 87–90.

Venter, P. A., Hof, J. O., Coetzee, D. J., Van der Walt, C., & Retief, A. E. (1984). No marker (x) syndrome in autistic children. *Human Genetics, 67,* 107.

Waldrop, M. F., & Halverson, C. F. (1971). Minor physical anomalies and hyperactive behavior in young children. In J. Helmuth (Ed.), *Exceptional infant: Studies in abnormalities* (Vol 2). New York: Brunner/Mazel.

Watson, M. S., Leckman, J. F., Annex, B., Breg, W. R., Boles, D., Volkmar, F. R., Cohen, D. J., & Carter, C. (1984). Fragile X in a survey of 75 autistic males. *New England Journal of Medicine, 310,* 1462.

Williams, R. S., Hauser, S. L., Purpura, D., DeLong, R., & Swisher, C. N. (1980). Autism and mental retardation: Neuropathological studies performed in four retarded persons with autistic behavior. *Archives of Neurology, 37,* 749–753.

Wing, J. K., O'Connor, N., & Lotter, V. (1967). Autistic conditions in early childhood: A survey in Middlesex. *British Medical Journal, 3,* 389–392.

Wing, L. (1981). Asperger's syndrome: A clinical account. *Psychological Medicine, 11,* 115–130.

Wing, L., & Gould, J. (1979). Severe impairments of social interactions and associated abnormalities in children: Epidemiology and classification. *Journal of Autism and Developmental Disorders, 9,* 11–30.

Wing, L., Yeates, S. R., Brierley, L. M., & Gould, J. (1976). The prevalence of early childhood autism: Comparison of administrative and epidemiological studies. *Psychological Medicine, 6,* 89–100.

Wolff, S., & Barlow, A. (1979). Schizoid personality in childhood: A comparative study of schizoid, autistic and normal children. *Journal of Child Psychology and Psychiatry, 20,* 19–46.

Wolff, S., & Chick, J. (1980). Schizoid personality in childhood: A controlled follow-up study. *Psychological Medicine, 10,* 85–100.

Woolf, L. I., Griffiths, R., & Moncrieff, A. (1955). Treatment of phenylketonuria with a diet low in phenylalanine. *British Medical Journal, 1,* 57–64.

Young, J., Kavanagh, M. E., Anderson, G. M., Shaywitz, B. A., & Cohen, D. J. (1982). Clinical neurochemistry of autism and associated disorders. *Journal of Autism and Developmental Disorders, 12,* 147–166.

Yule, W., & Rutter, M. (1985). Reading and other learning difficulties. In M. Rutter & L. Hersov (Eds.), *Child and adolescent psychiatry: Modern approaches* (2nd ed., chap. 27). Oxford: Blackwell Scientific.

Cerebral–Brainstem Relations in Infantile Autism

MARCEL KINSBOURNE

In infantile autism, many higher mental functions of the cerebrum are grossly abnormal, and yet direct evidence of cerebral damage has proven elusive. I shall attempt to resolve this contradiction by arguing that the functional cerebral deficiencies are secondary to impairments of ascending activation. I first consider ascending activation, then hemisphere function, and finally relations between them.

OVERACTIVATION IN AUTISM: BEHAVIORAL OBSERVATIONS

Hutt, Hutt, Lee, and Ounsted (1964) introduced the idea that autistic children are habitually in a state of maladaptively high arousal. According to the Yerkes–Dodson (1908) function, performance is optimal at intermediate arousal levels. If so, overarousal would impair these children's cognitive efficiency. On the basis of Easterbrook's (1959) theorizing, attention during overarousal would be hyperselective. According to the theory of stimulation level homeostasis (Zentall & Zentall, 1983), overaroused people would generally avoid external stimulation.

Lovaas, Schreibman, Koegel, and Rehm (1971) reinforced autistic children for responding to a stimulus simultaneously incorporating visual, auditory, and tactile features. When, after they had reached criterion, the children were presented with individual features of the stimulus one at a time, they responded to one only of the three features. Koegel and Wilhelm (1973) similarly elicited stimulus overselectivity using a visual stimulus that incorporated two features, and Reynolds, Newsom, and Lovaas (1974) found the same with a complex auditory stimulus. Although mentally retarded children also exhibit stimulus overselectivity (Koegel & Lovaas, 1978; Zeaman & House, 1979), autistic children do so to a greater extent than mental age-matched controls (Boucher, 1977; Hermelin & Frith, 1971; Prior, 1977). So they exhibit restricted cue utilization, perhaps because they are overaroused.

MARCEL KINSBOURNE • Eunice Kennedy Shriver Center for Mental Retardation, Waltham, Massachusetts 02254; and Harvard Medical School, Boston, Massachusetts 02115.

Not only can many aspects of autistic behavior be reasonably regarded as representing avoidance of stimulation, but experimental evidence supports this interpretation. Hutt, Hutt, and Ounsted (1965) found that autistic children display a preference for blanks or animals as opposed to human faces in pictures. Hermelin and O'Connor (1970) found that, whereas autistic children attended for long periods of time to a simple task, they failed to attend even briefly to a novel task.

Hutt and Hutt (1965) observed children in each of four different situations: (1) an empty familiar room, (2) with a box of colored blocks, (3) with an adult sitting quietly in a corner, and (4) with an adult attempting to engage the child in playing with the blocks. Between situations (1) and (3) the percentage of time spent in stereotypy rose from 28 to 52. In situation (4) the children did play with the blocks and the bouts of stereotypy, though shorter, were more frequent. Hutt (1967) placed children in a room that contained five familiar and one novel toy. Unlike normal and brain-damaged children, who readily approached the novel toy, the autistic children initially ignored it. The prolonged bouts of stereotypic behavior that are so characteristic of autism may serve a dearousing function (Kinsbourne, 1980a). Hutt, Hutt, Lee, and Ounsted (1965) found stereotypies to increase as environmental novelty or complexity increased. Similar findings had been reported with novelty (Stroh & Buick, 1968) and increasing stress. Furthermore, Hutt and Hutt (1968) reported that autistic children displayed a higher rate of stereotypy at a given level of environmental stimulation than mentally retarded children, and the stereotypic bout lasted longer. For them, stereotypies increased with stimulation, whereas for the retarded children they decreased (Davies, Sprague, & Werry, 1969; Hutt & Hutt, 1968; compare also Berkson & Davenport, 1962; Berkson & Mason, 1963, 1964; Gardner, Cromwell, & Foshee, 1959). Heart rate abnormalities documented by Kootz and Cohen (1981) are consistent with the view that autistic subjects are in a state of sensory rejection.

Some autistic symptoms can be simulated in normal people by imposing sensory overload. Sensory overload disorganizes thinking (Gottschalk, Haer, & Bates, 1972) as well as behavior (Ludwig & Stark, 1973). It generates social alienation and withdrawal (Gottschalk et al., 1972). The range of cue utilization (Easterbrook, 1959) shrinks in response to arousal caused both by external stimuli and by anxiety state and stimulant drugs (Duffy, 1962; Hockey, 1970). The overaroused state is accompanied by stereotyped repetitive movements of head and voice and by tics (Rago & Case, 1978; Zentall, 1980). This stereotyped behavior is analogous to "displacement behaviors" seen in animals in response conflict and state of frustration (Kinsbourne, 1980a).

Experimental animals reared in environmental deprivation exhibit stereotypies, as do mentally retarded and autistic individuals when alternative activities are not available and after the completion of tasks. In the absence of goal-directed responding, the set point for optimal stimulation appears to drift lower.

The relationship between stereotypies and high arousal levels is most directly illustrated by so-called amphetamine stereotypic behavior. Given a high dose of amphetamine, animals engage in repetitive behavior. As the effect gathers strength (Randrup & Munkvad, 1967) it first takes the form of a coordinated behavior—for instance, locomotion—but becomes, at the highest level of drug effect, quite primitive. Rats, for instance, typically gnaw the wire of the cage at a high and regular rate. In more ecologically valid situations, animals emit bouts of high-frequency behaviors—chicks peck and cats groom when thwarted or in response to conflict relative to reinforcers such as food (Delius, 1967, 1969). These "displacement activities" appear to be motivated not by an external goal but by an internal need to dispel excessive arousal (which they sometimes do even to the point of driving the animal into a sleepy state) (Hutt & Hutt, 1968). Some reactions of normal human adults to high levels of stimulation can be similarly interpreted (Ludwig & Stark, 1973; Rago & Case, 1978; Zentall, 1980). Displacement activities in normal animals and humans are usually quite short-lived, whereas in amphetamine stereotypic behavior and in autistic people it may be quite prolonged. Arousal may be more difficult to dispel when it arises from enduring psychologic or pharmacologic abnormality than when it occurs in reaction to the environment. A degree of support for this view of the function of stereotypic behavior derives from reported beneficial effects on autistic behavior of reducing ambient stimulation (Charny, 1963; Fassler & Bryant, 1971; Gardner et al., 1959; Koegel & Egel, 1979; Margolies, 1977; Schechter, Shurley, Towssieng, & Maier, 1969).

OVERACTIVATION IN AUTISM: PSYCHOPATHOLOGICAL OBSERVATIONS

Predictions of the overarousal hypothesis are not always borne out by psychophysiological study. Hutt, Hutt, and Ounsted (1965) reported desynchronized EEG indicative of arousal. They found the arousal to be striking during, but less after, a bout of stereotypies. However, the effect of the movements themselves on the EEGs complicates the interpretation of this finding. Also, stereotypies at times occur when no external sources of arousal are apparent. However, if stereotypies result in relief from dysphoria then this might reinforce their appearance at other times also. Contradictions also complicate the literature on other parameters presumed sensitive to arousal levels, such as average evoked potentials, contingent negative variation, heart rate, skin conductance, and measures of cerebral metabolism. Much of the contradiction is perhaps due to methodological difficulties. The complicating presence of minor nonspecific neurological abnormality obscures such measures as EEG. It is difficult to enlist the cooperation and control the state of autistic subjects. There are yet unresolved questions as to whether given abnormalities are specific to autistic individuals or more generally apply to mentally retarded or immature individuals (see James & Barry, 1980, for a review).

On the face of it, the hyperarousal model of autistic behavior should be amenable to objective evaluation by measurement of psychophysiological indices of arousal. Indeed, in their pioneering work, the Hutts and their colleagues felt they had accomplished this by documenting EEG desynchronization in their patients, increasing in degree with increasing novelty and complexity of the environment. The finding is similar to that accompanying compulsive behavior in adults, which occurs at high levels of autonomic activity and reduces them to resting levels (Walton & Mather, 1964). Subsequent work has tended to complicate and confuse this straightforward position, though not necessarily to refute it.

Some of these complicating factors are simply irrelevant to the issue. Numerous studies have documented a miscellany of electroencephalographic abnormalities in autistic samples, paralleling the miscellany of clinical and radiological abnormalities also found in autistic groups (Caparulo et al., 1982). It is clear that autistic children include many with minor neurological abnormalities that perhaps render them vulnerable to the full-blown syndrome of infantile autism but are not a condition of its appearance. Such findings are tangential to the Hutts' hypothesis or could even obscure the predictions of that hypothesis.

More serious are straightforward failures of competent attempts to confirm predictions of the Hutts' hypothesis (Creak & Pampiglione, 1969; Hermelin & O'Connor, 1970; Ritvo, Ornitz, Walker, & Hanley, 1970). If children can exhibit prolonged stereotypic behavior during periods of little sensory stimulation (Sorosky, Ornitz, Brown, & Ritvo, 1968) and not increase their stereotypies when environmental complexity increases (Ornitz, Brown, Sorosky, Ritvo, & Dietrich, 1970), then overarousal as detected by Hutt, Hutt, and Ounsted (1965) could be epiphenomenal, and one would have to turn elsewhere for an explanation of the behavior in question. However the alternative explanation need not discredit, but might merely qualify, the overarousal hypothesis.

Perhaps the overarousal hypothesis should be qualified. Autistic variability is just as characteristic as autistic symptomatology. Autistic children at times seem quite insensitive even to powerful stimulation (being in a state of sensory rejection), and yet at other times they are hypersensitive to minimal external change. In the cognitive domain, at least among higher-functioning autistic people, variability is extreme. Some autistic children manifest skills at certain times and yet seem to lack the same skills at other times. The control system that is biased toward generating overarousal may also be unstable, permitting arousal levels to swing to both maladaptive extremes (Hermelin & O'Connor, 1970). A single case study has suggested that an autistic subject swung between a state in which he sought maximal stimulation and one in which he sought sensory isolation (Leventhal, Kinsbourne, & Reichler, 1972). A clear case exists for performing single case repeated-measure studies, noting arousal status in the subjects when they exhibit overfocused autistic behavior (e.g., hyperselective attention) and when they do not. If a tight coupling exists between the degree of autistic attending and the level of arousal in these children, then such work would reveal it.

If activating systems are unstable rather than simply functioning at an inappropriate level, it becomes understandable why the use of agents that simply raise or lower the levels of particular neurotransmitters has been disappointing. One should search instead for means of stabilizing control systems. In other contexts there is some reason to suppose that stress, and in particular electroconvulsive shock (Ploog, 1950) and amphetamines (Kinsbourne, 1985), can have a stabilizing action. However, the manipulation that might have such an effect on autistic children remains to be discovered.

THE VARIETIES OF HEMISPHERIC DYSFUNCTION

Human cerebral hemisphere functioning can be abnormal in the following instances: (1) The hemisphere is structurally imperfect (lesioned or maldeveloped). It continues to control the functions for which it is specialized, but the performance that results is impaired. (2) The hemisphere is structurally imperfect, and functions that it normally represents are assumed by the other hemisphere. Contralateral compensation could then (a) be complete, tantamount to normality, or (b) be incomplete, leaving behavior impaired. (3) The hemisphere is structurally intact, but not efficiently activated when called upon to process. Activation can be either deficient or excessive, each being detrimental to performance, though in a different manner.

Subcategory 1 yields the wide range of classical acute clinical neuropsychological symptomatology. More often than is currently realized, subcategory 2a is responsible for recovery from cognitive deficit, and subcategory 2b generates much clinical phenomenology. But in psychopathology one is rarely able to invoke any of these mechanisms, although on occasion diseases causing structural lesions do in part simulate the major psychopathological entities. Nevertheless, one does observe, usually indirectly, through the overdevelopment of some behaviors (Hutt, Hutt, & Ounstead, 1965) evidences of an imbalance in the patient's use of the various cortical mechanisms. Certain processors are underused, and, by default or disinhibition, others are overused. Both underuse and overuse contribute to the maladaptive behavioral style that describes and even defines the psychopathological syndrome. Such imbalance may be primary or secondary.

ACTIVATIONAL PATHOLOGY

Those people who are mentally disturbed on account of environmental rigors may simply not make use of some of the cerebral facilities available to them. This may be apparent on behavioral laterality or on cerebral metabolic or electrophysiological investigation. In other cases the anomaly of usage is brain-based and in that sense primary. There is a continuity between personality type and personality disorder of that type in the case of autism, from overfocused attention (Kinsbourne & Caplan, 1979), through schizotypal personality disorder, Asperger syndrome, to pervasive developmental disorder and early infantile autism. Laterality and psychophysiological findings cannot distinguish between primary and secondary deviances in the use of cerebral facilities.

It is perhaps sufficient for the neural facilities to be in place for the automatic behavior to result. In effortful (voluntary) processing this cannot be so. The appropriate processor has to be in a state of selective activation, and competing unwanted responses must be inhibited. This selective activation appears to be under the control of brainstem centers, which by their activity implement the categorical mental set that is called for by the nature of the problem. Insufficient activation results in inadequate selectivity, leaving the appropriate form of processing in competition with irrelevant responding. In terms of Easterbrook's (1959) formulation, an inappropriately wide range of cues is being used. To the contrary, overactivation narrows the range of cue use unduly, leaving the person attentive to only a few or only one of the multiple cues relevant in any complex human mental activity. Overactivation can result from high drive states, but also from centrally acting influences, such as stimulant drugs. Instability of activating influences will cause the individual to fluctuate between these extreme opposite states.

In developmental psychopathology, it is the spectrum of developmental personality disorder that best lends itself to categorization under heading 3, activational pathology. Externalizing conditions such as attention deficit, hyperactivity, conduct disorder, and psychopathy conform to a construct involving deficient activation in certain behavioral control or behavioral inhibition systems. Internalizing conditions, and particularly the condition of infantile autism, can be described in terms of excessive ascending activation of cortex by brainstem structures. We will proceed to consider possible effects on cortical function, and specifically hemisphere use of the hypothesized excess of ascending activation and the extent to which clinical and experimental data on autism support such expectations.

NEUROLOGICAL FINDINGS IN AUTISM

Infantile autism is considered to result from a genetically transmitted vulnerability (Folstein & Rutter, 1977). This is discussed in Chapter 5. In high "dose" this is sufficient in itself to generate the clinical syndrome. In low dose it requires potentiation by nonspecific early brain damage (Gillberg & Gillberg, 1983). Thus many, but not all, autistic children manifest a miscellany of signs of neurological deficit comprising soft signs on examination, psychophysiological abnormality, and deviant appearances on both static (ventriculography, CT scan) and dynamic (regional cerebral blood flow, positron emission tomography) radiological investigation. In general, hallmarks of neurological deficit, to the extent that they pertain to the cerebral cortex, implicate the left hemisphere somewhat more than the right, perhaps because its arterial blood supply is less direct. Nevertheless, left hemisphere insult is neither necessary nor sufficient to set up the autistic syndrome. Thus we may conclude no more from the wide range of neurological findings in autistic samples than that nonspecific neurological damage increases the risk of autism. Although in unusual and well-documented cases a specific distribution of cortical damage (e.g., bitemporal; DeLong, Bean, & Brown, 1981) can simulate idiopathic infantile autism, it is clear that no particular pattern of structural cerebral involvement is a necessary condition for autistic symptomatology to emerge. This point of view is confirmed by the few anatomical studies that exist, which find the cerebral cortex remarkably free of both gross and microscopic pathology (Baumann & Kemper, 1985; Darby, 1976; Williams, Hauser, Purpura, DeLong, & Swisher, 1980). This finding is corroborated by measurement of cerebral metabolism in autism, which revealed none of the local diminution to be expected in the presence of damaged or underdeveloped brain (Rumsey et al., 1985). If anything, there was variable hypermetabolism, as would be expected on the basis of the overarousal theory. Nor can we use neuropsychological test data to implicate with confidence a particular area of cerebrum such as one hemisphere. Fein, Humes, Kaplan, Lucci, and Waterhouse (1984) could find no convincing evidence at the behavioral level, either, for specifically implicating the left hemisphere in autism. Autistic individuals manifest a wealth of cognitive deficits and thus are clearly not using their cerebral hemispheres normally, but attempts to specifically identify their abnormalities with classical neuropsychological syndromes (Damasio & Maurer, 1978) failed to convince (Fein et al., 1983), and in any case the dissociations are only relative and often quite variable within an individual patient. But even if the left hemisphere does exhibit more dysfunction than the right (see Chapter 12), this cannot be taken to imply left hemisphere deficit in the classical neuropsychological sense. We therefore turn to laterality findings in an attempt to cast further light on whether either the organization or the utilization of the cerebral hemispheres is in some consistent or systematic way abnormal in infantile autism.

Two hypotheses can be entertained. One, within the class of 2b, is that lateralization is deviant in autistic subjects and that this deviance somehow results in behavioral deficit. The other, in class 3, is that autistic subjects improperly activate their cerebrum and that this is what the laterality findings are indirectly indicating.

Before attempting to interpret laterality findings in autism we must consider some methodological issues relative to both peripheral and central laterality.

PERIPHERAL LATERALITY

The best developed account of hand preference is that of Annett (1973). She posits a "right shift factor" in dextrals. In its absence, hand preference comes under control of subsidary determinants, and the phenotype that results varies across individuals from right-handedness through ambidexterity to left-handedness. We have argued that this right shift tendency is not limited to asymmetry of hand preference and proficiency but involves a rightward turning bias manifested in biased orientation of head, eyes, and body, even in infancy, before hand preference proper could be entertained as a developmentally appropriate construct (Kinsbourne & Hiscock, 1983a). This turning bias is strikingly evident at birth and even at premature birth (Turkewitz, Moreau, & Birch, 1977) and thus has to be a product of brainstem mechanisms. These presumably activate the cortex in a correspondingly asymmetrical fashion and, when the cortex has sufficiently matured, influence its functional differentiation so as to establish central lateralization. In the absence of the right shift factor, ascending activation is presumably not laterally biased, and it is perhaps for this reason that some 70% of sinistrals are, based on the best available evidence, bilateralized for language (Gloning, Gloning, Haub, & Quatember, 1969; Satz, 1979) and also for spatial function. (In almost all of the remaining 30% lateralization is not, as used to be believed, the mirror image of that in the dextral, but rather the same as in the dextral majority, left for language, right for spatial function.) It is among left-handed individuals showing evidence of early brain damage that right hemisphere language representation appears to be frequent (Rasmussen & Milner, 1975).

In dextrals a developmental sequence can be traced, beginning with rightward orientation and culminating in stable right-hand preference and superior right-hand proficiency several years later. Left-handedness also emerges developmentally and ultimately achieves stability. Ambidextrous individuals use one hand for some activities and another for others, but in each case they do so in a reliable fashion. It is only in the earliest years of normal development that the hand used for a particular activity fluctuates. We would attribute such fluctuation to a combination of greater susceptibility to environmental determinants of hand use of the very young and an as yet not fully consistent asymmetry of ascending activation. It is from this perspective that we shall consider hand preference of autistic individuals.

EVIDENCE ON PERIPHERAL LATERALITY IN INFANTILE AUTISM

The incidence of non-right-handedness is much greater in autistic than in normal samples (Colby & Parkinson, 1977). This in itself is not revealing since it holds for mentally retarded individuals in general (Hicks & Barton, 1975; Bradshaw-McAnulty, Hicks, & Kinsbourne, 1984). But the effect is greater in autism than in any other developmental disability. Furthermore, the bulk of non-right-handed autistic individuals, who may exceed 50% of the sample, are not firmly sinistral or indeed reliably ambidextrous, but ambiguously handed. Like certain very young normal children, they vary in which hand they use for a given activity (Soper & Satz, 1984). Furthermore, when autistic individuals were subdivided into dextral, sinistral, and ambidextrous, the sinistrals were found to be the highest functioning and the ambidextrous (ambiguous?) the lowest (Fein, Waterhouse, Lucci, Pennington, & Humes, 1985).

A persuasive explanation for the excess of sinistrality among the mentally retarded (Bradshaw-McAnulty et al., 1984; Hicks & Barton, 1975) and other putatively brain-damaged categories, such as patients with focal epilepsy of early origin (Silva & Satz, 1979), is based on the concept of pathological left-handedness (PLH; Satz, 1972). This proposes that early left brain damage overlapping the motor strip causes a functional impairment of the right-sided limbs that, though subtle, is sufficient to overcome the genotypic instruction for dextrality by some unknown mechanism and results instead in a sinistral phenotype. In far fewer cases in which the genotype is sinistral, right hemisphere damage could correspondingly induce pathological dextrality. Satz, Orsini, Saslow and Henry (1985), have further characterized the syndrome of PLH. In contrast to genotypic sinistrals, pathological sinistrals would not be expected to show any excess of sinistrals in their families, and their hand preference would not show the usual approximately 0.3 correlation with mid-parent hand preference, but instead should not correlate significantly at all. In addition, the pathological left-hander might show some minor smallness of right-sided limbs, presumably due to trophic disadvantage induced by the hypothesized left hemisphere damage. Autistic individuals who are non-right-handed conform quite well to these stipulations. Several studies (Boucher, 1977; Tsai, 1982) have found no excess of familial sinistrality among autistic individuals. Thus it would be reasonable to infer the deviant hand preference of many autistic individuals to be pathological in origin. Satz *et al.* (1985) have argued that left-handed autistic individuals have left hemisphere dysfunction, whereas ambiguously handed autistic individuals have bilateral cerebral dysfunction. This is plausible, but it does not explain why the hand preference of so many autistic individuals—namely, the ones presumably bilaterally damaged— is not ambidextrous but ambiguous.

Ambiguous hand preference may simply reflect maturational lag. But although it may be less frequent in older autistic cohorts, many autistic individuals certainly manifest it toward the end of the first decade and in the second. Thus the "lag" may often be permanent. The question remains, what exactly is lagging (or arrested) in development of hand preference?

Lateral cerebral damage or delayed maturation is unlikely to be responsible for the left hemisphere dysfunction in pathological left-handedness in the autistic population. Hand preference is resistant even to quite severe contralateral damage, as has been found in animals (Olmstead & Villablanca, 1979) as well as in humans (Rasmussen & Milner, 1975), and there is no direct evidence of even slight left hemisphere damage in autistic individuals. Another explanation appears to be needed.

In the immature nervous system the ascending activational systems, although asymmetric in their action, are not able consistently to override other determinants of hand use (such as the reluctance to reach across the midline normally seen in infants). This immaturity may persist later in autism. But the hyperarousal hypothesis suggests a different solution. Lateral asymmetry may prevail at moderate levels of activation. But when bilateral ascending activation is maximal, this overrides activational asymmetry. Overarousal could obstruct the establishment of a consistent relationship between a preferred hand and a given activity. The cases most subject to such hyperarousal could therefore both be the ones who are most severely autistic and the ones most likely to have ambiguous hand preference. In contrast, the excess of strong sinistrality could represent a more isolated left hemisphere underactivation.

HEMISPHERE DYSFUNCTION: LESS IS MORE?

Hemisphere specialization in the young child represents an early stage in the differential specialization that characterizes the hemisphere in maturity. Lateralized functions have precursors in the same hemisphere (not bilaterally, as Lenneberg, 1967, supposed). This is the invariance hypothesis of cerebral lateralization (Kinsbourne, 1975). It has been overwhelmingly supported by studies of both early lateralized pathology and the ontogeny of laterality effects in normal development (reviewed by Kinsbourne & Hiscock, 1983b). Nevertheless even the effectively total loss of a hemisphere early in life may leave the child capable of impressive cognitive development within the hemisphere's domain. After left hemispherectomy, children's language skills may reach a plateau well within the normal range. It has been claimed that such children nevertheless exhibit recalcitrant syntactic difficulties not found after right hemispherectomy (Dennis & Kohn, 1975), but even these relatively subtle findings are undermined by sampling bias and statistical error (Bishop, 1984). Indeed, it is supposed that the right hemisphere is far better able to compensate for left hemisphere change implicating the language area than the left hemisphere can compensate for right hemisphere lesions implicating visuospatial skills (Milner, 1974). Thus even if there were gross structural damage of the left hemisphere in autism, this would not suffice to explain the severity of an autistic person's language problem.

Not only is right hemisphere compensation for left hemisphere deficit impressive in children (Milner, 1974) and even in adults (Czopf, 1972, Kinsbourne, 1971) but the pattern and pragmatics of right-hemisphere-based language use are indistinguishable from those generated by the left hemisphere. The language derived from right hemisphere shows no trace of alleged right hemisphere strategies (Prizant, 1983, notwithstanding), and the aphasic syndromes that result when right hemisphere compensation is incomplete are indistinguishable from those where the left hemisphere retains control. There is no clinically distinctive right hemisphere aphasia. It therefore makes no sense to label the way autistic individuals speak as "right hemispheric."

EVIDENCE ON CENTRAL LATERALITY IN INFANTILE AUTISM

It is generally agreed that laterality effects index hemisphere specialization. Thus right ear advantage for dichotic listening to verbal material derives from the left hemisphere specialization for language, and left ear advantages for identifying certain musical and environmental sounds correspondingly suggest a right hemisphere specialization for the decoding of such input. But the relationship between hemisphere specialization and laterality effect is probably indirect. Though the mechanism that sets up these asymmetries remains controversial, there is much evidence that the selective activation of the hemisphere specialized for the task in question contributes to the laterality effect (Kinsbourne, 1970). An important consequence of this concept is that laterality effects may change or be deviant not only if the underlying structural specialization is deviant but also if the way in which the cerebral cortex is activated at the time of the task performance is unusual (even though hemispheric specialization itself may conform to the conventional pattern). Thus we have shown that a left visual field advantage for nonsense shape identification (in normal adults) can be abolished by imposing manipulations calculated to enhance activation of the left hemisphere (Kinsbourne & Bruce, in press; Kinsbourne & Byrd, 1985). So even in the intact brain, the pattern of task-related hemisphere activation (which generates the laterality effect) may not correspond to the task-relevant specialization of hemispheric activation. Taking into account the evidence for unusual patterns of laterality findings in infantile autistic subjects (e.g., Dawson, Warrenburg, & Fuller, 1982; also see Chapter 12), we must decide whether to follow these authors in interpreting them as indicating unusual patterns of underlying structural cerebral specialization, or whether they indicate abnormalities in how the cerebral hemispheres are activated in these patients.

For there to be a substantial developmental language deficit, both hemispheres probably have to be involved. The lack of right ear advantage on verbal dichotic testing that characterizes the language-delayed child (Rosenblum & Dorman, 1978) is not evidence for a left hemisphere deficit. Only a substantial and consistent left ear advantage would indicate this, as it does in some cases of left hemispherectomy (Nebes & Nashold, 1980; Netley, 1972). Lack of perceptual asymmetry suggests either bilateralization of language representation or lack of selective left hemisphere activation during language activity. Autistic language disorders also would have to be referred to dysfunction of both hemispheres because one has to explain not only why the left hemisphere is not working but also why the right is not compensating. The available evidence conclusively excludes gross bilateralized cerebral damage as a necessary condition for the emergence of the autistic syndrome. Instead we hypothesize a failure of selective activation that may be somewhat variable and even task-specific, permitting the diversity of pattern of cognitive deficit found in individuals who exhibit autistic behavior.

Laterality testing in autistic children is applicable only to the higher-functioning children who are able to cooperate in the procedures. Such samples exhibited either the same asymmetries as normal controls (Arnold & Schwartz, 1983) or, more commonly, little or no asymmetry at all (Prior & Bradshaw, 1979; Wetherby, Koegel, & Mendel, 1981). The same is generally true of electrophysiological measures of cerebral activation (i.e., desynchronization of rhythms) when autistic samples are given particular tasks. In general, the evidences of activation are more bilateralized in the autistic than in the control group. Test-retest reliability of such measures has not been reported, so that one is unable to judge whether this bilateralization is relatively stable, at least to the extent that it might be in a normal group, or whether it varies as much as does manual behavior of those individuals with ambiguous hand preference. Also, little is known about the relationship between peripheral and central laterality within autistic samples.

A literal structuralist interpretation of these findings might be that many, if not most, autistic individuals are bilateralized in cerebral representation, and this would fit reasonably well with the prevalence of non-right-handedness in this condition. But such bilateralization explains nothing whatever about autistic symptomatology or cognitive deficit. As has already been noted, representation of cerebral function is bilateralized in a substantial minority of normal individuals (i.e., genetic sinistrals), and strenuous efforts have failed to demonstrate any substantial difference in the mental skills of presumptively bilateralized and unilateralized individuals from the normal population (Hardyck & Petrinovitch, 1977). Thus there is little reason to suppose that bilateralization of cerebral function *per se* incurs any significant penalty in adaptive behavior. It may occasion some difficulty in doing two different things at the same time for reasons that are of theoretical interest (Berry, Hughes, & Jackson, 1980; Kinsbourne, 1980b) but it appears to have minimal impact on activities of daily living. Certainly there is nothing about bilateralization of cerebral representation that would help explain why autistic individuals fail and what they fail in or why they go about tasks in the uniquely peculiar way that they do.

Another aspect of laterality that has been studied is ear preference. Blackstock (1978) has reported that autistic children tend to use their left ear to listen both to music and to speech (whereas normals used the right ear more for speech and, to a slight extent, the left ear more for music). According to hemisphere activation theory, this would indicate a predisposition to activate the right hemisphere during cognitive activity, thereby causing attention to deviate leftward. However, age, hand preference, and length of exposure of stimuli appear not to have been balanced between groups. It remains to be determined whether an autistic sample would differ in this way from a mental age-matched younger normal control. The most one can say is that the behavioral lateral asymmetry in the autistic sample was less than that in the particular normal control group used. Also, Kuttner (1983) was unable to confirm Blackstock's finding. He found a right ear preference to an equal degree both for speech and musical stimuli in autistic, retarded, and normal subjects. On the Halstead-Reitan neuropsychological battery applied by Dawson (1984) to autistic individuals, abnormalities referable to left brain outnumbered those referable to right brain. But as we have already remarked, that is generally true of minor early brain damage. What is definite is that there is less lateral asymmetry in autistic than in normal samples for the behaviors measured.

An alterative explanation of the pervasive bisymmetry of laterality findings could be based on an activational model. There is some evidence from experimental animal work that bears upon this view.

ASCENDING ACTIVATION AND LATERALITY

Animals suffering from unilateral neglect of space due to contralateral lesions of the lateral hypothalamus or nigrostriatal bundle transiently show remarkable improvement when they are activated by stressful stimuli or stimulant drugs. When their tails are pinched, laterally lesioned cats orient normally to stimuli that they previously neglected (Teitelbaum & Wolgin, 1975; Wolgin & Teitelbaum, 1978). A similar improvement is noted in rats when they are immersed in cold water or an ice bath or placed together in a cage with cats or other rats (Levitt & Teitelbaum, 1975; Marshall, Turner, & Teitelbaum, 1971; Robinson & Wishaw, 1974). Injection of stimulant drugs also counteracts neglect in brain-damaged animals (Butterworth, Belanger, & Barbeau, 1978; Wolgin, Hein, & Teitelbaum, 1980; Wolgin & Teitelbaum, 1978). Thus, stimulation resulting in diffuse ascending activation corrects imbalances between cortically based opponent systems (Kinsbourne, 1977). If one can think of lateral specialization as conferring an advantage on the specialized hemisphere in an opponent interaction, then one can see how with extreme ascending bilateral activation, the hemisphere normally not involved in a given cognitive activity (i.e., nondominant) might become involved to an extent comparable to that of the customarily leading hemisphere. Thus chronic or repeated phasic-intense bilateral ascending activation could account not only for the ambiguous hand preference that is so common in autistic individuals but also for evidences of bilateralization of cerebral activation when they undertake cognitive tasks.

OVERACTIVATION AND AUTISTIC SYMPTOMATOLOGY

Autistic symptomatology can be classified into that which exemplifies the effects of hyperarousal and that which represents an attempt to escape from such effects or fend them off. Notably, the shallow verbal encoding of echolalia suggests the overaroused individual (e.g., stressed) who can only repeat but not understand what is said to him or her. The well-known "hyperselective" attention (propensity to attend to minutiae) of autistic individuals could be an extreme case of constricted cue utilization in the sense of Easterbrook. In general, their overfocus (Kinsbourne & Caplan, 1979) suggests that autistic individuals are more comfortable when the range of cues to be used is limited. Their very individual and even idiosyncratic predilections may reflect those activities that they can undertake without experiencing dysphoria due to excessive ascending activation. Other autistic behaviors, such as the stereotypies and mannerisms, appear to correspond to displacement activities that have the function of decreasing arousal when it has exceeded a comfortable level (Kinsbourne, 1980a). Gaze avoidance, isolation, and need for sameness obviously could be, and have often been, interpreted as being defensive, minimizing the possibility of encountering a novel and therefore arousing input.

The hypothesized hyperarousal is not necessarily tonic (though it has certainly been repeatedly inferred from electroencephalographic data and is consistent with such findings as that of an increased heart rate in autistic individuals [Kootz & Cohen, 1981]). An unstable control system for ascending activation could oscillate between extremes of over- and under-arousal. Apparently endogenous state changes had been repeatedly reported in autistic individuals. The puzzling underreactivity and overreactivity to environmental stimuli (Goldfarb, 1961, 1963; Ornitz, 1971) could represent shifts between extremes of overarousal and underarousal for endogenous reasons or in relation to triggering factors. Bouts of inconsolable crying could similarly be explained.

Ascending activation may be abnormal not only in amount but also in direction. In an evoked potential study, Dawson and Galpert (1986) found N1 amplitudes to correlate with language abilities over the right but not the left hemisphere. She suggests that deficient language in autism is associated with overactivation of the right hemisphere. This is not incompatible with left lateralization of language. Misdirected activation might leave left hemisphere language processes inactivated in situations calling for speech, and thus mute or reduced to automatic (e.g., echolalic) functioning.

A brainstem dysfunction at the level of the vestibular complex has been invoked, based on abnormalities of postural reflexes in autistic children, notably the absence of postrotary nystagmus (Ornitz, 1974; Pollack & Krieger, 1958). However, both the specificity and the localizing significance of this finding are open to question. Deficient postrotary nystagmus is also prevalent among "emotionally disturbed" (Piggott, Purcell, Cummings, & Caldwell, 1976) and minimally brain-dysfunctional (Steinberg & Rendle-Short, 1977) children. Given that most autistic children exhibit multiple signs of minimal brain dysfunction, the postrotary nystagmus deficit could well be nonspecific, and an unreliable basis for theories attempting to explain phenomenology peculiar to autistic children.

Regardless of etiology, postrotary nystagmus can be suppressed by dysfunction cephalad to the vestibular complex. Maurer and Damasio (1979) have drawn attention to the finding that experimental lesions of the frontal lobe and striatum can cause a similar nystagmic deficit (Mettler & Mettler, 1940). Striatal dysfunction is a more plausible explanation than vestibular. The oscillation of some autistic individuals between tonic immobility and whirling activity (Ornitz, 1974) is reminscent of Sacks's (1973) description of postencephalitic Parkinsonian patients: immobile, yet with lightening speed responsive to certain stimuli. Perhaps autistic individuals' notorious "need for sameness" and external structure is relevant here. Dopamine-deficient individuals are volitionally impoverished and have to use features of the environment to help them initiate activities. Correspondingly they are at the mercy of the environment. Much of their avoidant behavior can be construed as an attempt to minimize contact with unpredictable environmental change capable of taking control of their behavior. But in other respects autistic individuals behave as if flooded with dopamine: fearful, hyper-vigilant, and limited in range of cue utilization (Agnew & Agnew, 1963; Easterbrook, 1959). Damasio and Maurer (1978) have cogently attributed autistic phenomenology to mesial frontal lobe and striatal impairment, including the (intermittent or pervasive) failure to speak and the dystonic posturing. Ritualistic behaviors they regard as secondary adaptations by the patients to their primary disabilities. Their account could be complemented by an attribution of stereotypies to hyperfunction of the same system that Damasio and Maurer incriminate as relatively inactive. This suggests, not a static deficit, but an oscillating dysregulation, due to undampened swings of frontal dopaminergic activity. Hyperalert states alternate with hypoalert, the latter yielding deficient response even to usually arousing stimuli.

In hyperactivation, there should be other evidences of dopamine excess (such as an increased blink rate; Stevens, 1978). In hypoactivation, signs of dopamine deficiency—for example, movements resembling tardive dyskinesias—should be apparent. In hyperactivation there should be excessive startle, in hyperactivation failure to respond. High activation states should usher in stereotypic sequences and low activation states should supervene at their conclusion.

An intriguing aspect of the neuropsychology of infantile autism is the suggested relationship of that syndrome and the amnesic syndrome of acquired forgetting in adults (Boucher & Warrington, 1976). They and DeLong (1978) have remarked on poor performance of autistic individuals on memory tests, and there is at least anecdotal evidence of impairment of episodic memory in individuals recovering from autistic states (in contrast to preservation of factual knowledge). In this issue cause and effect are particularly hard to disentangle. A congenital amnesic syndrome in autism would account for habituation failures and would explain why repeatedly encountered stimuli could appear perpetually novel, and therefore hyperarousing, to the autistic individual. It would also explain why the sensory (i.e., hyper-arousal) manifestations of autism recede after the preschool years (Ornitz, 1971). Presumably over many trials the congenital amnesic, like his acquired counterpart, does become familiar with much of what impinges upon him in his activities of daily living (Wood, Ebert, & Kinsbourne, 1982). Alternatively, continual state change in an autistic person might restrict learning by state dependence. By this account the memory problems of an autistic person would be secondary to an activation disorder.

In summary, the evidences of cerebral abnormality in autism are interpretable as indicating deviant utilization (i.e., activation) at this highest level of the brain rather than specific pathology inherent in its structure. Presumably an investigation of the characteristics of human and animal behavior in chronically overaroused states will clarify whether this point of view is a profitable one.

APPROACH VERSUS WITHDRAWAL AND THE BALANCE OF HEMISPHERIC ACTIVATION

Some years ago I introduced a formulation of hemispheric specialization in terms of approach (left hemisphere) versus withdrawal (right hemisphere), relying on Schneirla's (1959) exposition of this basic dichotomy in animal behavior. This formulation had two major advantages. It placed hemispheric specialization in contact with a biologically more general principle, and it embraces both cognitive and emotional differentiation of each hemisphere. The approach formulation for the left hemisphere accommodates both the propensity of the left hemisphere to subserve skilled action routines and plans, including language, which arises from naming objects within selective attention (Lempert & Kinsbourne, 1985), and the positive affect associated with the left hemisphere (Davidson & Fox, 1982). The withdrawal concept accommodates aspects of right hemisphere specialization in the sense that one withdraws into a space, defined by visuospatial processors. It clearly conforms to the right hemisphere's specialization for various forms of negative affect. I argued (Kinsbourne, 1979) that autistic individuals have a preponderance of withdrawal tendency (a formulation recently adopted by Dawson, see Chapter 12). The reticence of autistic individuals and their reluctance to confront or expose themselves to new experiences is quite consistent with a preponderantly withdrawal tendency. A recent reformulation of this proposed dichotomy (Kinsbourne & Bemporad, 1984) enables one to make this proposal more specific. The approach tendency of the left hemisphere is seen as the continuing of ongoing behavior (primitively continuing approach toward a target, but in humans at a higher level of abstraction any coordinated action sequence in pursuit of a goal). The right hemisphere is seen as specialized for the detection of the incongruous and unexpected. Its proximate function is to generate an orienting response in the presence of an unexpected event ("mismatch" to expectation) that arrests ongoing behavior and prepares the organism for a reformulation of its action plan in view of the changed circumstance. Consistent with this point of view is evidence that the right hemisphere better reflects than the left the organism's changing arousal states (Heilman, Schwartz, & Watson, 1977). If either the organism's arousal in response to the orienting were excessive, or the right hemisphere oversensitive to such changes, the same consequences would ensue, as follows. Novelty and change would elicit an excessive withdrawal response, and individuals would learn to shield themselves to the extent possible from such events, and also to discharge the excessive activation when it builds up to an uncomfortable level (by displacement activities). The relative overactivation of the right hemisphere that would result would modify the outcomes of behavioral and electrophysiological laterality tests so as to neutralize or even reverse expected left hemisphere advantages. The overactivation of the right hemisphere would not necessarily be tonic and therefore need not be reflected in cerebral metabolism studies. A phasic overactivation would suffice to set up the symptomatology in question.

This model suggests three possible origins for autistic symptomatology: excessive ascending activation, manifested as extreme arousal swings; a hypersensitivity of the right hemisphere to arousal and arousing events; and perhaps left hemisphere impairment, causing the right hemisphere to be disinhibited. Chronic readiness of the right hemisphere for function would presumably also favor right hemisphere types of processing, perhaps to the detriment of left, thus leading to "right hemispheric" profiles of psychometric findings repeatedly discovered in high-functioning autistic individuals.

REFERENCES

Agnew, N., & Agnew, M. (1963). Drive level effects on tasks of narrow and broad attention. *Quarterly Journal of Experimental Psychology, 15*, 58–62.

Annett, M. (1973). Handedness in families. *Annals of Human Genetics, 37*, 93–105.

Arnold, G., & Schwartz, S. (1983). Hemispheric lateralization of language in autistic and aphasic children. *Journal of Autism and Developmental Disorders, 13*, 129–139.

Bauman, M., & Kemper, T. L. (1985). Histoanatomic observations of the brain in early infantile autism. *Neurology, 35*, 866–874.

Berkson, G., & Davenport, R. K. (1962). Stereotyped movements of mental defectives: Initial survey (I). *American Journal of Mental Deficiency, 66*, 849–852.

Berkson, G., & Mason, W. A. (1963). Stereotyped movements of mental defectives: Situation effects (III). *American Journal of Mental Deficiency, 68*, 409–416.

Berkson, G., & Mason, W. A. (1964). Stereotyped movements of mental defectives: Effects of toys and the character of the acts (IV). *American Journal of Mental Deficiency, 68*, 511.

Berry, G. A., Hughes, R. V., & Jackson, L. D. (1980). Sex and handedness in simple and integrated task performance. *Perceptual and Motor Skills, 51*, 807–812.

Bishop, D. V. M. (1984). Linguistic impairment after left hemidecortification for infantile hemiplegia? A reappraisal. *Quarterly Journal of Experimental Psychology, 35A*, 199–207.

Blackstock, E. G. (1978). Cerebral asymmetry and the development of infantile autism. *Journal of Autism and Childhood Schizophrenia, 8*, 339–353.

Boucher, J. (1977). Hand preference in autistic children and their parents. *Journal of Autism and Childhood Schizophrenia, 7*, 177–187.

Boucher, J., & Warrington, E. K. (1976). Memory deficits in early infantile autism: Similarities to the amnesic syndrome. *British Journal of Psychology, 67*, 73–87.

Bradshaw-McAnulty, G., Hicks, R. E., & Kinsbourne, M. (1984). Pathological left-handedness and familial sinistrality in relation to degree of mental retardation. *Brain and Cognition, 3,* 349–356.

Butterworth, R. F., Belanger, F., & Barbeau, A. (1978). Hypokinesis produced by anterolateral hypothalamic 6-hydroxydopamine lesions and its reversal by some antiparkinson drugs. *Pharmacology, Biochemistry and Behavior, 8,* 41–45.

Caparulo, B. K., Cohen, D. J., Rothman, S. L., Young, J. G., Katz, J. D., Shaywitz, S. E., & Shaywitz, B. A. (1982). Computed tomographic brain scanning in children with developmental neuropsychiatric disorders. In S. Chess & A. Thomas (Eds.), *Annual progress in child psychiatry and child development.* New York: Brunner/Mazel.

Charny, I. W. (1963). Regression and reorganization in the "isolation treatment" of children: A clinical contribution to sensory deprivation research. *Journal of Child Psychology and Psychiatry, 4,* 47–60.

Colby, K. M., & Parkinson, C. (1977). Handedness in autistic children. *Journal of Autism and Childhood Schizophrenia, 7,* 3–9.

Creak, E. M., & Pampiglione, G. (1969). Clinical and EEG studies on a group of 35 psychotic children. *Developmental Medicine and Child Neurology, 11,* 218–227.

Czopf, J. (1972). Uber die Rolle der nicht dominanten Hemisphare in der Restitution der Sprache der Aphasischen. *Archiv für Psychiatrie und Nervenkrankheiten, 216,* 162–171.

Damasio, A. R., & Maurer, R. G. (1978). A neurological model for childhood autism. *Archives of Neurology, 35,* 777–786.

Darby, J. K. (1976). Neuropathologic aspects of psychosis in children. *Journal of Autism and Childhood Schizophrenia, 6,* 339–352.

Davidson, R. J., & Fox, N. A. (1982). Asymmetrical brain activity discriminates between positive and negative affective stimuli in human infants. *Science, 21,* 1235–1237.

Davis, K. V., Sprague, R. L., & Werry, J. S. (1969). Stereotyped behavior and activity level in severe retardates: The effects of drugs. *American Journal of Mental Deficiency, 73,* 721–727.

Dawson, G. (1984). Lateralized brain dysfunction in autism: Evidence from the Halstead–Reitan neuropsychological battery. *Journal of Autism and Developmental Disorders, 13,* 269–286.

Dawson, G., & Galpert, L. (1986). A developmental model for facilitating the social behavior of autistic children. In E. Schopler & G. Mesibov (Eds.), *Social behavior in autism.* New York: Plenum Press.

Dawson, G., Warrenburg, S., & Fuller, D. (1982). Cerebral lateralization in individuals diagnosed as autistic in early childhood. *Brain and Language, 15,* 353–368.

Delius, J. D. (1967). Displacement activities and arousal. *Nature, 214,* 1259–1260.

Delius, J. D. (1969). Irrelevant behavior, information processing and arousal hemeostasis. *Psychologische Forschung, 33,* 65–185.

DeLong, G. R. (1978). A neuropsychological interpretation of infantile autism. In M. Rutter & E. Schopler (Eds.), *Autism: A reappraisal of concepts and treatments.* New York: Plenum Press.

DeLong, G. R., Bean, S. C., & Brown, F. R. (1981). Acquired reversible autistic syndrome in acute encephalopathic illness in children. *Archives of Neurology, 38,* 191–194.

Dennis, M., & Kohn, B. (1975). Comprehension of syntax in infantile hemiplegics after cerebral hemidecortication: Left hemisphere superiority. *Brain and Language, 2,* 475–486.

Duffy, E. (1962). *Activation and behavior.* New York: Wiley.

Easterbrook, J. A. (1959). The effect of emotion on cue utilization and the organization of behavior. *Psychological Review, 66,* 183–201.

Fassler, J., & Bryant, D. N. (1971). Disturbed children under reduced auditory input: A pilot study. *Exceptional Children, 38,* 197–204.

Fein, D., Humes, M., Kaplan, E., Lucci, D., & Waterhouse, L. (1984). The question of left hemisphere dysfunction in autism. *Psychological Bulletin, 95,* 258–281.

Fein, D., Waterhouse, L., Lucci, D., Pennington, B., & Humes, M. (1985). Handedness and cognitive functions in pervasive developmental disorders. *Journal of Autism and Developmental Disorders, 15,* 323–333.

Folstein, S., & Rutter, M. (1977). Genetic influence and infantile autism. *Nature, 205*, 726–728.

Gardner, W. I., Cromwell, R. L., & Foshee, J. G. (1959). Studies in activity level: II. Effects of distal visual stimulation in organics, familials, hyperactives, and hypoactives. *American Journal of Mental Deficiency, 63*, 1028–1033.

Gillberg, C., & Gillberg, I. C. (1983). Infantile autism: A total population study of reduced optimality in the pre-, peri-, and neonatal period. *Journal of Autism and Developmental Disorders, 13*, 153–166.

Gloning, I., Gloning, K., Haub, G., & Quatember, R. (1969). Comparison of verbal behavior in right-handed and non right-handed patients with anatomically verified lesions of one hemisphere. *Cortex, 5*, 43–52.

Goldfarb, W. (1961). *Childhood schizophrenia*. Cambridge, MA: Harvard University Press.

Goldfarb, W. (1963). Self-awareness in schizophrenic children. *Archives of General Psychiatry, 8*, 47–60.

Gottschalk, L. A., Haer, J. L., & Bates, D. E. (1972). Effect of sensory overload on psychological state. *Archives of General Psychiatry, 27*, 451–457.

Hardyck, C., & Petrinovitch, L. F. (1977). Left-handedness. *Psychological Bulletin, 84*, 385–404.

Heilman, K. M., Schwartz, H., & Watson, R. T. (1977). Hypoarousal in patients with the neglect syndrome and emotional indifference. *Neurology, 28*, 229–232.

Hermelin, B., & Frith, V. (1971). Psychological studies of childhood autism: Can autistic children make sense of what they see and hear? *Journal of Special Education, 5*, 107–117.

Hermelin, B., & O'Connor, N. (1970). *Psychological experiments with autistic children*. Oxford: Pergamon.

Hicks, R. E., & Barton, A. K. (1975). A note on left-handedness and severity of mental retardation. *Journal of Genetic Psychology, 127*, 323–324.

Hockey, G. R. J. (1970). Effects of loud noise on attentional selectivity. *Quarterly Journal of Experimental Psychology, 22*, 28–36.

Hutt, C. (1967). Exploration, arousal, and autism. *Psychologische Forschung, 33*, 1–8.

Hutt, C., & Hutt, S. J. (1965). Effects of environmental complexity on stereotyped behaviours of children. *Animal Behaviour, 13*, 1–4.

Hutt, S. J., & Hutt, C. (1968). Stereotypy, arousal, and autism. *Human Development, 11*, 277–286.

Hutt, C., Hutt, S. J., Lee, D., & Ounsted, C. (1964). Arousal and childhood autism. *Nature, 204*, 908–909.

Hutt, C., Hutt, S. J., Lee, D., & Ounsted, C. (1965). A behavioral and electroencephalographic study of autistic children. *Journal of Psychiatric Research, 3*, 181–198.

Hutt, C., Hutt, S. J., & Ounsted, C. (1965). The behavior of children with and without upper CNS lesions. *Behavior, 24*, 246–268.

James, A. L., & Barry, R. J. (1980). A review of psychophysiology in early onset psychosis. *Schizophrenia Bulletin, 6*, 506–525.

Kinsbourne, M. (1970). The cerebral basis of lateral asymmetries in attention. *Acta Psychologica, 33*, 193–201. In A. F. Sanders (Ed.), *Attention and performance* (Vol. 3). Amsterdam: North-Holland.

Kinsbourne, M. (1971). The minor cerebral hemisphere as a source of aphasic speech. *Archives of Neurology, 25*, 302–306.

Kinsbourne, M. (1975). The ontogeny of cerebral dominance. *Annals of the New York Academy of Sciences, 263*, 244–250. (Reprinted in R. Rieber (Ed.), *Neuropsychology of language—Essays in honor of Eric Lenneberg*. New York: Academic Press, 1976).

Kinsbourne, M. (1977). Hemi-neglect and hemisphere rivalry. In E. A. Weinstein & R. P. Friedland (Eds.), *Hemi-inattention and hemisphere specialization. Advances in Neurology, 18*, 41–49. New York: Raven Press.

Kinsbourne, M. (1979). The neuropsychology of infantile autism. In L. A. Lockman, K. F. Swaiman, J. S. Drage, K. B. Nelson, & K. M. Marsden (Eds.), *Workshop on the neurobiological basis of autism* (NINCDA Monograph No. 23). Bethesda, MD: U.S. Department of HEW.

Kinsbourne, M. (1980a). Do repetitive movement patterns in children and animals serve a dearousing function? *Journal of Developmental and Behavioral Pediatrics. 1*, 39–42.

Kinsbourne, M. (1980b). A model for the ontogeny of cerebral organization in non-right-handers. In J. Herron (Ed.), *Neuropsychology of left handedness*. New York: Academic Press. (Reprinted in Japanese translation, Tokyo, Nihimura, 1983)

Kinsbourne, M. (1985). Base-state dependency of stimulant effects on the cognitive performance of hyperactive children. In L. M. Bloomingdale (Ed.), *Attention deficits disorder (II): Identification, course and treatment rationale*. New York: Spectrum.

Kinsbourne, M., & Bemporad, B. (1984). Lateralization of emotion: A model and the evidence. In N. Fox & R. J. Davidson (Eds.), *The psychobiology of affective disorder*. Hillsdale, NJ: Erlbaum.

Kinsbourne, M., & Bruce, R. (in press). Shift in visual laterality within blocks of trials. *Acta Psychologica*.

Kinsbourne, M., & Byrd, M. (1985). Word load and visual hemifield shape recognition: Priming and interference effects. In M. I. Posner, & O. S. M. Marin (Eds.), *Mechanisms of attention: Attention and performance XI*. Hillsdale, NJ: Erlbaum.

Kinsbourne, M., & Caplan, P. J. (1979). *Children's learning and attention problems*. Boston: Little, Brown.

Kinsbourne, M., & Hiscock, M. (1983a). Asymmetries of dual-task performance. In J. Hellige (Ed.), *Cerebral hemisphere asymmetry: Method, theory and application*. New York: Praeger.

Kinsbourne, M., & Hiscock, M. (1983b). The normal and deviant development of functional lateralization of the brain. In P. Mussen, Haith, M. & J. Campos (Eds.), *Handbook of child psychology* (4th ed., Vol. 2, Chap. 4). New York: Wiley.

Koegel, R. L., & Egel, A. L. (1979). Motivating autistic children. *Journal of Abnormal Psychology, 88*, 418–426.

Koegel, R. L., & Lovaas, O. I. (1978). Comments on autism and stimulus overselectivity. *Journal of Abnormal Psychology, 87*, 563–565.

Koegel, R. L., & Wilhelm, H. (1973). Selective responding to the components of multiple visual cue by autistic children. *Journal of Experimental Child Psychology, 15*, 442–453.

Kootz, J. P., & Cohen, D. J. (1981). Modulation of sensory intake in autistic children: Cardiovascular and behavioral indices. *Journal of the American Academy of Child Psychology, 20*, 692–701.

Kuttner, K. C. (1983). *Left hemisphere dysfunction in early infantile autism*. Doctoral dissertation, University of Chicago.

Lempert, H., & Kinsbourne, M. (1985). Possible origin of speech in selective orienting. *Psychological Bulletin, 97*, 62–73.

Lenneberg, E. H. (1967). *Biological foundations of language*. New York: Wiley.

Leventhal, D., Kinsbourne, M., & Reichler, R. (1972). *Periodic stimulus seeking and avoiding by an autistic patient*. Unpublished manuscript.

Levitt, D. R., & Teitelbaum, P. (1975). Somnolence, akinesia and sensory activation of motivated behavior in the lateral hypothalamic syndrome. *Proceedings of the National Academy of Sciences, 72*, 2819–2823.

Lovaas, O. I., Schreibman, L., Koegel, R. L., & Rehm, R. (1971). Selective responding by autistic children to multiple sensory input. *Journal of Abnormal Psychology, 77*, 211–222.

Ludwig, A. M., & Stark, L. H. (1973). Schizophrenia, sensory deprivation and sensory overload. *Journal of Nervous and Mental Disease, 157*, 210–216.

Margolies, P. J. (1977). Behavioral approaches to the treatment of early infantile autism: A review. *Psychological Bulletin, 84*, 249–264.

Marshall, J. F., Turner, B. H., & Teitelbaum, P. (1971). Sensory neglect produced by lateral hypothalamic damage. *Science, 90*, 536–546.

Maurer, R. G., & Damasio, A. R. (1979). Vestibular dysfunction in autistic children. *Developmental Medicine and Child Neurology, 21*, 656–658.

Mettler, F. A., & Mettler, C. C. (1940). Labyrinthine disregard after removal of the caudate. *Proceedings of the Society of Experimental Biology and Medicine, 45*, 473–475.

Milner, B. (1974). Hemispheric specialization: Scope and limits. In F. O. Schmitt & F. G. Worden (Eds.), *The neurosciences third study program* (pp. 742–775). Cambridge, MA: MIT Press.

Nebes, R. D., & Nashold, B. S. (1980). A comparison of dichotic and visuo-acoustic competition in hemispherectomized patients. *Brain and Language, 9*, 246–254.

Netley, C. (1972). Dichotic listening performance of hemispherectomized patients. *Neuropsychologia, 10*, 233–240.

Olmstead, C. E., & Villablanca, J. R. (1979). Effects of caudate nuclei on frontal cortical ablations in cats and kittens: Paw usage. *Experimental Neurology, 63*, 559–572.

Ornitz, E. M. (1971). Childhood autism: A disorder of sensori-motor integration. In M. Rutter (Ed.), *Infantile autism: Concepts, characteristics and treatment*. London: Churchill-Livingstone.

Ornitz, E. M. (1974). The modulation of sensory input and motor input in autistic children. *Journal of Autism and Childhood Schizophrenia, 4*, 197–216.

Ornitz, E. M., Brown, M. B., Sorosky, A. D., Ritvo, E. R., & Dietrich, L. (1970). Environmental modification of autistic behavior. *Archives of General Psychiatry, 22*, 560–565.

Piggott, L., Purcell, G., Cummings, G., & Caldwell, D. (1976). Vestibular dysfunction in emotionally disturbed children. *Biological Psychiatry, 11*, 719–729.

Ploog, D. (1950). Psychische Gegon regulation dargestellr am Verlaufe von Elektroschock behandlungen. *Archiv für Psychiatrie und Zeitschrift Neurologie, 183*, 617–663.

Pollack, M., & Krieger, H. P. (1958). Ocularmotor and postural patterns in schizophrenic children. *Archives of Neurology and Psychiatry, 79*, 720–726.

Prior, M. R. (1977). Conditional matching learning set performance in autistic children. *Journal of Child Psychology and Psychiatry, 18*, 183–189.

Prior, M., & Bradshaw, J. (1979). Hemisphere functioning in autistic children. *Cortex, 1*, 73–81.

Prizant, B. M. (1983). Language acquisition and communicative behavior in autism: Toward an understanding of the whole of it. *Journal of Speech and Hearing Disorders, 48*, 296–307.

Rago, W. V., & Case, J. C. (1978). Stereotyped behavior in special education teachers. *Exceptional Children, 44*, 342–344.

Randrup, A., & Munkvad, I. (1967). Behavioral stereotypes induced by pharmacological agents. *Pharmakopsychiatry, 1*, 18–26.

Rasmussen, T., & Milner, B. (1975). Clinical and surgical studies of the cerebral speech areas in man. In K. Zulch, O. Creutzfeld, & G. Galbraith (Eds.), *Otfrid Foerster symposium on cerebral localization*. Heidelberg: Springer.

Reynolds, B. S., Newsom, C. D., & Lovaas, O. I. (1974). Auditory overselectivity in autistic children. *Journal of Abnormal Child Psychology, 2*, 253–263.

Ritvo, E. R., Ornitz, E. M., Walker, R. D., & Hanley, J. (1970). Correlation of psychiatric diagnoses and EEG findings: A double-blind study of 184 hospitalized children. *American Journal of Psychiatry, 126*, 988–996.

Robinson, T. E., & Wishaw, I. Q. (1974). Effects of posterior hypothalamic lesions on voluntary behavior and hippocampal electroencephalograms in the rat. *Journal of Comparative and Physiological Psychology, 86*, 768–786.

Rosenblum, D. R., & Dorman, M. F. (1978). Hemispheric specialization for speech perception in language deficient kindergarten children. *Brain and Language, 6*, 378–389.

Rumsey, J. M., Duara, R., Grady, C. G., Rapoport, J. L., Margolin, R. A., Rapoport, S. F., & Cutler, N. R. (1985). Brain metabolism in autism: Testing cerebral glucose utilization rates as measured with positron emission tomography (PET). *Archives of General Psychiatry, 42*, 448–455.

Sacks, O. (1973). *Awakenings*. London: Duckworth.

Satz, P. (1972). Pathological left-handedness: An explanatory model. *Cortex, 8*, 121–135.

Satz, P. (1979). A test of some models of hemisphere speech organization in the left- and right-handed. *Science, 203*, 1131–1133.

Satz, P., Orsini, D., Saslow, E., & Henry, R. (1985). The pathological left-handedness syndrome. *Brain and Cognition, 4*, 27–46.

Schechter, M. D., Shurley, J. T., Towssieng, P. W., & Maier, W. J. (1969). Sensory isolation therapy of autistic children: A preliminary report. *Journal of Pediatrics, 74,* 564–569.

Schneirla, T. C. (1959). An evolutionary and developmental theory of biphasic processes underlying approach and withdrawal. In M. R. Jones (Ed.), *Nebraska symposium on motivation.* Lincoln: University of Nebraska Press.

Silva, D. A., & Satz, P. (1979). Pathological left-handedness: Evaluation of a model. *Brain and Language, 7,* 8–16.

Soper, H. V., & Satz, P. (1984). Pathological left-handedness and ambiguous handedness: A new explanatory model. *Neuropsychologia, 22,* 511–515.

Sorosky, A. D., Ornitz, E. M., Brown, M. B., & Ritvo, E. R. (1968). Systematic observations of autistic behavior. *Archives of General Psychiatry, 18,* 439–449.

Steinberg, M., & Rendle-Short, J. (1977). Vestibular dysfunction in young children with minor neurological impairment. *Developmental Medicine and Child Neurology, 19,* 639–651.

Stevens, J. (1978). Eye blink and schizophrenia: Psychosis or tardive dyskinesia? *American Journal of Psychiatry, 135,* 223.

Stroh, G., & Buick, D. (1968). The effect of relative sensory isolation on the behavior of two autistic children. In S. J. Hutt & C. Hutt (Eds.), *Behavior studies in psychiatry.* New York: Pergamon Press.

Teitelbaum, P., & Wolgin, D. L. (1975). Neurotransmitters and the regulation of food intake. In W. H. Gispen, Tj. B. van Wimersma Greidanus, B. Bohus, & D. deWied (Eds.), *Progress in brain research, Vol. 42. Hormones, homeostasis and the brain.* Amsterdam: Elsevier.

Tsai, L. Y. (1982). Handedness in autistic children and their families. *Journal of Autism and Developmental Disorders, 12,* 421–423.

Turkewitz, G., Moreau, T., & Birch, H. G. (1968). Relation between birth condition and neurobehavioral organization in the neonate. *Pediatric Research, 2,* 243–249.

Walton, D., & Mather, M. D. (1964). The application of learning principles to the treatment of obsessive compulsive states in the acute and chronic phases of illness. In H. J. Eysenck (Ed.), *Experiments in behavior therapy.* Oxford: Pergamon Press.

Wetherby, A. M., Koegel, R. L., & Mendel, M. (1981). Central auditory nervous system dysfunction in echolalic autistic individuals. *Journal of Speech and Hearing Research, 24,* 420–429.

Williams, R. S., Hauser, S. L., Purpura, D. P., DeLong, G. R., & Swisher, C. N. (1980). Autism and mental retardation: Neuropathological studies performed in four retarded persons with autistic behavior. *Archives of Neurology, 37,* 749–753.

Wolgin, D. L., Hein, A., & Teitelbaum, P. (1980). Recovery of forelimb placing after lateral hypothalamic lesions in the cat: Parallels and contrasts with development. *Journal of Comparative and Physiological Psychology, 94,* 795–807.

Wolgin, D. L., & Teitelbaum, P. (1978). Role of activation and sensory stimuli in recovery from lateral hypothalamic damage in the cat. *Journal of Comparative and Physiological Psychology, 92,* 474–500.

Wood, F., Ebert, V., & Kinsbourne, M. (1982). The episodic–semantic memory distinction in memory and amnesia: Clinical and experimental observations. In L. Cermak (Ed.), *Human memory and amnesia.* Hillsdale, NJ: Erlbaum.

Yerkes, R. M., & Dodson, J. D. (1908). The relation of strength of stimulus to rapidity of habit formation. *Journal of Comparative Psychology, 18,* 459–482.

Zeaman, D., & House, B. J. (1979). A review of attention theory. In N. R. Ellis (Ed.), *Handbook of mental deficiency, psychological theory, and research* (2nd ed.). Hillsdale, NJ: Erlbaum.

Zentall, S. S. (1980). Behavioral comparisons of hyperactivity and normally active children in natural settings. *Journal of Abnormal Child Psychology, 8,* 93–109.

Zentall, S. S., & Zentall, T. R. (1983). Optimal stimulation: A model of disordered activity and performance in normal and deviant children. *Psychological Bulletin, 94,* 446–471.

Implications of Social Deficits in Autism for Neurological Dysfunction

DEBORAH FEIN, BRUCE PENNINGTON, and
LYNN WATERHOUSE

INTRODUCTION

In this chapter, we will consider some of the implications of the social deficits in autism for neurological dysfunction. In the first section, we will consider the nature of the social deficit, and the arguments for considering it a primary and not a secondary manifestation of neurological disorder. In the second section, we will review some of the evidence for specific neurological systems involved in social and attachment behavior, and in the third section, we will consider whether any clinical evidence supports the involvement of these systems in autism. Finally, we will suggest some implications for future research.

SOCIAL DEFICITS IN AUTISM

Social unrelatedness is the hallmark of the autistic syndrome. The prototypic view of the autistic child captured in many moving clinical descriptions (Cohen, Caparulo, & Shaywitz, 1978; DeLong, 1978; Kanner, 1943; Park, 1967; Rimland, 1964; Rutter, 1968; Wing, 1981) is of a child who acts as if other people are of no special interest, or are objects of active avoidance. In their unresponsiveness they seem "in a glass ball" or "behind a veil" (Rimland, 1964). They do not intentionally communicate their feelings, nor are they interested in the feelings of others. They do not willingly meet the gaze of others and appear to "look through" or "beyond" people. They may respond to others' hands or arms or hair in a way that suggests that they do not regard them as parts of another being who has feelings or intentions. Many autistic children do become interested in social interactions at a later point

DEBORAH FEIN • Laboratory of Neuropsychology, Boston University Medical Center, Boston, Massachusetts 02118.   BRUCE PENNINGTON • University of Colorado Health Sciences Center, Denver, Colorado 80262.   LYNN WATERHOUSE • Child Behavior Study, Trenton State College, Trenton, New Jersey 08625.

in their development. But even these children remain profoundly socially impaired, insensitive to others' nonverbal social cues, and unaware of their own socially inappropriate behavior. Analyses of language in verbal autistic children (see Tager-Flusberg, 1981, for review) suggest that linguistic features *per se* are often relatively intact, but that pragmatics and communicative intent are deviant. Autistic children differ from equally language-impaired aphasic children in being less communicative nonverbally (Bartak, Rutter, & Cox, 1975).

More systematic observations or experimental investigations of specific social behaviors (e.g., Ornitz, Guthrie, & Farley, 1978; Sigman & Ungerer, 1981) are much fewer. One such behavior that has been documented is gaze aversion, an unwillingness to make eye contact with others (Richer & Coss, 1976; Rutter, 1968; Wing, 1976). Other early developmental signs include delayed or absent development of imitation, pointing, and reciprocal play, as well as lack of interest in the human voice or human speech (Wing, 1974). Unexpectedly, however, early appearance of the social smile appears to be normal in many cases (DeLong, 1978; Park, 1967), although it may be lost at a later age.

Ornitz *et al.* (1978) examined specific social behaviors in young autistic children. They report that 85% of their sample ignored people, 76% showed gaze aversion, and 90% seemed unresponsive, hard to reach. Preliminary evidence from Hobson suggests that some autistic children may differ from normal children in which areas of the face they use for face recognition (Hobson, 1981). Boucher (1981) had autistic and retarded children perform 10 cognitive tasks, including a face recognition task. At a later time, she asked the children to remember what tasks they had performed for her. She found that unlike the normal retarded control groups, none of the autistic group recalled that there had been a face recognition task (all other tasks were recalled by at least 3 out of 10 autistic children).

Abnormalities in other areas such as language, motor functions, and adaptability, are widespread—to the point where some investigators have made them defining criteria or have based etiological theories upon them. Nevertheless, deviance in social relations is the only feature included in every set of diagnostic criteria (see, for example, the diagnostic criteria of Delong, 1978; Eisenberg & Kanner, 1956). A very experienced clinician and head of a school for autistic children, Fred Krell, once remarked to one of the authors (D. F.) that he had one major criterion for autism: If he was alone in the room with the child and felt as if he were alone, he considered the child autistic. This is not to imply that the unrelatedness must be pervasive and the autistic child totally asocial. Nor does it imply that social disinterest must be lifelong in the autistic child. But it does imply that if a child, early in life, shows an interest in and empathy for other people that is commensurate with his mental age (and infants show selective interest in other people from the earliest weeks of life), then that child should not be considered autistic.

It has been argued that the social difficulties, although universal in autistic children, stem from more basic impairments in perception, attention, or cognition. The impetus for these arguments, which have dominated the field for almost 20 years, have interesting historical roots.

Early theories held that autism was a disorder of the child's emotional life, and professionals in the late 1940s through the 1960s tended to put the blame for the condition on faulty child-rearing or emotional problems in the parents (although these opinions were couched in more subtle language). Indeed, we are repeatedly startled to learn from parents how widely this view is still held by child psychiatrists, especially in Europe.

Probably beginning with the publication of Rimland's classic work in 1964, and furthered by the elegant arguments of Rutter (1968) and others, the pendulum began to swing from seeking the cause in early experiences to searching for neurological abnormalities. This revolt against blaming parental practices carried with it a shift in emphasis from the social to the cognitive aspects of autistic behavior. Partly because the cognitive aspects of brain damage are better understood than the social or behavioral aspects, and partly because the field of child development in the 1960s and 1970s was heavily centered on the study of language and cognitive development, research on autism has focused almost exclusively on analyzing cognitive features and searching for their neurological underpinnings.

However, the last 5 to 10 years have seen the burgeoning of interest in the neurological substrates of social behavior in animals and humans, and the application of psychological research methods to the study of social and affective development. Consequently, research interest has begun to return to the social unrelatedness in autism, but with a neuropsychological rather than a psychoanalytic/environmental orientation.

It is our contention that the social deficits in autism cannot be reasonably attributed to more primary cognitive deficits, but should be regarded as primary manifestations of the neurological disorder. There are several reasons for this assertion (discussed in detail by Fein, Pennington, Markowitz, Braverman, & Waterhouse, 1986).

First, if social unrelatedness is due to a cognitive impairment, there should be a close correlation between the two areas of deficiency. This does not seem to be the case in the autistic population. Clinically, one can observe quite retarded children who are only mildly asocial, and profoundly asocial children who are almost at a normal level in many areas of intellectual functioning. Experimentally, cognitive and social/emotional functioning have also been shown to be at least partly independent (Bartak & Rutter, 1976; Fein, Waterhouse, Lucci, & Snyder, 1985; Sigman & Ungerer, 1984). The severely retarded autistic child may not discriminate among people and may have no communicative language, while the normal IQ autistic child may discriminate among and talk to people but be unable to read social cues or understand what the other is feeling. Though the behaviors differ, the lack of social/emotional connectedness may be as profound in the high-functioning autistic child.

The dissociation between social and cognitive development can be seen in even more striking form in different clinical groups. Social relatedness is usually intact in even the severely retarded Down syndrome child (Emde, Katz, & Thorpe, 1978), while, on the other hand, severe emotional deprivation can disturb interpersonal relations but have little effect on cognition (Rutter, 1979, who concludes: "To an important extent, intellectual growth and social growth have their main influences from rather different sources").

Second, the specific cognitive deficits put forth as possible bases for the social problems seem unconvincing. Areas of deficiency include auditory and language processing, perceptual dysfunction, and memory. It is undoubtedly true that these deficits and others are widespread in autistic children. However, it has never been demonstrated that any of these deficits are found in all autistically aloof children, that the severity of these cognitive deficits correlates with the severity of the autistic aloofness, or that they cannot be found in as severe a form in sociable retarded children. A retarded child with an IQ as low as 20 will undoubtedly have poor memory, language, and higher perceptual processes but may be very sociable, suggesting that a very low cognitive level may suffice for a primitive and undifferentiated sociability.

Third, many of the cognitive functions, especially language, do not appear early enough in normal development to account for the failure of sociability in the first 6 months so frequently reported in autism (DeLong, 1978).

The fourth point concerns the cognitive strengths and weaknesses found most often in autism. Although no one pattern is found in all autistic children, visuospatial and sensorimotor processes are most often spared (Tanguay, 1984) while language and symbolic play are most often impaired (Rutter, 1983; Sigman & Ungerer, 1984; Wing, 1981). One could argue that the areas most often deficient are just those that rest most clearly on a base of shared meaning, communicative intent, and reciprocal interaction—the products of early sociability.

A fifth, perhaps most convincing, argument for the primacy of the social deficit is the specific difficulty autistic children have on cognitive tasks that depend on understanding social or emotional information. Research in this area is just beginning, but some studies suggest that autistic children are much more impaired on tasks with social content than on tasks without social content, even when the apparent cognitive demands are closely parallel.

In a dissertation study, Jennings (1973), using Izard's (1971) facial affect photographs with 11 autistic, and matched retarded and normal children, found that autistic children, more than the control groups, preferred to match photographs on the basis of accessories rather than affect. In addition, they performed more accurately on tasks that required the use of nonemotional cues than on tasks that required discrimination between emotional facial expressions. The autistic children, however, did not differ significantly from the other groups in ability to accurately identify different emotions from facial expressions, although their scores were lower. Wolff and Barlow (1979) found that autistic children used fewer emotional constructs and more physical ones when describing photographs of strangers, but not when describing their mothers, while schizoid children were more concrete and physical in their descriptions of both strangers and mothers.

Hobson (1982) asked autistic and matched normal and retarded children to match 10-inch videotape sequences of four real facial expressions to schematic facial expressions. He then had the children match these schematics to tapes of affective vocalizations, gestures, and situations. He found that autistic children were more impaired on these tasks than on tasks of matching inanimate objects to their movements or sounds. Some of these matching tasks were cross-modal, but since some control tasks were also cross-modal, deficits in matching across modalities cannot explain the autistic deficit on the affective material. Thus, these studies are consistent in suggesting a specific deficit in the processing of affective and social stimuli.

A last point in this argument is that lack of social interest, as in early autism, is extremely rare in severe brain damage, retardation, or environmental deprivation. The attachment system in normal development is evidently highly protected against disturbance, and forms a framework for further cognitive and emotional growth. In normal development,

> what a partner does, shows, or offers is immediately interesting because a person has done it . . . highly specialized innate mental processes for perceiving the particular interests and intentions of other persons, and for cooperating with them in experience and action . . . . Immediately after the neonate period, in the second month, babies orient selectively and preferentially to persons who attend to their vocalizations, facial expressions, gestures, and movements in discriminating ways. . . . in neonates there is a set of fairly automatic responses to perception of others' expressive acts. More complete analysis of the communicative interactions shows, however, that the baby is not just reacting reflexively or performing conditioned responses. The infant is both decoding elaborate facial and vocal signals from the mother and generating complementary communicative movements that are organized into patterns. . . . (Trevarthen, 1983, p. 69)

In sharp contrast to this prewired social receptivity, the social disinterest in autism is very pronounced and very resistent to therapeutic intervention. Social behaviors are hard to train and easy to extinguish, do not readily generalize, and usually continue to appear "hollow."

If the social deficits in autism are considered to be primary and to have their roots in the autistic neurological dysfunction(s), then it is useful to examine some of the experimental and clinical literature on the neurological basis of social and attachment behavior, to look for cues about which neurological systems we might expect to be compromised in the autistic child.

NEUROLOGICAL BASIS OF SOCIAL BEHAVIOR

In this section, we will attempt to review what is known about the neurological basis of social behavior and use those findings to speculate about the possible neurological basis of the social deficits in autism. The preliminary and speculative nature of both enterprises needs to be emphasized at the ouset for three reasons:

1. Our current ability to objectively measure different aspects of social and emotional functioning is much less well developed than our ability to measure discrete cognitive and linguistic skills.
2. There is much less clinical and experimental work on the neurological basis of social behavior, partly because focal lesions occur less frequently in some of the main parts of the brain believed to subserve social behavior (i.e., limbic and frontal areas) than in areas that subserve most cognitive and linguistic skills.
3. What little is known is based almost entirely on work with adult animals or humans. Thus, almost nothing is known about the developmental neuropsychology of social behavior, especially in humans.

The third point is particularly important because, as indicated earlier, the social deficits in autism appear before many neocortical systems are thought to be fully functioning. Therefore, a neurological theory of the social deficits in autism that was based entirely on a neocortical system (e.g., prefrontal areas) would be improbable developmentally. Moreover, there is evidence (Francis, Self, & McCaffree, 1984) to suggest that anencephalic babies possess normal social drive at a rudimentary level, which is often lacking in autistic infants. Similarly, hamsters whose neocortices are removed at birth develop normally with respect to social behavior and daily routines (Murphy, MacLean, & Hamilton, 1981). It may well be that regulation of social behavior undergoes a developmental shift from mainly subcortical to cortical control, as has been elegantly demonstrated by Goldman-Rakic, Isseroff, Schwartz, and Bugbee (1983) for the control of delayed alternation behavior in rhesus monkeys. In that example, control of this complex problem-solving behavior is first mediated in immature animals by portions of the caudate nucleus in the basal ganglia and then shifts to control by the dorsolateral portion of the prefrontal areas.

Given these caveats, what is known about the neurological basis of social behavior in primates? There is fairly broad consensus that several brain areas are more specifically involved in social functioning than others; these are principally the limbic system and its projections in the orbital and medial portions of the frontal lobes. It is also important to mention that in humans the right hemisphere appears to have a preferential role in the perception and production of affective and social cues (Bryden & Ley, 1983; Heilman, Watson, & Bowers, 1983), that disease of the basal ganglia can produce affective changes, particularly depression (Mayeux, 1983), and that bilateral inferior occipital lesions can impair facial recognition (i.e., prosopagnosia), as reviewed by Benton (1979).

We will first briefly discuss prosopagnosia, right hemisphere processing of social cues, and the emotional aspects of basal ganglia function and dysfunction, none of which appears to provide an adequate model for autism. We will then discuss in more detail the social functions of the limbic and frontal lobes, which currently appear to be the most promising candidates for a neurological model of the social deficits in autism.

Prosopagnosia

This intriguing syndrome in humans is an acquired defect in the ability to recognize familiar faces in the presence of intact person identification on the basis of other cues. Clinicoanatomical correlations indicate that right inferior occipital involvement is necessary but not sufficient, since virtually all autopsied cases evidence bilateral involvement (Benton, 1979). Geschwind (1979) reported a case with bilateral inferior-medial occipital and temporal lobe involvement in which there was a specific prosopagnosia with few other deficits. The importance of prosopagnosia for autism is that, as previously mentioned, autistic children may have impaired facial recognition. Obviously, prosopagnosia cannot provide a comprehensive neurological model for autism because both person identification and social drive more generally are preserved in patients with prosopagnosia. The facial recognition deficit in autism may well be secondary to more basis deficits in social drive, which could deprive the facial recognition system of necessary developmental inputs. Clearly, however, more systematic empirical investigation of facial recognition in autistic children is needed.

Right Hemisphere Processing of Social Cues

A number of human studies in both normal individuals (for a review, see Bryden & Ley, 1983) and adults with acquired lesions (Heilman *et al.*, 1983; E. D. Ross, 1981, 1983) support the general conclusion that emotional cues are preferentially perceived and produced in the right hemisphere. For instance, there appears to be a left visual field superiority for matching emotional faces (Ley & Bryden, 1979), a left ear superiority for identifying the affective value of both musical tone sequences and speech (Bryden, Ley, & Sugarman, 1982; Ley & Bryden, 1982), and greater involvement of the left side of the face in expressing affect (Borod, Koff, & Caron, 1983). On the basis of clinical studies, E. D. Ross (1981, 1983) has proposed that different right hemisphere lesions disrupt the comprehension, repetition, or production of emotion in a manner parallel to that observed for the acquired aphasias. Although this comprehensive proposal needs further empirical support, the general finding that right hemisphere lesions are more likely to impair emotional reception or expression is generally accepted.

Again, there is some correspondence with symptoms in autism (Fein, Humes, Kaplan, Lucci, & Waterhouse, 1984). The speech of autistic children who have developed language is often described as flat, robotlike, and generally deficient at the pragmatic and prosodic levels rather than the phonological or syntactic levels. However, a right hemisphere model of the social deficits in autism faces a number of problems. One is that children with early right hemispherectomies do not become autistic (Dennis, 1980). A second is the apparent paradox of usually preserved (or even enhanced) visuospatial skills in nonretarded autistic children, skills that presumably reflect intact right hemisphere functioning.

Emotional Aspects of Basal Ganglia Function and Dysfunction

While the basal ganglia have traditionally been viewed as part of the motor system under control of the motor cortex, both animal studies and human diseases of the basal ganglia suggest other functions. MacLean (1978; Greenberg, MacLean, and Ferguson, 1979) has found that particular lesions in the striatum of lizards and squirrel monkeys disrupt conspecific displays, a primitive form of social signal.

Human diseases of the basal ganglia also offer some parallels to autistic symptomatology. In Parkinson disease, there is an enormous variety of rigid and involuntary movements as well as blocking of movements (which are richly described by Sacks, 1973). Some of these are reminiscent of the motor stereotypies observed in autism, and it is on this basis that Damasio and Maurer (1978) included the basal ganglia in their neurological model of autism, which is one of the most comprehensive models yet presented.

However, MacLean (1985) speculates that the basal ganglia and related structures may subserve fairly primitive social and adaptive behaviors that are found in both reptiles and mammals, whereas the limbic thalamocingulate complex is important for specifically mammalian social adaptations (maternal behavior, audiovocal communication, and play). If this division between basal ganglia and limbic contributions to social behavior proves correct, a limbic deficit would seem more relevant to the social deficits in autism, although basal ganglia disorder could be a contributor in some cases. In addition, patients with Parkinson disease and other basal ganglia disorders frequently show depression, apathy, and irritability, and, less frequently, lability of emotion and psychosis (Mayeux, 1983), but not a lack of social interaction.

To summarize to this point, neither prosopagnasia, right hemisphere dysfunction, nor basal ganglia dysfunction seems adequate to explain the core deficit in autism: a profound asociability that can appear quite early in development. We will next consider the limbic system.

Limbic System

Although discussions of human brain evolution usually emphasize the enormous increases in neocortical, especially frontal, areas, there is evidence that humans also have the highest level of limbic system evolution (Douglas & Marcellus, 1975).

Attention was refocused on the limbic system ("visceral brain") by MacLean (1952), who later described the limbic system as one of the components of his triune brain (MacLean, 1973). Recently, MacLean (1985) has presented evidence suggesting that the development of three crucial mammalian social behaviors—nursing and maternal care; audiovocal communication, including the separation call; and play—depended on the evolution of the thalamocingulate portion of the limbic system. Similarly, Lamendella (1977) has also proposed that the limbic system is really a center for mammalian social communication, which in humans is elaborated in a specifically linguistic way by the neucortical speech and language structures. Thus, in his view, these neocortical structures are but the latest evolutionary "layer" added on to a more fundamental mammalian and premammalian communication center. While these neocortical structures provide the complex technical facility necessary for human speech, they do not provide the basis for its "underlying communication motives, strategies and content" (Lamendella, 1977, p. 158).

The limbic system in mammals controls communicative behavior sequences that are signs for basic internal motivational states such as fear, alarm, surprise, and rage. It also controls more specifically social messages, including those involved in territoriality, dominance, sexuality, and attachment. Thus, generally the limbic system can be said to provide the basis for "communicative intent." More specifically, in early infant development, it may mediate the various communicative behaviors that are involved in the development of the attachment of the infant to the mother (Konner, 1982). There is also evidence that the limbic frontal lobe (i.e., cingulate cortex) is important, at least in rats, in the attachment to the infant. Stamm (1955) found that cingulate, but not adjacent neocortical, lesions disrupted virtually all aspects of maternal behavior, which led to a considerably reduced survival rate of the infant rat pups.

There is an extensive literature on experimental lesions of the limbic system in animals (Isaacson, 1982). Two such lesions deserve comment here: bilateral temporal lobectomy (which produces the Kluver–Bucy syndrome) and combined limbic and orbital frontal lesions.

The Kluver–Bucy syndrome has been discussed as a model for autism (see Boucher & Warrington, 1976; DeLong, 1978). Kluver and Bucy (1939) did their pioneering work on adult monkeys, which possessed both the benefit and the liability of mature, organized central nervous systems and ample experience in the domains of socialization and interpersonal interactions. In these adult monkeys, bilateral ablations of the temporal lobes, including the hippocampus and amygdala, produced visual agnosia, strong oral tendencies, hypervigilance, absence of emotional response, and an increase in sexual activity. Only absence of emotional response and perhaps the oral tendencies seem similar to autistic symptoms.

The behavioral effects of experimental ablation of orbitofrontal and anterior temporal cortex and the amygdala are summarized and discussed by Kling and Steklis (1976), who propose that these brain regions bilaterally subserve primate social behavior. Lesions in juvenile or mature animals of various primate species have characteristically resulted in aberrant behavior typified by social withdrawal and isolation, cessation of grooming and other behaviors that subserve social contact, and abolition of infant caretaking activity. Other changes that have been noted are reduced and inappropriate vocal activity, alterations in the quantity and quality of facial expressivity, and locomotor stereotypies, such as wandering or circling. These behaviors are similar to those seen in autism. These effects have occurred in both artificial and naturalistic settings, and so, unlike those in the Kluver–Bucy syndrome, do not appear to be situation-specific. This evidence implicates these regions as a neuroanatomical substrate for primate social and affiliative behavior. Recent findings (Bachevalier & Mishkin, personal communication) and older data (Mirsky, 1960) suggest that amygdala involvement alone may produce some of these effects on social behavior.

Overall, the work of MacLean, Lamendella, Kling and Stecklis, Mishkin, and Mirsky supports the view of the limbic system as an important substrate for social behavior in primates. Unfortunately, there are few human data because of the rarity of focal limbic lesions in man. However, Damasio and Van Hoesen (1983) have discussed the effects of focal lesions in the anterior cingulate cortex, the medial portion of the frontal lobe directly adjacent to the limbic system; these are discussed in the next section.

Despite this lack of human data, the limbic system is an appealing candidate for a neurological system underlying the social deficits in autism because of its central role in affect and social communication and because it appears to be a system that matures early enough to explain the early onset of the deficits in autism. Damasio and Van Hoesen (1983) have said that the limbic system "probably exerts a specific affect related influence on functional areas and systems that are relevant to the larger functions of these areas and systems" (page 94). They have also discussed the many afferent and efferent connections between the limbic system and the cortex, including higher association areas. Thus it is not hard to imagine how dysfunction in the limbic system early in life could disrupt many aspects of cognitive and linguistic development. It is important, however, not to compartmentalize the limbic system too much, since it is intimately connected with many other parts of the brain, especially the portions of the frontal lobes (i.e., orbital and medial) most involved in social functioning.

Frontal Lobes

Since the frontal lobes are both large and functionally heterogeneous, it is important to specify the parts of the frontal lobes discussed here. We will not be concerned with primary motor or premotor cortex, but rather with prefrontal cortex, of which there are three divisions: dorsolateral, orbital, and medial.

Damasio (1979) and Lishman (1978) have discussed the social and emotional deficits in human adults with prefrontal lesions. These include lack of initiative and spontaneity, diminished sexual and exploratory drives, diminished ability to experience pleasure and possibly pain, decreased social awareness and judgment, and inappropriate mild euphoria and boastfulness.

Although deficits in social functioning can accompany lesions in any of the three areas of prefrontal cortex, there is broad agreement that orbital and medial frontal cortex is more specifically involved in social processes than dorsolateral cortex, but less involved in complex cognitive processes (Stuss & Benson, 1983). Long-term follow-up of leukotomy patients, who have focal orbital frontal lesions, found them to have deficits on tasks of social cognition but fewer deficits than patients with dorsolateral lesions on pure cognitive tasks such as tests of perseveration. For instance, the leukotomy patients could correctly perceive emotions in a face but were unable to pick the appropriate emotional reaction to a social situation (Stuss & Benson, 1983). Similarly, there was a dissociation in the leukotomy patients' physical expression of emotion and their verbal labeling of their own emotion (Stuss & Benson, 1983). Thus, what appears to be impaired in these patients is social judgment and the planning of socially appropriate actions, not the perception of social cues *per se*.

Although there is less evidence regarding medial frontal lesions in humans, what there is provides some interesting parallels to autism. Damasio and Van Hoesen (1983) review previous cases and discuss in detail two cases in which there were focal lesions in the anterior cingulate gyrus. These lesions produced an overall decreased drive for action and communication and a decreased experience and expression of affect. The acute phase of these lesions was marked by akinetic mutism, followed by a more chronic aspontaneity of behavior. In contrast, verbal repetition was preserved in all phases of the illness (which is reminiscent of some cases of autism), as was verbal comprehension (which contrasts sharply with autism); hence, the social deficits cannot be attributed to an aphasic syndrome.

Summary

What should be clear from this brief review is both the complexity of the brain systems subserving social behavior and the complexity of the social deficits to be explained in autism (not to mention their variability across patients). An adequate neurological theory needs to address, at the minimum, the following deficits in autism: reduced social drive and communicative intent, faulty perception of faces and other social cues, faulty expression of social cues, and a generalized comprehension deficit for both social and nonsocial information. Specific syndromes, such as anterior cingulate or amygdala lesions, provide intriguing models for understanding reduced social drive and affective expression, while inferotemporal and right hemisphere deficits may provide models for understanding the deficits in perception and expression of social cues and face recognition but cannot explain the deficits in social drive.

We should be cautious about simple neurological explanations of the social deficits of autism. An early failure in limbic system functioning could perhaps lead to failures in other systems, but total or widespread limbic involvement is problematic because a locus that lesioned both the hippocampus and the amygdala bilaterally would presumably cause a more profound memory deficit than is compatible with the behavioral data in autism (Fein *et al.*, 1985). It is important to remember that the limbic system contains a set of complex and highly differentiated structures. Therefore, a limbic model of autism will need to focus more precisely on specific structures and connections.

NEUROLOGICAL INVOLVEMENT IN AUTISM

Is there any evidence for dysfunction of occipital or inferotemporal cortex, right hemisphere, basal ganglia, limbic system, or prefrontal cortex in autistic children? Four major types of research have been conducted to explore possible neurophysiological or anatomical abnormalities in autistic individuals: (1) neuropathologic studies, (2) neuroradiologic studies (including PEG, CAT, and PET studies), (3) EEG studies, and (4) evoked potential or EP studies.

Abnormalities in EEGs are common in autistic children (see review by Deykin & MacMahon, 1979) but so far have provided little in the way of autism-specific localizing findings. Similarly, brainstem evoked potential studies (Fein, Skoff, & Mirsky, 1981; Rumsey, Grimes, Pikus, Duara, & Ismond, 1984; Skoff, Mirsky, & Turner, 1980; Tanguay, Edwards, Buchwald, Schwafel, & Allen, 1982) and cortical evoked potential studies (Courchesne, Lincoln, Kilman, & Galambos, 1985) frequently find abnormalities but ones that may be nonspecific to autism.

Pathologic and radiologic studies are reviewed in detail in Chapter 13 by DeLong and Bauman. Our reading of this literature suggests to us that findings are mixed. What is clearly suggested is that there must be a wide variety of neurological deficits underlying the cardinal features of the autistic syndrome; investigators have been unable to show any neurological deficit shared by all "autistic" children, even when they have been diagnosed by the same system. Furthermore, among subgroups of autistic patients who do show a given neurological symptom, no unique behavioral pattern has yet emerged.

Positive anatomical findings are as diverse as cell degeneration in the hippocampal formation (1 case, Schain & Yannet, 1960); degeneration in the reticular formation (1 case, I. S. Ross, 1959); possible hemorrhagic infarct in the left hemisphere—frontal and parietal lobes (1 case, Weir & Salisbury, 1980); abnormalities in the hippocampal complex, subiculum, entorhinal cortex, septal nuclei, mammillary body, selected nuclei of the amygdala, neocerebellar cortex, roof nuclei of the cerebellum, and inferior olivary nucleus (1 case, Bauman & Kemper, 1985); intraparenchymal lesions (2 of 17 cases, Damasio, Maurer, Damasio, & Chui, 1980); abnormalities in the right frontal lobe (Aarkrog, 1968); reversed cerebral asymmetry (9 of 16 cases, Hier, LeMay, & Rosenberger, 1979); and abnormalities of the ventricular system (25 of 46 cases, Aarkrog, 1968; 16 of 19 cases, Bauman, LeMay, Bauman, & Rosenberger, 1985; 11 of 45 cases, Campbell et al., 1982; 3 of 22 cases, Caparulo et al., 1981; 5 of 17 cases, Damasio et al., 1980; 2 of 16 cases, Harcherik et al., 1985; 13 of 18 cases, Hauser, DeLong, & Rosman, 1975; 2 of 13 cases, Rosenbloom et al., 1984).

Darby (1976) surveyed the autopsies done on individuals diagnosed as having childhood psychosis. This survey included eight cases of autistic symptomatology, and in six of these cases evidence of diverse neuropathological change was indicated. More recently, Williams, Hauser, Purpura, DeLong, and Swisher (1980) reported autopsies on four patients who displayed autistic behavior. The authors examined sections of the hippocampus, parahippocampal gyrus, thalamus, hypothalamus, striatum, and midbrain tectum. They found no gross abnormalities, and they suggested that the neurological abnormality in autism may be metabolic, or may be structural but not detectable by current commonly available neuropathological techniques.

Most recently Bauman and Kemper presented a report (1985) in which they examined the brain of a 29-year-old autistic man and found morphological abnormalities in the hippocampal complex, subiculum, entorhinal cortex, septal nuclei, mammillary body, selected nuclei of the amygdala and neocerebellar cortex, and deep cerebellar nuclei and inferior olive.

Caparulo et al. (1981) and Harcherik et al. (1985) both compared various groups of children with developmental delay. In the 1981 study the authors report that of 22 children with primary childhood autism, 2 had clearly abnormal CT scans involving increased ventricular size and 2 autistic children, in addition, had mildly abnormal scans, 1 with a prominent fourth ventrical and 1 with a very large cisterna magnum. In the 1985 study the group reports similarly that 2 out of 16 individuals diagnosed as autistic, or 13% of the sample, showed evidence of ventricular asymmetry. Both studies, however, taken together found no significant differences across diagnostic groups, including infantile autism, attention deficit disorder, Tourette disorder, and language disorder. It is the authors' contention that ventricular abnormalities are not specifically associated with the syndrome of autism.

In a similar fashion Campbell et al. (1982) and Rosenbloom et al. (1984) replicated their own findings. In 1982, 45 children with autism were studied by means of CT scan. For 11 of the 45 children, evidence of ventricular enlargement was found. In 1984, Rosenbloom et al. reported that a study of 13 autistic children replicated the findings of the 1982 study in showing that a small proportion of the sample of 13 autistic children had ventricular enlargement. Prior, Tress, Hoffman, & Boldt (1984) have recently reported that CT scans on 9 autistic boys showed no sign of any abnormality.

As is apparent from this abbreviated review, there is no clear single deficit or pattern of deficit associated with autism.

Findings of deficit in one study are often not replicated in subsequent studies conducted on other samples. For example, while Hauser et al. (1975) and Damasio et al. (1980) found evidence of ventricular abnormalities, Prior et al. (1984) did not. And while Tanguay et al. (1982) and Skoff et al. (1980) found significant BAEP abnormalities in autistic subjects, Rumsey et al. (1984) did not. Furthermore, while Hier et al. (1979) found evidence for reversed cerebral asymmetry, Tsai and Stewart (1982) and Prior et al. (1984) did not.

The failure to replicate findings has been variously attributed to shifts or problems in diagnostic practice, to methodological differences across studies, to limitations of sample size, and to sample heterogeneity. While it is widely accepted that the behavioral syndrome of autism may have multiple etiologies, it is nonetheless still widely believed that there is likely to be some physiological commonality leading to the behavioral syndrome (Damasio, 1984).

The unity of the clinical or behavioral syndrome itself is rarely questioned except in terms of diagnostic criteria (Waterhouse, Fein, Nath, & Snyder, in press).

Moreover, most findings cannot be considered unique to autistic symptoms or the autistic syndrome but are found in other developmentally disordered or neurological populations as well.

In addition to the problem of paucity of autism-specific findings and failures of replication, a third problem is that few studies have found an association between specific symptoms or behaviors (within the autistic syndrome) and specific neurological deficits. This may be largely due to the fact that few studies explore such possible links.

For example, Aarkrog found that very early evidence of psychotic symptoms occurred more frequently in the group of children he saw who had abnormal PEGs than in the group with normal PEGs who are also autistic. However, Aarkrog also found that the most severe symptomatology coupled with loss of previously acquired speech occurred in the group of children who have normal PEGs. Neither of these findings, however, showed significance on a chi-square test. Fein *et al.* (1981) found an association between abnormalities in BAEP and the psychopathology of social relatedness found in the autistic syndrome. Small's review of EEG data (1975) suggested an association between abnormal EEG and lower verbal performance and lower full-scale IQs, and an association between abnormal EEG findings and greater neurological impairment and poorer long-term outcome.

More typical of findings is Campbell *et al.* (1982), where the authors report that *t* tests failed to show any relationship between indices of ventricular size in autistic patients and measured clinical variables such as language development, adaptive behaviors, severity of withdrawal, stereotypies, and the like. Rumsey *et al.* (1985) also found no relationship between PET scan abnormalities and measures of cognitive or social impairment. Courchesne also reported that there was no connection between smaller amplitudes and various components of the ERPs shown for the autistic subjects he studied and their performance accuracy in classifying targets (a behavioral index).

Despite these serious limitations, one may examine the neurological studies as a whole for consistent trends. The only results that appear across several studies and have been documented in a reasonable number of cases are (1) ventricular enlargement and (2) a variety of EEG and EP abnormalities. The EEG and EP abnormalities (except perhaps for BAEP findings) are fairly nonspecific to autism and often nonlocalizing, as well as being quite diverse. The ventricular enlargements found in an impressive number of cases may produce, or be secondary to, mesial cortical destruction. In either case, the finding is consistent with dysfunction in the mesial temporal and frontal structures of the limbic system (see discussion of this point in Chapter 13). In addition, the most technically sophisticated serial section study of an autistic brain recently performed by Bauman and Kemper shows clear evidence of problems in exactly the areas indicated (see Chapter 13). The circuitry that they outline as impaired and abnormal in the brain they studied is circuitry that certainly would be implied as part of any system controlling the emotional and social behavior suggested by current theoretical models. As Bauman and Kemper report, lesions in the regions they have explored can produce prominent effects on motivation, emotion, memory, and learning. It is also true that bilateral amygdalectomy in monkeys leads the monkeys to no longer fear normally aversive stimuli and to withdraw from rewarding social interactions. Mishkin and Bachevalier (personal communication, 1985) have begun a study of monkeys with bilateral ablation of the hippocampus and amygdala. Their research to date suggests that autisticlike behaviors in social-tactile avoidance of other monkeys may be generated by such ablations.

One thing that emerges clearly is the need for further investigation of the character of memory deficit in autistic individuals. There has been very little work done to date (Boucher, 1981; Boucher & Warrington, 1976; Frith, 1970a, 1970b), and the work that has been done leaves pertinent questions unanswered. If the limbic system is implicated, then memory must be impaired in autistic individuals. One puzzle is what *types* of memory are affected in autistic individuals. At present there is no clear or comprehensive answer.

If the limbic system deficit model of autism is to be explored, then both imaging studies and studies of the relationships between memory and social deficit need to be conducted on populations of autistic individuals. While Bauman and Kemper's single case neuropathologic findings suggest to them (1985) that memory deficits may underlie all other deficits in autism, neuropsychological research suggests that this is unlikely.

It is possible that the severe learning deficits shown by their severely retarded case resulted from bilateral involvement of both amygdala and hippocampus. Perhaps in other cases, where the autistic child is more high functioning and has islands of presevered ability, the hippocampus is spared but the amygdala affected, resulting in social impairment but some intact learning capacity. Clearly, more work needs to be done to outline these crucial relationships within autistic individuals.

CONCLUSIONS

There is a set of fundamental limitations affecting the inferences that can be drawn from the research findings to date. These limitations, however, also suggest crucial directions for research:

1. We don't yet know what the crucial set of defining deficits are for the syndrome of autism—there is currently debate about which aspects of the syndrome are the key or defining aspects.
2. We currently do not have an adequate formal structural analysis of normal or abnormal social behavior.
3. We don't yet know the links between relatively more primitive social functions (gaze, touch, attachment, emotions) and social cognition.
4. We don't know the true nature of different emotions in terms of cognitive labeling and arousal states.
5. We don't know the specific developmental course of social behaviors.
6. We don't have knowledge of those brain systems that may be sources for social and emotional behavior, although we have evidence concerning some aspects of these systems.
7. We don't adequately understand the developmental course of the brain systems that may be hypothesized to underlie or control aspects of social behavior and emotion.
8. A final caveat is that much work in this area is essentially argument by analogy. For example, Hauser *et al.* (1975) argue that autistic children's deficits are like those of individuals with Korsakoff syndrome. Hetzler and Griffin (1981) have similarly argued that the deficits of autistics are analogous to the deficits found in the Kluver–Bucy syndrome. Bauman and Kemper (1985) have supported the

theoretical modeling of Hetzler and Griffin and have suggested that the findings from their single autopsy case do suggest damage in the areas that might be damaged in Kluver–Bucy syndrome. Arguments by analogy are potent and provocative, but a direct chain of relationship in any series of cases has yet to be proven.

While the knowledge of social impairments in autism has existed clinically since Kanner's first report in 1943, the notion that social deficits are key to the syndrome is just now being accepted (Denckla, 1986), and the notion that the social deficits have a direct organic basis is just beginning to be outlined (Fein et al., 1986). While the nature of the relationship between cognitive and social behaviors is not yet well elucidated (Rutter, 1983), work on the question continues.

Because of the lack of consistent positive findings for neuropathology or inferred brain structure deficit, and because of the presence of great clinical heterogeneity in the manifestation of symptoms (Waterhouse et al., in press) in autistic populations, the issue of the unity of the syndrome is still under question (Damasio, 1984). Thus it is important not only that future work focus on the relationship of memory deficits to social deficits, and focus on more refined versions of imaging studies on larger populations, but also that populations to be studied in these designs include both autistic individuals and individuals who have autisticlike symptoms of social impairment, but who fail to meet currently determined diagnostic criteria.

ACKNOWLEDGMENTS

This work was supported by NIMH Research Scientist Development Awards to authors Fein and Pennington and project awards from NIMH (MH00250-06 and MH40162-01) and NINCDS (NS20489-01A1 to the Child Neurology Society—International Neuropsychological Society Joint Task Force on Nosology of Higher Cortical Dysfunction in Children) to Drs. Waterhouse and Fein. We are grateful to Drs. Martha Denckla and Marlene Oscar Berman for theoretical and moral support, to Dr. Thomas Anders, Dr. Lorna Wing, Dorothy Lucci, Mark Braverman, Linda Wiesner, and the Developmental Psychobiology Research Group at the University of Colorado for stimulating theoretical discussions, and to Rose Razzino for editoral assistance and manuscript preparation.

REFERENCES

Aarkrog, T. (1968). Organic factors in infantile psychoses and borderline psychosis. Danish Medical Bulletin, November, 283–287.
Bartak, L., & Rutter, M. (1976). Differences between mentally retarded and normally intelligent autistic children. Journal of Autism and Childhood Schizophrenia, 6, 109–120.
Bartak, L., Rutter, M., & Cox, A. (1975). A comparative study of infantile autism and specific developmental receptive language disorder. I. The children. British Journal of Psychiatry, 126, 127–145.
Bauman, M. L., & Kemper, T. L. (1985). Histoanatomic observations of the brain in early infantile autism. Neurology, 35, 866–874.
Bauman, M. L., & LeMay, M., Bauman, R. A., & Rosenberger, P. B. (1985). Computerized tomographic (C.T.) observations of the posterior fossa in early infantile autism. Neurology, 35, 247.

Benton, A. L. (1979). Visuoperceptive, visuospatial, and visuoconstructive disorders. In K. M. Heilman & E. Valenstein (Eds.), *Clinical neuropsychology* (pp. 186–232). New York: Oxford University Press.

Borod, J., Koff, E., & Caron, H. (1983). Right hemispheric specialization for the expression and appreciation of emotion: A focus on the face. In E. Perecman (Ed.), *Cognitive processes in the right hemisphere*. New York: Academic Press.

Boucher, J. (1981). Memory for recent events in autistic children. *Journal of Autism and Developmental Disorders, 11*, 293–302.

Boucher, J., & Warrington, E. K. (1976). Memory deficits in early infantile autism: Some similarities to the amnesic syndrome. *British Journal of Psychology, 67*, 73–87.

Bryden, M. P., & Ley, R. G. (1983). Right hemisphere involvement in the perception and expression emotion in normal humans. In K. M. Heilman & P. Satz, (Eds.), *Neuropsychology of human emotion* (pp. 6–44). New York: Guilford Press.

Bryden, M. P., Ley, R. G., & Sugarman, J. H. (1982). A left ear advantage for identifying the emotional quality of tonal sequences. *Neurologia, 20*, 83–87.

Campbell, M., Rosenbloom, S., Perry, R., George, A. J., Kirchell, I. I., Anderson, L., Small, A. M., & Jennings, S. J. (1982). Computerized axial tomography in young autistic children. *American Journal of Psychiatry, 139*, 510–512.

Caparulo, B. K., Cohen, D. J., Rothman, S. L., Young, J. G., Katz, J. D., Shaywitz, S. E., & Shaywitz, B. A. (1981). Computed tomographic brain scanning in children with developmental neuropsychiatric disorders. *Journal of the American Academy of Child Psychiatry, 20*, 338–357.

Cohen, D. J., Caparulo, B., & Shaywitz, B. A. (1978). Neurochemical and developmental models of childhood autism. In G. Serban, (Ed.), *Cognitive defects in the development of mental illness* (pp. 66–102). New York: Brunner/Mazel.

Courchesne, E., Lincoln, A., Kilman, B., & Galambos, R. (1985). Event-related brain potential correlates of the processing of novel visual and auditory information in autism. *Journal of Autism and Developmental Disorders, 15*, 55–76.

Damasio, A. R. (1979). The frontal lobes. In K. M. Heilman, & E. Valenstein, (Eds.), *Clinical neuropsychology*. (pp. 360–412). New York: Oxford University Press.

Damasio, A. R. (1984). Autism. *Archives of Neurology, 41*, 481.

Damasio, A., & Maurer, R. (1978). A neurological model for childhood autism. *Archives of Neurology, 35*, 777–786.

Damasio, H., Maurer, R. G., Damasio, A. R., & Chui, H. C. (1980). Computerized tomographic scan findings in patients with autistic behavior. *Archives of Neurology, 37*, 504–510.

Damasio, A. R., & Van Hoesen, G. W. (1983). Emotional disturbances associated with focal lesions of the limbic frontal lobe. In K. M. Heilman, & P. Satz, (Eds.), *Neuropsychology of human emotion*. (pp. 85–110). New York: Guilford Press.

Darby, J. (1976). Neuropathologic aspects of psychology in children. *Journal of Autism and Childhood Schizophrenia, 6*, 339–352.

DeLong, G. R. (1978). A neuropsychologic interpretation of infantile autism. In M. Rutter, & E. Schopler, (Eds.), *Autism: A reappraisal of concepts and treatment* (pp. 207–219). New York: Plenum Press.

Denckla, M. (1986). New diagnostic criteria for autism and related behavioral disorders—guidelines for research protocols. (Editorial). *Journal of American Academy of Child Psychiatry, 25*, 221–224.

Dennis, M. (1983). The developmentally dyslexic brain and the written language skills of children with one hemisphere. In U. Kirk, (Ed.), *Neuropsychology of language, reading, and spelling* (pp. 185–208). New York: Academic Press.

Deykin, E. Y., & MacMahon, B. (1979). The incidence of seizures among children with autistic symptoms. *American Journal of Psychiatry, 136*, 1310–1312.

Douglas, R. J., & Marcellus, D. (1975). The ascent of man: Deductions based on a multivariate analysis of the brain. *Brain, Behavior and Evolution, 2*, 179–213.

Eisenberg, L., & Kanner, L. (1956). Early infantile autism, 1943–1955. *American Journal of Orthopsychiatry, 26*, 556–566.

Emde, R. N., Katz, E. L., & Thorpe, J. K. (1978). Emotional expression in infancy: II. Early deviations in Down's syndrome. In M. Lewis, & L. A. Rosenblum, (Eds.), *The development of affect.* (pp. 351–359). New York: Plenum Press.

Fein, D., Humes, M., Kaplan, E., Lucci, D., & Waterhouse, L. (1984). The question of left hemisphere dysfunction in infantile autism. *Psychological Bulletin, 95*, 258–281.

Fein, D., Pennington, B., Markowitz, P., Braverman, M., & Waterhouse, L. (1986). Towards a neuropsychological model of autism. *Journal of the American Academy of Child Psychiatry, 25*, 198–212.

Fein, D., Skoff, B., & Mirsky, A. F. (1981). Clinical correlates of brainstem dysfunction in autistic children. *Journal of Autism and Developmental Disorders, 11*, 303–315.

Fein, D., Waterhouse, L., Lucci, D., & Snyder, D. (1985). Cognitive subtypes in developmentally disabled children: A pilot study. *Journal of Autism and Developmental Disorders, 15*, 77–95.

Francis, P. L., Self, P. A., & McCaffree, M. A. (1984). Behavioral assessment of a hydraencephalic infant. *Child Development, 55*, 262–266.

Frith, U. (1970a). Studies in pattern detection in normal and autistic children: I. Immediate recall of auditory sequences. *Journal of Abnormal Psychology, 76*, 413–420.

Frith, U. (1970b). Studies in pattern detection in normal and autistic children: II. Reproduction and production of color sequences. *Journal of Experimental Child Psychology, 10*, 120–135.

Geschwind, N. (1979). Specializations of the human brain. *Scientific American, 241*(3), 180–202.

Goldman-Rakic, P., Isseroff, A., Schwartz, M. L., & Bugbee, N. M. (1983). The neurobiology of cognitive development. in M. M. Haith, & J. Campos, (Eds.), *Infancy and developmental psychobiology*, Vol. 2, of P. H. Mussen, (Ed.), *Handbook of child psychology* (4th ed., pp. 282–344). New York: Wiley.

Greenberg, N., MacLean, P. D., & Ferguson, J. L. (1979). Role of the paleostriatum in species-typical display behavior of the lizard (*anolis carolinensis*). *Brain Research, 172*, 229–241.

Harcherik, D., Cohen, D., Ort, S., Paul, R., Shaywitz, B., Volkmar, F., Rothman, S. & Leckman, J. (1985). Computed tomographic brain scanning in four neuropsychiatric disorders of childhood. *American Journal of Psychiatry, 142*, 731–734.

Hauser, S., DeLong, R., & Rosman, P. (1975). Pneumographic findings in the infantile autism syndrome. *Brain, 98*, 667–688.

Heilman, K. M., Watson, R. T., & Bowers, D. (1983). Affective disorders associated with hemispheric disease. In K. M. Heilman, & P. Satz, (Eds.), *Neuropsychology of human emotion* (pp. 45–64). New York: Guilford Press.

Hetzler, B., & Griffin, J. (1981). Infantile autism and the temporal lobe of the brain. *Journal of Autism and Developmental Disorders, 11*, 317–330.

Hier, D. B., LeMay, M., & Rosenberger, P. B. (1979). Autism and unfavorable left-right asymmetries of the brain. *Journal of Autism and Developmental Disorders, 9*, 153–160.

Hobson, R. P. (1981). The autistic child's concepts of person. *International conference on autism.* Boston: National Society for Autistic Children.

Hobson, R. P. (1982, September 17–20). *The autistic child's knowledge of persons.* Invited paper for a symposium on affective and social understanding, BPS Developmental Section Conference, Durham, England.

Isaacson, R. L. (1982). *The limbic system* (2nd ed.). New York: Plenum Press.

Izard, C. E. (1971). *The face of emotion.* New York: Appleton-Century-Crofts.

Jennings, W. (1973). A study of the preference for affective cues in autistic children. *Dissertation Abstracts International, 34*(8-B), 4045–4046.

Kanner, L. (1943). Autistic disturbances of affective contact. *Nervous Child, 2*, 217–250.

Kling, A., & Steklis, H. D. (1976). A neural substrate for affiliative behaviors in non-human primates. *Brain Behavior and Evolution, 13*, 126–238.

Kluver, H., & Bucy, P. C. (1939). Preliminary analysis of functions of the temporal lobes in monkeys. *Archives of Neurological Psychology, 42*, 979–1000.

Konner, M. (1982). Biological aspects of the mother–infant bond. In R. Emde, & R. Harmon, (Eds.), *The development of attachment* (pp. 31–54). New York: Plenum Press.

Lamendella, J. (1977). The limbic system. In M. Whitaker, & H. Whitaker, (Eds.), *Studies in neurolinguistics* (Vol. 3, pp. 157–222). New York: Academic Press.

Ley, R. G., & Bryden, M. P. (1979). Hemispheric differences in recognizing faces and emotions. *Brain and Language, 7*, 127–138.

Ley, R. G., & Bryden, M. P. (1982). A dissocation of right and left hemispheric effects for recognizing emotional tone and verbal content. *Brain and Cognition, 1*, 3–9.

Lishman, W. A. (1978). *Organic psychiatry*. Oxford: Blackwell Scientific.

MacLean, P. D. (1952). Some psychiatric implications of physiological studies on fronto-temporal portion of limbic system (visceral brain). *Electroencephalography and Clinical Neurophysiology, 4*, 407–418.

MacLean, P. D. (1973). *A triune concept of the brain and behavior*. Toronto: Toronto University Press.

MacLean, P. D. (1978). Effects of lesions of globus pallidus on species-typical display behavior of squirrel monkeys. *Brain Research, 149*, 175–196.

MacLean, P. D. (1985). Brain evolution relating to family, play and the separation call. *Archives of General Psychiatry, 42*, 405–417.

Mayeux, R. (1983). Emotional changes associated with basal ganglia disorders. In K. M. Heilman, & P. Satz, (Eds.), *Neuropsychology of human emotion* (pp. 141–164). New York: Guilford Press.

Mirsky, A. F. (1960). Studies of the effects of brain lesions on social behavior in macaca mulatta: Methodological and theoretical considerations. *Annals of the New York Academy of Sciences, 85*, 785–794.

Murphy, M. R., MacLean, P. D., & Hamilton, S. C. (1981). Species-typical behavior of hamsters deprived from birth of the neocortex. *Science, 213*, 459–461.

Ornitz, E., Guthrie, D., & Farley, A. J. (1978). The early symptoms of childhood autism. In G. Serban, (Ed.), *Cognitive defects in the development of mental illness* (pp. 24–42). New York: Brunner/Mazel.

Park, C. (1967). *The seige*. Boston: Little, Brown.

Prior, M. R., Tress, B., Hoffman, W. L., & Boldt, D. (1984). Computed tomographic study of children with classic autism. *Archives of Neurology, 41*, 482–484.

Richer, J. M., & Coss, R. G. (1976). Gaze aversion in autistic and normal children. *Acta Psychologica, 53*, 193–210.

Rimland, B. (1964). *Infantile autism: The syndrome and its implications for a neural theory of behavior*. New York: Appleton-Century-Crofts.

Rosenbloom, S., Campbell, M., George, A. E., Kircheff, I. I., Taleporos, E., Anderson, L., Reuben, R. N., & Korein, J. (1984). High resolution CT scanning in infantile autism: A quantitative approach. *Journal of the American Academy of Child Psychiatry, 23*, 72–77.

Ross, E. D. (1981). The aprosodias. Functional-anatomic organization of the affective components of language in the right hemisphere. *Archives of Neurology, 38*, 745–748.

Ross, E. D. (1983). Right-hemisphere lesions in disorders of affective language. In A. Kertesz, (Ed.), *Localization in neuropsychology* (pp. 493–508). New York: Academic Press.

Ross, I. S. (1959). An autistic child. *Pediatric Conferences, 2*, 1–13.

Rumsey, J., Duara, R., Grady, C., Rapoport, J., Margolin, R., Rapoport, S., & Cutler, N. (1985). Brain metabolism in autism. *Archives of General Psychiatry, 42*, 448–455.

Rumsey, J., Grimes, A., Pikus, A., Duara, R., & Ismond, D. (1984). Auditory brain stem responses in pervasive developmental disorders. *Biological Psychiatry, 19*, 1403–1418.

Rutter, M. (1968). Concepts of autism: A review of research. *Journal of Child Psychiatry, 9*, 1–25.

Rutter, M. (1979). Maternal deprivation, 1972–1978: New findings, new concepts, new approaches. *Child Development, 50*, 283–305.

Rutter, M. (1983). Cognitive deficits in the pathogenesis of autism. *Journal of Child Psychology and Psychiatry, 24*, 513–531.

Sacks, O. (1973). *Awakenings*. London: Duckworth.

Schain, R., & Yannet, H. (1960). Infantile autism, an analysis of 50 cases and a consideration of certain relevant neurophysiological concepts. *Journal of Pediatrics, 57*, 550–567.

Sigman, M., & Ungerer, J. (1981). Sensorimotor skills and language comprehension in autistic children. *Journal of Abnormal Child Psychology, 9*, 149–165.

Sigman, M., & Ungerer, J. (1984). Cognitive and language skills in autistic, mentally retarded and normal children. *Developmental Psychology, 20*, 293–302.

Skoff, B. F., Mirsky, A. F., & Turner, D. (1980). Prolonged brainstem transmission time in autism. *Psychiatric Research, 2*, 151–166.

Small, J. G. (1975). EEG and neurophysiological studies of early infantile autism. *Biological Psychiatry, 10*, 385–397.

Stamm, J. S. (1955). The function of the median cerebral cortex in maternal behavior in rats. *Journal of Comparative and Physiological Psychology, 48*, 347–356.

Stuss, D. T., & Benson, D. F. (1983). Frontal lobe lesions and behaviors. In A. Kertesz (Ed.), *Localization in neuropsychology* (pp. 429–454). New York: Academic Press.

Tager-Flushberg, H. (1981). On the nature of linguistic functioning in early infantile autism. *Journal of Autism and Developmental Disorders, 11*, 45–56.

Tanguay, P. E. (1984). Toward a new classification of serious psychopathology in children. *Journal of the American Academy of Child Psychiatry, 23*, 373–384.

Tanguay, P. E., Edwards, R. M., Buchwald, J., Schwafel, J., & Allen, V. (1982). Auditory brainstem evoked responses in autistic children. *Archives of General Psychiatry, 39*, 174–180.

Trevarthen, C. (1983). Development of the cerebral mechanisms for language. In U. Kirk, (Ed.), *Neuropsychology of language, reading and spelling* (pp. 45–80). New York: Academic Press.

Tsai, L. Y., & Stewart, M. A. (1982). Handedness and EEG correlation in autistic children. *Biological Psychiatry, 17*, 595–598.

Waterhouse, L., Fein, D., Nath, J., & Snyder, D. (in press). PDD and SOC: A review of critical commentary. In G. Tischler, (Ed.), *Diagnosis and classification in psychiatry*. New York: Cambridge University Press.

Weir, K., & Salisbury, D. (1980). Acute onset of autistic features following brain damage in a ten-year-old. *Journal of Autism and Developmental Disorders, 10*, 185–191.

Williams, R. S., Hauser, S. L., Purpura, P. D., DeLong, G. R., & Swisher, C. N. (1980). Autism and mental retardation: Neuropathologic studies in four retarded persons with autistic behavior. *Archives of Neurology, 37*, 749–753.

Wing, L. (1974). Language development and autistic behaviors in severely mentally retarded children. *Proceedings of the Royal Society of Medicine, 67*, 1031–1032.

Wing, L. (1976). Diagnosis, clinical description and prognosis. In L. Wing, (Ed.), *Early childhood autism* (pp. 15–48). New York: Pergamon Press.

Wing, L. (1981). Language, social and cognitive impairments in autism and severe mental retardation. *Journal of Autism and Developmental Disorders, 11*, 31–44.

Wolff, S., & Barlow, A. (1979). Schizoid personality in childhood: A comparative study of schizoid, autistic and normal children. *Journal of Child Psychology and Psychiatry, 20*, 29–46.

The Neurochemical Basis of Symptoms in the Lesch–Nyhan Syndrome
Relationship to Central Symptoms in Other Developmental Disorders

GEORGE R. BREESE, ROBERT A. MUELLER, and
STEPHEN R. SCHROEDER

INTRODUCTION

There have been a number of investigations in adult patients that have associated neurological symptoms with neurochemical alterations in brain. For example, lesions to specific neural systems have been described for such conditions as Parkinsonism (Bernheimer, Birkmayer, Hornykiewicz, Jellinger, & Seitelberger, 1973; Grafe, Forno, & Eng, 1985; Hornykiewicz, 1973; Javoy-Agid et al., 1984; Scatton, Javoy-Agid, Montfort, & Agid, 1984; Taquet et al., 1983; Tenovuo, Rinne, & Viljanen, 1984; Uhl, Whitehouse, Price, Tourtelotte, & Kuhar, 1984), Huntington chorea (Bird & Iversen, 1974; Enna et al., 1976; Enna, Stern, Wastek, & Yamamura, 1977; Rossor & Emson, 1982), and Alzheimer disease (Candy et al., 1983; Coyle, Price, & DeLong, 1983; Gottfries et al., 1983; Nemeroff, Youngblood, Manberg, Prange, & Kizer, 1983). However, few studies have attempted to relate symptoms observed in developmental disorders of the central nervous system—such as autism, mental retardation, or motor disabilities—to deficiencies in specific neurotransmitter systems. An exception to this general thesis is a report by Lloyd et al. (1981), who examined the neurotransmitter deficiencies found in Lesch–Nyhan disease—a developmental syndrome associated with a genetic deficiency of the enzyme hypoxanthine-guanine phosphoribosyltransferase (HGPRT) (Gutensohn, 1984; Kelley & Wyngaarden, 1983; Patel & Caskey, 1985; Wilson, Young, & Kelley, 1983).

GEORGE R. BREESE • Departments of Psychiatry and Pharmacology, Child Development Institute and Mental Health Clinical Research Center, University of North Carolina, Chapel Hill, North Carolina 27514. ROBERT A. MUELLER • Departments of Anesthesiology and Pharmacology, and STEPHEN R. SCHROEDER • Department of Psychiatry, Child Development Institute, University of North Carolina, Chapel Hill, North Carolina 27514.

Information concerning the basic neurobiology of the Lesch–Nyhan syndrome could have particular relevance to understanding symptoms in autism. Both syndromes have considerable overlap of symptoms, including movement disorder, stereotypes, intellectual impairment, interpersonal difficulties, and behavioral problems (Schopler, Reichler, DeVellis, & Daly, 1980). In this chapter, the symptoms found in Lesch–Nyhan disease will be reviewed and related to the neurochemical findings about this childhood disorder. In addition, symptoms of the Lesch–Nyhan syndrome will be compared to those in Parkinson disease, an adult neurological disorder with a comparable neurochemical deficiency. We will also discuss our effort to develop an animal model of the neurological deficiency observed in children with Lesch–Nyhan disease and indicate how results from this work have allowed conclusions about the neurobiology of the behavioral and motor disturbances in these children. Finally, the relationship of these findings to the possible involvement of neurotransmitters observed in other developmental disorders with central symptoms similar to the Lesch–Nyhan syndrome (e.g., autism, self-injurious behavior) will be discussed.

NEUROLOGICAL SYMPTOMS

The Lesch–Nyhan syndrome is an inborn error of purine metabolism that is expressed exclusively in males (Lesch & Nyhan, 1964). As a result of a deficiency of the enzyme HGPRT, these patients cannot reuse certain purines. Instead, these purine building blocks are metabolized to uric acid for excretion. The high levels of this purine metabolite are responsible for some of the somatic clinical findings that resemble gout (Kelley & Wyngaarden, 1983; Seegmiller, Rosenbloom, & Kelley, 1967). Neurological manifestations of Lesch–Nyhan disease, which are not observed in patients with gout, include choreoathetosis, hypertonicity, opisthotonus, aggression, and compulsive self-biting (Lesch & Nyhan, 1964; Nyhan, 1976). Patients with Lesch–Nyhan disease appear normal at birth, and the severe central neurological abnormalities of this syndrome are not apparent until about 5 months of age. By 1 year of age, chorea and writhing movements of the extremities are usually noted and muscular hypertonicity is invariably observed (Kelley & Wyngaarden, 1983). These symptoms associated with motor function are sufficiently severe that older children cannot stand without assistance (Kelley & Wyngaarden, 1983; Lesch & Nyhan, 1964). While mental retardation is usual in Lesch–Nyhan patients (Nyhan, 1976), there are cases where normal intelligence is observed (Christie et al., 1982; Nyhan, personal communication). The self-biting observed in Lesch-Nyhan syndrome has a variable onset, but it always occurs (Christie et al., 1982; Nyhan, 1976). In children with this disorder, tissue loss about the mouth and amputation of digits are commonly observed (Lesch & Nyhan, 1964). Since sensory modalities appear intact, a lack of pain perception cannot explain this behavior (Nyhan, 1976).

NEUROCHEMICAL ASSESSMENT

The motor dysfunction noted in patients with Lesch–Nyhan disease suggests an involvement of the basal ganglia. The basal ganglia are a group of subcortical structures which make up a portion of the extrapyramidal system in the central nervous system and which integrate voluntary movements. Parkinsonism and Huntington disease are central disorders of basal ganglia structures. Particularly important to the function of the basal ganglia is the pathway that originates in the substantia nigra and terminates in the corpus striatum.

This system is known to be made up of dopamine-containing neurons and has been demonstrated to be deficient in Parkinson disease.

Regarding basal ganglia involvement in Lesch–Nyhan disease, Lloyd *et al.* (1981) recently reported that biochemical measures of the function of central dopamine-containing neurons at autopsy are deficient in Lesch–Nyhan patients. Dopamine content is reduced by 80 to 90% in areas of the basal ganglia of affected patients, as are activities for dopa decarboxylase and tyrosine hydroxylase, enzymes found in dopaminergic neurons. These latter data suggest that dopaminergic fibers largely disappear or do not develop normally. Markers for other neurotransmitters in brain were also examined. Glutamic acid decarboxylase (GAD) and dopamine-beta-hydroxylase activities are not reduced, indicating that gamma-aminobutyric acid (GABA)ergic and noradrenergic fibers, respectively, are not affected. However, plasma dopamine-beta-hydroxylase, a marker for peripheral noradrenergic neurons, is reduced (Lake & Ziegler, 1977). Serotonin content, an index of serotonin-containing neurons, is increased in the striatum of patients with Lesch–Nyhan disease, and choline acetyltransferase (CAT) activity, the marker for cholinergic neurons, is reduced in only one area of the striatum (i.e., putamen) of these children. These data indicate that patients with Lesch–Nyhan disease have a primary deficit in central dopaminergic pathways, with the possibility that the site-specific changes in central cholinergic and serotonergic neurons may contribute to their neurological symptoms. While the reduced content of plasma dopamine-beta-hydroxylase may account for the diminished peripheral sympathetic responses in Lesch–Nyhan disease (Lake & Ziegler, 1977), this change does not likely contribute to the central symptoms associated with this disorder.

The very fact that dopaminergic neurons are deficient in children with Lesch–Nyhan disease, who also have a deficiency of HGRPT preventing a means to conserve purines, suggests some link between purine metabolism and the survival or development of these neurons. In Parkinson patients, however, even though dopaminergic fibers are absent, changes in purine metabolites are not observed. Therefore, it appears more likely that abnormal purine metabolism is merely one way to reduce dopamine content, as opposed to the less likely possibility that a deficiency of dopaminergic neurons invokes abnormal purine metabolism in brain. However, it is unclear whether the neurochemical deficiency of dopamine observed in Lesch–Nyhan patients and their HGPRT deficiency are causally linked or if they are simply separate sequelae of the genetic defect.

Because dopamine-containing neurons and HGPRT are both deficient in brain in Lesch–Nyhan disease, one could argue that HGPRT activity is particularly important for the appropriate ontogenesis or survival of dopaminergic neurons. HGPRT activity in the CNS is normally highest in the basal ganglia, which also is the richest area for dopaminergic neurons, and is higher in other brain areas than in peripheral tissues (Howard, Kerson, & Appel, 1970; Krenitsky, 1969). Like the neurotransmitters, HGRPT rises rapidly in brain during early development. While the products of this enzyme, guanilyic acid (GMP) and inosinic acid (IMP), can be synthesized through alternate pathways (which could possibly prevent cell death), the enzyme activity of these alternate pathways is low and is not increased in Lesch–Nyhan patients (Kelley & Wyngaarden, 1983). These findings suggest that neurons in brain may be unusually dependent upon the HGPRT salvage pathway for normal cellular function. It is not known whether the destructive process associated with dopaminergic neurons in Lesch–Nyhan patients is due to the loss of products of HGRPT (e.g., GMP, IMP, and their phosphorylated derivatives) or to the abnormally elevated purine metabolites that accumulate (e.g., hypoxanthine, xanthine, and uric acid) as a result of the absence of HGRPT. Also unknown is whether a deficiency of the products of HGPRT alters the ability of cells in brain to form cyclic nucleotides (e.g., ATP, GTP, binding protein), which may play a role in a variety of cellular processes, including neurotransmitter synthesis and transfer of information from neurotransmitter receptors. Regardless of the exact involvement of HGPRT, the HGPRT deficiency likely has its effect during the period of ontogenesis, disrupting arborization and synaptogenesis of dopaminergic neurons.

COMPARISON WITH PARKINSONISM AND HUNTINGTON CHOREA

Parkinsonism is an adult affliction associated with the loss of dopamine-containing fibers in brain (Hornykiewicz, 1973). Since dopamine-containing fibers are also reduced in the brain of patients with Lesch–Nyhan disease, one might suppose that the motor dysfunctions would resemble those of Parkinson patients. However, in spite of their common biochemical deficiency, the symptoms in these two afflictions are not comparable. Lesch–Nyhan patients have choreoathetoid movements and hypertonicity rather than the tremor, bradykinesia, stooped posture, and stiffness associated with Parkinsonism. Further, Parkinson patients do not have self-biting associated with their syndrome, as do children with the HGRPT deficiency. Both syndromes can have impairment of intellect (Benson, 1984; Lesch & Nyhan, 1964), suggesting that reduced dopaminergic function could contribute to such mental deficiency in both diseases. It is well documented that Parkinson patients have their motor symptoms improved when treated with a dopamine agonist. There is anectodal evidence that symptoms of patients with Lesch–Nyhan disease are worsened when given such drug therapy. In addition to these differences in symptoms, there is one major neurochemical difference. In Lesch–Nyhan disease, serotonin content in the striatum is elevated (Lloyd et al., 1981), whereas content of this neurotransmitter is reduced in Parkinsonism.

The fact that cholinergic function is reduced in the basal ganglia of Lesch–Nyhan patients could also contribute to their symptoms (Lloyd et al., 1981). There is considerable literature that documents influences of dopamine on the function of cholinergic fibers (Butcher,, 1977; Lloyd, 1975; Nose & Takemoto, 1974). Motor symptoms in children with Lesch–Nyhan disease are reminiscent of those observed in the adult form of Huntington chorea. However, while Huntington disease patients have deficiencies of acetylcholine as well as GABA in the striatum, they are without changes in markers for dopaminergic function (Bird & Iversen, 1974; Eckernas, 1977). The similarity of Lesch–Nyhan motor dysfunction to the choreic movements in Huntington disease and the observation that this symptom is exacerbated by dopaminergic agonists is compatible with a similar neural mechanism (Klawans, Paulson, Ringel, & Barbeau, 1972). However, self-biting has not been described in Huntington disease, even when these patients were challenged with L-dopa. Therefore, by inference, it could be suggested that the reduction in acetylcholine in the Lesch–Nyhan syndrome is not responsible for self-biting, because this symptom is not observed in Huntington disease. Thus, the susceptibility for self-biting that is associated with the Lesch–Nyhan disorder is logically attributable to the absence of dopaminergic fibers observed in this syndrome (Lloyd et al., 1981). Again by inference, symptoms such as the mental retardation observed in the Lesch–Nyhan syndrome may well be attributable to loss of cholinergic fibers because juvenile as well as adult patients with brain acetylcholine dysfunction are reported to demonstrate learning and memory deficits (Coyle et al., 1983). However, as pointed out earlier, an involvement of the dopamine deficiency in the mental deficiency cannot be excluded, because Parkinson patients can demonstrate loss of mental capacity (Benson, 1984). The relationship of the altered cholinergic function in Lesch–Nyhan syndrome to the motor dysfunction cannot be defined at this time.

Another important difference between Parkinsonism and Lesch–Nyhan disease is the age of onset of the symptoms. In this regard, it is important to note that motor dysfunction in the juvenile form of Huntington disease is characterized by bradykinesia—a symptom similar to that described for Parkinson disease (Enna *et al.*, 1976, 1977). This is an obvious shift in the character of the motor symptoms observed in the adult form of Huntington disease. Thus, the different motor dysfunctions observed in Parkinsonism and Lesch–Nyhan patients or in the adult and juvenile forms of Huntington disease strongly suggest that *the age at which neural function is disrupted is an important factor in the type of motor symptoms observed after a neural insult to basal ganglia structures.*

MODELING THE NEUROCHEMICAL DEFICIT

The goal of neurological research is to understand the etiology and neural mechanisms of disorders of the CNS. Such knowledge should permit development of appropriate protocols for corrective treatment of these diseases. For obvious reasons, achievement of this goal would be hampered if all basic research had to be performed in humans. To overcome this disadvantage, neurobiologists have sought to produce animal models that are sufficiently homologous to the human disease to permit definition of underlying neurochemical abnormalities (Breese, Mueller, Mailman, Frye, & Vogel, 1978). This general approach has led investigators to take several strategies to "model" the self-biting in the Lesch–Nyhan syndrome (Casas-Bruce *et al.,* 1985; Minana, Portoles, Jorda, & Grisolia, 1984; Mueller, Saboda, Palmour, & Nyhan, 1982). In spite of these investigations, understanding of the central dysfunctions in Lesch–Nyhan disease has been limited.

The report by Lloyd *et al.* (1981) that dopamine is reduced in brain of Lesch–Nyhan patients provided evidence that at least some of the symptoms may be associated with this neurochemical change. It is rare to find a single specific neurotransmitter dysfunction implicated in a disease state or even with specific symptoms. The discovery that dopamine is deficient in the basal ganglia of patients with Parkinson disease marked a major breakthrough in the understanding and subsequent treatment of this neurological disorder (see Hornykiewicz, 1973). The knowledge of the human neurochemical pathology in Lesch–Nyhan disease clearly provides a strategy by which the neurochemical deficiency can be duplicated in animals. In regard to this strategy to produce an animal model of the dopamine deficiency in Lesch–Nyhan disease, pharmacological means are available to destroy catecholamine-containing pathways (Breese & Traylor, 1970, 1971) and to preferentially reduce brain dopamine (Breese & Traylor, 1972; Smith, Cooper, & Breese, 1973) in developing rats. We have previously shown that adult rats can be treated with 6-hydroxydopamine (6-OHDA) to produce the neurochemical deficiency associated with Parkinsonism (Breese *et al.*, 1978). Thus, comparison of adult and neonatally adult treated rats might resolve why symptoms in Parkinson and Lesch–Nyhan syndromes differ, even though the two have a similar neurochemical deficit.

In previous work with 6-OHDA-treated developing rats (Smith *et al.*, 1973), we demonstrated prominent functional deficits, including reduced body weight, learning disabilities, deficits in ingestive behavior, and altered responses to dopamine-mimetics (Breese, Cooper, & Smith, 1973). These deficits are similar to certain dysfunctions seen in Parkinsonism and Lesch–Nyhan patients. However, neither rats treated as adults nor those treated neonatally with 6-OHDA spontaneously show self-biting (Breese *et al.*, 1973).

Some years ago, workers in our laboratory observed that self-mutilation of forepaws is commonly observed in mature rats lesioned neonatally with 6-OHDA when their dopamine receptors were activated by administration of L-dihydroxyphenylalanine (L-dopa), data consistent with the report of Creese and Iversen (1973). Ungerstedt (1971b) reported self-biting in adult rats with bilateral 6-OHDA lesions to the nigrostriatal pathways when high doses of the dopamine receptor agonist apomorphine are administered. Other investigators (Herrera-Marschitz & Ungerstedt, 1984; Kuga & Goldstein, 1984; Ungerstedt, 1971a) also reported that unilateral 6-OHDA lesions in young rats can result in self-biting after dopamine receptor activation with apomorphine treatment. Treatment of rats with various dopamine agonists with a normal complement of dopamine-containing nerve terminals does not produce self-mutilation.

When postsynaptic receptors are deprived of stimulation, a compensatory increase in the sensitivity of these receptors occurs. In this regard, the loss of dopamine-containing neurons induces a functional supersensitivity of dopamine receptors. Data with dopamine agonists in neonatally lesioned rats suggest that activation of supersensitive dopamine receptors is essential to produce self-biting behavior. On the basis of clinical data in patients with Parkinsonism or Lesch–Nyhan disease, we postulated that the incidence of self-biting following L-dopa administration would be greater in neonatally 6-OHDA-treated rats compared to adult 6-OHDA-treated rats because of the age at which the dopaminergic fibers were destroyed. Similarly, motor function would be expected to differ between these 6-OHDA treatment groups.

Recently, we obtained direct evidence for this hypothesis. When challenged with L-dopa, self-biting is not observed in control rats or in adult 6-OHDA-treated rats, but it is observed in adult rats lesioned neonatally with 6-OHDA (Breese, Baumeister, McCown, Emerick, Frye, Crotty, & Mueller, 1984; Breese, Baumeister, McCown, Emerick, Frye, & Mueller, 1984). In addition to the increased susceptibility for self-biting observed when dopaminergic fibers are destroyed neonatally, the character of certain behavioral responses to dopamine agonists is found to differ between neonatally and adult 6-OHDA-lesioned rats (Breese et al., 1984 [both]). In addition, the locomotor response to apomorphine is significantly greater in adult 6-OHDA-lesioned rats than in those rats with dopamine-containing fibers destroyed neonatally (Breese, Baumeister, McCown, Emerick, Frye, Crotty, & Mueller, 1984). Moreover, the striatum is found to have serotonin elevated in neonatally 6-OHDA-lesioned rats, just as seen in Lesch–Nyhan disease (Breese, Baumeister, McCown, Emerick, Frye, Crotty, & Mueller, 1984). Thus, on the basis of these findings in 6-OHDA-lesioned rats, it seems appropriate to attribute the behavioral and biochemical differences to the age at which the dopamine-containing neurons were destroyed. Thus, these data support our view that the neonatal 6-OHDA treatment can serve as a neurochemical model of the deficiency of brain dopamine in Lesch–Nyhan disease.

AGE-DEPENDENT RESPONSES: NEUROBIOLOGICAL CONSIDERATIONS

It seemed particularly important to define the basis of the behavioral differences between adult and neonatally 6-OHDA-lesioned rats since this might allow clues as to therapies for treating symptoms in children with Lesch–Nyhan disease. It is clear that supersensitive dopamine receptors are important for the drug-induced precipitation of self-mutilation. However, this view appears inconsistent with the failure of neuroleptic drugs, such as thioridiazine and haloperidol, which antagonize dopamine function, to decrease self-mutilation behavior in Lesch–Nyhan disease or other types of self-injurious behavior (Singh & Millichamp, 1985).

Recently, it has become clear that there are at least two types of dopamine receptors in brain that have been designated D-1 and D-2 subtypes (Kebabian & Calne, 1979). In recent years, several drugs have been developed that interact with these dopamine receptor subtypes. Setler, Serau, Zirkle, and Saunders (1978) introduced a compound, SKF-38393, with properties consistent with an agonist action on D-1 dopamine receptors. While SKF-38393 produces only minor behavioral changes in control rats, it facilitates turning in rats with unilateral 6-OHDA lesions of the nigrostriatal dopamine pathway. Iorio, Barnett, Leitz, Houser, and Korduba (1983) introduced a compound, SCH-23390, which is believed to be a D-1 dopamine antagonist, and LY-171555 is a dopamine agonist with primary actions on D-2 receptors (Tsuruta et al., 1981). Many neuroleptics, including haloperidol, antagonize D-2 dopamine receptors (Seeman, 1980). Thus, specific D-1 and D-2 receptor agonists and antagonists for dopamine receptor subtypes are available to explore the relative contribution of each to behavioral changes observed in neonatally and adult 6-OHDA-lesioned rats after L-dopa administration.

In our original publication contrasting the behaviors of adult and neonatally 6-OHDA-treated rats after L-dopa challenge, it was observed that the dopamine antagonist, cis-flupentixol, was more potent than haloperidol as an antagonist of the self-biting induced by L-dopa in neonatally 6-OHDA-lesioned rats. Because cis-flupentixol is a neuroleptic that inhibits adenylate cyclase activated by dopamine (Christensen, Arnt, Hytell, Larson, & Svendsen, 1984; Hyttel, 1978), it is believed to have greater effects on D-1 dopamine receptors than haloperidol, which has potent effects on D-2 dopamine receptors (Seeman, 1980). On the basis of this observation, it was postulated that D-1 dopamine receptors might be more responsible for the self-biting behavior after L-dopa administration than D-2 dopamine receptors (Breese, Baumeister, McCown, Emerick, Frye, Crotty, & Mueller, 1984).

Subsequent investigations supported this hypothesis that functionally supersensitive D-1 dopamine receptors are specifically involved in the self-mutilation behavior observed after L-dopa administration to neonatally 6-OHDA-lesioned rats (Breese, Baumeister, Napier, Frye, & Mueller, 1985). This conclusion is based upon (1) the antagonism of this behavior by SCH-23390, a D-1 dopamine receptor antagonist, (2) induction of self-mutilation behavior in neonatally 6-OHDA-treated rats by the D-1 dopamine receptor agonist (SKF-38393), (3) a high correlation between the supersensitive locomotor responses to the D-1 receptor agonist with the occurrence of L-dopa-induced self-mutilation, and (4) the inability of the D-2 agonist, LY-171555, to induce self-mutilation behavior. Previous investigations demonstrated that haloperidol does not block self-mutilation behavior in patients with Lesch–Nyhan syndrome (Watts, McKeran, Brown, Andrews, & Griffiths, 1974)—an observation consistent with the inability of even high doses of this drug to completely antagonize self-mutilation behavior induced by L-dopa in neonatally 6-OHDA-lesioned rats (Breese et al. 1984 [both]; Breese, Baumeister, Napier, et al., 1985).

Additional investigations indicated that other motor responses induced by the D-1 and D-2 agonists differed between adult and neonatally 6-OHDA-lesioned rats (Breese, Baumeister, Napier, et al., 1985; Breese, Napier, & Mueller, 1985). Administration of the D-1 dopamine agonist resulted in a major locomotor increase in neonatally 6-OHDA-lesioned rats, with a smaller response observed with adult 6-OHDA-treated rats (Breese, Napier, & Mueller, 1985). These data suggest that a primary increase in the functional sensitivity of D-1 dopamine receptors is responsible for locomotor activity induced by L-dopa in neonatally

6-OHDA-lesioned rats. In rats lesioned with 6-OHDA as adults, the D-2 dopamine agonist produces a dose-related increase in locomotor activity that is several times that of normal. In neonatally 6-OHDA-treated rats, the locomotor response to the D-2 dopamine agonist (LY-171555) is less than one-third that seen in adult-lesioned rats (Breese, Napier, & Mueller, 1985). This finding with the specific D-2 dopamine agonist is similar to that for apomorphine reported earlier (Breese, Bauemeister, McCown, Emerick, Frye, Crotty, & Mueller, 1984). Behaviors other than locomotor activity were also examined after D-1 and D-2 dopamine agonist administration (Breese, Baumeister, Napier, et al., 1985). In this case, except for the incidence of self-biting, the two agonists produce similar behaviors in neonatally 6-OHDA-treated rats, but some motor responses differ from those observed in adult 6-OHDA-lesioned rats (Breese, Baumeister, Napier, et al., 1985). These observations provide convincing evidence that behavioral responses could indeed be attributed to the D-1 dopamine receptor subtype in the neonatally lesioned rats, but that this alteration alone does not account for the age-dependent differences in behavior.

INVESTIGATION OF DOPAMINE RECEPTOR SUPERSENSITIVITY

It is well documented that a unilateral lesion to dopamine-containing neurons in adult rats causes an increase in the number of receptor sites, as indicated by ^{3}H-spiperone binding in striatum ipsilateral to the side of the lesion. This procedure is a standard biochemical method for quantifying receptors for neurotransmitters. This increase in ^{3}H-spiperone binding sites is suggested to be responsible for the functional supersensitivity observed with dopamine agonists after such lesions (Creese, Burt, & Snyder, 1977). For this reason, we explored whether such a change in receptor number is present in our 6-OHDA-lesioned rats. In this case, binding of ^{3}H-spiperone and ^{3}H-Sch-23390, antagonist ligands for D-2 (Seeman, 1980) and D-1 dopamine receptors (Billard, Ruperts, Crosby, Iorio, & Barnett, 1984), respectively, were chosen to explore this question. In contrast to results after unilateral lesions to a dopaminergic pathway, binding of these ligands is not altered by the adult or neonatal 6-OHDA lesions (Breese, Duncan, et al., 1986; Breese, Mueller, et al., 1986), which would destroy dopaminergic systems bilaterally. In view of these results, a change in receptor number for dopamine antagonists does not appear to account for the functional supersensitivity of dopamine agonists after these treatments. This absence of an association of behavioral supersensitivity and receptor binding suggests that future experiments will need to resolve what appear to be discrepancies in our present understanding of dopamine receptor mechanisms as related to their functional supersensitivity. If an alteration in receptor number is not responsible for the enhanced responses after dopamine agonists, it would seem likely that a postreceptor mechanism that converts receptor occupation to cellular change is responsible for the functional hypersensitivity after destruction of dopamine-containing neurons. Previous work (Breese, Mueller, & Mailman, 1979) indicates that generation of cAMP, a second messenger for certain receptors, is not involved in the supersensitivity to dopamine agonists with primary actions on D-2 dopamine receptors in adult 6-OHDA-lesioned rats. This latter observation appears consistent with the recent finding that D-2 receptors inhibit dopamine-stimulated adenylate cyclase (Onali, Olianas, & Gessa, 1985). It has yet to be determined whether this second messenger is involved in the supersensitive responses to D-1 dopamine receptor activation in neonatally 6-OHDA-lesioned rats.

PURINERGIC MECHANISMS ASSOCIATED WITH SELF-BITING

Because a deficiency of HGRPT alters several enzymes associated with purine metabolism (Kelley & Wyngaarden, 1983), it is only natural that the relationship of such changes to the self-biting seen in Lesch–Nyhan patients has been investigated. One possible link between self-biting, purine metabolism, and dopamine may be adenosine—a purine compound proposed to be directly involved in neurotransmission (Snyder, 1985), producing an inhibition of spontaneous firing of neurons. Urinary excretion of adenosine has been found to be decreased in Lesch–Nyhan patients (Sweetman & Nyhan, 1970). Further, Wojcik and Neff (1983a, 1983b) have recently observed that striatal adenosine is decreased after destruction of GABA-containing neurons in the striatum, whereas destruction of dopamine-containing neurons did not alter adenosine content, release, or receptor binding. These observations provide additional evidence that purines may influence dopaminergic neurons, rather than reduced dopamine release affecting purinergic mechanisms.

There is further evidence for this latter conclusion. Previous data have demonstrated interactions between adenosine receptor antagonists such as the methylxanthines and dopamine responses (Anden & Jackson, 1975). Furthermore, chronic administration of high doses of methylxanthines (e.g., theophylline and caffeine) results in self-mutilation in unlesioned rats (Mueller et al., 1982). This methylxanthine-induced behavior could be due to blockade of adenosine receptors (Snyder, 1985). It has also been reported that the unilateral reduction of dopamine in striatum enhances the ability of theophylline to produce self-injury in rats (Casas-Bruce et al., 1985), and we have observed such behavior after theophylline treatment of neonatally 6-OHDA-treated rats (Criswell, Mueller, & Breese, 1986). In addition, we recently observed that bilateral administration of an adenosine analogue into the striatum blocks the self-mutilation and associated behaviors induced by L-dopa in neonatally 6-OHDA-lesioned rats (Criswell et al., 1986). However, an excess of an adenosine analogue placed into one striatum induces self-mutilation when administered with apomorphine (Green, Proudfit, & Young, 1982). Since local application of the adenosine analogue would be expected to decrease dopamine function, it is possible that this paradigm may in fact resemble mechanistically the unilaterally lesioned rats given apomorphine (Ungerstedt, 1971a). Thus, given the reduced level of adenosine in children with a deficiency of HGPRT, it is possible that this alteration increases further the sensitivity of dopamine receptors to dopamine or allows additional amounts of dopamine to be released from remaining dopaminergic fibers in these patients. Either of these possibilities could contribute to the abnormal behaviors and motor dysfunction observed in Lesch–Nyhan disease (see next section).

POSSIBLE TREATMENT STRATEGIES

The basic findings in the neurochemical model of Lesch–Nyhan disease provide important strategies for treatment. Even though brain dopamine is reduced in Lesch–Nyhan disease, the usual replacement therapy for the motor dysfunction in Parkinsonism, L-dopa, would appear to be contraindicated in the childhood disorder. This view is based upon the remarkable sensitivity neonatally 6-OHDA-treated rats have for exhibiting self-biting and skin lacerations after L-dopa treatment (Breese, Baumeister, McCown, Emerick, Frye, Crotty, & Mueller,

1984). Therefore, it would appear advisable to antagonize D-1 dopamine receptors before initiating any dopamine agonist therapy in Lesch–Nyhan patients. D-2 dopamine receptor agonists are useful in Parkinsonism (Lieberman, Shopsin, Lebruth, Boal, & Zolfaghari, 1975) and do influence motor function of neonatally 6-OHDA-lesioned rats (Breese, Napier, & Mueller, 1985). Nevertheless, it is not known whether administration of a D-2 dopamine receptor agonist would be beneficial to the motor dysfunction in the Lesch–Nyhan syndrome or would exacerbate the choreic symptoms, as observed with L-dopa in Huntington chorea (Klawans et al., 1972).

The data in neonatally 6-OHDA-lesioned rats do not permit conclusions whether activation of dopamine receptors is the mechanism by which self-biting is induced in Lesch–Nyhan disease. It is possible that other neural mechanisms can precipitate self-biting once the susceptibility for this response is increased by the neonatal destruction of dopamine-containing fibers. However, recent clinical reports from patients with Lesch–Nyhan disease are relevant to this question. Silverstein, Johnston, Hutchinson, and Edwards (1985) reported that homovanillic acid (HVA), the major metabolite of dopamine, is reduced, but not absent, in spinal fluid of children with Lesch–Nyhan disease. Further, Goldstein, Anderson, Reuben, and Dancis (1985) reported that fluphenazine, but not haloperidol, antagonized or attenuated the self-biting observed in patients with Lesch–Nyhan disease. Since fluphenazine antagonizes both D-1 and D-2 dopamine receptors (Breese, Mueller, Napier, & Duncan, 1986), these latter results suggest that activation of dopamine receptors is responsible for, or contributes to, the self-mutilation in these patients. Further, it supports the hypothesis (Breese, Baumeister, McCown, Emerick, Frye, Crotty, & Mueller, 1984) that the D-1 dopamine receptor subtype is more important than the D-2 dopamine receptor for initiating this behavior. Once a specific D-1 dopamine receptor blocker is available clinically, it will be possible to determine with certainty whether activation of D-1 dopamine receptors alone is critical for the incidence of self-biting in Lesch–Nyhan patients or whether other neural mechanisms contribute to this symptom.

In addition to the potential of administering drugs that affect dopaminergic function directly to modify neurological symptoms associated with Lesch–Nyhan disease, it should be investigated whether alterations in neurotransmitter systems that modify dopaminergic function may be an alternative for treating their neurological symptoms. The potential for drugs that activate adenosine receptors has been mentioned. Recent data suggest that endogenous opiate systems may be involved in self-injurious behavior (Richardson & Zaleski, 1983) and these systems are known to influence dopaminergic function (Algeri, Calderimi, Consolazione, & Garattini, 1977; Van Loon & Kim, 1978; Wood, Stotland, Richard, & Rackham, 1980). Withdrawal from chronic opiate treatment can result in self-biting in rodents, implicating endogenous opiates in this abnormal behavior (Leander, McMillan, & Harris, 1975; Lucot, McMillan, & Leander, 1979). In this regard, several investigators have recently described the effectiveness of naloxone, an opiate antagonist, to reduce self-injurious behavior in mentally retarded persons (Richardson & Zaleski, 1983; Sandman et al., 1983; Sandyk, 1985); others have failed to find this therapeutic advantage (Beckwith, Couk, & Schumacher, 1986; Davidson, Kleene, Carroll, & Rockowitz, 1983). These preliminary clinical observations will need to be extended before the general utility of this latter treatment can be assessed. While neurotransmitters other than the examples provided can influence dopaminergic function, additional animal experiments are necessary to determine whether these neural systems contribute to symptoms in Lesch–Nyhan disease or if their influence can be applied to a strategy for treating symptoms in Lesch–Nyhan disease.

RELEVANCE OF NEUROCHEMICAL FINDINGS TO OTHER DEVELOPMENTAL DISORDERS

Many children with developmental disorders have symptoms common with the Lesch–Nyhan syndrome. Therefore, data being collected in this defined genetic disease may provide important clues for the basis of symptoms in other developmental disorders of the CNS. For example, some children with autism have mental retardation, choreiform movements, and self-injurious and aggressive behaviors reminiscent of symptoms in Lesch–Nyhan disease (Nyhan, 1976). Could a deficiency of dopamine or a change associated with a specific purinergic defect (other than HGPRT) account for these symptoms in autism or other developmental disorders as they appear to in the Lesch–Nyhan disorder? As already indicated, information defining the neurochemical basis of symptoms in adult-onset disorders may not be applicable to childhood disorders. It is our belief that information available concerning the neurochemical basis of symptoms in Lesch–Nyhan disease can provide a new strategy for dissecting the neurochemical basis of motor symptoms, mental deficiencies, and perhaps self-mutilation associated with other developmental diseases of the CNS. Similarly, the symptoms and neurochemistry associated with early onset of Huntington chorea during childhood may provide an equally important avenue for exploration of the neurochemical basis of symptoms associated with other central disorders in pediatric patients that resemble those seen in this early-onset form of Huntington disease. Certainly, these examples provide support for the often stated view that "children are not small adults." Belief in this view and the emerging information concerning the neurochemical basis of symptoms in Lesch–Nyhan disease and childhood Huntington chorea should provide a rational basis to explore the neurobiology of symptoms in developmental disorders of the CNS with symptomatology like those observed in these defined genetic disorders.

SUMMARY

There are few studies in autism or other developmental disabilities where a specific set of symptoms can be related to deficiencies in specific neurotransmitter systems. A noted exception is the Lesch–Nyhan syndrome, a sex-linked genetic disorder of purine metabolism in which dopamine is found to be deficient. Recent animal and human studies suggest that Lesch–Nyhan syndrome may be a neurobiological window for conceptualizing the ontogenesis and treatment of self-injurious behavior and other symptoms observed in this childhood disorder. It is hypothesized that susceptibility for self-biting is selectively related to a neonatal deficiency of dopamine and a compensatory increase in D-1 dopamine receptor functional sensitivity. A critical principle is that the age at which the neural insult to dopamine-containing neurons occurs can have an important influence on the motor symptoms manifested. Therefore, careful evaluation of the symptoms observed in Lesch–Nyhan disease may allow differentiating the neural basis of symptoms in other developmental disorders of the central nervous system that resemble those seen in Lesch–Nyhan disease.

ACKNOWLEDGMENTS

The authors wish to acknowledge the excellent typing assistance of Carolyn Reams. The work was supported by USPHS grants MH-33127, HD-03110, and HL-31424.

REFERENCES

Algeri, S., Calderini, G., Consolazione, H., & Garattini, S. (1977). The effect of methionine-enkephalin and d-alanine methione-enkephalinamide on the concentration of dopamine metabolites in rat striatum. *European Journal of Pharmacology, 45,* 207–209.

Anden, N-E., & Jackson, D. M. (1975). Locomotor activity stimulation in rats produced by dopamine in the nucleus accumbens: Potentiation by caffeine. *Journal of Pharmacy and Pharmacology, 27,* 666–670.

Beckwith, B., Couk, D., & Schumacher, K. (1986). Effectiveness of naloxone in reducing self-injurious behavior in two developmentally disabled females. *Applied Research in Mental Retardation 7,* 183–188.

Benson, D. F. (1984). Parkinsonian dementia: Cortical or subcortical. *Advances in Neurology, 40,* 235–240.

Bernheimer, H., Birkmayer, W., Hornykiewicz, O., Jellinger, & Seitelberger, F. (1973). Brain dopamine and the syndromes of Parkinson and Huntington: Clinical, morphological and neurochemical correlates. *Journal of Neurological Science, 20,* 415–455.

Billard, W., Ruperts, V., Crosby, G., Iorio, L. S., & Barnett, A. (1984). Characterization of the binding of ^{3}H-SCH-23390, a selective D-1 receptor antagonist ligand, in rat striatum. *Life Sciences, 35,* 1885–1893.

Bird, E. D., & Iversen, L. L. (1974). Post-mortem measurement of glutamic acid decarboxylase, choline acetyltransferase and dopamine in basal ganglia. *Brain, 97,* 457–472.

Breese, G. R., Baumeister, A. A., McCown, T. J., Emerick, S. G., Frye, G. D., Crotty, K., & Mueller, R. A. (1984). Behavioral differences between neonatal and adult-6-hydroxydopamine treated rats to dopamine agonists: Relevance to neurological symptoms in clinical syndromes with reduced brain dopamine. *Journal of Pharmacology and Experimental Therapeutics, 231,* 343–354.

Breese, G. R., Baumeister, A. A., McCown, T. J., Emerick, S. G., Frye, G. D., & Mueller, R. A. (1984). Neonatal-6-hydroxydopamine treatment: Model of susceptibility for self-mutilation in the Lesch–Nyhan syndrome. *Pharmacology, Biochemistry and Behavior, 21,* 459–461.

Breese, G. R., Baumeister, A., Napier, T. C., Frye, G. D., & Mueller, R. A. (1985). Evidence that D-1 dopamine receptors contribute to the supersensitive behavioral responses induced by L-dihydroxyphenylalanine in rats treated neonatally with 6-hydroxydopamine. *Journal of Pharmacology and Experimental Therapeutics, 235,* 287–295.

Breese, G. R., Cooper, B. R., & Smith, R. D. (1973). Biochemical and behavioral alterations following 6-hydroxydopamine administration into brain. In E. Usdin & S. Snyder (Eds.)., *Frontiers in catecholamine research* (pp. 701–706). New York: Pergamon Press.

Breese, G. R., Duncan, G., Napier, T. C., Bondy, S. C., Emerick, S., Iorio, L. C., & Mueller, R. A. (1986). 6-Hydroxydopamine treatments enhance behavioral responses to intra-cerebral microinjection of D-1 and D-2 dopamine agonists into nucleus accumbens and striatum without changing dopamine antagonist binding. *Journal of Pharmacology and Experimental Therapeutics.*

Breese, G. R., Mueller, R. A., & Mailman, R. B. (1979). Effect of dopaminergic agonists and antagonists on *in vivo* cyclic nucleotide content: Relation of guanosine 3′:5′monophosphate (cGMP) changes in cerebellum to behavior. *Journal of Pharmacology and Experimental Therapeutics, 209,* 262–270.

Breese, G. R., Mueller, R. A., Mailman, R. B., Frye, G. D., & Vogel, R. A. (1978). An alternative to animal models of central nervous system disorders: Study of drug mechanisms and disease symptoms in animals. *Progress in neuropsychopharmacology, 2,* 313–325.

Breese, G. R., Mueller, R. A., Napier, T. C., & Duncan, G. E. (1986). Neurobiology of D-1 dopamine receptors after neonatal 6-OHDA treatment: Relevance to Lesch–Nyhan disease. In G. Breese & I. Creese (Eds.), *Neurobiology of central D-1 dopamine receptors* (pp. 197–216). New York: Plenum Press.

Breese, G. R., Napier, T. C., & Mueller, R. A. (1985). Dopamine agonist-induced locomotor activity in rats treated with 6-hydroxydopamine at differing ages: Functional supersensitivity of D-1 dopamine receptors in neonatally lesioned rats. *Journal of Pharmacology and Experimental Therapeutics, 234,* 447–455.

Breese, G. R., & Traylor, T. D. (1970). Effects of 6-hydroxydopamine on brain norepinephrine and dopamine: Evidence for selective degeneration of catecholamine neurons. *Journal of Pharmacology and Experimental Therapeutics, 174,* 413–420.

Breese, G. R., & Traylor, T. D. (1971). Depletion of brain noradrenaline and dopamine by 6-hydroxydopamine. *British Journal of Pharmacology, 42,* 88–89.

Breese, G. R., & Traylor, T. D. (1972). Developmental characteristics of brain catecholamines and tyrosine hydroxylase in the rats: Effects of 6-hydroxydopamine. *British Journal of Pharmacology, 44,* 210–222.

Butcher, L. L. (1977). Nature and mechanisms of cholinergic-monoaminergic interactions in the brain. *Life Sciences, 21,* 1207–1226.

Candy, J. M., Perry, R. H., Perry, E. K., Irving, D., Blessed, G., Fairbairn, A. F., & Tomlinson, B. E. (1983). Pathological changes in the nucleus of Meynert in Alzheimer's and Parkinson's diseases. *Journal of Neurological Science, 59,* 277–289.

Casas-Bruce, M., Almenar, C., Grau, I. M., Jane, J., Herrera-Marschitz, M., & Ungerstedt, U. (1985). Dopaminergic receptor supersensitivity in self-mutilatory behaviour of Lesch–Nyhan disease. *Lancet, 1,* 991–992.

Christensen, A. V., Arnt, J., Hytell, J., Larson, J. J., & Svendsen, O. (1984). Pharmacological effects of a specific dopamine D-1 antagonist SCH-23390 in comparison with neuroleptics. *Life Sciences, 34,* 1529–1540.

Christie, R., Bay, C., Kaufman, I. A., Bakay, B., Borden, M., & Nyhan, W. L. (1982). Lesch–Nyhan disease: Clinical experience with nineteen patients. *Developmental Medicine and Child Neurology, 24,* 293–306.

Coyle, J. T., Price, D. L., & DeLong, M. R. (1983). Alzheimer's disease: A disorder of cortical cholinergic innervation. *Science, 219,* 1184–1190.

Creese, I., Burt, D. R., & Snyder, S. H. (1977). Dopamine receptor binding enhancement accompanies lesion-induced behavioral supersensitivity. *Science, 197,* 596–598.

Creese, I., & Iversen, S. D. (1973). Blockade of amphetamine-induced motor stimulation and stereotypy in the adult rat following neonatal treatment with 6-hydroxydopamine. *Brain Research, 55,* 369–382.

Criswell, H. B., Mueller, R. A., & Breese, G. R. (1986). Evidence for adenosine–dopamine interactions in the CNS. *Society for Neuroscience Abstracts, 12,* 10027.

Davidson, P. W., Kleene, B. M., Carroll, M., & Rockowitz, R. J. (1983). Effects of naloxone on self-injurious behavior: A case study. *Applied Research in Mental Retardation, 4,* 1–4.

Eckernas, S.-A. (1977). Plasma choline and cholinergic mechanisms in the brain. *Acta Physiologica Scandinavica Supplementum, 449,* 1–62.

Enna, S. J., Bird, E. D., Bennett, J. P., Jr., Bylund, D. B., Yamamura, H. I., Iversen, L. L., Snyder, S. H. (1976). Huntington's chorea–Changes in neurotransmitter receptors in the brain. *New England Journal of Medicine, 294,* 1305–1309.

Enna, S. J., Stern, L. Z., Wastek, G. J., & Yamamura, H. I. (1977). Neurobiology and pharmacology of Huntington's disease. *Life Sciences, 20,* 205–212.

Goldstein, M., Anderson, L. T., Reuben, R., & Dancis, J. (1985). Self-mutilation in Lesch–Nyhan disease is caused by dopaminergic denervation. *Lancet, 1,* 338–339.

Gottfries, C-G., Adolfsson, R., Aquilonius, S-M., Carlsson, A., Eckernas, S-A., Nordberg, A., Oreland, L., Svennerholm, L., Wiberg, A., & Winblad, B. (1983). Biochemical changes in dementia disorders of Alzheimer type. *Neurobiology of Aging, 4,* 261–271.

Grafe, M. R., Forno, L. S., & Eng, L. F. (1985). Immunocytochemical studies of Substance P and Met-Enkephalin in the basal ganglia and substantia nigra in Huntington's, Parkinson's and Alzheimer's disease. *Journal of Neuropathology and Experimental Neurology, 44,* 47–59.

Green, R. D., Proudfit, H. K., & Yeung, S-M. H. (1982). Modulation of striatal dopaminergic function by local injection of 5'-N-ethylcarboxamide adenosine. *Science, 218*, 58–61.

Gutensohn, W. (1984). Inherited disorders of purine metabolism—Underlying molecular mechanisms. *Klinische Wochenschrift, 62*, 953–962.

Herrera-Marschitz, M., & Ungerstedt, U. (1984). Evidence that striatal efferents relate to different dopamine receptors. *Brain Research, 323*, 269–278.

Hornykiewicz, O. (1973). Parkinson's disease: From brain homogenate to treatment. *Federation Proceedings, 32*, 183–190.

Howard, W. J., Kerson, L. A., & Appel, S. H. (1970). Synthesis denovo of purines in slices of rat brain and liver. *Journal of Neurochemistry, 17*, 121–123.

Hyttel, J. (1978). A comparison of the effect of neuroleptic drugs on binding of ^{3}H-flupenthixol and adenylate cyclase activity in rat striatal tissue *in vitro*. *Progress in Neuropsychopharmacology, 2*, 239–335.

Iorio, L. C., Barnett, A., Leitz, F. H., Houser, V. P., & Korduba, A. (1983). SCH-23390, a potential benzazepine antipsychotic with unique interactions on dopaminergic systems. *Journal of Pharmacology and Experimental Therapeutics, 226*, 462–468.

Javoy-Agid, F., Taquet, H., Cesselin, F., Epelbaum, J., Grouselle, D., Mauborgne, A., Studler, J. M., & Agid, Y. (1984). Neuropeptides in Parkinson's disease. In *Catecholamines: Neuropharmacology and central nervous system—Therapeutic aspects* (pp. 34–42).

Kebabian, J. W., & Calne, D. B. (1979). Multiple receptors for dopamine. *Nature (London), 227*, 93–96.

Kelley, W. N., & Wyngaarden, J. B. (1983). Clinical syndromes associated with hypoxanthine-guanine phosphoribosyl-transferase deficiency. In J. B. Stanberry, Y. B. Wyngaarden, D. S. Frederickson, J. L. Goldstein, & M. S. Brown (Eds.)., *The metabolic basis of inherited disease* (pp. 1115–1143). New York: McGraw Hill.

Klawans, W. L., Paulson, G. W., Ringel, S. P., & Barbeau, A. (1972). Use of L-dopa in the detection of presymptomatic Huntington's chorea. *New England Journal of Medicine, 286*, 1332–1334.

Krenitsky, T. A. (1969). Tissue distribution of purine ribosyl- and phosphoribosyltransferases in the rhesus monkey. *Biochimica et Biophysica Acta, 179*, 506–509.

Kuga, S., & Goldstein, M. (1984). Effect of dopamine agonists on compulsive self-mutilation behavior in monkeys and rats with lesions of the nigro-striatal dopamine neurons. *Federation Proceedings, 1984, 43*, 585.

Lake, C. R., & Ziegler, M. G. (1977). Lesch–Nyhan syndrome: Low dopmaine-B-hydroxylase activity and diminished sympathetic responses to stress and posture. *Science, 196*, 905–906.

Leander, J. D., McMillan, D. E., & Harris, L. S. (1975). Schedule induced oral narcotic administration: Acute and chronic effects. *Journal of Pharmacology and Experimental Therapeutics, 195*, 279–287.

Lesch, M., & Nyhan, W. L. (1964). A familial disorder of uric acid metabolism and central nervous system function. *American Journal of Medicine, 36*, 561–570.

Lieberman, A. N., Shopsin, B., Lebruth, Y., Boal, D., & Zolfaghari, M. (1975). Studies on Piribedil in Parkinsonism. *Advances in Neurology, 9*, 339–413.

Lloyd, K. G. (1975). Special chemistry of the basal ganglia 2. Distribution of acetylcholine, choline acetyltransferase and acetylcholinesterase. *Pharmacology and Therapeutics Bulletin*, part B, *1*, 63–77.

Lloyd, K. G., Hornykiewicz, O., Davidson, L., Shannak, K., Farley, I., Goldstein, M., Shibuya, M., Kelly, W. N., & Fox, I. H. (1981). Biochemical evidence of dysfunction of brain neurotransmitters in the Lesch–Nyhan syndrome. *New England Journal of Medicine, 305*, 1106–1111.

Lucot, L. B., McMillan, D. E., & Leander, J. D. (1979). The behavioral effects of d-amphetamine alone and in combination with acute and chronic morphine treatments in rats. *Journal of Pharmacology and Experimental Therapeutics, 210*, 158–165.

Minana, M. D., Portoles, M., Jorda, A., & Grisolia, S. (1984). Lesch–Nyhan syndrome, caffeine model: Increase of purine and pyrimidine enzymes in rat brain. *Journal of Neurochemistry*, 1984, *43*, 1556–1560.

Mueller, K., Saboda, S., Palmour, R., & Nyhan, W. L. (1982). Self-injurious behavior produced in rats by daily caffeine and continuous amphetamine. *Pharmacology, Biochemistry and Behavior*, *17*, 613–617.

Nemeroff, C. B., Youngblood, W. W., Manberg, P. J., Prange, A. J., Jr., & Kizer, J. S. (1983). Regional brain concentrations of neuropeptides in Huntington's chorea and schizophrenia. *Science*, *221*, 972–155.

Nose, T., & Takemoto, H. (1974). Effect of oxotremorine on homovanillic acid concentration in the striatum of the rat. *European Journal of Pharmacology*, *25*, 51–55.

Nyhan, W. (1976). Behavior in the Lesch–Nyhan syndrome. *Journal of Autism and Childhood Schizophrenia*, *6*, 235–252.

Onali, P., Olianas, M., & Gessa, G. L. (1985). Characterization of dopamine receptors mediating inhibition of adenylate cyclase activity in rat striatum. *Molecular Pharmacology*, *28*, 138–145.

Patel, P. I., & Caskey, C. T. (1985). HPRT and the Lesch–Nyhan syndrome. *Bioessays*, *2*, 4–7.

Richardson, J. S., & Zaleski, W. A. (1983). Naloxone and self-mutilation. *Biological Psychiatry*, *18*, 99–101.

Rossor, M. N., & Emson, P. C. (1982). Neuropeptides in degenerative disease of the central nervous system. *Trends in Neuroscience*, *5*, 399–401.

Sandman, C. A., Datta, P. C., Barron, J., Hochler, F. K., Williams, C., & Swanson, J. W. (1983). Naloxone attenuates self-abusive behavior in developmentally disabled clients, *Applied Research in Mental Retardation*, *4*, 5–11.

Sandyk, R. (1985). Naloxone abolishes self-injuring in a mentally retarded child. *Annals of Neurology*, *17*, 520.

Scatton, B., Javoy-Agid, F., Montfort, J. C., & Agid, Y. (1984). Neurochemistry of monoaminergic neurons in Parkinson's disease. In *Catecholamines: Neuropharmacology and central nervous system—Therapeutic aspects* (pp. 43–52). New York: Alan R. Liss.

Schopler, E., Reichler, R. J., DeVellis, R. F., & Daly, K. (1980). Toward objective classification of childhood autism: Childhood autism rating scale. *Journal of Autism and Developmental Disorders*, *10*, 91–103.

Seegmiller, J. E., Rosenbloom, F. M., & Kelley, W. N. (1967). An enzyme defect associated with a sex-linked human neurological disorder and excessive purine synthesis. *Science*, *155*, 1682–1684.

Seeman, P. (1980). Brain dopamine receptors. *Pharmacological Reviews*, *32*, 229–313.

Setler, P. E., Sarau, H. M., Zirkle, C. L., & Saunders, H. L. (1978). The central effects of a novel dopamine agonist. *European Journal of Pharmacology*, *50*, 419–430.

Silverstein, F. S., Johnston, M. V., Hutchinson, R. J., & Edwards, N. L. (1985). Lesch–Nyhan syndrome: CSF neurotransmitter abnormalities. *Neurology*, *35*, 907–911.

Singh, N. N., & Millichamp, C. J. (1985). Pharmacological treatment of self-injurious behavior in mentally retarded persons. *Journal of Autism and Developmental Disorders*, *15*, 257–267.

Smith, R. D., Cooper, B. R., & Breese, G. R. (1973). Growth and behavioral changes in developing rats treated intracisternally with 6-hydroxydopamine: Evidence for involvement of brain dopamine. *Journal of Pharmacology and Experimental Therapeutics*, *85*, 609–619.

Snyder, S. H. (1985). Adenosine as a neuromodulator. *Annual Review of Neuroscience*, *8*, 103–24.

Sweetman, L., & Nyhan, W. L. (1970). Detailed comparison of the urinary excretion of purines in a patient with the Lesch–Nyhan syndrome and a control subject. *Biochemical Medicine*, *4*, 121–134.

Taquet, H., Javoy-Agid, F., Hamon, M., Legrand, J. C., Agid, Y. & Cesselin, F. (1983). Parkinson's disease affects differently Met^5-and Leu^5-enkephalin in the human brain. *Brain Research*, *280*, 379–382.

Tenovuo, O., Rinne, U. K., & Viljanen, K. (1984). Substance P immunoreactivity in the post-mortem Parkinsonian brain. *Brain Research*, *303*, 113–116.

Tsuruta, K., Frey, E. A., Grewe, C. W., Cote, T. E., Eskay, R. L., & Kebabian, T. W. (1981). Evidence that LY-141865 specifically stimulates the D-2 dopamine receptor. *Nature (London)*, *292*, 463–465.

Uhl, G. R., Whitehouse, P. J., Price, D. L., Tourtelotte, W. W., & Kuhar, M. J. (1984). Parkinson's disease: Depletion of substantia nigra neurotensin receptors. *Brain Research, 308*, 186–190.

Ungerstedt, U. (1971a). Post-synaptic supersensitivity after 6-hydroxydopamine induced degeneration of the nigro-striatal dopamine system. *Acta Physiologica Scandinavica Supplementum, 367*, 69–93.

Ungerstedt, U. (1971b). Adipsia and aphagia after 6-hydroxydopamine induced degeneration of the nigro-striatal dopamine system. *Acta Physiologica Scandinavica Supplementum, 367*, 95–122.

Van Loon, G. R., & Kim, C. (1978). Beta-endorphin-induced increase in striatal dopamine turnover. *Life Sciences, 23*, 961–970.

Watts, R., McKeran, R. O., Brown, E., Andrews, T. M., & Griffiths, M. I. (1974). Clinical and biochemical studies on treatment of Lesch–Nyhan syndrome. *Archives of Disease in Childhood, 49*, 693–702.

Wilson, J. M., Young, A. B.,& Kelley, W. N. (1983). Hypoxanthine-guanine phosphoribosyl transferase deficiency: The molecular basis of the clinical syndromes. *New England Journal of Medicine, 309*, 900–910.

Wojcik, W. J., & Neff, N. H. (1983a). Location of adenosine release and adenosine A-2 receptors to rat striatal neurons. *Life Sciences, 33*, 755–763.

Wojcik, W. J., & Neff, N. H. (1983b). Differential location of adenosine A1 and A2 receptors in striatum. *Neuroscience Letters, 41*, 55–60.

Wood, P. L., Stotland, M., Richard, J. W., & Rackham, A. (1980). Actions of Mu, Sigma, Delta, and agonist/antagonist opiates on striatal dopaminergic function. *Journal of Pharmacology and Experimental Therapeutics, 215*, 697–703.

Neurological and Genetic Issues
Empirical Basis

9

The Search for Neurological Subgroups in Autism

MARY COLEMAN

INTRODUCTION

An autistic child is a sensitive, emotionally fragile human being. Starting in infancy, these babies fail to relate well to their parents and other people around them and appear lost in their own world. Language is late and unusual in its development or does not come at all. The children have elaborate repetitive routines or form bizarre attachments to certain objects. Stones, a fragment of metal, pieces of a plastic toy, or a rag in its last stages may be carried around by the child, who becomes frantic if anybody tries to remove his prized object (Figure 1). Still other children line up toys in neat rows for hours on end or sit fascinated as they endlessly spin wheels of a toy car or watch the rotations of music records or fans.

It is no wonder that when these children were first described clinically, it was thought that they had a psychiatric illness probably based on the failure of the adults around them to introduce them to the world all the rest of us share. However, after more than 40 years of clinical description and medical research, we now realize that these children have innate difficulties in the functioning of their brains. The disease is primarily in the child, not in the parents.

Is autism a single disease? Or is it the clinical expression (through damage to a common system in the brain) of many different disease entities? Originally, Kanner and other early investigators thought it was one disease; today, we know that autism is a syndrome with many different etiologies. In this chapter, the search for the neurological subgroups that can present with a clinical picture of an autistic child will be reviewed. We will trace, through the chapter, the thoughts of a doctor seeing an autistic child for the first time and questions that the doctor asks herself or himself. Is the disease genetic in this child? Is it due to infectious illness? Was birth injury a factor? etc., etc., etc.

The importance of going through this differential diagnosis of autism cannot be overstated. Accurate medical diagnosis is the first step of developing a successful medical treatment

MARY COLEMAN • Children's Brain Research Clinic, Washington, DC 20008; and Georgetown University School of Medicine, Washington, DC 20007.

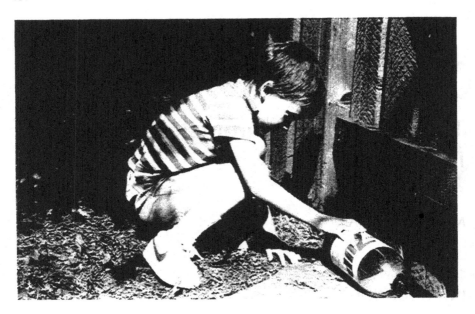

Figure 1. An autistic boy constantly rolling a bottle from the trash rather than playing with his toys.

for a patient. The medical therapies that exist for the subgroups of autistic patients are all in their infancy (Coleman & Gillberg, 1985). But they can only be developed and new ones created on the basis of accurate diagnostic information.

GENETIC DISORDERS

Kanner (1971) was the first author to suggest some sort of constitutional predisposition in autistic children. Such a predisposition could, of course, be genetic.

Except for a literature survey by Rimland (1964), who found case reports of 11 monozygotic twins reported to be concordant for autism, there was little serious investigation of possible genetic factors in autistic patients until the last decade.

One approach to the study of genetic predisposition is a comparison of monozygotic and dizygotic twins. In Great Britain in 1977, Folstein and Rutter identified 21 sex-matched pairs in which at least one twin was autistic. In 11 monozygotic twin pairs, 4 were concordant for typical or atypical autism while another 5 showed either a speech language disorder or unusual intelligence quotient profile with low verbal scores or general intellectual retardation. These authors concluded that autism often requires a heritable cognitive defect involving language to develop but that it can occur on the basis of brain damage alone.

In 1985, Ritvo, Freeman, Mason-Brothers, Mo, and Ritvo studied 40 pairs of twins in the United States who were enrolled after an advertisement in a newsletter. In this study, concordance for autism was seen in 22 of the 23 of the monozygotic pairs (or 96%). And concordance also was found in 4 of the 17 dizygotic pairs (or 24%).

A Scandinavian study that encompassed a total screening population of some 20 million children and adolescents identified 36 matched pairs of twins in which at least one twin had a childhood psychosis. Again, high concordance was seen in the monozygotic pairs, with a very much lower rate in the dizygotic pair (Gillberg, 1984).

Population-based family studies, attempting to sort out possible genetic and constitutional factors, have indicated a 50- to 100-fold increase in the risk rate for developing autism in siblings of autistic children (Gillberg & Wahlstrom, 1985; Lotter, 1967).

In 1976, Coleman and Rimland found that 8% of the families who came for a special research study on the biochemistry of autism had other family members who met the criteria of classic Kanner autism. The pattern seen was compatible with autosomal recessive autism, and there was one family where a sex-linked recessive pattern appeared possible (Coleman & Rimland, 1976).

A great deal has been learned in the 10 years since that study was first performed, and we now know that there are several autosomal recessive forms of autism (see section on metabolic diseases) and that a sex-linked subgroup also exists.

Since 1969, it has been known that there is a familial syndrome of mental retardation found only in males that is characterized by hypertrophy of secondary sex characteristics after puberty, large ears, and minor malformations of the hands and feet (Lubs, 1969). It was found that these patients had a fragile site of the long arm of the X chromosome at the location of q27. The syndrome was originally reported in mentally retarded boys but, in 1982, Brown *et al.* and Meryash, Szymanski, and Gerald reported on the concordance of infantile autism and the fragile X syndrome (Figure 2). Since then additional studies have confirmed the presence of the fragile X chromosomal abnormality in a small but significant percent of male autistic children. With increasing age, it becomes more difficult to demonstrate the fragile X chromosome abnormality. In a recent study by Blomquist *et al.* (1985), a study of autistic children up to 24 years of age was conducted and 16% of 102 cases were found to have the fragile X syndrome.

In order to ascertain the fragile X syndrome, a chromosome culture must be grown

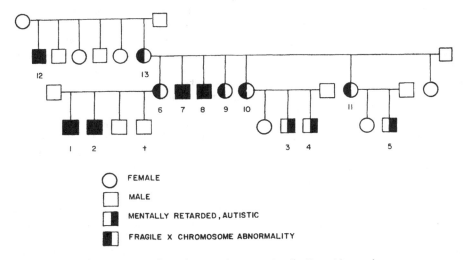

Figure 2. Family with several autistic fragile-X-positive males.

in a medium that is deficient in folic acid. This observation has led to several double-blind crossover studies that are currently in process, comparing the value of folic acid and placebo as a possible pharmacological therapy for this subgroup of autistic boys. It is still too early to evaluate the results.

INFECTIOUS DISORDERS

One of the questions that has been raised about autism is the possibility of an infectious etiology to the syndrome. Could infection of the central nervous system either prenatally or in the first year of life cause autistic symptoms? A study of the monthly distribution of birth of autistic children has disclosed a statistically significant increase in the months of March and August—a finding compatible with, but certainly not establishing, possible infectious causes (Bartlik, 1981).

To study the possibility of an infectious etiology in autism, Deykin and MacMahon (1979) did a retrospective epidemiological study of 163 cases of autism and 355 unaffected siblings using parent interviews and medical records. The number of cases where an infectious etiology could be established was small, indicating that the viruses studied were unlikely to have played a major role in any substantial portion of the autistic patients.

One virus that appears to be established as an etiology in autistic children is the rubella virus (Chess, 1977; Chess, Korn, & Fernandez, 1971; Desmond et al., 1967; Deykin & MacMahon, 1979; Freedman, Fox-Kolenda, & Brown, 1970; Rimland, 1964). One of the last documented epidemics of rubella occurred in 1964. It has been estimated that at least 20,000 children in the United States alone were born damaged as a result of the 1964 rubella epidemic. At New York University Medical Center, a rubella birth-defect evaluation project was established in which 243 children were studied, and it was found that 18 of these patients had a psychiatric disorder compatible with either an autistic syndrome or a partial syndrome of autism (Chess et al., 1971).

In 1977, Chess published a follow-up longitudinal study of the children with congenital rubella. Four new cases, one of the full and three of the partial, were identified on follow-up. It was very interesting that of the original 18 cases, 6 had recovered and 1 had improved with respect to autistic symptomology. Four new cases that were unexpected point out that, although rubella is thought of as a virus that causes prenatal damage, there may be continuing damage after birth owing to the chronic and persistent nature of many viral infections. This follow-up study suggests that in those very rare cases where autistic symptomology develops after 30 months of age, the underlying presence of the congenital rubella syndrome should be considered in the differential diagnosis.

Attempts to establish other prenatal viral infections are in their infancy. Cytomegalovirus (Markowitz, 1983; Stubbs, 1978; Stubbs, Ritvo, & Mason-Brothers, 1985) and syphilis (Knobloch & Pasamanick, 1975; Rutter & Bartak, 1971) have both been reported in more than one autistic case, but their concurrence with the autistic symptomology has yet to be firmly established as etiological.

Postnatal infections may also be an occasional rare factor in the autistic syndrome. In 1981, Delong, Beau, and Brown identified three cases with striking autistic features that had developed in previously normal children in the course of an acute encephalopathic illness. In two of the children the specific etiology was not identified and the children eventually made a complete recovery, while in the third, herpes simplex infection was confirmed and extensive necrosis of the left temporal lobe was found on CT scans. Another documented case of herpes encephalopathy was described by Gillberg (1986) in a 14-year-old girl who, after quite normal development, was suddenly taken ill and left with many classic symptoms of autism after she recovered from the acute phase of the encephalopathy.

Other infectious agents such as bacteria and fungi have very little documentation as etiological agents in autism, although Knobloch and Pasamanick (1975) have described an autistic patient who had a hydrocephalic picture secondary to meningitis.

Thus, there is evidence in a few patients suggesting that infectious agents in both the prenatal and the postnatal period may be a factor in the development of autistic symptoms. The mechanism appears to be a direct affect on brain cells (encephalitis), but there is a second possibility of indirect damage resulting from altered pressure relationships within the brain (mild hydrocephalus).

BIRTH INJURY

In any individual case the question of birth injury may be raised when a child is diagnosed later on as autistic. Attempts to examine this question in conjunction with all types of brain injury of children have been confusing. Many children who have difficulty in the birth process are children who enter the birth canal already at risk because of previous central nervous system lesions (subject reviewed in Coleman, 1981).

In the case of autistic children, there have been several recent studies that attempt to look carefully at this question. Campbell, Hardesty, and Burdock (1978) published a perinatal profile on 105 autistic children. In their study the infant weights ranged from normal values to as low as 1.33 kg, suggesting that the sampling included some preterm or small-for-date infants. They also found maternal hypertension in 6.7% of their population.

In 1980, Deykin and MacMahon investigated the prenatal delivery and neonatal histories of 145 autistic children matched with 330 unaffected siblings. Problems during gestation and neonatal problems were noted more frequently in the autistic children, but the difference between the autistic children and their unaffected siblings was found to be statistically significant only when all complications were grouped together with no one complication standing out as predictive of autism.

Gillberg and Gillberg (1983) applied the neonatal Prechtl optimality score as adapted to Swedish obstetrical and neonatal records to a group of 25 autistic children (Gillberg & Gillberg, 1983; Prechtl, 1980). The score was compared with controls of the same sex born at the same time in the same obstetrical department in Sweden. In this study, autistic children showed statistically significantly increased scores for reduced optimality, although individual items in the perinatal period were not statistically significant except for lower gestational age. The greatest rate of reduced optimality was in the prenatal rather than in the perinatal period.

Thus, in the present state of knowledge, it is difficult to attribute to birth injury an etiological factor in most cases of autism, although there is evidence of both prenatal and perinatal difficulty in the medical histories of some autistic children.

METABOLIC DISEASES

In 1969, a paper was published by Friedman, who pointed out that children had been given the diagnosis of autism who, in fact, had a metabolic disease called phenylketonuria. This observation raised a question about the possibility of other metabolic diseases underlying autism, and a search for such disease entities has been under way by a few investigators during the last decade.

At the time of this writing, errors in metabolism have been found in autistic children that arise from three sections of the metabolic system. These three sections are amino acid metabolism, purine synthesizing pathways, and carbohydrate metabolic pathways.

The first metabolic disease that was discovered to present with autistic symptoms was phenylketonuria, a disease entity based on error in amino acid metabolism. Since that time, many centers specializing in autism have checked many autistic patients looking for other amino acidurias, without success. To date, phenylketonuria remains the only error in amino acid metabolism demonstrated to present with autistic symptomology.

In 1934, Folling identified an unusual compound—excessive phenylpyruvic acid—in the urine of a group of retarded patients. It is now understood that a block of phenylalanine-4-hydroxylase in the amino acid step between phenylalanine and tyrosine results in a backup of minor metabolites such as phenylpyruvic acid spilling over into the urine. Dietary therapy for phenylketonuria consists of a special formula for babies containing a very low amount of phenylalanine—thus preventing a backup of unused phenylalanine in the child and its conversion into large amounts of otherwise minor metabolites. When minor metabolites rise to high levels they can interfere with the functioning of neighboring metabolic pathways. The successful treatment of phenylketonuria depends upon early identification of the abnormality in a small infant. Since it is virtually impossible to detect it by a clinical examination, newborn screening laboratories exist for the purpose of testing every baby for this inborn error of metabolism. All states in the United States and most countries in Europe test newborns for phenylketonuria. If the patients are not started on treatment in the early weeks of life, the central nervous system starts to deteriorate, which results in delayed psychomotor milestones and a loss of approximately 50 IQ points during the first year of life.

The majority of patients with phenylketonuria are retarded and neurologically damaged individuals without a preponderance of autistic symptomology. However, a significant number of these children do have autistic symptoms, as is demonstrated by the literature (Bliumina, 1975; Friedman, 1969; Knobloch & Pasamanick, 1975; Lowe, Tanaka, Seashore, Young, & Cohen, 1980).

In the initial evaluation of an autistic patient, a test for phenylketonuria should always be done even if the child is born in the United States or in a country that tests for newborn phenylketonuria. The paper by Lowe et al. (1980) from the Yale University School of Medicine found 3 children with this disease while screening 65 children with autism and atypical childhood psychosis. One child, age 2 years, had been tested for PKU in the newborn period and had been reported as negative. The second, age 7 months, had not been screened at all as a newborn. The third child, age 4 years, had been born in a state that at that time did not require testing.

How could these children have been missed? A study by Sepe, Levy, and Mount (1979) indicates that as many as 20% of all newborn infants may not receive first screening even if they are born in states or countries where laboratories are doing newborn screening. This may be due to nurse's error, laboratory error, or screening of the infant too early (before the placental compensation for the phenylalanine level ceases to have an effect).

To the clinician finding the diagnosis of phenylketonuria in an older autistic child, the question arises, "Is there any value in starting treatment past early infancy?" In the medical literature, L-dopa has been used to treat the extrapyramidal manifestations of these children (Macleod, Munro, Ledingham, & Farquhar, 1983). Although there is relatively little experience with starting the diet at later ages, a few studies (Gruter, 1963; Lewis,

1959; Lowe *et al.*, 1980) do suggest that dietary treatment of the disorder can prevent further progression of the disability and might even have some behavioral benefit to the child. This question needs evaluation by a large collaborative study.

At this time the most promising area for development in identifying metabolic etiologies of autism appears to be the purine metabolic pathways. Already three of the enzymes in those pathways have been found to be abnormal in one or more patients with autism (Figure 3).

In 1969, Nyhan, James, Teberg, Sweetmen, and Nelson described a 3-year-old boy with unusual autistic behavior, failure to cry with tears, absence of speech, hypoplastic discolored teeth, and persistently pink urine. Later studies also indicated that the child was deaf. In 1980, Becker, Raivio, Bakay, Adams, and Nyhan demonstrated that the excessive rate of uric acid synthesis in this child could be explained by an increase in the purine enzyme—phosphoribosylpyrophosphate synthetase (PRPP synthetase) in his fibroblasts.

In 1974, a large research project was conducted at the Children's Brain Research Clinic of Washington, D.C., on 69 patients, and 22% were found to have increased excretion of uric acid in the urine. Uric acid is the end product of the multiple purine pathways. Recently, Gruber, Jansen, Willis, and Seegmiller (1985) have demonstrated that two of these patients had abnormal levels of inosinate dehydrogenase in their lymphoblasts.

A third enzyme error has been identified by Belgian investigators in two siblings whose

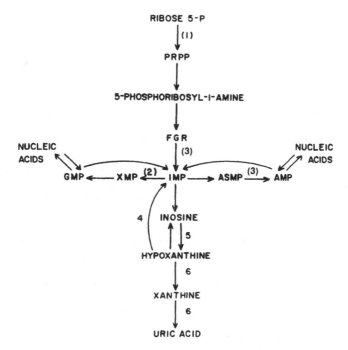

Figure 3. Schematic drawing of the purine pathways in humans. The three enzymes found abnormal in autistic children are (1) 5-phosphoribosyl-1-pyrophosphate (PRPP synthetase), (2) inosinate dehydrogenase, and (3) adenylosuccinase or adenylsuccinate lyase. Enzymes 4 to 6 are associated with other types of brain diseases in humans.

grandparents were first cousins, and also in another autistic child (Jaeken & Van den Berghe, 1984). These patients had an error in the purine enzyme-adenylosuccinate lyase.

The understanding of these metabolic errors of purine metabolism in autistic patients is in its early stages. As further knowledge is gained, there is still the possibility that these may be secondary rather than primary errors. Thus, treatment approaches for purine autism are also extremely preliminary at this time.

The area of carbohydrate metabolism in autistic children has had very little study. In 1971, DeMyer, Schwier, Bryson, Solow, and Roeske studied plasma-free fatty acid metabolism in a mixed group of autistic and schizophrenic children, who demonstrated greater variability than controls. Recently, Coleman and Blass (1985) described four patients who have the coexisting syndrome of autism and lactic acidosis. Lactic acidosis or hyperlactatemia without acidosis indicates some abnormality in the utilization of sugar, which increases the rate of lactate production relative to the rate of lactate utilization. Thus, hyperlactatemia is not a specific biochemical abnormality itself but rather an indication that a particular patient may have an inborn error of metabolism in the family of disorders of carbohydrate metabolism.

In the patients described by Coleman and Blass one of the four patients had motor delay, a finding that is seen in patients with lactic acidosis and other neurological syndromes. Preliminary evidence in this patient indicates that she may have a deficiency of one portion of the pyruvate dehydrogenase complex (PDHC).

Additional patients with evidence of hyperlactatemia are also known to the author, so carbohydrate metabolism may also turn out to be a fruitful area for investigation in autism.

STRUCTURAL CHANGES IN THE BRAIN ASSOCIATED WITH AUTISTIC SYMPTOMS

In 1960, Schain and Yannet published the first case of an autistic child with a high blood serotonin level. The child's diagnosis from a neurological point of view was arrested hydrocephalus. Knobloch and Pasamanick (1975) also published some cases of autistic children who had hydrocephalus caused either by the Dandy Walker syndrome or by papilloma of the chroid plexus. They also had a hydrocephalic patient with autistic features whose problem had been secondary to a case of meningitis. Damasio, Maurer, Damasio, and Chui (1980) and Garreau, Barthelemy, Sauvage, Leddet, and Lelord (1984) also reported autistic children with hydrocephalus. Coleman and Gillberg (1985) described a 9-year-old boy who had a shunt at 3-month stage because of a diagnosis of hydrocephalus. In a CT study utilizing special volumetric measurements of the ventricles of subarachnoid spaces, the presence of an occasional child with ventricular enlargement again has been confirmed (Rosenbloom et al., 1984).

It needs to be noted that the patients with autism and a diagnosis of hydrocephalus tend to have either arrested, mild, or moderate hydrocephalus—not the severe types. Because of the numbers of autistic patients, it could be coincidence that a number of cases have been described in the literature. However, it is also possible that a mild hydrocephalus syndrome puts pressure in areas of the brain that are particularly susceptible to a type of malfunction leading to autistic symptomology.

Porencephaly and other gross abnormalities of the brain are occasionally seen in autistic patients. They are found in all areas of the brain, neither consistently on one side or another nor in one section or another (Coleman & Gillberg, 1985). Imaging of the brain today has been disappointing in terms of localizing the lesions that could be consistently found in association with autistic symptoms. With the development of magnetic resonance imaging, perhaps a great deal more information will be gathered in the future about structural changes in the brain associated with autistic symptoms.

OTHER DISEASE ENTITIES

In addition to the classic autistic syndrome, autistic symptomology is often seen in patients who have other known disease entities. Sometimes the patient is labeled "autistic" until the underlying disease entity is discovered. These diseases tend to fall into two groups: those with a static encephalopathy and those with progressive degenerative disease of the brain. However, the distinction between these two groups sometimes is obscured, as is seen in children with birth defects and autistic symptoms who may appear to have increasing difficulties with age.

The Moebius syndrome has been described in several cases of autism (Coleman & Gillberg, 1985; Gillberg & Winnergard, 1984; Ornitz et al., 1972). Although there is a myopathic form of the Moebius syndrome, most cases result from aplastic, hypoplastic, or necrotic cranial nerve nucleii. The presence of undeniable brainstem involvement in these children with autistic symptoms is of theoretical interest regarding the discussion of the possible anatomical location of lesions that cause autistic symptoms.

Other congenital syndromes where patients with autistic symptoms have been reported are the deLange syndrome (Knobloch & Pasamanick, 1975), Noonan syndrome (Paul, Cohen, & Volkmar, 1983), Coffin Siris syndrome (Hersh, Bloom, & Weisskopf, 1982), fetal alcohol syndrome (Hauser, DeLong, & Rosman, 1975), Biedl-Bardet syndrome (Gillberg & Wahlstrom, 1985), achondroplasia (Gillberg & Andersson, 1984), Williams syndrome (Knobloch & Pasamanick, 1975; Reiss, Feinstein, Rosenbaum, Borengasser–Caruso, & Goldsmith, 1985) and the chromosomal syndromes of trisomy 21, trisomy 22, and XYY (Gillberg & Wahlstrom, 1985; Knobloch & Pasamanick, 1975; Turner & Jennings, 1961). It is also possible that fragile sites on other chromosomes—other than the X chromosome—may be found to be associated with autistic symptomology in some patient groups.

Several of the neurocutaneous syndromes appear to have subgroups of patients with autistic symptoms. Tuberous sclerosis is a disease characterized by tubers in the brain, which frequently occur within the gyrii but can also be imbedded in the thalamus or caudate or elsewhere in the brain. Such patients have been described by Coleman and Gillberg (1985), Lotter (1974), Valente (1971), and Wing (1975).

Neurofibromatosis, or von Recklinghausen disease, is another neurocutaneous syndrome marked by a proclivity to tumor formation. The tumors in this case are not usually in the central nervous system. However, occasionally it has been described as having autistic symptomology (Coleman & Gillberg, 1985; Crowe, Schull & Neil, 1956; Gillberg & Forsell, 1984).

In contrast to the fragile X syndrome, which is seen almost exclusively in males, there is another syndrome that is seen almost exclusively in females and has a developmental phase that can easily be characterized as autistic. In Vienna in 1966 and again in 1968, Rett described a syndrome in girls characterized by autistic behavior between the years of 1 and 4, apraxia of gait, loss of facial expression, and stereotypical wringing of the hands, and loss of use of the hands. Unaware of Rett's description, Hagberg (1980) reported a similar pattern in girls in Sweden. Recent good reviews of the syndrome have been published by

Hagberg, Aicardi, Dias, and Ramos (1983), Hagberg (1985), Holm (1985), Nomura, Segawa, and Hasegawa (1984), and in Supplement 1 of the American Journal of Medical Genetics (1986) (Figure 4).

Rett syndrome may be more frequent than one would think from the delay in recognition of the syndrome. The Hagberg (1985) paper gives a prevalence of 0.65 per 10,000 girls, which makes it about twice as common as phenylketonuria (PKU) in the same area of Sweden where this epidemiologic study was undertaken. The girls appear to have normal physical and psychomotor development up to the age of 7 to 18 months. Then psychomotor development slows and is followed by rapid deterioration. Eighteen months after the onset of the disease, acquired microcephaly, loss of purposeful use of the hands, jerky trunk ataxia, and severe dementia are seen. Bouts of hyperpnea and loss of ambulation may develop later.

This spectrum of children with autistic symptoms and other diagnosable disease entities reminds the clinician that each child showing autistic symptomology must have a thorough clinical and laboratory evaluation. Autism is not a final diagnosis. This is a syndrome of

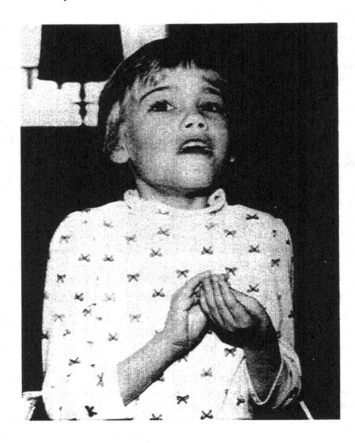

Figure 4. Classical hand posture of girl with Rett syndrome who has no use of her hands and is constantly wringing them.

many etiologies. When a known disease entity affecting the brain is then identified in a child with autistic symptoms, the question arises as to whether the concomitant disease entity is relevant to the child's autistic condition or is an incidental finding. This can be determined only on a case-by-case basis.

BLINDNESS AND DEAFNESS

It has been known for some time that the autistic syndrome is sometimes seen in children with congenital blindness and congenital deafness. An excellent review of the effects of early blindness and deafness on cognition by Rapin (1979) emphasizes that the majority of these children do become competent adults when the severity of the handicap is taken into consideration. She points out that the blind are viewed as having few barriers to full cognitive competence but the situation with the deaf child is different. The detrimental consequences of deafness intensify in age for all children because communication about events remote in time and place and about abstract principles and sophisticated ideas is contingent upon the availability of a common symbolic system.

Patients with a congenital rubella syndrome with associated deafness would be an example of children at risk for autistic symptomology. However, in spite of numerous studies, it is far from clear what distinguished one deaf child from another in the development of autism. In a preliminary clinical study of autistic blind children in Sweden it has been suggested that the underlying brain damage rather than the blindness itself may be etiologically responsible for autistic symptoms (Bensch & Gillberg, manuscript in preparation).

In the case of a child who is both deaf and autistic, there is a profound sensory deprivation occurring. For a child having no auditory contact with the environment, failure to maintain visual contact through good eye contact is the equivalent of noninteraction and is completely isolating for such a deaf child. Thus, autistic symptoms add a major handicap to such children and are a great challenge to teachers dealing with multihandicapped children (Meadow, 1984).

In the same way, a blind child with the autistic syndrome who has difficulty tolerating sound and "appears deaf" at times also has a major compounding variable that challenges the most resourceful educator in terms of teaching such a child. Konstantareas, Hunter, and Sloman (1982) have reported on a successful program relying primarily on tactile kinesthetic and auditory modalities for teaching sign language to such a blind autistic child.

In such children the physician has a particularly significant responsibility to do everything possible from a medical point of view to decrease tactile defensiveness, lack of eye contact, and poor attention span so that the child may benefit from educational programming. These children present one of the ultimate challenges to those working in the field of autism.

CONCLUSION

In this chapter, various subgroups of the autistic syndrome have been discussed. It is encouraging that subgroups have started to be defined so that their etiology and diagnosis can be specifically addressed.

However, most children with autism still remain without a specific diagnosis. A number of areas of research are currently under way that may elucidate further subgroups of autistic children.

One such possible subgroup is the children with autism and hypocalcinuria originally described in 1976 (Coleman, Landgrebe, & Landgrebe, 1976). Multiple attempts to identify the cause for hypocalcinuria have failed. Extensive testing for calcitonin, parathormone, 1,25 dihydroxy vitamin D_3, jejunal bowel biopsy with gluten priming, and kidney studies in this patient group have all been nonproductive.

Another unsolved problem that may affect the subgroup of autistic patients is the finding of statistically lowered serum magnesium level in the large 1976 Children's Brain Research Clinic study. Attempts to account for this depletion to date have been unsuccessful since only one enzyme so far described as abnormal in an autistic child (PRPP synthetase) uses magnesium in the enzyme complex.

An area of intensive research at the present time is a study of urinary peptide patterns (Gillberg, Trygstad, & Foss, 1982; Lis, McLaughlin, McLaughlin, Lis, & Stubbs, 1976; Trygstad et al., 1980). Whether such studies will eventually identify subgroups of autistic children is unknown at this time.

Studies of endorphin levels in autistic children have been very interesting. Gillberg, Terenius, and Lönnerholm (1985) examined 20 autistic children and found evidence of raised CSF levels of endorphin fraction II in those children who were self-destructive and appeared to have a relative insensitivity to pain. In contrast, Weizman et al. (1984) have found significantly reduced levels in the blood of autistic children.

One of the most exciting leads at the moment is studies of immunological and autoimmunological disease in autistic children. In 1982, Weizman, Weizman, Szekely, Wijsanbeek, and Livni studied cell-mediated immune response to human myelin basic protein by the macrophage migration inhibition factor test. Of 17 autistic children, 13 demonstrated inhibition of macrophage migration, while none of the control group who suffered from other mental disorders showed such a response. More recently, Todd and Ciaranello (1985) have reported that about one-third of autistic children they have examined have an unusual antibody circulating in their blood and spinal fluid. This antibody appears to attack the receptor for serotonin, an important neurotransmitter. Thus it is possible that a subgroup of autistic children will be determined in the future to have an autoimmune disease.

As it is becoming increasingly clear that there are many different subgroups within the autistic syndrome, each autistic child is now evaluated with an eye toward a specific diagnosis. At the present time, the majority of such children still do not have definite etiological factors established.

But it is an exciting time to be doing research in the field of autism. We have come a long way from the guilty, despairing parents of the early years to the neurobiological laboratory of today.

REFERENCES

Bartlik, B. D. (1981). Monthly variation in births of autistic children in North Carolina. *Journal of the American Medical Women's Association, 36*, 363–368.

Becker, M. A., Raivio, K. O., Bakay, B., Adams, W. B., & Nyhan, W. L. (1980). Variant human phosphoribosylpyrophosphate synthetase altered in regulatory and catalytic functions. *Journal of Clinical Investigation, 65*, 109–120.

Bensch, A., & Gillberg, C. (Manuscript in preparation). *A study of blind autistic children in Sweden.*

Bliumina, M. G. (1975). A schizophrenic-like variant of phenylketonuria. *Zhurnal Nevropatologii Psikhiatrii, 75,* 1525–1529.

Blomquist, H. K., Bohman, M., Edvinsson, S. O., Gillberg, C., Gustavson, K. H., Holmgren, G., & Wahlstrom, J. (1985). Frequency of the fragile X syndrome in infantile autism. *Clinical Genetics, 27,* 113–117.

Brown, W. T., Jenkins, E. C., Friedman, E., Brooks, J., Wisniewski, K., Raguthu, S., & French, J. (1982). Autism is associated with the fragile X syndrome. *Journal of Autism and Developmental Disorders, 12,* 303–308.

Campbell, M., Hardesty, A. S., & Burdock, E. I. (1978). Demographic and perinatal profile of 105 autistic children: A preliminary report. *Psychopharmacology Bulletin, 14,* 36–39.

Chess, S. (1977). Follow-up report on autism in congenital rubella. *Journal of Autism and Childhood Schizophrenia, 7,* 68–81.

Chess, S., Korn, S. J., & Fernandez, P. B. (1971). *Psychiatric disorders of children with congenital rubella.* New York: Brunner/Mazel.

Coleman, M. (1981). Congenital brain syndromes. In M. Coleman (Ed.), *Neonatal neurology* (pp. 371–384). Baltimore: University Park Press.

Coleman, M., & Blass, J. P. (1985). Autism and lactic acidosis. *Journal of Autism and Developmental Disorders, 15,* 1–8.

Coleman, M., & Gillberg, C. (1985). *The biology of the autistic syndrome, 1985.* New York: Praeger.

Coleman, M., & Rimland, B. (1976). Familial autism. In M. Coleman (Ed.), *The autistic syndromes* (pp. 175–182). Amsterdam: North-Holland.

Coleman, M., Landgrebe, M. A., & Landgrebe, A. R. (1976). Purine autism. Hyperuricosuria in autistic children: Does this identify a subgroup of autism? In M. Coleman (Ed.), *The autistic syndromes* (pp. 183–185). Amsterdam: North-Holland.

Crowe, F. W., Schull, W. J., & Neil, J. W. (1956). *A clinical pathological and genetic study of multiple neurofibromatosis.* Springfield, IL: Charles C Thomas.

Damasio, H., Maurer, R. G., Damasio, A. R., & Chui, H. C. (1980). Computerized tomographic scan findings in patients with autistic behavior. *Archives of Neurology, 37,* 504–510.

DeLong, G. R., Beau, S. C., & Brown, F. R., III. (1981). Acquired reversible autistic syndrome in acute encephalopathic illness in children. *Archives of Neurology, 38,* 191–194.

DeMyer, M. K., Schwier, H., Bryson, C. Q., Solow, E. B., & Roeske, N. (1971). Free fatty acid response to insulin and glucose stimulation in schizophrenic, autistic, and emotionally disturbed children. *Journal of Autism and Childhood Schizophrenia, 1,* 436–452.

Desmond, M. M., Wilson, G. S., Melnick, J. L., Singer, D. B., Zion, T. E., Rudolph, A. J., Pineda, R. G., Ziai, M. H., & Blattney, R. J. (1967). Congenital rubella encephalitis. *Journal of Pediatrics, 71,* 311–331.

Deykin, E. Y., & MacMahon, G. (1979). Viral exposure and autism. *American Journal of Epidemiology, 109,* 628–638.

Deykin, E. Y., & MacMahon, G. (1980). Pregnancy, delivery and neonatal complications among autistic children. *American Journal of Diseases of Children, 134,* 860–864.

Folling, A. (1934). Uber Ausscheidung von Phenylbenztraubensaure in den Haarn als Stoffwechselanomalie in Verbindung mit Imbessillitat. *Hoppe Seylers Zeitschrift für Physiologische Chemie, 227,* 169.

Folstein, S., & Rutter, M. (1977). Infantile autism: A genetic study of 21 twin pairs. *Journal of Child Psychology and Psychiatry, 18,* 297–321.

Freedman, D. A., Fox-Kolenda, B. J., & Brown, S. L. (1970). A multihandicapped rubella baby: The first 18 months. *Journal of the American Academy of Child Psychiatry, 9,* 298–317.

Friedman, E. (1969). The autistic syndrome and phenylketonuria. *Schizophrenia, 1,* 249–261.

Garreau, B. C., Barthelemy, C., Sauvage, D., Leddet, I., & Lelord, G. (1984). A comparison of autistic syndromes with and without associated neurological problems. *Journal of Autism and Developmental Disorders, 14,* 105–111.

Gillberg, C. (1984). Infantile autism and other childhood psychoses in a Swedish urban region. Epidemiological aspects. *Journal of Child Psychology and Psychiatry, 25,* 35–43.

Gillberg, C. (1986). Onset at age 14 of a typical autistic syndrome: A case report of a previously normal girl with herpes encephalitis. *Journal of Autism and Developmental Disorders, 16,* 369–375.

Gillberg, C., & Andersson, L. (1984). Autism and achondroplasia: A case study. Unpublished manuscript.

Gillberg, G., & Forsell, C. (1984). Childhood psychosis and neurofibromatosis—More than a coincidence? *Journal of Autism and Developmental Disorders, 14,* 1–8.

Gillberg, C., & Gillberg, I. C. (1983). Infantile autism: A total population study of reduced optimality in the pre-, peri-, and neonatal period. *Journal of Autism and Developmental Disorders, 13,* 153–166.

Gillberg, C., Rasmussen, P., & Wahlstrom, J. (1982). Minor neurodevelopmental disorders in children born to older mothers. *Developmental Medicine and Child Neurology, 24,* 437–447.

Gillberg, C., Terenius, L., & Lönnerholm, G. (1985). Endorphin activity in childhood psychosis. *Archives of General Psychiatry, 42,* 780–783.

Gillberg, C., Trygstad, O. E., & Foss, I. (1982). Childhood psychosis and urinary excretion of peptides and protein-associated peptide complexes. *Journal of Autism and Developmental Disorders, 12,* 229–241.

Gillberg, C., & Wahlstrom, J. (1985). Chromosome abnormalities in infantile autism and other childhood psychoses. A population study of 66 cases. *Developmental Medicine and Child Neurology, 27,* 293–304.

Gillberg, C., & Winnergard, I. (1984). Childhood psychosis in a case of Moebius syndrome. *Neuropaediatrics, 15,* 147–149.

Gruber, H. E., Jansen, I., Willis, R. C., & Seegmiller, J. E. (1985). Regulation of the inosinate branchpoint enzymes in cultured human lymphoblasts. *Biochimica et Biophysica Acta, 846,* 135–144.

Gruter, W. (1963). *Angeborene Stoffwechselstorungen und Schwachsinn am Beispiel der Phenylketonurie.* Stuttgart, Germany: Verlag, F. Enke.

Hagberg, B. (1980). *Infantile autism, dementia and loss of hand use: A report of 16 Swedish girl patients.* Paper presented at the Research Session of the European Federation of Child Neurology Societies, Manchester, England.

Hagberg, B. (1985). Rett's syndrome: Prevalence and impact on progressive severe mental retardation in girls. *Acta Paediatrica Scandinavica, 74,* 405–408.

Hagberg, B., Aicardi, J., Dias, K., & Ramos, O. (1983). A progressive syndrome of autism, dementia, ataxia and loss of purposeful hand use in girls: Rett's syndrome: report of 35 cases. *Annals of Neurology, 14,* 471–479.

Hauser, S., DeLong, G., & Rosman, N. (1975). Pneumographic findings in the infantile autism syndroms: A correlation with temporal lobe disease. *Brain, 98,* 667–688.

Hersh, L., Bloom, A., & Weisskopf, B. (1982). Childhood autism in a female with Coffin Siris syndrome. *Developmental and Behavioral Pediatrics, 3,* 249–251.

Holm, V. A. (1985). Rett's syndrome: A progressive developmental disability in girls. *Developmental and Behavioral Pediatrics, 6,* 32–35.

Jaeken, J., & Van den Berghe, G. (1984). An infantile autistic syndrome characterised by the presence of succinylpurines in body fluids. *Lancet, 2,* 1058–1061.

Kanner, L. (1971). Follow-up study of 11 autistic children originally reported in 1943. *Journal of Autism and Childhood Schizophrenia, 1,* 119–145.

Knobloch, H., & Pasamanick, B. (1975). Some etiologic and prognostic factors in early infantile autism and psychosis. *Journal of Pediatrics, 55,* 182–191.

Konstantareas, M. M., Hunter, D., & Sloman, L. (1982). Training a blind autistic child to communicate through signs. *Journal of Autism and Developmental Disorders, 12,* 1–12.

Lewis, E. (1959). The development of concepts in a girl after dietary treatment for phenylketonuria. *British Journal of Medical Psychology, 32,* 282–287.

Lis, A. W., McLaughlin, D. I., McLaughlin, R. K., Lis, E. W., & Stubbs, E. G. (1976). Profiles of ultraviolet-absorbing components of urine from autistic children, as obtained by high-resolution ion-exchange chromatography. *Clinical Chemistry, 22*, 1528–1532.

Lotter, V. (1967). Epidemiology of autistic conditions in young children. I. Prevalence. *Social Psychiatry, 1*, 163–173.

Lotter, V. (1974). Factors related to outcome in autistic children. *Journal of Autism and Childhood Schizophrenia, 4*, 263–277.

Lowe, T. L., Tanaka, K., Seashore, M. R., Young, J. G., & Cohen, D. J. (1980). Detection of phenylketonuria in autistic and psychotic children. *Journal of the American Medical Association, 243*, 126–128.

Lubs, H. A. (1969). A marker X-chromosome. *American Journal of Human Genetics, 2*, 231–244.

Macleod, M. D., Nunro, J. F., Ledingham, J. G., & Farquhar, J. W. (1983). Management of the extrapyramidal manifestations of phenylketonuria with L-dopa. *Archives of Diseases in Childhood, 58*, 457–466.

Markowitz, P. I. (1983). Autism in a child with congenital cytomegalovirus infection. *Journal of Autism and Developmental Disorders, 13*, 249–253.

Meadow, K. (1984). Social adjustment of preschool children: Deaf and hearing, with and without other handicaps. In F. Fewell (Ed.), *Topics in early childhood special education* (pp. 27–40). Austin, TX.

Meryash, D. L., Szymanski, L., & Gerald, P. (1982). Infantile autism associated with fragile X syndrome. *Journal of Autism and Developmental Disorders, 12*, 295–301.

Nomura, Y., Segawa, M., & Hasegawa, M. (1984). Rett syndrome—clinical studies and pathophysiological consideration. *Brain and Development, 6*, 475–486.

Nyhan, W. L., James, J. A., Teberg, A. J., Sweetmen, L., & Nelson, L. G. (1969). A new disorder of purine metabolism with behavioral manifestations. *Journal of Pediatrics, 74*, 20–27.

Ornitz, E. M., Tanguay, P. E., Lee, J. C. M., Ritvo, E. R., Silvertsen, B., & Wilson, C. (1972). The effect of stimulus interval on the auditory evoked responses during sleep in autistic children. *Journal of Autism and Childhood Schizophrenia, 2*, 140–150.

Paul, R., Cohen, D. J., & Volkmar, F. R. (1983). Autistic behaviors in a boy with Noonan syndrome (Letter). *Journal of Autism and Developmental Disorders, 13*, 433–434.

Prechtl, H. F. R. (1980). The optimality concept. *Early Human Development, 4*, 201–205.

Rapin, I. (1979). Effects of early blindness and deafness on cognition. In R. Katzman (Ed.), *Congenital and acquired cognitive disorders* (pp. 189–245). New York: Raven Press.

Reiss, A. L., Feinstein, C., Rosenbaum, K. N., Borengasser-Caruso, M. A., & Goldsmith, B. M. (1985). Autism associated with Williams syndrome. *Journal of Pediatrics, 106*, 247–249.

Rett, A. (1966). *Uber ein cerebral-atrophisches Syndrom bei Hyperammonamie.* Vienna: Bruder Hollinek.

Rett, A. (1968). Uber ein eigenartiges hirnatrophisches Syndrom bei Hyperammoniamie in Kindesalter. *Wiener Medizinische Wochenschrift, 116*, 723–738.

The Rett syndrome. (1986). *American Journal of Medical Genetics*, (Suppl. 1), pp. 1–403.

Rimland, B. (1964). *Infantile autism.* Englewood Cliffs, NJ: Prentice-Hall.

Ritvo, E. R., Freeman, B. J., Mason-Brothers, A., Mo, A., & Ritvo, A. M. (1985). Concordance of the syndrome of autism in 40 pairs of afflicted twins. *American Journal of Psychiatry, 142*, 74–77.

Rosenbloom, S., Campbell, M., George, A., Kricheff, I., Taleporos, E., Anderson, L., Reuben, R., & Korein, J. (1984). High resolution CT scanning in infantile autism: A quantitative approach. *Journal of the American Academy of Child Psychiatry, 23*, 72–77.

Rutter, M., & Bartak, L. (1971). Causes of infantile autism: Some considerations from recent research. *Journal of Autism and Childhood Schizophrenia, 1*, 20–32.

Schain, R., & Yannet, H. (1960). Infantile autism: An analysis of 50 cases and a consideration of certain relevant neuropsychological concepts. *Journal of Pediatrics, 57*, 560–567.

Sepe, J., Levy, H. L., & Mount, F. W. (1979). An evaluation of routine follow-up blood screening of infants for phenylketonuria. *New England Journal of Medicine, 300*, 606–609.

Stubbs, E. G. (1978). Autistic symptoms in a child with congenital cytomegalovirus infection. *Journal of Autism and Childhood Schizophrenia, 8*, 37–43.

Stubbs, E. G., Ritvo, E. R., & Mason-Brothers, A. (1985). Autism and shared parental HLA antigens. *Journal of the American Academy of Child Psychiatry, 24*, 182–185.

Todd, R. D., & Ciaranello, R. D. (1985). Demonstration of inter- and intraspecies differences in serotonin binding sites by antibodies from an autistic child. *Proceedings of the National Academy of Sciences, USA, 82*, 612–616.

Trygstad, O. E., Reichelt, K. L., Foss, F. Edminson, P. D., Saelid, G., Bremer, J., Hole, K., Orbeck, H., Johansen, J. H., Boler, J. B., Titlestad, K., & Opstad, P. K. (1980). Patterns of peptides and protein-associated peptide complexes in psychiatric disorders. *British Journal of Psychiatry, 136*, 59–72.

Turner, B., & Jennings, A. N. (1961). Trisomy for chromosome 22. *Lancet, 2*, 49–50.

Valente, M. (1971). Autism: Symptomatic and idiopathic—and mental retardation. *Pediatrics, 48*, 495–496.

Weizman, A., Weizman, R., Szekely, G. A., Wijsenbeek, H., & Livni, E. (1982). Abnormal immune response to brain tissue antigen in the syndrome of autism. *American Journal of Psychiatry, 139*, 1462–1465.

Weizman, R., Weizman, A., Tyano, S., Szekely, G., Weissman, B. A., & Sarne, Y. (1984). Humoral-endorphin blood levels in autistic, schizophrenic and healthy subjects. *Psychopharmacology, 82*, 368–370.

Wing, L. (1975). A study of language impairments in severely retarded children. In N. O'Conner (Ed.), *Language, cognitive deficits and retardation* (pp. 87–116). London: Butterworths.

10

Pre-, Peri-, and Neonatal Factors in Autism

LUKE Y. TSAI

It is clear from previous chapters that autism is now considered a syndrome due to a neuropathology of the central nervous system, which, in turn, may have a variety of etiologies. Studies have found that many autistic children suffer from organic brain disorders, ranging from 30 to 100%, depending on whether the children were selected from psychiatric or pediatric-neurologic cohorts (Fish & Ritvo, 1979). A wide variety of neurologic disorders have been reported, including cerebral palsy, maternal rubella, toxoplasmosis, tuberous sclerosis, cytomegalovirus infection, demyelinating disease, lead encephalopathy, meningitis, encephalitis, severe brain hemorrhage, phenylketonuria, and many types of epilepsy.

There are also studies that show autistic children exhibiting substantial excess of congenital minor physical anomalies (Campbell, Geller, Small, Petti, & Ferris, 1978) as well as soft neurological signs such as hypotonia or hypertonia, disturbance of body schema, clumsiness, choreiform movements, pathological reflexes, myoclonic jerking, drooling, abnormal posture and gait, dystonic posturing of hands and fingers, tremor, ankle clonus, emotional facial paralysis, and strabismus (reviewed by Ornitz & Ritvo, 1976).

Since many of these neurological disorders and/or congenital physical anomalies tend to derive from unfavorable pre-, peri-, and neonatal complications, it has been suggested that pre- or perinatal insults to the brain are the biological causation of autism for children whose autistic symptoms are manifested from birth, and that postnatal cerebral infections or injuries have been suggested as the etiology for children whose autism is manifested after a period of apparent normal development.

The pre-, peri-, or postnatal etiology of autism can stem from genetic defects and/or vulnerability, or from conditions in the uterine environment that make for physical anomalies in the fetus and neonate. The genetic aspect of autism is discussed in Chapter 5. This chapter is concerned primarily with the relationship between autism and pre-, peri-, and neonatal complications.

Many investigators have evaluated pre-, peri-, and neonatal complications in children classed as psychotic or autistic in their early years (Bender, 1973; Bender & Faretra, 1961;

LUKE Y. TSAI • Department of Psychiatry, University of Kansas, Kansas City, Kansas 66103.

DeMyer, 1979; Deykin & MacMahon, 1979, 1980; Finegan & Quarrington, 1979; Funderburk, Carter, Tanguay, Freeman, & Westlake, 1983; Gillberg, 1980; Gillberg & Gillberg, 1983; Gittleman & Birch, 1967; Harper & Williams, 1974; Hinton, 1963; Knobloch & Pasamanick, 1975; Kolvin, Ounsted, & Roth, 1971; Lobascher, Kingerlee, & Gubbay, 1970; Osterkamp & Sands, 1962; Rutt & Offord, 1971; Taft & Goldfarb, 1964; Terris, Lapouse, & Monk, 1964; Torrey, Hersh, & McCabe, 1975; Tsai & Stewart, 1983; Vorster, 1960; Whittam, Simon, & Mitter, 1966; Wing, O'Connor, & Lotter, 1967). However, one must interpret the results of earlier studies with caution. These studies used different diagnostic criteria, the obstetrical history information was often based on the rather unreliable or inaccurate maternal reports (Harper & Williams, 1974; Kolvin *et al.*, 1971; Wing *et al.*, 1967), or the source of the data was not reported (Knobloch & Pasamanick, 1975; Lobascher *et al.*, 1970). The present chapter, therefore, reviews mainly those studies published since 1975, with the exception of that by Knobloch and Pasamanick (1975). These studies have applied well-defined and internationally accepted operational diagnostic criteria in order to distinguish between autistic and schizophrenic children. Furthermore, their data sources were less questionable; that is, original medical records were the source of the obstetrical and postnatal data.

Nevertheless, the interpretation of the results of these selected studies is not easy because these studies have used heterogeneous comparison groups, such as siblings (Deykin & MacMahon, 1980; Finegan & Quarrington, 1979), both mentally retarded and normal nonautistic children (Torrey *et al.*, 1975), same-sex nonautistic children (Gillberg & Gillberg, 1983), and general population data (Finegan & Quarrington, 1979; Gillberg, 1980; Tsai & Stewart, 1983). Furthermore, these studies did not report uniform or comparable types of pre-, peri-, and neonatal complications. The studies that reported relatively comparable types of obstetrical and postnatal complications are listed in Table 1. Blank spaces in the table indicate that no information was available. The diversity among these investigations is immediately apparent.

PRENATAL FACTORS

Maternal Age

It has been suggested that there is a greater risk of birth stress, and associated brain damage, to those infants born to older mothers (Birch & Gussow, 1970). In their investigation of 14 autistic children, Torrey *et al.* (1975) prospectively collected 26 aspects of obstetrical histories, including age of mother at delivery. These authors failed to identify any significant association between maternal age and autism.

Finegan and Quarrington (1979), in a Canadian study of 23 autistic children, found 47.8% of the mothers to be in the age range of 30 to 39 at the time of each child's birth, as compared with 30.9% mothers in the general population. However, the difference was not statistically significant. The same finding was also noted in the comparison between the 15 autistic subjects and their age-closest siblings (i.e., 40% vs. 33%).

DeMyer (1979) reported that the mothers of autistic children in her intensive interview study were significantly older than the mothers of normal controls at the birth of the index child (mean age of the autistic mothers, 28.1 years; mean age of the normal mothers, 24.6 years). Since general population data were not used for comparison, sampling bias may exist in the control group.

Table 1. A Three-Study Comparison between Autistic Children and Controls for Frequency of Pre-, Peri-, and Neonatal Problems

Authors:	Study 1 (Finegan, 1979)		Study 2 (Deykin & MacMahon, 1980)		Study 3 (Gillberg & Gillberg, 1983)	
Groups:	Aut[a] (N = 15)	Sib[a] (N = 15)	Aut (N = 118)	Sib (N = 246)	Aut (N = 25)	Cont[a] (N = 25)
Factors						
Prenatal						
Bleeding	3 (20%)	1 (7%)	15 (13%)	23 (9%)	11 (44%)	2 (8%)
Infection/illness	1 (7%)	0 (0%)	19 (16%)	37 (15%)	7 (27%)	2 (8%)
Edema			21 (18%)	45 (18%)	12 (48%)	6 (24%)
Toxemia			4 (3%)	10 (4%)		
Accident/injury	1 (7%)	0 (0%)	5 (4%)	3 (1%)		
Use of medication	3 (20%)	0 (0%)	52 (44%)	90 (37%)	10 (40%)	4 (16%)
Weeks gestation < 37	3 (20%)	2 (13%)			12 (48%)	3 (12%)
< 36						
Perinatal						
Malposition	2 (13%)	0 (0%)	15 (13%)	22 (9%)	1 (4%)	2 (8%)
General anesthesia	10 (67%)	6 (40%)				
Forceps/vacuum extraction	6 (40%)	8 (53%)	71 (60%)	146 (59%)	3 (12%)	4 (16%)
Cesarean section	1 (7%)	1 (7%)	10 (8%)	4 (2%)		
Cord complications	1 (7%)	1 (7%)	21 (18%)	35 (14%)	3 (12%)	4 (16%)
Amniotic fluid	4 (27%)	0 (0%)				
Prolonged labor	1 (7%)	0 (0%)	18 (15%)	21 (9%)	6 (24%)	1 (4%)
Neonatal						
Low birth weight	3 (20%)	1 (7%)	8 (7%)	7 (3%)	1 (4%)	1 (4%)
Respiratory distress	3 (20%)	0 (0%)			1 (4%)	0 (0%)
Oxygen treatment	2 (13%)	0 (0%)	24 (20%)	35 (15%)		
Low Apgar score or poor condition	3 (20%)	1 (7%)	16 (14%)	20 (8%)	6 (24%)	1 (4%)
Jaundice	3 (20%)	0 (0%)	10 (8%)	21 (9%)	1 (4%)	0 (0%)

[a] Aut = autistic subjects, Sib = siblings, Cont = controls.

Gillberg (1980), in a Swedish study of 20 autistic children identified in a total population survey, compared the observed distribution of mean maternal age according to the year of birth of each autistic child with the corresponding figures in the general population. It is necessary to do so because the distribution of maternal age in the general population varies with location and year (Barry, 1945). Gillberg (1980) reported a significantly higher mean maternal age at the time of birth of the autistic child compared with that of the general population (30.7 vs. 26.0 years, $p < .001$). In a further study of 25 autistic children, Gillberg and Gillberg (1983) reported that 7 mothers (28%) were 35 years of age or older.

Tsai and Stewart (1983) compared the maternal ages of 113 Iowa autistic patients with the figures for mean maternal age in the general population of Iowa according to the year of birth of each autistic child. They found that the mean maternal age for the whole group (25.3 years) was very similar to that of the general population (24.6 years). They also found that the proportion of mothers of 30 years of age or older was about the same in the two groups (25% vs. 17%). However, there was an excess (9%) over the expected (4.5%) for mothers aged 35 or older in the autistic group.

The results seem to suggest some association between maternal age and autism, particularly in the group with mothers aged 35 or older. This suggestion can be supported by Gillberg and Gillberg's (1983) finding of a tendency toward more reduced optimality with high maternal age in cases when the mother was 35 years of age or older at the time of the birth of the child. It is, however, unclear how much "older mother" contributes to the development of autism.

Birth Order

Brain insult during pregnancy has been suggested to be most likely to occur during high-risk (first- and fourth- or later-born) pregnancies (Bakan, 1971). There is some evidence from earlier studies suggesting an excess of firstborn among autistic children (Creak & Ini, 1960; Kanner, 1954; Rimland, 1964; Rutter & Lockyer, 1967). Wing (1966) found that while there was no overall association between autism and birth order, there was a clear one between primacy of birth order in two-child families and later birth order in multiple-child families.

Recently, Deykin and MacMahon (1980) also observed an excess of autistic children in the first, fourth, and higher birth orders. Since more pregnancy and birth complications can occur during first pregnancies, they adjusted ratios (between autistics and their sibs) for the effect of birth order. However, they found no difference from the unadjusted ratios with regard to the various complications. They concluded that the first birth order carries a true elevated and independent risk of autism. Their study of birth order, however, has a shortcoming. They used the Greenwood–Yule method (1914), which is not suitable for analysis of data when some sibships are still incomplete, such as in the case of the autistic population. The method may cause an overrepresentation of subjects in the later birth order (McKeown & Record, 1956).

Tsai and Stewart (1983), using the Slater method (1958), which is useful for studying birth order of incomplete sibships, also observed more firstborn autistic children in two-child families, more fourth- or higher born autistic children in large families, and a corresponding lack of secondborn autistic children.

These results seem to suggest some association between autism and at-risk pregnancy. However, as the at-risk pregnancies are also observed in a relatively high proportion of the general population, the lack of specificity suggests that other factors are also involved in the causation of autism.

Bleeding in Pregnancy

Bleeding during pregnancy has been said to be associated with a wide range of subsequent abnormalities in children. Torrey *et al.* (1975) found that 9 of the 14 mothers (64%) in the autistic group had some bleeding, compared with 5 of the low-IQ control group (36%) and 4 of the normal-IQ control group (29%). There was a striking amount of early, and especially mid-trimester, bleeding among mothers who subsequently delivered autistic children. However, there was neither apparent cause of the bleeding nor any consistent relationship between bleeding and other events during pregnancy. Nonetheless, the authors found that out of the 26 aspects of the obstetrical histories examined, "maternal uterine bleeding during pregnancy" is the only one event that appeared to be significantly associated with the subsequent development of autism. There are three other studies (Deykin & MacMahon, 1980; Finegan & Quarrington, 1979; Gillberg & Gillberg, 1983) that also reported bleeding in pregnancy as more common in the autistic than in the control group (Table 1).

Maternal Infectious Disease of Any Kind during Pregnancy

As described earlier, Deykin and MacMahon (1980) noted a proportionate overrepresentation of autistic children in the first, fourth, and higher birth orders. They speculated that, in the three cases, maternal infection may be the cause because the mothers tended to have work and recreational activities in the community during their first pregnancy and tended to be exposed to their school-age children's infectious diseases during later pregnancies. Such a birth order distribution has been found, for example, in the victims of congenital rubella. In fact, Chess (1971), in a behavioral study of 243 children with congenital rubella, found that 10 children presented a picture of autism corresponding in most respects to Kanner's classical infantile autism, and an additional 8 children showed a significant number of symptoms of autism. The findings lead Deykin and MacMahon (1979) to evaluate a number of infectious agents (e.g., measles, rubella, mumps, and chickenpox) as possible etiological factors of autism. The authors, however, found that not more than 5% of autism could be attributable to prenatal rubella or influenza infection. Their data also showed that the presence of other infectious agents during pregnancy was equally low for the autistic children and their normal siblings. Two other studies (Finegan & Quarrington, 1979; Gillberg & Gillberg, 1983) also found a low rate of maternal infections during pregnancy in both the autistic and control groups (Table 1). Although these results do not seem to support the notion of infectious agent(s) in the development of autism, they suggest that should such an agent(s) exist, it is likely to be a rare or difficult-to-recognize infection(s).

Preeclampsia and Toxemia

Gillberg and Gillberg (1983) noted that "generalized edema" was more common in the autistic than in the control group, but the difference fell short of statistical significance (Table 1). Torrey *et al.* (1975) and Deykin and MacMahon (1980), however, did not find any increased risk of such a factor for their autistic group.

Gillberg and Gillberg (1983) noted a similarly low incidence of having both albuminuria and raised blood pressure in the autistic (8%) and in the control (4%) groups. Deykin and MacMahon (1980) also observed a similar finding (Table 1).

Maternal Accident/Injury during Pregnancy

Torrey *et al.* (1975) reported that there was no significant association between maternal physical trauma and autism; Finegan and Quarrington (1979) noted a low rate of "physical injury" in both the autistic and control groups. Deykin and MacMahon (1980) also observed a low frequency of prenatal trauma requiring medical attention (falls, auto collisions, burns, or cuts) in both the autistic and sibling groups (Table 1). The data showed that, should the prenatal trauma cause autism, it involves only a very small proportion of autistic persons.

Use of Physician-Prescribed Drugs

While the type and quantity of medication taken were not described, there were three studies (Deykin & MacMahon, 1980; Finegan & Quarrington, 1979; Gillberg & Gillberg, 1983) that found the autistic group using more medications than the control group (Table 1). Furthermore, Deykin and MacMahon (1980) found that "use of medication" was the only prenatal variable in their study that significantly differentiated the autistic group from the sibling group.

A recent study by Funderburk *et al.* (1983) specifically investigated the incidence of early gestational exposure to progesterone/estrogen compounds in 61 children evaluated for major childhood psychoses. Of the 61 patients, 42 met the criteria for infantile autism. The authors reported that the incidence of hormone exposure (10.7%) in their total sample was approximately double that reported for the general population, though it was not possible to determine from their data whether the gestational hormones contributed to abnormal fetal cerebral development.

Other Prenatal Factors ,

The following prenatal factors have also been investigated for their association with autism: previous X rays, history of stillbirths and spontaneous abortion prior to the birth of the study child, frequency of intercourse during pregnancy, smoking during pregnancy, psychiatric specialist care, maternal diabetes or epilepsy, premature rupture of the membranes, and gestational age. Since these variables were not investigated across the studies, comparable data were not available. However, the general conclusion has been that none of these factors shows any clear relationship with autism.

PERINATAL FACTORS

Malposition of Fetus

Studies of Finegan and Quarrington (1979), Deykin and MacMahon (1980), and Gillberg and Gillberg (1983) reported a low incidence of abnormal presentation in both the autistic and control groups (Table 1).

Use of General Anesthesia

The use of general anesthesia was quite common in both the autistic and the sibling group (Finegan & Quarrington, 1979) (Table 1). However, there is no statistically significant difference between the two groups. Torrey *et al.* (1975) also failed to identify any significant association between such an event and the development of autism.

Use of Forceps or Other Instruments

Use of forceps during deliveries was also quite common in both the autistic and the sibling group (Deykin & MacMahon, 1980). There was, however, no difference between the two groups in terms of the use of forceps (Finegan & Quarrington, 1979). Gillberg and Gillberg (1983) found the "use of vacuum extraction" was also similarly common in both the autistic and control group (Table 1).

Cesarean Section

Finegan and Quarrington (1979) reported an equally low incidence of cesarean section in the autistic and the sibling groups. Deykin and MacMahon (1980) also reported a similar observation (Table 1).

Cord Complications

Both prolapse of cord and wrapping the cord around the newborn's neck were observed to be equally infrequent in the autistic and the sibling group (Deykin & MacMahon, 1980; Finegan & Quarrington, 1979; Gillberg & Gillberg, 1983) (Table 1).

Meconium in Amniotic Fluid

Finegan and Quarrington (1979) found that the autistic group had a significantly higher ($p = .05$) incidence of "meconium in amniotic fluid" (a sign of fetal distress) than did the sibling group. This finding was supported by Gillberg and Gillberg's (1983) study (Table 1).

Prolonged First-Stage Labor

Both Finegan and Quarrington (1979) and Deykin and MacMahon (1980) reported that prolonged first-stage labor was similarly infrequent in both the autistic and the sibling group (Table 1).

Other Perinatal Factors

Each of the following factors was examined by only one of the above studies: weight of the placenta (Torrey *et al.*, 1975), placental infarcts/calcification (Finegan & Quarrington,

1979), and twins/multiple birth (Gillberg & Gillberg, 1983). The role of these factors in the development of autism is not clear.

NEONATAL FACTORS

Low Birth Weight

For many years it was generally believed that most low-birth-weight infants either were born prematurely or were abnormal. However, there have been many recent reports of low incidents of handicaps (10% or less) among very-low-birth-weight survivors cared for with methods designed to prevent handicaps. Nevertheless, the relationship between low birth weight and autism has been investigated. Two of these studies (Deykin & MacMahon, 1980; Finegan & Quarrington, 1979) observed a similarly low incidence of low birth weight in both the autistic and the sibling group (Table 1).

Respiratory Distress and Oxygen Treatment

The main autistic symptoms have been postulated to be manifestations of bilateral dysfunction of the temporal lobes, which are especially vulnerable to damage during pre-, peri-, and neonatal episodes of anoxia (Hetzler & Griffin, 1981). Gillberg and Gillberg (1983) reported that the incidence of respiratory distress and oxygen treatment was very low in both the autistic and the control group. However, Finegan and Quarrington (1979) found that such an event was not rare as compared to the sibling group (Table 1).

Apgar Score

The Apgar score is a useful discriminator of risk for poor neurological outcome. The study by Torrey et al. (1975) did not describe the incidence of a low Apgar score in either the autistic or the control group. Their results, however, implied that there was no significant association between a low Apgar score and autism. Finegan and Quarrington (1979) and Gillberg and Gillberg (1983) reported that the incidence of a low Apgar score was low in both the autistic and the sibling group. In the study of Deykin and MacMahon (1980), data on an Apgar score were not collected; however, they have a rating on the "newborn's condition" based on strength of cry and color. They found that similarly few newborns of both the autistic and control groups were rated as having a "poor condition at birth" (Table 1).

Hyperbilirubinemia

High serum bilirubin level has been related with encephalopathy. Deykin and MacMahon (1980) and Gillberg and Gillberg (1983) reported that jaundice occurred with similarly low frequency among autistic subjects, their siblings, and controls. Finegan and Quarrington (1979) noted that jaundice was significantly more common in their autistic sample than it was in the general population, but the rate of jaundice was similar in the autistics and their siblings (Table 1).

Other Neonatal Factors

Deykin and MacMahon (1980) found that more of the autistic children (20%) were in need of medical intervention in the first month of life than were their siblings (15%). Gillberg and Gillberg (1983) also noted that the incidence of septicemia or meningitis in the neonatal phase was higher in the autistic group than in the control group.

CONCLUSIONS

From the current review we conclude that unfavorable pre-, peri-, and neonatal factors seem to be more frequent in autistic children than in their siblings or in controls. Particularly, older mother, first- and fourth- or later born, bleeding after the first trimester, use of medication, and meconium in amniotic fluid appear to occur more frequently in the autistic groups than in the sibling or control groups. In Deykin and MacMahon's study (1980), the autistic children were significantly more likely than their siblings to have at least one of the listed prenatal complications. They also found that when all perinatal complications were grouped together, the autistic group had a significantly higher frequency of unfavorable events than that of their siblings. On the other hand, Gillberg and Gillberg (1983) noted that the autistic children showed greatly increased scores for reduced optimality, especially with regard to prenatal factors.

As most of the data analyzed were obtained from medical records established long before the autism diagnosis was made, it is unlikely that these findings are subject to bias of ascertainment. On the other hand, the interpretation of the findings should be cautious because of the following reasons. First, although many of the symptoms or factors in these studies did not appear as statistically significant, it could be that each one might occur so infrequently that it cannot show up as statistically significant. It is possible that in the future, with larger sample size studies, these factors may turn out to be clinically important. Second, the highest-risk pre-, peri-, and neonatal factors were observed in only small proportions of autistic children in the studies. Finally, the obstetrical and postnatal factors found to be associated with autism have been rather heterogeneous in type across studies (Rutter, 1985). No single variable or combination of variables could either reasonably account for a large number of cases of autism (Deykin & MacMahon, 1980) or discriminate between the autistic and control groups.

It seems that, in some instances, unfavorable pre-, peri-, and neonatal factors may be associated with autism. However, the data reviewed so far do not suggest a unifying pathologic process in autism. This lack of specificity indicates either that various types of physical damage may produce autism (Deykin & MacMahon, 1980) or that there is (are) yet unidentified unifying obstetric and/or postnatal variable(s) responsible for all cases of autism, or that factors (e.g., genetic factor) other than obstetrical and postnatal complications may also be responsible for the subsequent development of autism. In future studies it will be necessary to consider all of these aspects.

REFERENCES

Bakan, P. (1971). Handedness and birth order. *Nature, 229,* 195.
Barry, H. (1945). Incidence of advanced maternal age in mothers of one thousand state hospital patients (A.M.A.). *Archives of Neurology and Psychiatry, 54,* 186–191.

Bender, L. (1973). The life course of children with schizophrenia. *American Journal of Psychiatry,* *130,* 783–786.

Bender, L., & Faretra, G. (1961). Pregnancy and birth histories of children with psychiatric problems. *Proceedings of the Third World Congress of Psychiatry, 2,* 1329–1333.

Birch, H. G., & Gussow, J. D. (1970). *Disadvantaged children: Health, nutrition and school failure.* New York: Harcourt, Brace and World.

Campbell, M., Geller, B., Small, A. M., Petti, T. A., & Ferris, S. H. (1978). Minor physical anomalies in young psychotic children. *American Journal of Psychiatry, 135,* 573–575.

Chess, S. (1971). Autism in children with congenital rubella. *Journal of Autism and Childhood Schizophrenia, 1,* 33–47.

Creak, M., & Ini, S. (1960). Families of psychotic children. *Journal of Child Psychology and Psychiatry. 1,* 156–175.

DeMyer, M. K. (1979). *Parents and children in autism,* Washington, D.C.: Winston.

Deykin, E. Y., & MacMahon, B. (1979). Viral exposure and autism. *American Journal of Epidemiology, 109,* 628–638.

Deykin, E. Y., & MacMahon, B. (1980). Pregnancy, delivery, and neonatal complications among autistic children. *American Journal of Diseases of Children, 134,* 860–864.

Finegan, J-A., & Quarrington, B. (1979). Pre-, peri-, and neonatal factors and infantile autism. *Journal of Child Psychology and Psychiatry, 20,* 119–128.

Fish, B., & Ritvo, E. R. (1979). Psychoses of childhood. In J. D. Noshpitz (Ed.), *Basic handbook of child psychiatry.* New York: Basic Books.

Funderburk, S. J., Carter, J., Tanguay, P., Freeman, B. J., & Westlake, J. R. (1983). Parental reproductive problems and gestational hormonal exposure in autistic and schizophrenic children. *Journal of Autism and Developmental Disorders, 13,* 325–332.

Gillberg, C. (1980). Maternal age and infantile autism. *Journal of Autism and Developmental Disorders, 10,* 293–297.

Gillberg, C., & Gillberg, I. C. (1983). Infantile autism: A total population study of reduced optimality in the pre-, peri-, and neonatal period. *Journal of Autism and Developmental Disorders, 13,* 153–166.

Gittleman, M., & Birch, H. G. (1967). Childhood schizophrenia. *Archives of General Psychiatry, 17,* 16–25.

Greenwood, M., & Yule, G. U. (1914). On the determination of size of family and of the distribution of characters in order of birth. *Journal of the Royal Statistical Society, 77,* 179–197.

Harper, J., & Williams, S. (1974). Early environmental stress and infantile autism. *Medical Journal of Australia, 1,* 341–346.

Hetzler, B. E., & Griffin, J. (1981). Infantile autism and the temporal lobe of brain. *Journal of Autism and Developmental Disorders, 13,* 317–330.

Hinton, G. G. (1963). Childhood psychosis or mental retardation: A diagnostic dilemma. *Canadian Medical Association Journal, 89,* 1020–1024.

Kanner, L. (1954). To what extent is early infantile autism determined by constitutional inadequacies. *Proceedings of the Association for Research in Nervous and Mental Diseases, 33,* 378–385.

Knobloch, H., & Pasamanick, B. (1975). Some etiologic and prognostic factors in early infantile autism and psychosis. *Pediatrics, 55,* 182–191.

Kolvin, I., Ounsted, C., & Roth, M. (1971). Studies in the childhood psychoses—V. Cerebral dysfunction and childhood psychoses. *British Journal of Psychiatry, 118,* 407–414.

Lobascher, M. E., Kingerlee, P. E., & Gubbay, S. S. (1970). Childhood autism: An investigation of aetiological factors in twenty-five cases. *British Journal of Psychiatry, 117,* 525–529.

McKeown, T., & Record, R. G. (1956). Maternal age and birth order as indices of environmental influence. *American Journal of Human Genetics, 14,* 25–30.

Ornitz, E. M., & Ritvo, E. R. (1976). The syndrome of autism: A critical review. *American Journal of Psychiatry, 133,* 609–621.

Osterkamp, A., & Sands, D. J. (1962). Early feeding and birth difficulties in childhood schizophrenia: A brief study. *Journal of Genetic Psychology, 101,* 363–366.

Rimland, B. (1964). *Infantile autism.* New York: Appleton-Century-Crofts.

Rutt, C. N., & Offord, D. R. (1971). Prenatal and perinatal complications in childhood schizophrenia and their sibships. *Journal of Nervous and Mental Disease, 152,* 324–331.

Rutter, M. (1985). Infantile autism and other pervasive developmental disorders. In M. Rutter & L. Hersov (Eds.), *Child and adolescent psychiatry: Modern approaches.* Oxford: Blackwell Scientific.

Rutter, M., & Lockyer, L. (1967). A five to fifteen year follow-up study of infantile psychosis—I. Description of the sample. *British Journal of Psychiatry, 113,* 1169–1182.

Slater, E. (1958). The sibs and children of homosexuals. In D. R. Smith & W. M. Davidson (Eds.), *Symposium on nuclear sex.* London: Heinemann.

Taft, L. T., & Goldfarb, W. (1964). Prenatal and perinatal factors in childhood schizophrenia. *Developmental Medicine and Child Neurology, 6,* 32–43.

Terris, M., Lapouse, R., & Monk, M. (1964). The relation of prematurity and previous fetal loss to childhood schizophrenia. *American Journal of Psychiatry, 121,* 476–481.

Torrey, E. F., Hersh, S. P., & McCabe, K. D. (1975). Early childhood psychosis and bleeding during pregnancy: A prospective study of gravid women and their offspring. *Journal of Autism and Childhood Schizophrenia, 5,* 287–297.

Tsai, L. Y., & Stewart, M. A. (1983). Etiological implication of maternal age and birth order in infantile autism. *Journal of Autism and Developmental Disorders, 13,* 57–65.

Vorster, D. (1960). An investigation into the part played by organic factors in childhood schizophrenia. *Journal of Mental Science, 106,* 494–522.

Whittam, H., Simon, G. B., & Mittler, P. J. (1966). The early development of psychotic children and their sibs. *Developmental Medicine and Child Neurology, 8,* 552–560.

Wing, J. K. (1966). Diagnosis, epidemiology, and etiology. In J. K. Wing (Ed.), *Early childhood autism.* Oxford: Pergamon Press.

Wing, J. K., O'Connor, N., & Lotter, V. (1967). Autistic conditions in early childhood: A survey of Middlesex. *British Medical Journal, 3,* 389–392.

11

Neurobiological Implications of Sex Differences in Autism

CATHERINE LORD and ERIC SCHOPLER

The nature and meaning of sex differences in autism present a paradox for researchers. On the one hand, one of the most well-established facts about autism is that it occurs with much greater frequency in males than in females. On the other hand, two difficulties quickly become apparent when one tries to move beyond the sex difference in the incidence of autism to its neurobiological implications. First, the theoretical links between sex differences, possible etiologies, and organic mechanisms underlying autism are far from straightforward. While there have been numerous failures to confirm specific hypotheses, few positive findings have emerged. Because of small sample sizes, nonepidemiological samples, and difficulties in balancing factors such as sex and degree of mental retardation within autism, negative findings cannot be taken as conclusive.

Second, there is almost no information available about females with autism. Females have been excluded from many of the more carefully controlled studies of autism (e.g., Bartak, Rutter, & Cox, 1975). In other studies, the numbers of females have been so low that it has been inappropriate to analyze them separately (August, Stewart, & Tsai, 1981; Schopler, Andrews, & Strupp, 1979; Wing, 1981b). Because of these difficulties, a chapter covering research on autism and sex differences must necessarily be as much a discussion of what we would like to know about sex differences, and why, as it is a description of what is already known.

Altogether, three goals underlie this chapter: (1) to describe sex differences in autism that have already been identified and those that have been hypothesized but remain unconfirmed, (2) to discuss the neurobiological implications of these differences, and (3) to outline needs for future research.

CATHERINE LORD • Department of Pediatrics, University of Alberta, and Department of Psychology, Glenrose Hospital, Edmonton, Alberta T5G 0B7, Canada.   ERIC SCHOPLER • Division TEACCH, University of North Carolina, Chapel Hill, North Carolina 27514.

SEX DIFFERENCES IN INCIDENCE

Sex Differences in the Incidence of Autism

The largest and most carefully controlled epidemiological study of the incidence of autism (Lotter, 1966) showed ratios of between 2.4 and 2.8 autistic males for every autistic female in Middlesex County in England. This result has been replicated with minor variations in several other epidemiological studies (Brask, 1972, cited in Wing, 1981b; Treffert, 1970). Perhaps most well known is the research of Wing (Wing, 1981b; Wing, Gould, Yeates, & Brierly, 1977), who found a sex ratio of 2.6 males to 1 female for a combined group of typically autistic and more broadly defined socially impaired, language-delayed, mentally retarded children in the London borough of Camberwell. Both the Camberwell and Middlesex studies included children with all degrees of retardation, some of whom had known organic conditions, as long as the children met diagnostic criteria for autism or, in Wing's case, for a triad of social, language, and cognitive impairments.

Sex ratios of autistic samples in studies of clinic populations have generally, though not always, been somewhat higher than those in epidemiological samples. For example, Rutter and Lockyer (1967) reported a ratio of 4.25 to 1 for a sample collected from a London-based clinic, while Lord and Schopler (1985) reported a ratio of 3.6 to 1 for a large clinic-based sample in North Carolina, in the United States. Ratios ranging from 2.3 to 1 (Tsai & Beisler, 1983) to 4.8 to 1 (Baird & August, 1985) have been reported in other studies (e.g., Lord, Schopler, & Revicki, 1982; Tsai, Stewart, & August, 1981).

Sources of difference between studies, both epidemiological and clinic-based, are multiple. These include referral biases (which vary according to the nature of the clinic), selection and interpretation of diagnostic criteria, method of diagnosis (i.e., direct assessment vs. review of medical records), proportion of subjects with severe mental retardation (see below), and the size of the total sample. Epidemiological studies, particularly the studies of Lotter (1966) and Wing (Wing, 1981b; Wing et al., 1977), where the autistic children were seen firsthand, have the advantage of avoiding referral biases, but the disadvantage of yielding small samples. In general, epidemiological studies have tended to include more severely retarded subjects and to use somewhat broader diagnostic criteria than clinic-based research. These two factors have been associated with lower sex ratios (Lord, 1984; Wing, 1981b, 1984). Overall, if one excludes profoundly retarded children with autistic features, the fairest estimate seems to be about 3 to 4 autistic males for every female (Rutter, 1985; Rutter & Schopler, in press).

Sex Differences in the Incidence of Related Disorders

Males are more frequently affected than females with almost all behavioral disorders (Eme, 1979), mental handicaps (Rutter, Tizard, & Whitmore, 1970/1981), and learning problems (Finucci & Childs, 1981). The significance of the sex ratio in autism lies, therefore, not in the direction of the effect but in its size. The difference between the high male-to-female sex ratio in autism and the roughly equal incidence of schizophrenia in the two sexes has been used to support claims of the discreteness of the two disorders (Eme, 1979; Rutter & Garmezy, 1983). In fact, the high male:female ratio in autism has been one of the most clearcut distinguishing features differentiating autism from schizophrenia (Eme, 1979; Lewine, 1981).

In other childhood disorders, very high male:female ratios (greater than 3 to 1) have been associated with three general areas of handicap or pathology: language dysfunction (Cantwell, Baker, & Mattison, 1979), activity level/behavior problems (Richman, Stevenson, & Graham, 1985), and criminality/antisocial behavior (Cloninger, Christiansen, Reich, & Gottesman, 1978). High sex ratios in criminality seem unlikely to have any bearing on autism since the association between antisocial or criminal behavior and autistic patterns of development is rather minimal (although recent discussions of Asperger syndrome may eventually call this statement into question; see Wing, 1981a). On the other hand, the association between early restlessness and high activity level (whether considered separately or as a single "attention deficit"), language delay, and later learning difficulties (Richman et al., 1985) could perhaps be more easily related to autism. One could speculate about high activity level/restlessness as an indicator of greater male vulnerability to cognitive and/or mild neurological dysfunction, although at this point the links between early behavior problems and cognitive development are not well understood. Their relevance to autism is therefore not clear.

The association between high male:female ratios and language disorders is more interesting, especially given findings from several studies of a higher incidence than expected of language and cognitive delay in families of autistic children (August et al., 1981; Folstein & Rutter, 1977; Minton, Campbell, Green, Jennings, & Samit, 1982). The suggestion has been made that less specific cognitive dysfunctions than autism, such as speech and language disorders and general cognitive delay (Folstein & Rutter, 1977; Minton et al., 1982), are aggregated in some families. Male:female ratios appear to be particularly high for stuttering (Gualtieri & Hicks, 1985; Reinisch, Gandelman, & Spiegel, 1979) and severe, specific reading retardation (Berger, Yule, & Rutter, 1975; Finucci & Childs, 1981). For other language-related disorders, males usually exceed females, but the ratios tend to be much lower, as in reading backwardness or milder reading problems (Finucci & Childs, 1981; Rutter et al., 1970/1981) or early expressive language delay (Cantwell et al., 1979; Fundudis, Kolvin, & Garside, 1979). Sometimes sex ratios appear to be equal, such as in severe receptive language disorders (Bartak et al., 1975). In their epidemiological study of the Isle of Wight, Rutter and colleagues (Rutter et al., 1970/1981) found that verbally based intelligence tests produced a higher male:female ratio of children scoring below average than did nonverbal tests. Two other studies of children with broadly defined language delays found smaller sex differences (2:1 or less than in autism) or no differences at all in the incidence of broadly defined language delays (Cantwell et al., 1979; Fundudis et al., 1979).

Rutter et al., (1970/1981) also found greater male:female ratios for severe mental retardation than for mild to moderate retardation. This finding was replicated in Wing's (1981b) Camberwell study. Both Wing and Rutter speculated that this difference reflected greater male vulnerability to organic brain damage, as well as greater environmental stress in males than in females.

Vulnerability to organic brain damage may vary in initial cause or etiology, in pathophysiology (i.e., the physiological processes that are affected), and in the nature of the resulting handicap(s). For example, in a group of *socially impaired*, severely mentally retarded children, Wing (1981b) found that, of children with well-defined organic conditions (e.g., cerebral palsy), 78% of girls but only about 33% of boys were profoundly retarded. This sex difference could not be accounted for by differences in the incidence of Down syndrome, because most of those children were not socially impaired beyond their cognitive delays. The difference suggests that there are differential associations involving social impairment, overall level of intellectual retardation, and certain forms of brain dysfunction in the two sexes. Because of the necessarily small size of the sample and the heterogeneity of documented organic conditions, however, more information is needed before conclusions can be drawn.

A similar finding from a different perspective occurs in reports of unusually good skills in otherwise mentally retarded persons. While not epidemiological, such case reports have been much more common for males than for females (Hermelin & O'Connor, 1983). However, the methodological dilemma that occurs for sex ratios in autism is also relevant to sex ratios in severe and profound retardation, for neurological disabilities such as cerebral palsy, and for general mental retardation co-occurring with unusual abilities. Epidemiological samples usually yield such small numbers of these low-incidence disorders that sex ratios can fluctuate dramatically on the basis of one subject. On the other hand, clinic samples are open to numerous biases, discussed earlier and again below.

Finally, neither speech and language problems nor mental retardation are homogeneous syndromes etiologically, pathophysiologically, or phenomenologically. As discussed below, factors that may contribute to sex differences of a few points in verbal IQ within a normal population, to mild reading difficulties or to expressive language delay measurable at age 3 but overcome by age 7, may be entirely different from factors accounting for sex differences in severe mental retardation, specific reading retardation, or stuttering (Childs & Finucci, 1983). On the other hand, the possibility of common transmittable factors associated with a not-too-large number of potentially identifiable cognitive or learning-related disorders is also intriguing (Folstein & Rutter, 1977), especially given the variation of language disorder and IQ even within autism.

SEX RATIOS, AUTISM, AND MENTAL RETARDATION

As for other speech and language disorders, the IQ range for autism is very broad. While most autistic persons also have general mental retardation to some degree, autism occurs in persons with average or above-average intelligence as well. It has been suggested that sex ratios in autism are systematically related to these variations in intelligence (Wing, 1981b, 1984). It is now well established that, on the average, mean IQ scores for groups of autistic females are slightly lower than for groups of autistic males (Lord et al., 1982; Lord & Schopler, 1985; Tsai et al., 1981). This finding of lower IQs in females and males has been replicated in epidemiological as well as clinic-based studies (Wing, 1981b).

Several models have been proposed to account for the distribution of IQ across the sexes. One possibility is that females all along the IQ range score slightly lower than males. This was the case in the research of Lord and Schopler (1985; Lord et al., 1982). Another possibility, not necessarily in contradiction to the first, is that there is an excess of autistic females in the mentally retarded ranges of intelligence compared to the number of autistic females of normal intelligence, which does not occur to such a large degree in males. This possibility has also been confirmed in several studies (Tsai & Beisler, 1983; Tsai et al., 1981; Wing, 1981b).

The question still remains of where, within the ranges of mental retardation, this excess of females occurs. Detailed analysis of a large sample indicated that the sex ratio shifted most markedly from about 4:1 for children with IQs 35 and above to 2.5–3.0:1 for children with IQs of 34 and under (Lord & Schopler, 1985). Thus the excess of autistic females was located in *very* severe to profound ranges of retardation. These autistic persons with severe and profound mental retardation have the highest incidence of other disabilities;

for many of them, autism or severe social and language impairments are just one of multiple handicaps (Wing, 1981b). Within this group of children, the theoretical and practical usefulness of giving an additional diagnosis of autism has been questioned by numerous authors (see Wing & Gould, 1979). How specific any genetic or familial patterns in this group are to the syndrome of *autism* (Baird & August, 1985), rather than to mental retardation and/ or other disorders, is almost impossible to assess. What is particularly problematic is when large numbers of these children are combined with higher-functioning groups of children with autism and, for research purposes, referred to as "autistic," when in fact the findings about them could be related to many other factors than the autism *per se*.

A third way to account for differences in mean IQs of autistic males and females would be through an excess of autistic males at the high end of the distribution of intelligence. Thus, it could be the case that sex ratios steadily rise with IQ, indicating proportionately greater numbers of autistic males as IQ increases. Both Lotter (1966) and Symmes (1976) provided early reports of failures to find *any* high-functioning autistic females in contrast to several males. Wing (1981b) found only one social- and language-impaired female with an IQ greater than 55 in her epidemiological sample, compared to 15 males. Several authors reported ratios of 5:1 or more males to females in high-functioning samples, in contrast to ratios of 3 or 4 to 1 for children with IQs under 50 (Tsai & Beisler, 1983; Tsai *et al.*, 1981; Wing, 1981a,b).

However, when "high-functioning" is defined as an IQ over 70, findings of extremely high male:female ratios have generally not been reported (Baird & August, 1985; Lord *et al.*, 1982; Lord & Schopler, 1985). One early paper reported ratios of nearly 5 to 1 males to females for subjects with IQs over 70 (Tsai *et al.*, 1981). However, in a later paper including these subjects and others, higher-functioning children were grouped with those with lower IQs, suggesting that the particularly high ratio was not replicated. Altogether, given the small numbers of females and the small numbers of subjects of either sex with IQs over 70 (even in the largest sample, that of Lord & Schopler, 1985, there were only 19 females with IQs over 70), whether or not there is a particularly high ratio of autistic males to females of near-normal intelligence must remain an open question.

In earlier papers, Wing (1981b) and Tsai and colleagues (Tsai *et al.*, 1981; Tsai & Beisler, 1983) suggested that two of the possible trends in distributions just described (that is, an excess of low-functioning females and an excess of high-functioning males) resulted in a linear relationship between IQ and sex ratio in autism. If a linear relationship had been identified, it would have provided support for some kind of homogeneous factor in autism that related to sex. A model suggesting sex differences in "threshold" (on a yet unspecified biological dimension, that could be either etiological or pathophysiological) would have been supported.

From current data, however, it seems likely that there is *not* a linear relationship between sex ratio and IQ (Lord, 1984). Rather, there are differences in sex ratios for broadly defined IQ ranges, such that the sex ratio for autistic children with IQs below 35 is significantly lower than for children with IQs of 35 or above. At this point, no consistent differences between sex ratios in high-functioning (IQ greater than 70) and mildly to moderately retarded (IQ = 35–69) autistic youngsters have been identified (Lord & Schopler, 1985). Given the likelihood of etiologically and possibly pathophysiologically distinct types of autism, findings of different sex ratios associated with different levels of retardation are still of great interest. However, the characterization of subtypes of autism will require careful consideration and validation of many factors, in addition to sex and IQ ranges, in order to arrive at useful conceptualizations (see Lord & Schopler, 1985, for more discussion of this issue).

GENETIC IMPLICATIONS OF DIFFERENCES IN SEX RATIOS

The initial reaction of many people to the high male:female ratio in autism is that the sex difference must be related to genetic factors. In one way, this of course is true since sex itself is inherited. Sex is transmitted in the form of two X chromosomes in females or an X and a Y chromosome in males. However, it is not *necessarily* the case that autism is genetically transmitted at all, or if so, in the same way as sex—that is, on a sex chromosome. Genetic and environmental factors may interact with the sex of an individual child in many different ways such that the overall result is a higher incidence of autism in males than in females.

Although the relationship between the genetic transmission of autism and sex is not yet understood, it seems highly likely that, at some level, genetic factors figure in the etiologies of at least some cases of autism (Folstein & Rutter, 1977; Spence, Ritvo, Marazita, Funderbunk, Sparkes, & Freeman, 1985). Families with more than one autistic child occur more often than one would expect from estimates of the incidence of autism (Folstein & Rutter, 1977). These families include autistic siblings of both sexes. This finding suggests that genetic factors, perhaps even the same factors, may at least in *some* cases contribute to autism in both males and females (Ritvo, Spence, *et al.*, 1985). Still, at present, the proportion of autistic individuals who come from multiple-incidence families appears to be rather small. Given the proposed heterogeneity of etiology in autism, there is certainly room for several different patterns of familial transmission, as well as cases where environmental factors predominate. These familial patterns may or may not be related to sex, may or may not be specific to autism, and may or may not require environmental occurrences as well. In fact, the multiplicity of possible factors can leave one feeling as if it is impossible to prove or disprove any specific hypotheses, a feeling that may in fact be justified.

In addition, it is important to remember that genetic differences must be manifested somehow physiologically or anatomically. On what level these differences occur—whether in brain structure, hormones, other aspects of neurochemistry or neurophysiology, other single biologic factors, or a multiplicity of factors—is not clear at this point from genetic analyses. Because of our relatively unsophisticated understanding of the causes and roots of autism, models may be generated for genetic transmission and for "pathophysiology" quite independently. At this point in our knowledge, it is not surprising or inappropriate that sometimes these models are entirely different from each other. The ultimate goal, however, is to identify links between patterns of transmission and the pathophysiology and phenomenology of whatever is transmitted that would have implications for treatment or prevention.

X-Linked Disorders

The first reaction of many people with an introductory knowledge of genetics to the high male:female ratio in autism is that autism must be a sex-linked disorder. That is, autism must be transmitted from generation to generation on one of the two sex chromosomes, X or Y. To date, this possibility has been assumed to be unlikely for most individuals with autism, except for a subset of autistic children with fragile X. However, it is raised so frequently that it seems worthwhile to outline why it is unlikely to be the case, at least for most autistic individuals.

To date, no human disorders have been clearly identified as transmitted on the Y chromosome, so for all intents and purposes, sex-linked disorders are those transmitted through the X chromosome (Carter, 1972). Autism could be an X-linked disorder inherited as a dominant trait. That is, it would be inherited on the X chromosome, and, taking a simple perspective, anyone who inherited it would manifest the symptoms of autism. Three characteristics should then be present in family histories: (1) It should appear in each successive generation, (2) only affected individuals should have affected offspring, and (3) females should be affected twice as often as males (since, having received an X chromosome from each parent, they would have twice the opportunity to inherit the disorder as would males, who can only receive an X chromosome from their mothers). These patterns have not typically been found in families of autistic individuals.

Although the consistent lack of support for these predictions sounds straightforward, there are several other factors that mean that a hypothesis of X-linked dominant transmission in some cases cannot yet be rejected completely. One of these factors is *lyonization*, which refers to the process in females (who always have two X chromosomes) during which one or the other of these chromosomes may be inactive in any given cell. Thus, a female may have an X-linked dominant gene but appear to be unaffected because a high proportion of the X chromosomes with the responsible gene may be inactive. This occurrence could result in generations of females who, according to theory, should have autism but who do not manifest the behavioral symptoms of the disorder.

A second factor adding to confusion is variation in *penetrance*, which is the frequency with which a trait is manifest (in some measurable way) by those who possess the gene responsible for it. *Epistasis* is the process whereby one gene modifies another gene at a different locus. It is one possible explanation for variable penetrance. Penetrance is also affected by the female's possession of two X chromosomes. Thus, in some known genetic disorders such as neurofibromatosis or tuberous sclerosis, a group of individuals may all have the gene but vary greatly among themselves in number and severity of symptoms associated with the genetic disorder.

For autism to be a disorder with a dominant pattern of transmission, its penetrance would have to be very low in some families, since *most* family members of autistic individuals clearly do not have autism. On the other hand, if one broadens the notion of what is transmitted from autism only to include mild language and cognitive disorders, *and* if one allows for low penetrance, then the possibility of dominant patterns must still remain open. At this point, though, there is no evidence in favor of an *X-linked* dominant pattern occurring with any frequency in autism.

Finally, a third factor that makes rejection of hypotheses of X-linked dominant transmission more difficult is the possibility that the responsible gene could be lethal for males, though not for females (where lyonization might be expected to moderate the effect somewhat). There would be no male-to-male or male-to-female transmission since affected males would not survive. If females with the gene could reproduce, then their surviving offspring would be expected to consist of affected daughters, unaffected daughters, and unaffected sons. If females with the gene could not reproduce, the disorder would appear only in females and each case would appear as a new mutation. The possibility of this pattern has been raised for Rett syndrome (Hagberg, Aicardi, Dias, & Rasmos, 1983).

An X-linked *recessive* mode of inheritance is a bit more plausible in accounting for some cases of autism in males, but it would not easily account for the presence of the disorder in most females with autism. Except for cases of fragile X, which is discussed in detail in Chapter 5, family histories of autistic persons do not seem to follow an X-linked recessive pattern (Ritvo, Spence, *et al.*, 1985; Spence, *et al.*, 1985). Such a pattern would require that one-half the male offspring of female carriers and none of the female offspring of female carriers would be affected. This pattern has also not been typical of most families of autistic children (Hanson & Gottesman, 1976). Lyonization in female carriers and variable penetrance might account for some of the failures to find support for this pattern, but they seem unlikely to make much difference.

In general, genetic models of autism are made more complicated than models of many other disorders because few autistic individuals bear children. Thus, in autism, assessment of successive generations always needs to work "up" from the autistic proband rather than working "down" to the proband's children. Genetic studies of autism require consideration of unaffected relatives (since parents of autistic children are not usually autistic) or inclusion of persons with nonautistic, cognitive deficits, if family patterns are to be identified.

If autism in some males was the result of X-linked recessive transmission, one would expect a higher incidence of related disorders in the siblings of these males than in the siblings of autistic females (most of whom would presumably have the disorder because of other etiologies). To date, this prediction has not been supported (August et al., 1981; Baird & August, 1985), though the series of papers on multiple incidence families by Ritvo, Spence, and colleagues (Ritvo, Freeman, et al., 1985; Ritvo, Spence, et al., 1985; Spence et al., 1985) were based on a sample with an excess of males. It is also interesting that all of the monozygotic twins concordant for autism in the Folstein and Rutter (1977) study were male (4/8 male pairs). All of the female monozygotic pairs (3/8) were concordant for cognitive and socioemotional disorder (but not for autism), compared to 2 of the 8 male monozygotic pairs (concordant for cognitive/socioemotional disorder but not for autism). Altogether, however, sample sizes have been small, and not necessarily equivalent across sex in risk factors. Furthermore, X-linked patterns are known to be frequent in families of nonautistic children with nonspecific mental retardation (Herbst & Miller, 1980). Thus, the question of the role of X-linkage and autism remains open.

Autosomal Disorders and Sex-Limited Patterns

A third possibility, besides the two forms of X-linked or sex-linked patterns of inheritance, is autosomal (i.e., involving nonsex chromosomes) patterns of transmission that are sex-limited. In sex-limited disorders, the gene may be inherited from a parent of either sex, but the sex of the proband or individual receiving the gene determines whether the trait appears, such as in baldness in males (Carter, 1972). Autosomal *dominant* patterns are somewhat unlikely in autism because then the disorder should appear in successive generations and one-half of the siblings of an affected individual should be affected. However, variability in penetrance might account for some apparently skipped generations.

Autosomal recessive patterns (Ritvo, Spence, et al., 1985; Spence et al., 1985) are somewhat more plausible, since the disorder would not necessarily occur in each generation, and unaffected individuals may have affected offspring according to this pattern. These patterns would be the simplest way to account for mixed-sex sibships with autism. However, the high male:female ratio in autism would not be accounted for by autosomal recessive inheritance unless sex-limited constraints are posited. To date, no serious attempt has been made to identify or study such constraints.

The recent genetic studies of multiplex families by Ritvo, Spence, and colleagues (Ritvo, Spence, et al., 1985; Spence et al., 1985) are discussed in detail in Chapter 5. What is relevant in these studies to sex differences in autism is that, while autosomal recessive patterns may account for some cases of autism in males and females, another mode of transmission, or at least additional factors, is required to account for the greater number of autistic males than autistic females. Autosomal recessive patterns *alone* cannot account for the excess of males. Adding fragile X into the equation may help account to some extent for the sex ratio. However, though fragile X may play a role in some cases of autism in males, it probably does not occur with sufficient frequency to account completely for the 3 to 4:1 male-to-female ratio. The general trend for fragile X to occur in probands who are both autistic and moderately to severely mentally retarded (Fryns, 1984; Sherman, Morton, Jacobs, & Turner, 1984) is also somewhat in contradiction with findings that the sex ratio in autism is *lowest* for autistic individuals who are the most profoundly retarded (with IQs below 35).

Polygenic, Multifactorial Threshold Models of Transmission

Another type of transmission that has been suggested at a conceptual level to account for high male:female ratios in autism is a multifactorial, polygenic threshold model of inheritance (Tsai *et al.*, 1981; Wing, 1981b). This is a *mathematical* model interposed on frequency and severity data for disorders. It is used to explain higher-than-expected incidences in families whose histories do not follow Mendelian (i.e., single-gene) patterns of transmission. To date, polygenic threshold models typically have been proposed for disorders that show significant variations in severity, and that are defined in behavioral rather than biologic terms (e.g., stuttering or schizophrenia as opposed to hemophilia or phenylketonuria). In contrast to the single-gene autosomal and sex-linked theories discussed earlier, polygenic theories of autism propose that more than one gene would be involved in each case of autism. Multifactorial threshold models also allow the inclusion of environmental factors, and hypotheses about differences in threshold levels for the appearance of the actual disorder in predictions of incidence. For example, sex differences in a theoretical "threshold for autism"[1] could be hypothesized.

Multifactorial models pertain to autism because they can account for variations in the occurrence of a disorder in the sexes, without the constraints (discussed earlier) that are part of single-gene models of transmission. Given the elevated incidence of autism in males as opposed to females, a polygenic, multifactorial model that proposes a higher threshold for autism in females than males would yield three predictions. First, the severity of autism should be greater in the least-affected sex, because presumably it should take "more" defective genes and/or environmental factors to produce autism in females than males, if females have a higher threshold of vulnerability. Second, there should be a higher incidence of autism, or whatever disorder is transmitted, in the *families* of autistic females than males; again because it should take "more" defective genes to produce autism in females who have higher thresholds than in males who have lower thresholds. Thus, autistic females should have a greater number of affected relatives than should autistic males. Third, relatives of autistic females should be affected more severely (that is, should be more severely autistic or mentally retarded or language-handicapped) than relatives of autistic males, because more severe disorder should be required to exceed the hypothetical threshold for females than for males.

Difficulties in evaluating the first prediction—that is, of greater severity of autism in females than in males—are obvious right from the start. Rating the severity of autism independent of the severity of general cognitive deficits has been a goal of many investigators for years (Bartak & Rutter, 1976; Freeman *et al.*, 1981; Rimland, 1968; Schopler, Reichler, DeVellis, & Daly, 1980). In almost all cases, severity ratings of autism are closely correlated with degree of mental retardation. While this correlation frequently reflects the reality of the greater impairment(s) suffered by mentally retarded autistic children as compared to those with more normal intelligence, it makes it difficult to separate the genetic transmission of severe autism from the transmission of mental retardation without autism.

Studies purporting to support polygenic models have generally worked around this difficulty by assuming that the liability in families of autistic children is not for autism but rather for cognitive or language dysfunction at a more general level (August et al., 1981; Tsai et al., 1981). Severity of dysfunction is then operationally defined as severity of mental retardation (August et al., 1981; Lord et al., 1982; Tsai et al., 1981). This is not an unreasonable operational definition, but it is clearly one of convenience, rather than one based on empirical findings. It is important to note that when this argument has been proposed, what is assumed to be transmitted is not necessarily autism of any specific type but a more general form of autism/mental retardation.

As discussed earlier in this chapter, autistic females are, on the average, more severely mentally retarded than autistic males, when one includes in the sample persons with IQs below 35. It is not known whether, at equivalent levels of intelligence, females show more severely debilitating autistic behaviors or a greater number of autistic characteristics than males. In the one study where IQ was controlled, few sex differences appeared in behaviors associated with autism. When differences did occur, males were rated as more autistic (i.e., in sensory abnormalities and unusual object use) than females (Lord et al., 1982). Further study of the range of severity of autistic symptoms in males and females within well-defined IQ ranges is needed. Meanwhile, the finding that autistic females have lower intelligence, on the average, than autistic males lends support to polygenic, multifactorial models of transmission.

The second prediction of a multifactorial threshold model, and the one deemed most important from a genetic point of view (Gottesman, Shields, & Hanson, 1982; Merikangas, Weissman, & Pauls, 1985), is that there should be a higher incidence of cognitive dysfunction (or of the liability factor, however defined) in families of females than of males. This prediction allows differentiation of the question of whether the sex differences in autism are due to genetics at any level (which is probable) from whether the sex differences are due to the same genetics that underlie the condition of autism (Childs & Finucci, 1983; Merikangas et al., 1985). A prediction of higher incidence of autism and/or cognitive dysfunction in the families of autistic females than of autistic males has generally not been supported (Spence, Simmons, Brown, & Wikler, 1973; Tsai & Beisler, 1983).

Baird and August (1985) recently reported a greater incidence of cognitive disorder in families of severely retarded autistic persons (again, with IQs below 35) than in families of less severely retarded autistic individuals. These investigators did not find sex differences in incidence of cognitive dysfunction in families. However, given the small size of their sample and its somewhat unusual characteristics (including a very high male:female ratio even at very low levels of intelligence), their failure to find a sex difference cannot be considered conclusive.

Evaluation of the third prediction—that is, of greater severity of autism or related cognitive disorder in relatives of females than of males—is clearly dependent on identification and definition of the disorder in the first place, and so has not yet been forthcoming.

Altogether, of the three predictions generated by a multifactorial, polygenic model, only one has received any real support. While it would be premature to reject these models on the basis of the current lack of information, one certainly cannot automatically accept them, at least without serious reservations for many cases of autism. It is also important to remember that, in the long run, these polygenic models are dependent on the identification of some number of specific genes that, in combination with each other and with or without environmental effects, determine autism. So far, the identity or loci of these genes has not been proposed in even a tentative fashion, so that these models remain primarily abstract, mathematical formulas to account for patterns of distribution in the sexes. A further difficulty in these models is that the number of different mathematical formulas is infinite. Often, when data support one mathematical formulation, the same data can be used to support several other models as well (Freire-Maia, Freire-Maia, & Morton, 1974; Spence *et al.*, 1985).

Multifactorial polygenic models are important because, except for X-linked models (which have generally not been supported) and sex-limited patterns of inheritance (which have to date not yet been proposed in any detail), they are the only *genetic* models that could account for the sex difference in the incidence of autism for a large number of cases. With the emergence of several very large-scale family studies, it may be possible to identify what clearly are heterogeneous patterns of genetic transmission, both within a sex and between the sexes, and to evaluate the different theories empirically.

Summary of Genetic Implications of Sex Differences

Altogether, sex differences in incidence have the potential to yield very important genetic information for several different models of inheritance. Many of the necessary studies require access to very rare populations and have not yet been attempted in a well-designed fashion. It also must be recognized that, though there is much evidence suggesting a genetic component in some cases of autism (Folstein & Rutter, 1977; Ritvo, Freeman, *et al.*, 1985) and some evidence that this component might differ by sex (Spence *et al.*, 1985), to date, autism has not yet been consistently shown to fall clearly into any *well-defined* pattern or patterns of familial transmission (Gottesman *et al.*, 1982), with the exception of fragile X and a few rare disorders such as tuberous sclerosis (see Chapter 5).

Comparison of the incidence of autism and cognitive dysfunction in female and male monozygotic twins, their male and female nontwin siblings, and their siblings' children should yield important information about X-linked and sex-limited autosomal disorders. Differential effects of consanguinity across the sexes has direct implications for modes of transmission as well. However, these and the other predictions discussed earlier all require sufficient numbers of autistic females to yield reliable data. Factors such as mental retardation, which may be differentially associated with certain genetic patterns, must be controlled across sexes.

Sex differences play a potentially significant role in genetic studies. Assuming that autism is an etiologically and, even within genetics, a genetically heterogeneous condition, the sex ratio of a particular sample may be governed by the subtypes, both genetic and other, within that sample. At one level, until we know the loci of the relevant genes, and what it is that they do (or fail to do) that results in autism, we are still many steps away from pinpointing particular etiologies. On the other hand, it may be possible to identify one or several patterns of inheritance with sufficiently careful examination of families and large enough samples. These patterns of inheritance would allow more accurate genetic counseling. Further studies, such as linkage analyses (see Chapter 5) may help elucidate specific causes of autism in males and females.

RELEVANCE OF SEX DIFFERENCES IN NORMAL DEVELOPMENT TO AUTISM

From the moment of conception, males and females follow different patterns of development (Hutt, 1972). Documenting these differences is a task pursued on many levels. Differences can be categorized according to when they are precipitated (e.g., during fetal development), when they are most obviously manifested (e.g., sterility, which becomes apparent only after puberty), the level of etiology if known (e.g., genetic), or the level of pathophysiology (e.g., structural differences in the brain accompanied by differences in neurochemistry). Since autism is present by age 3 years or younger, it is assumed that differences in neurobiological functioning proposed to account for sex differences in the occurrence of autism must be present at least by age 3. Thus, most relevant for this chapter are sex differences in normal embryological, fetal, and infant development.

Differences Related to Sex Hormones

Differences mediated by sex hormones (e.g., androgens, estrogens) are present from very early in fetal development (Hines, 1982). The results of differential amounts of sex hormones in females and males are most obvious in sexual differentiation, such as the development of genitalia, eventual fertility, and sexual behavior (Hines, 1982). Much of the scientific knowledge in this area arises from anomalies in the availability of sex hormones, such as those seen either in congenital syndromes such as congenital adrenal hyperplasia, or from the administration of exogenous hormones, such as in the sons of mothers receiving synthetic progestins during pregnancy.

Besides sexual differentiation, fetal hormones have also been implicated in some behavioral sex differences. In rats, these differences include patterns of juvenile play, activity level, and aggression (Hines, 1982; Hutt, 1972). Similar differences postulated in humans are discussed below in the section on skills and behavior because, in humans, environmental as well as biological factors require consideration. It is worth noting, however, that even in rats, general behavioral differences related to hormones have been found much less consistently than differences in genitalia (Hines, 1982). None of these differences (except those discussed below) seem particularly relevant to autism, where, so far at least, there has been no evidence of frequent genital abnormalities similar to those associated with hormone-related syndromes. Differences in sexual behavior in autistic adults have not been studied systematically. In most cases, adult development of sexual behavior has been assumed to be very limited in autistic persons (Wing, 1976).

Differences in Neurological Development

Sex differences in brain structure and function, some clearly related to sex hormones and others with less clear or more complex relationships, are also present from fetal development (Brawer & Naftolin, 1979; Swaab & Hofman, 1984). Male brains weigh more than female brains; head circumference in males is typically greater than in females, although this latter finding may be due to stature. Sex differences in the *appearance* of the human brain have been reported so far in the preoptic areas, ventromedial hypothalamus, amygdala, cerebellum, and septum (Reinisch *et al.*, 1979). Most of these differences are relatively small and have to do with lateralization (Swaab & Hofman, 1984). For example, females are more likely to have unusual ratios of length of left to right temporal lobes than males (Wada, Clark, & Hamm, 1975). Females seem to require more extensive bilateral brain damage to develop receptive aphasia and so have been assumed to be less lateralized than males for some language functions (Kimura & Harshman, 1984; Lansdell, 1962). Sex differences in the neurological connections between the hypothalamus and other parts of the brain, in the size of the nucleus cells in certain parts of the hypothalamus, and in oxidative metabolism of RNA related to serotonin levels have also been reported (Brawer & Naftolin, 1979; Swaab & Hofman, 1984). The finding that profound general retardation is more common in females than in males with autism is compatible with some of these differences in functional and/or structural lateralization/localization, postulated to occur in normal males and females (Lord *et al.*, 1982).

Thus, growing evidence supports small but real, basic structural and possibly neurochemical differences in male and female brains (Springer & Deutsch, 1981). The problem is that relationships between anatomical and functional aspects of CNS development are often not clear, with implications for differences in skill and behavior even less well understood. For example, EEG patterns have often been directly opposite to those predicted from structural differences (Springer & Deutsch, 1981); greater lateralization has been linked to slower maturation in attempts to account for both strengths (Buffery & Gray, 1972) and deficits (Waber, 1977) in visuospatial skills.

One possibility is that some of the structural or neurochemical differences in brain development associated with sex are not solely a function of sex *per se* but are related to other factors, such as rate of maturation, which may differ for the sexes. Ounsted (1972) and Taylor and Ounsted (1972) suggested that the greater frequency of infantile spasms in males and the combination of more frequent febrile convulsions in males with more adverse outcomes in affected females are related to slower development in males. It has also been suggested that fetal hormones interact with maternal hormones to increase the likelihood of implantation for males, speed the rate of growth in male fetuses, and perhaps increase the probability of spontaneous abortion, placenta abruptio, and maternal toxemia for male fetuses (Taylor & Ounsted, 1972).

Maternal–fetal immune reactions have been suggested to play a role in sex differences in the incidence of many developmental disorders, including autism (Gualtieri & Hicks, 1985). This hypothesis is based on the assumption that mothers may accumulate male-specific antigens over a series of pregnancies with male fetuses. These antigens could be detrimental to fetal development in subsequent offspring, although neither the nature of the immune reaction nor specific consequences are delineated. However, on the basis of this theory, one can predict that affected (e.g., autistic) males should have more antecedent male siblings than unaffected males. These predictions have not yet been evaluated on appropriately large and stratified samples.

Similarly, studies of general populations have found that males are more vulnerable to effects of perinatal and birth difficulties than females (Ounsted & Taylor, 1972; Rutter *et al.*, 1970/1981). It is theoretically possible (and not necessarily incompatible with genetic models discussed earlier) that the higher incidence of autistic males than females is related to a greater frequency of perinatal insult or "nonoptimal" pregnancy and birth characteristics in males than in females. However, sex differences in these occurrences in the general population are not sufficiently high to account for the high male:female ratio in autism.

Of the several studies of pregnancy and birth factors in autism, none have reported sex differences (Deykin & MacMahon, 1980; Finegan & Quarrington, 1979; Gillberg & Gillberg, 1983). However, given the variety of perinatal problems studied, possible differences in IQ levels of autistic subjects across sex, and relatively small numbers of females, statistically significant findings would be unlikely even if clinically significant differences existed. The high likelihood of heterogeneity in the occurrence and source of perinatal problems means that samples of females will need to be considerably larger than available in the past in order to properly evaluate whether there are sex differences in these factors.

Sex differences in vulnerability to specific infections, such as congenital cytomegalovirus or toxoplasmosis, are also a possibility (see Chapter 5), although the small proportion of cases of autism associated with identifiable infections means that the number of individuals accounted for would be very low. Data concerning the association of such infections with autism in the two sexes are not yet generally available. Again, factors such as developmental rates, which might be studied in terms of age of onset, certainly offer one potential lead to sex differences.

Differences in Skills and Behavior

Although relationships between sex differences in skills and behavior and basic neurobiological differences in structure and function are far from clear, several authors have observed that the pattern of skills associated with autism include skills in which normal sex differences have traditionally been reported (Wing, 1981b). This observation has been a tantalizing source of speculation, even if one is not always certain what the neurobiological implications of the speculations are.

Wing (1981b) used evidence that normal females are often superior to males on verbal measures to suggest that males ("normal" and "abnormal") may have greater susceptibility to certain kinds of communication disorder. In combination with hypothesized male superiority in visuospatial skills, Wing proposed that the particular pattern of deficits in communication and relative strengths in visuospatial skills that characterizes many autistic individuals may be viewed as an exaggeration of "normal" sex differences. From a neurobiological point of view, these differences could be located at any point in pathophysiology but, as discussed earlier, would not be incompatible with normal sex differences proposed in brain localization or lateralization of specific skills (Lord et al., 1982).

As Wing (1981b) herself points out, however, there are several major difficulties with this hypothesis. First, sex differences in normal populations in both visuospatial and verbal skills are still controversial for somewhat different reasons (Caplan, McPherson, & Tobin, 1985). Often, what have been treated as sex differences in skill have been highly confounded with differences in interest and experience (Childs & Finucci, 1983; Jacklin, 1979). The distinction between sex differences in ability versus sex differences in motivation relates to whether the sex differences are biologically based or a product of culture and learning. Clearly, differences in motivation and ability *could* both be biologically determined or at least influenced by neurobiologic factors. However, sex differences in skill that could be accounted for primarily by motivation (often compounded by experience) would have far less clear neurobiological implications for autism than sex differences in ability *per se*, if motivational differences were also highly culture-specific.

Although often no differences are found, when they do occur, sex differences in visuospatial skills have shown male superiority across several different tasks (Vandenberg & Kuse, 1979). Although present to some degree from early childhood, these differences in skill are most clearly seen after puberty (Maccoby & Jacklin, 1975), which makes their relevance to autism, where peak visuospatial skills are most obvious during preschool years, rather questionable (Wing, 1981b). The size of these sex differences has also decreased in studies performed in the last 10 years compared to studies carried out 20 to 30 years ago (Kimball, 1980). In many cases, differences have also been abolished when girls are given quite brief training programs with the materials typically employed in such research (Connor, Schackman, & Serbin, 1978; Jacklin, 1979). Thus, the question of whether "normal" sex differences in visuospatial skill and ability are biologically based or are more related to experience still remains open.

Evidence for sex differences in verbal ability is even more problematic. Which sex has been shown to be superior has varied according to the aspect of language studied, the age of subjects, the culture (even within Western society), and ability groups (Dwyer, 1979; Jacklin, 1979). For example, in the United States, adult females typically outscore males on verbal comprehension tests, whereas the reverse is true in Great Britain, Germany, and India (Dwyer, 1979). Sex differences are most obvious on verbal tests at the low end of ability (Jacklin, 1979), which may be most relevant to autism but limits analogies between autism and "normal development."

Overall, even at their most obvious, sex differences in performance on cognitive tasks have typically not been greater than one-quarter of a standard deviation (Springer & Deutsch, 1981). The amount of overlap within normal populations is far greater than the divergence. Individual differences are typically much greater than sex differences.

This is not to argue against the existence of any neurobiologically based sex differences in skill or behavior in normally developing populations. Instead, our point is that *simple* analogies between sex differences in normal populations and sex differences in the incidence of autism are not yet appropriate. More specific and perhaps more complex analogies may be in order. For example, girls do seem to begin to speak at earlier ages than do boys, even though sex differences in language skills at later ages are in dispute (Dwyer, 1979). Thus, a relationship between sex differences in autism and earlier onset of expressive language in females may be a possibility, even though female superiority in language across development may not be sufficiently simple or well established to use it as an argument for a protective factor against autism/severe communication disorders in females.

Similarly, sex differences in interest in certain activities and materials have been found from very early in childhood. These differences include both social areas, such as interest in caretaking (e.g., interacting with a baby) (Berman & Goodman, 1984) and interest in same-sex playmates (Hinde, Titmus, Easton, & Tamplin, 1985; Jacklin & Maccoby, 1978), and cognitive areas, such as toddlers' selection of toys (Eisenberg, Tryon, & Cameron, 1984). It is likely that these differences are strongly influenced by culture. However, it is also possible that analogies to autistic children's presumably biologically based, avid interest in visuospatial phenomena and early pronounced lack of interest in social interaction may be possible. This speculation clearly needs more thought, however, and careful testing.

Summary of Implications of Sex Differences in Normal Development

Neurobiological implications from "normal" sex differences that initially appeared straightforward are actually very complex. Yet what is even more striking is the paucity of information about autistic females that could be potentially related to development in non-autistic females and males. Other than differences in mean IQ and differences in sex ratios across IQ level, virtually nothing beyond anecdotes is known about this subset of autistic individuals. In the one series of studies where IQ was controlled, the only sex differences that emerged were a higher frequency of unusual visual interests and a higher frequency of less appropriate play in males than in females (Lord *et al.*, 1982). Given the number of analyses performed in that particular study, it is difficult to know how seriously to take this finding. Samples of autistic females stratified by IQ and matched to males are clearly needed before conclusions about equivalent or differential patterns of skill and development across the sexes can be reached.

SEX DIFFERENCES IN IDENTIFICATION, DIAGNOSIS, AND REFERRAL

Sex biases in diagnosis and referral rates also need to be considered. As stated earlier, clinic samples have tended to yield higher male:female ratios than epidemiological ones (Baird & August, 1985; Rutter & Lockyer, 1967; Wing, 1981b, 1984). Higher male:female ratios have been reported even from clinics where many severely handicapped children are seen, as well as from clinics that would be likely to attract referrals of primarily higher-functioning autistic children (Lord, 1984; Lord *et al.*, 1982). Sex biases in reporting and referral for treatment/special education have been clearly documented for many disorders besides autism, including such diverse problems as reading difficulties (Childs & Finucci, 1983; Finucci & Childs, 1981) and depression (Merikangas *et al.*, 1985). For example, adult females report a greater number of depressive symptoms than males but do not differ from males in the duration of social impairment they suffer as a consequence of their "depression" (Merikangas *et al.*, 1985). The sex ratio of males to females in special schools for learning-disabled children is typically very high, in many cases exceeding the 4:1 ratio in autism (Finucci & Childs, 1981). Sex ratios of children from regular schools with equivalent degrees of impairment in reading and spelling are typically much lower, in fact under 2 to 1 (Berger *et al.*, 1975; Finucci & Childs, 1981). This is not to claim that sex differences in reading and reading problems, or in autism, do not exist, but rather to point out that factors other than simple measures of severity may be of importance in determining which children are identified as autistic and dyslexic and/or which children receive special services.

In autism, biases might occur at a number of points in the process of referral, diagnosis, and use of treatment and educational services. Professionals, particularly those not experienced with autistic children, might expect autism to occur only in males, fail to recognize it in a young female, and fail to refer the autistic girl on to more appropriate resources (which generally serve as the source of research populations). Referral biases might also occur if there are sex differences in behavior or in characteristics not specific to autism, such as aggression, hyperactivity, or physical size, that would influence the likelihood of a child's attracting the attention of teachers or specialists (this could be particularly the case both for severely retarded children and for those of near-normal skills). Concern about such behaviors would affect the probability of a child with either a milder form of autism or autism in conjunction with multiple handicaps receiving a psychiatric referral or a request for specific special educational services, and so be given a formal diagnosis of autism. On the other hand, incidence ratios of autism for males versus females remain higher than for other disorders, even in the well-controlled epidemiological samples discussed earlier. Thus, referral practices may exaggerate an already high male:female ratio but could not be responsible for it entirely. Hypotheses concerning possible sex biases could be tested in ways beyond counts of service statistics by asking professionals from various disciplines and with varying levels of experience to judge medical records, behavioral descriptions, or even videotaped interviews of males and females in order to make diagnoses of autism.

CONCLUSION

In conclusion, sex differences in the incidence of autism have been important in the conceptualization of the disorder as a discrete, although heterogeneous, syndrome that differs from adult psychoses (Lewine, 1981), mild communication delays (Fundudis et al., 1979), severe communication disorders (Bartak et al., 1975; Ingram, 1972), other childhood psychiatric disturbances (Eme, 1979), and mental retardation (see Chapter 5). Sex differences in the incidence of autism are evidence, in a simple way, of its neurobiological bases but at present do not yield specific information about etiologies or the pathophysiologies underlying the disorder. As interest has grown in identifying subsets of autistic individuals, the potential for using sex as one defining variable within the heterogeneity of autism has become apparent, as has the need to do so. However, practical difficulties in collecting samples of sufficient size, with controls for factors such as referral biases and differing intellectual distributions, currently limit the conclusions that can be drawn from individual research projects. On the other hand, starting from a position of mild skepticism, it seems possible that we will be able to reach important and reasonable conclusions when the evidence is in from large-scale family studies and from carefully designed investigations of individual autistic females and males.

REFERENCES

August, G. J., Stewart, M. A., & Tsai, L. (1981). The incidence of cognitive disabilities in the siblings of autistic children. *British Journal of Psychiatry, 138*, 416–422.

Baird, T. D., & August, G. J. (1985). Familial heterogeneity in infantile autism. *Journal of Autism and Developmental Disorders, 15*, 315–322.

Bartak, L., & Rutter, M. (1976). Differences between mentally retarded and normally intelligent autistic children. *Journal of Autism and Childhood Schizophrenia, 6*, 109–120.

Bartak, L., Rutter, M., & Cox, A. (1975). A comparative study of infantile autism and specific developmental receptive language disorder. I: The children. *British Journal of Psychiatry, 126*, 127–145.

Berger, M., Yule, W., & Rutter, M. (1975). Attainment and adjustment in two geographical areas. II. The prevalence of specific reading retardation. *British Journal of Psychiatry, 126*, 510–519.

Berman, P. W., & Goodman, V. (1984). Age and sex differences in children's responses to babies: Effects of adults' caretaking requests and instructions. *Child Development, 55*, 1071–1077.

Brawer, J. R., & Naftolin, F. (1979). The effects of oestrogen on hypothalamic tissue. In CIBA Foundation (Ed.), *Sex, harmones and behavior* (pp. 19–41). Amsterdam: Excerpta Medica.

Buffery, A. W. H., & Gray, J. A. (1972). Sex differences in the development of spatial and linguistic skills. *Gender differences: Their ontogeny and significance* (pp. 123–157). London: Churchill Livingstone.

Cantwell, D. P., Baker, L., & Mattison, R. E. (1979). The prevalence of psychiatric disorder in children with speech and language disorder. *Journal of the American Academy of Child Psychiatry, 18*, 450–461.

Caplan, P. J., McPherson, G. M., & Tobin, P. (1985). Do sex related differences in spatial abilities exist? *American Psychologist, 40*, 786–799.

Carter, C. O. (1972). Sex-linkage and sex limitation. In C. Ounsted & D. C. Taylor (Eds.), *Gender differences: Their ontogeny and significance* (pp. 1–12). London: Churchill Livingstone.

Childs, B., & Finucci, J. M. (1983). Genetics, epidemiology and specific reading disability. In M. Rutter (Ed.), *Developmental neuropsychiatry* (pp. 507–519). New York: Guilford Press.

Cloninger, C. R., Christiansen, K. O., Reich, T., & Gottesman, I. (1978). Implications of sex differences in the prevalence of antisocial personality, alcoholism and criminality for familial transmission. *Archives of General Psychiatry, 35,* 941–951.

Connor, J. M., Schackman, M., & Serbin, L. A. (1978). Sex-related differences in response to practice on a visual-spatial test and generalization to a related test. *Child Development, 49,* 24–29.

Deykin, E. Y., & MacMahon, B. (1980). Pregnancy, delivery, and neonatal complications among autistic children. *American Journal of Disordered Children, 134,* 860–864.

Dwyer, C. (1979). The role of tests and their construction in producing apparent sex-related differences. In M. A. Wittig & A. C. Peterson (Eds.), *Sex-related differences in cognitive functioning* (pp. 335–353). New York: Academic Press.

Eme, R. F. (1979). Sex differences in childhood psychopathology: A review. *Psychological Bulletin, 86,* 574–595.

Eisenberg, N., Tryon, K., & Cameron, E. (1984). The relation of preschoolers' peer interaction to their sex-typed toy choices. *Child Development, 55,* 1044–1050.

Finegan, J., & Quarrington, B. (1979). Pre-, peri- and neonatal factors and infantile autism. *Journal of Child Psychology and Psychiatry, 20,* 119–218.

Finucci, J. M., & Childs, B. (1981). Are there really more dyslexic boys than girls? In A. Anasona (Ed.), *Sex differences in dyslexia* (pp. 1–9). Towson, MD: Orton Dyslexia Society.

Folstein, S., & Rutter, M. (1977). Infantile autism: A genetic study of 21 twin pairs. *Journal of Child Psychology and Psychiatry, 18,* 297–321.

Freeman, B. J., Ritvo, E. R., Schroth, P. C., Tonick, I., Guthrie, D., & Wake, L. (1981). Behavioural characteristics of high and low IQ autistic children. *American Journal of Psychiatry, 138,* 25–29.

Freire-Maia, A., Freire-Maia, D. V., & Morton, N. E. (1974). Sex effect on intelligence and mental retardation. *Behavior Genetics, 4,* 269–272.

Fryns, J. P. (1984). The fragile X syndrome: A study of 83 families. *Clinical Genetics, 26,* 197–528.

Fundudis, T., Kolvin, I., & Garside, R. F. (Eds.). (1979). *Speech retarded and deaf children: Their psychological development.* London: Academic Press.

Gillberg, C., & Gillberg, I. C. (1983). Infantile autism: A total population study of reduced optimality in the pre-, peri-, and neonatal periods. *Journal of Autism and Developmental Disorders, 13,* 153–166.

Gottesman, I. I., Shields, J., & Hanson, D. R. (1982). *Schizophrenia: The epigenetic puzzle.* New York: Cambridge University Press.

Gualtieri, T., & Hicks, R. E. (1985). Immunoreactive theory of selective male affliction. *Behavioral and Brain Sciences, 8,* 427–477.

Hagberg, M. M., Aicardi, J., Dias, K., & Rasmos, O. (1983). A progressive syndrome of autism, dementia, ataxia, and loss of purposeful hand use in girls: Rett's syndrome: Report 35 cases. *Annals of Neurology, 14,* 471–479.

Hanson, D. R., & Gottesman, I. I. (1976). The genetics, if any, of infantile autism and childhood schizophrenia. *Journal of Autism and Childhood Schizophrenia, 6,* 209–234.

Herbst, D. S., & Miller, J. R. (1980). Nonspecific X-linked mental retardation II. The frequency in British Columbia. *American Journal of Medical Genetics, 7,* 461–469.

Hermelin, B., & O'Connor, N. (1983). The idiot savant: Flawed genius or clever Hans? *Psychological Medicine, 13,* 479–481.

Hinde, R. A., Titmus, G., Easton, D., & Tamplin, A. (1985). Incidence of "friendship" and behavior toward strong associates versus nonassociates in preschoolers. *Child Development, 56,* 234–245.

Hines, M. (1982). Prenatal gonadal hormones and sex differences in human behaviour. *Psychological Bulletin, 92,* 56–80.

Hutt, C. (1972). Neuroendocrinological, behavioural, and intellectual aspects of sexual differentiation in human development. In C. Ounsted & D. Taylor (Eds.), *Gender differences: Their ontogeny and significance* (pp. 73–122). London: Churchill Livingstone.

Ingram, T. T. S. (1972). The classification of speech and language disorders in young children. In M. Rutter & J. A. Martin (Eds.), *The child with delayed speech* (pp. 13–22). Clinics in Developmental Medicine No. 43. London: Heinemann Medical Books.

Jacklin, C. N. (1979). Epilogue. In M. A. Wittig & C. A. Peterson (Eds.), *Sex-related differences in cognitive functioning* (pp. 357–371). New York: Academic Press.

Jacklin, C. N., & Maccoby, E. E. (1978). Social behavior at thirty-three months in same-sex and mixed-sex dyads. *Child Development, 49,* 557–569.

Kimball, M. M. (1980). Women and science: A critique of biological theories. *International Journal of Women's Studies, 4,* 318–338.

Kimura, D., & Harshman, R. A. (1984). Sex differences in brain organization for verbal and nonverbal functions. In G. J. DeVries, J. P. C. DeBruin, H. B. M. Uylings, & M. A. Corner (Eds.), *Sex differences in the brain: Vol. 61. Progress in brain research* (pp. 423–441). Amsterdam: Elsevier.

Lansdell, H. (1962). A sex difference in effect of temporal lobe neurosurgery on design preference. *Nature, 194,* 852–854.

Lewine, R. R. J. (1981). Sex differences in schizophrenia: Timing or subtypes? *Psychological Bulletin, 90,* 432–444.

Lord, C. (1984). On the differences between the sexes. *Journal of Autism and Developmental Disorders, 14,* 212–214.

Lord, C., & Schopler, E. (1985). Differences in sex ratios in autism as a function of measured intelligence. *Journal of Autism and Developmental Disorders, 15,* 185–193.

Lord, C., Schopler, E., & Revicki, D. (1982). Sex differences in autism. *Journal of Autism and Developmental Disorders, 12,* 317-330.

Lotter, V. (1966). Epidemiology of autistic conditions in young children. I. Prevalence. *Social Psychiatry, 1966,* 124–137.

Maccoby, E. E., & Jacklin, C. N. (1975). *The psychology of sex differences.* London: Oxford University Press.

Merikangas, K. R., Weissman, M. M., & Pauls, D. L. (1985). Genetic factors in the sex ratio of major depression. *Psychological Medicine, 15,* 63–69.

Minton, J., Campbell, M., Green, W. H., Jennings, S., & Samit, C. (1982). Cognitive assessment of siblings of autistic children. *Journal of American Academy of Child Psychiatry, 21,* 256–261.

Ounsted, M. (1972). Gender and intrauterine growth. In C. Ounsted & D. C. Taylor (Eds.), *Gender differences: Their ontogeny and significance* (pp. 177–202). London: Churchill Livingstone.

Ounsted, C., & Taylor, D. C. (1972). *Gender differences: Their ontogeny and significance* (pp. 1–12). London: Churchill Livingstone.

Reinisch, J. M., Gandelman, R., & Spiegel, F. S. (1979). Prenatal influences on cognitive abilities: Data from experimental animals and human genetic and endocrine studies. In M. A. Wittig & A. C. Pedersen (Eds.), *Sex-related differences in cognitive functioning* (pp. 215–240). New York: Academic Press.

Richman, N., Stevenson, J., & Graham, P. J. (1985). Sex difference in the outcome of preschool behaviour problems. In A. R. Nicol (Ed.), *Longitudinal studies in child psychology and psychiatry* (pp. 75–90). Chichester: Wiley.

Rimland, B. (1968). On the objective diagnosis of infantile autism. *Acta Paedopsychiatrica, 35,* 146–161.

Ritvo, E. R., Freeman, B. J., Mason-Brothers, A., Mo, A., & Ritvo, A. M. (1985). Concordance for the syndrome of autism in 40 pairs of afflicted twins. *American Journal of Psychiatry, 142,* 74–77.

Ritvo, E. R., Spence, M. A., Freeman, B. J., Mason-Brothers, A., Mo, A., & Marazita, M. L. (1985). Evidence for autosomal recessive inheritance in 46 families with multiple incidence of autism. *American Journal of Psychiatry, 142,* 187–192.

Rutter, M. (1985). Infantile autism and other pervasive developmental disorders. In M. Rutter & L. Hersov (Eds.), *Child and adolescent psychiatry: Modern approaches* (pp. 545–566). London: Blackwell Scientific.

Rutter, M., & Garmezy, N. (1983). Developmental psychopathology. In P. H. Mussen (Ed.), E. M. Hetherington (Vol. ed.), *Handbook of child psychology. IV. Socialization, personality and social development* (pp. 775–912). New York/Chichester: Wiley.

Rutter, M., & Lockyer, L. (1967). A five to fifteen year follow-up study of infantile psychosis. I: Description of sample. *British Journal of Psychiatry*, 113, 1169–1182.

Rutter, M., & Schopler, E. (in press). Autism and pervasive developmental disorders: Concepts and diagnostic issues. *Journal of Autism and Developmental Disorders*.

Rutter, M., Tizard, J., & Whitmore, L. (1970/1981). *Education, health, and behavior.* London: Longman Group; New York: Krieger.

Schopler, E., Andrews, C. E., & Strupp, K. (1979). Do autistic children come from upper-middle-class parents? *Journal of Autism and Developmental Disorders*, 9, 139–152.

Schopler, E., Reichler, R., DeVellis, R., & Daly, K. (1980). Toward objective classification of childhood autism: Childhood Autism Rating Scale (CARS). *Journal of Autism and Developmental Disorders, 10,* 91–103.

Sherman, S. L., Morton, N. E., Jacobs, P. A., & Turner, G. (1984). The marker (X) syndrome: A cytogenetic and genetic analysis. *Annals of Human Genetics, 48,* 21–37.

Spence, M. A., Ritvo, E. R., Marazita, M. L., Funderburk, S. J., Sparkes, R. S., & Freeman, B. J. (1985). Gene mapping studies with the syndrome of autism. *Behavior Genetics, 15,* 1–13.

Spence, M. A., Simmons, J. Q., Brown, N. A., Wikler, L. (1973). Sex ratios in families of autistic children. *American Journal of Mental Deficiency, 77,* 405–407.

Springer, S., & Deutsch, G. (1981). *Left brain, right brain.* San Francisco: Freeman.

Swaab, D. F., & Hofman, M. A. (1984). Sexual differentiation of the human brain. A historical perspective. In G. J. DeVries, J. P. C. DeBruin, H. B. M. Uylings, & M. A. Corner (Eds.), *Sex differences in the brain. Vol. 61, Progress in brain research* (pp. 36–374)). Amsterdam: Elsevier.

Symmes, J. (1976). Evaluating competence and accessibility in autistic children. In M. Coleman (Ed.), *The autistic syndromes* (pp. 79–94). New York: Elsevier.

Taylor, D. C., & Ounsted, C. (1972). The nature of gender differences explored through ontogenetic analyses of sex ratios in disease. In C. Ounsted & D. Taylor (Eds.), *Gender differences: Their ontogeny and significance* (pp. 215–140). London: Churchill Livingstone.

Treffert, D. A. (1970). Epidemiology of infantile autism. *Archives of General Psychiatry, 22,* 431–438.

Tsai, L., & Beisler, J. M. (1983). The development of sex differences in infantile autism. *British Journal of Psychiatry, 142,* 373–378.

Tsai, L., Stewart, M. A., & August, G. (1981). Implications of sex differences in the familial transmission of infantile autism. *Journal of Autism and Developmental Disorders, 11,* 165–174.

Vandenberg, S. G., & Kuse, A. R. (1979). Spatial ability: A critical review of the sex-linked major gene hypothesis. In M. A. Wittig & A. C. Petersen (Eds.), *Sex-related differences in cognitive functioning* (pp. 67–95). New York: Academic Press.

Waber, D. P. (1977). Sex differences in mental abilities, hemispheric lateralization, and rate of physical growth at adolescence. *Developmental Psychology, 13,* 29–38.

Wada, J. A., Clark, R., & Hamm, A. (1975). Cerebral hemisphere asymmetry in humans. *Archives of Neurology, 32,* 239–246.

Wing, L. (1976). *Early childhood autism.* Oxford, England: Pergamon Press.

Wing, L. (1981a). Asperger's syndrome: A clinical account. *Psychological Medicine, 11,* 115–129.

Wing, L. (1981b). Sex ratios in early childhood autism and related conditions. *Psychiatry Research, 5,* 129–137.

Wing, L. (1984). Letter to the editor on the differences between the sexes. *Journal of Autism, 14,* 210–111.

Wing, L., & Gould, J. (1979). Severe impairments of social interaction and associated abnormalities in children: Epidemiology and classification. *Journal of Autism and Developmental Disorders, 9*, 11–29.

Wing, L., Gould, J., Yeates, S. R., & Brierly, L. M. (1977). Symbolic play in severely mentally retarded and in autistic children. *Journal of Child Psychology and Psychiatry, 18*, 425–427.

12

The Role of Abnormal Hemispheric Specialization in Autism

GERALDINE DAWSON

INTRODUCTION

In 1974 Rutter speculated that left hemisphere dysfunction may play a significant role in autistic symptomology. He based this supposition on the fact that autistic children often exhibit an uneven pattern of cognitive abilities suggestive of left hemisphere dysfunction. When the autistic child shows peak skills, they are usually in areas of functioning traditionally associated with the right hemisphere, such as visuospatial abilities and pattern recognition. In contrast, the autistic child's most pronounced deficiencies are in areas of functioning traditionally associated with the left hemisphere, such as the use of spoken and gestural language. Around the same time, Ricks and Wing (1975) made a similar speculation based on their finding that autistic children had specific difficulties in the use of symbols. In the last decade, several investigators have explored the role of abnormal hemisphere development in the syndrome of autism. Indeed, there now exist numerous studies of many aspects of brain functioning in autistic children. It is clear from these studies that, while left hemisphere dysfunction may play a role in autistic symptomology, it is only one piece in a complex and nonunitary neurological basis of autism. However, since many of the core symptoms of autism, such as impairments in the use of symbols, may involve dysfunction at the cortical level, it is important that this aspect of brain functioning be explored fully.

In the present chapter, a review of the existing research on hemispheric specialization in autistic children and adults is presented. Current theories regarding the role of abnormal hemispheric specialization in autism are discussed and evaluated in terms of the available data. Finally, several working hypotheses with respect to the possible role of abnormal hemispheric specialization in the affective and social deficits of autistic individuals are offered.

REVIEW OF THE EVIDENCE

This review will pertain only to those studies that *directly* assessed hemispheric specialization in autistic children. Studies of handedness, neuroanatomical asymmetries, and other indirect measures of hemispheric specialization in autistic children will not be included.

GERALDINE DAWSON • Department of Psychology, University of Washington, Seattle, Washington 98195.

Tanguay (1976) was the first to directly study hemisphere functioning in autistic children. He recorded cortical averaged evoked potentials to auditory stimuli from the right and left hemispheres of young autistic children while they were sleeping and compared them to similar recordings from normal children. He found that, in contrast to normal children, the autistic children showed an abnormal right–left amplitude ratio of the large N_1P_2 component during REM sleep. Whereas the normal children showed greater averaged evoked potentials over the right hemisphere than over the left, autistic children showed no consistent differences between the two hemispheres. Tanguay interpreted this finding to suggest that autistic children fail to develop normal hemispheric specialization. The notion that autism may be related to abnormal hemispheric specialization was especially intriguing in light of the proposed continuum between autism and other developmental receptive language disorders. A number of studies (Rosenblum & Dorman, 1978; Sommers & Taylor, 1972; Springer & Eisenson, 1977; Witelson & Rabinovitch, 1972) demonstrated that language-impaired children may exhibit reduced or reversed hemisphere dominance for speech stimuli.

A more traditional means of assessing hemispheric specialization was used with autistic children by Prior and Bradshaw (1979). They employed a dichotic listening technique in which a different speech sound was simultaneously presented to each ear over earphones and the child was asked to report which sound was heard. Their sample consisted of 19 autistic children between the ages of 8 and 13 years; MAs ranged from 3 years 2 months to 14 years 2 months. They found that, in contrast to a group of normal primary-school-age children, who showed a significant right ear advantage for speech perception, autistic children showed a great deal of variability in the direction of hemisphere dominance. Five autistic children showed a right ear advantage, 7 showed a left ear advantage, and 7 showed no preference. In addition, lateralized autistic subjects were more likely to have had speech before 5 years.

Two other studies have used dichotic listening to study hemispheric specialization in autistic children. Wetherby, Koegel, & Mendel (1981) studied six autistic subjects of a wide range of age and ability. Two of these subjects showed a left ear advantage, three showed a right ear advantage, and one showed no preference. Interestingly, one subject who was followed longitudinally exhibited a decrease in the degree of left ear advantage (right hemisphere dominance) as his language ability improved through treatment. In a more recent study, Arnold and Schwartz (1983) used a variation on the traditional dichotic listening technique with autistic children. Their sample consisted of eight autistic children, 6 to 14 years of age, whose MAs ranged from 3 years 6 months to 12 years 3 months. Consonant-vowel combinations were presented through earphones with a separation of 50 milliseconds. The autistic children were asked to "point to the ear you heard the sound in first." This technique was specifically designed to accommodate the autistic children's expressive language difficulties. However, it is possible that the relatively complex verbal instructions and pointing to a body part also were difficult for these children. These authors found that the autistic children performed similarly to the nomal controls, with seven of the eight pointing more often to the right ear.

Dawson, Warrenburg, and Fuller (1982, 1983) have employed electrophysiological techniques to study hemispheric specialization in autistic individuals. In the first of these studies, a sample of 10 autistic subjects, ranging from 9 to 34 years of age, with Full Scale IQs from 40 to 113, and a CA- and handedness-matched normal comparison group participated. The measure of hemispheric specialization was electroencephalographic (EEG) recordings of alpha rhythm (8–12 Hz) asymmetries from homologous parietal sites. These recordings were made during two verbal and two spatial tasks. This technique makes use of the well-documented EEG alpha-blocking phenomenon, which is considered to reflect cortical activation in underlying regions (e.g., Butler & Glass, 1974; Doyle, Galin, & Ornstein, 1974). Seven of the 10 autistic individuals were found to have an atypical pattern of cerebral lateralization, namely, right-hemisphere dominance for both verbal and spatial processing. This finding cannot be attributed to the autistic individuals' variability in handedness since the control group was matched for handedness; moreover, strongly right-handed autistic subjects were found to have the atypical pattern. Older autistic subjects were more strongly lateralized than younger subjects, suggesting that cerebral specialization increased with age. This was not found in the age-matched normal control subjects. Young normal subjects showed the same degree of lateralization as older subjects.

Using this same sample of autistic subjects, Dawson et al., (1983) explored whether these individuals showed abnormal patterns of hemispheric activation during a series of four motor imitation tasks (oral posture, oral movements, hand postures, hand movements). Our interest in motor imitation stemmed from the fact that young autistic children typically are impaired in the use of body imitation (Curcio, 1978; Dawson & Adams, 1984; Hammes & Langdell, 1981; Wing, 1981). This impairment appears to be fairly specific to autism in that most mentally retarded and dysphasic children actively use gesture and imitation (Bartak, Rutter, & Cox, 1975; DeMyer et al., 1972). Furthermore, autistic children's deficits in the use of body imitation may play a significant role in their impaired social functioning (Dawson & Adams, 1984; Dawson & Galpert, 1986). On the basis of EEG measures of alpha taken from the right and left hemispheres, we found that normal subjects, including elementary-school-age children, exhibited left hemisphere dominance during the four imitation tasks (Dawson, Warrenburg, & Fuller, 1985). Autistic subjects show greater right hemisphere activation than normal subjects during the four motor imitation tasks. Right hemisphere dominance was particularly pronounced during the oral imitation tasks. Older autistic subjects again showed more normal patterns than younger subjects.

Summary

Taken together, the evidence cited above points to two general findings. First, five of the six available studies suggest that, in comparison to normal individuals, autistic persons show more variability in their patterns of hemispheric specialization. They are more likely than normal individuals to show right hemisphere dominance for functions typically associated with the left hemisphere. Second, the possibility that there are changes in the pattern of hemispheric specialization with development is raised by the finding that older, higher-functioning, autistic children are more likely to show normal patterns than younger, more impaired children.

THEORIES REGARDING THE ROLE OF ABNORMAL HEMISPHERIC SPECIALIZATION IN AUTISM

Left Hemisphere Hypothesis

Several theories exist regarding the role of abnormal hemisphere specialization in autism. One theory is that autism is related to left hemisphere dysfunction, which may exist because of early brain trauma to the left hemisphere or functionally related brain structures, or because of genetic abnormality. According to this view, early left hemisphere dysfunction may lead to right hemisphere compensation for language functions. Such a compensatory process has been documented in cases of early left hemisphere brain trauma (Lansdell, 1962, 1969; Milner, 1974,) and could account for the abnormal patterns of hemisphere specialization reported above. The impairments in the use of spoken language and gesture, and in other areas of symbolic functioning such as imaginative play, are thought to arise from left hemisphere dysfunction. Social impairments may be secondary to early sensorimotor deficits such as in the use of motor imitation (Dawson & Galpert, 1986; DeMyer *et al.*, 1972) or directly attributed to inadequate left hemisphere functioning (this is discussed later in this chapter). Although left hemisphere dysfunction is given a central role in autistic symptomology in this theory, it is typically recognized that autistic children may suffer from a variety of accompanying impairments in brain functioning as well (e.g., Dawson *et al.*, 1982, 1983). For example, it is recognized that some children may additionally have subcortial dysfunction and/or right hemisphere dysfunction (Dawson, 1983). The most reasonable version of this theory, then, is that, while left hemisphere dysfunction may be necessary to cause autism, the disorder may be accompanied by various other deficits as well. (Indeed, the hemispheric dysfunction may be secondary to subcortical dysfunction.) Thus, this position would be consistent with the finding of considerable variability in both the types of neurological dysfunction found across autistic children, as well as with the finding of significant variability in the type and degree of behavioral impairments found in autism.

An interesting prediction arose from the left hemisphere hypothesis (Dawson *et al.*, 1982; Prior & Bradshaw, 1979): If, in fact, language development in autism depends on compensation by the right hemisphere for left hemisphere dysfunction, then it is possible that the failure to develop language occurs in those children with bilateral dysfunction. While this theory is a reasonable one, some evidence suggests this is not the case. In a study in which parts of the Halstead–Reitan Battery were administered to a group of 10 autistic individuals (Dawson, 1983), 5 of the subjects exhibited primarily right-sided (left hemisphere) motor deficits, 4 showed bilateral deficits, and 1 showed mild, left-sided (right hemisphere) deficits. The important finding with regard to the prediction described above was that language ability for this group of autistic subjects was not related to right hemisphere functional integrity. Language ability was significantly related to degree of left hemisphere impairment (right-sided motor deficits), however.

Reduced Hemispheric Specialization

Another interpretation of the finding of abnormal hemispheric specialization in autism recently was presented by Fein, Humes, Kaplan, Lucci, and Waterhouse (1984). These authors raised the possibility that the increased variability in patterns of hemispheric specialization in autism may reflect methodological artifacts. In particular, dichotic listening techniques usually require sustained attention, comprehension of verbal instructions, short-term memory of linguistic stimuli, and limited verbal comprehension. Since autistic children are likely to have difficulty with all of these requirements, it is possible that the data reflect performance deficits on the part of the autistic children. Arnold and Schwartz's (1983) finding, reported above, that autistic children showed the normal right ear advantage (pointing to right ear) for speech stimuli when the assessment technique involved little expressive language supports this contention.

Fein *et al.* (1984) proposed that autistic children's failure to develop clearly lateralized functions is better characterized as *delayed* or *reduced* cerebral lateralization for both verbal and nonverbal processing. They suggested that the reduced lateralization probably is secondary to generalized attentional and motivational deficits, and reflects developmental lag rather than specific left hemisphere pathology. To account for the excess number of autistic individuals with apparent left hemisphere dysfunction, Fein *et al.* (1984) suggested an inherent left hemisphere vulnerability that is not specific to autism.

Fein *et al.* (1984) further argued that "the notion of left hemisphere dysfunction is inadequate to explain the cardinal symptoms of infantile autism, and that left hemisphere dysfunction, which may occur disproportionately in the autistic population, probably produces the secondary symptoms found in some autistic children" (p. 258). In particular, these authors have suggested that the left hemisphere hypothesis is inadequate to explain some of the specific language characteristics and the social deficits of autistic children. With respect to language, it is often reported that some autistic adolescents may show adequate usage of syntax, semantics, and phonology (left hemisphere functions) while the social usage of language typically remains a problem (Baltaxe & Simmons, 1975). Since deficient pragmatic usage of language and impaired comprehension of emotional cues have been found in patients with *right* hemisphere damage (see Foldi, Cicone, & Gardner, 1983, for review), this pattern of impairment may be suggestive of right rather than left hemisphere dysfunction. Thus, these authors conclude that the left hemisphere dysfunction cannot be clearly related to either the specific language deficits or the social impairment found in autism.

There are a number of points to be made in response to the Fein *et al.* arguments. To begin with, it is important to keep in mind that autistic children typically exhibit impairment in most aspects of language, including semantics, syntax, and phonology, all of which are functions of the left hemisphere. Although it is true that a subgroup of autistic adolescents may show adequate usage of the formal aspects of language (Baltaxe & Simmons, 1975), *most* autistic individuals show severe and generalized impairments in the comprehension and expression of language throughout their entire lives, a sizable proportion remaining mute (Rutter, 1974). During early life, *all* autistic children show pervasive delays and/or deviances in language development. For this reason, the presence of gross language disturbances is considered one of the primary symptoms of autism and is included in the diagnostic criteria.

The question of whether left hemisphere dysfunction plays a role in the autistic child's social impairments is currently unanswered. As has been mentioned above, there is evidence from both brain-damaged (DeRenzi, Pieczuro, & Vignolo, 1966; Duffy, Duffy, & Pearson, 1975; Kimura & Archibald, 1974; Mateer & Kimura, 1977) and normal (Dawson *et al.*, 1985) populations to support left hemisphere mediation of facial and body imitation. Developmental research and theory (Bates, 1979; Piaget, 1962; Trevarthen, 1977; Uzgiris, 1981) suggest that imitation plays an important role in early social development, being one of the first means of communication. (This point will be elaborated on later in this chapter.) Furthermore, the failure to imitate others differentiates autistic children from children with closely related developmental disabilities in whom social deficits are not pronounced (for example, dysphasic and mentally retarded children) (Bartak *et al.*, 1975; DeMyer *et al.*, 1972).

Furthermore, the notion that all aspects of emotional expression and comprehension should be attributed to the right hemisphere may be overly simplistic. It is possible that the hemispheres have complementary involvement in emotional expression and perception. For example, it has been shown that amytal injections to the left hemisphere result in feelings of depression, whereas right hemisphere anesthesia is associated with euphoria (Homes & Pan-Huysen, 1971; Perrin, Rosadini, & Rossi, 1961; Terzian, 1964). Similarly, right-hemisphere-lesioned patients reportedly exhibit happiness and laughter while left-hemisphere-lesioned patients tend to become depressed and weepy (Benson, 1973; Gainotti, 1972). In a recent review of studies on hemisphere specialization, Trevarthen (1984) concluded the following: "Available evidence of hemispheric complementarity of moods and the evidence for lateralized facial and manual expression would indicate that the left hemisphere has an inherent tendency to control interpersonal approach behavior and the taking of initiative in cooperation, while the right is adapted to regulate withdrawal, avoidance, or retreat from initiative, and dependence" (p. 1174).

While Trevarthen's ideas are speculative at this time, they serve to underscore the point that, given the little available research on hemispheric control of emotions, it is premature to conclude that all emotions are predominantly mediated by the right hemisphere. Moreover, it may be inappropriate to use evidence obtained from brain-damaged adults to develop ideas regarding the basis of children's disabilities that have existed since birth or early childhood. The little information that exists on hemispheric specialization for emotional expression and perception in infancy and childhood has only recently become available (Davidson & Fox, 1982; Fox & Davidson, 1984). This information may be useful in developing theories regarding the neurological basis of autism.

Thus, while it is clear that the most extreme version of the left hemisphere hypothesis (that is, that all autistic symptoms can be explained in terms of left hemisphere dysfunction *or* that all autistic children suffer from selective left hemisphere dysfunction) is unacceptable, the role of abnormal left hemisphere development in autism is far from being understood. Moreover, the available evidence suggests that it may form a critical piece of the complex puzzle of autism.

Relationship to Subcortical Dysfunction

A third position regarding hemispheric specialization in autism was proposed by Tanguay, Edwards, Buchwald, Schwafel, and Allen (1982) and Ornitz (1983). Their studies, as well as those of others (Fein, Skoff, & Mirsky, 1981; Ornitz & Walter, 1975; Rosenblum *et al.*, 1980), have consistently found a subgroup of autistic children to show significant (although variable across subjects) brainstem abnormalities. As Tanguay *et al.* (1982) have pointed out, several possible relationships of brainstem deficit to autism should be considered. The first possibility is that brainstem deficits are not causally related to the autistic child's cognitive and behavioral impairments. According to this position, although there may exist disruption of brainstem functioning, it may not have a central role in causing autistic behavior. A second possibility is that the language and cognitive handicaps are directly caused by brainstem dysfunction that results in the distortion in sensory stimuli (Ornitz, 1983). Although impairments in cortical functioning are also likely to exist, subcortical dysfunction is given a central role in producing the autistic syndrome. Since the sensory distortion arising from brainstem dysfunction is likely to occur in all modalities, the pervasiveness of the autistic children's impairments can be explained.

The third possibility is that brainstem dysfunction itself may pathologically influence cortical development, resulting in atypical or incomplete hemispheric specialization. According to this position, the abnormal patterns of hemisphere specialization found in autistic children may be *secondary* to abnormalities in subcortical dysfunction. The autistic syndrome of social, cognitive, and language impairments may arise from a combination of both subcortical and cortical dysfunction. This idea has received some support from a study reported by Fein *et al.* (1981). They found that brainstem abnormalities were correlated with attentional and social deficits in autistic children, but not with language or cognitive impairments.

A TEST OF SOME PREDICTIONS

Dawson, Finley, Phillips, and Galpert (1986) recently conducted a study that tested some of the predictions, and also addressed some of the methodological issues discussed above. Cortical averaged evoked potentials were used to assess cerebral specialization for speech, since this technique previously had been used to detect hemispheric asymmetries in young human infants (Crowell, Jones, Kapuniai, & Nakagawa, 1973; Molfese, Freeman, & Palermo, 1975; Molfese & Molfese, 1979, 1980; Shucard, Shucard, Cummins, & Campos, 1981). This technique was specifically chosen to reduce the attentional and linguistic demands on the autistic children and thus to minimize this possible artifact. The study was designed to explore further the question of whether autism is associated with atypical (right hemisphere)versus simply reduced (Fein *et al.*, 1984) patterns of hemispheric specialization for speech. In addition, a sample of autistic children who varied widely in age and language ability was chosen in order to examine whether the direction or degree of hemispheric asymmetry is related to the level of language impairment and/or age in autism.

Cortical averaged evoked responses to speech (consonant-vowel sound, "Da") and nonspeech (musical chord) stimuli were recorded from left and right hemisphere scalp regions of 17 autistic children, 6 to 18 years of age, and 17 chronological age-matched normal subjects. Normal subjects showed consistent hemispheric asymmetries in the early components (N_1 and P_2) of the evoked response to speech. (Consistent hemisphere asymmetries were not found in the normal group for musical chord stimulus. Thus, meaningful group comparisons for this stimulus were not possible.)

A significant group difference in the direction of hemispheric asymmetry to speech stimuli was found. On the basis of two measures of cerebral asymmetry (N_1 amplitude and N_1 latency) autistic subjects were more likely to show the reversed direction of hemispheric asymmetry during speech processing from that characteristic of the normal subjects. The percentage of autistic subjects exhibiting reversed (right hemisphere) dominance for speech (approximately 68%) was similar to that found in a previous study of autistic individuals (Dawson *et al.*, 1982). Differences between normal and autistic children in absolute degree of hemispheric asymmetry were not found. In fact, autistic subjects with reversed asymmetries were more likely to show *greater* degrees of asymmetry than normal subjects and than those autistic subjects who showed the normal direction of asymmetry.

Normal children's pattern of hemispheric asymmetry did not differ as a function of age. Older autistic children, however, were more likely to show normal patterns of hemispheric asymmetry than were younger autistic children.

Significant relationships between the direction and magnitude of hemispheric asymmetry and language ability were also found. More advanced language abilities, in all aspects of language (articulation, syntax, semantics) were associated with a normal direction of hemispheric asymmetry for speech; children with poorer language abilities were more likely to show the reversed (right hemisphere) direction, as well as a greater degree of asymmetry. These correlations between cerebral asymmetry and language generally held even after age was partialed out.

These results do not support the Fein *et al.* (1984) argument that autism is associated with reduced, but otherwise normal, patterns of hemispheric specialization. Instead, it appears that a sizable percentage of these children, and, in particular, those children who are younger and more language-impaired, exhibit an atypical pattern of hemispheric specialization—that is, a greater degree of asymmetry and right hemisphere dominance for speech processing. If the hemispheres were equally dysfunctional in autism, such a pattern would not be expected. Moreover, these findings cannot be attributed to task-related artifacts since the procedure required minimal attentional and linguistic processing on the part of the children.

A Developmental Theory

The patterns of hemispheric specialization exhibited by autistic children are particularly interesting in light of what is known about the normal development of hemispheric specialization. In contrast to Lenneberg's (1967) theory, which assumed functional symmetry between the hemispheres until about 2 to 4 years of age, more recent investigations of hemisphere specialization in young infants suggest that functional cerebral asymmetries, similar to those found in adults, exist by at least 2 or 3 months of age, and possibly at birth (e.g., Best, Hoffman, & Glanville, 1982; Crowell *et al.*, 1973; Entus, 1977; Glanville, Best, & Levenson, 1977; Molfese *et al.*, 1975). Moreover, there is little evidence to suggest that major changes in brain organization occur with age (Bakker, Hoefkens, & VanderVlugt, 1979; Flaney & Balling, 1979; Hiscock & Kinsbourne, 1978; Hynd & Obrzut, 1977; Nava & Butler, 1977). Although the cortex becomes more specialized, and thus less plastic, as the child acquires cognitive and language skills (Witelson, 1977), there is little compelling evidence to suggest that the basic underlying organization, in terms of the functions of the right and left hemispheres, changes with development. In light of these general principles of normal development, it appears that autistic children are exhibiting an atypical, rather than a simply delayed, pattern of hemispheric specialization.* The data presented above suggest the possibility that, while the underlying cerebral organization of autistic children may be similar to that of normal children, their functional usage of the hemispheres may be abnormal.

The relationships found between pattern of hemispheric specialization and both age and language ability in the autistic group point to some interesting hypotheses regarding the development of hemispheric specialization in autism. It is possible that with increases in age and language ability, there occurs a shift in autistic children's pattern of hemispheric specialization for language. Data from the study reported above suggest that this shift is from atypical, right hemisphere speech processing, which is associated with a greater-than-normal degree of cerebral asymmetry, to normal, left hemisphere speech processing, which is

---

*The term *abnormal specialization* may not be entirely appropriate here, since it implies that an abnormality in underlying cerebral organization exists. In the model proposed here, it is the *functional usage*, rather than the intrinsic organization, of the hemispheres that is abnormal.

associated with a lesser, but more normal, degree of asymmetry. These age-related changes were not found in the normal group. Moreover, there was no evidence of sample selection bias that can easily account for these data (that is, younger autistic subjects did not differ from older subjects with respect to IQ, sex, handedness, or severity of autistic symptoms at time of diagnosis).

Interestingly, an atypical pattern of hemispheric specialization for speech, similar to that reported above for autistic children, has been documented in a presumably normal child who experienced an extremely deprived language and social environment (Fromkin, Krashem, Curtiss, Rigler, & Ringler, 1974). This finding suggests that postnatal hemispheric specialization for speech processing depends on the exercise of these processes in a facilitative social environment. The autistic child's severe linguistic and social impairments may, in effect, result in a degree of deprivation that would preclude normal development of the left hemisphere. At the same time, many autistic children spontaneously engage in object-related activities involving visuospatial relationships, such as puzzles. Thus it is possible that, for some children, asymmetric development of the hemispheres occurs early in life, resulting in overreliance on a right hemisphere processing mode for both verbal and nonverbal functions. As the autistic child begins to make use of language for communicative purposes, the left hemisphere, because of its inherent predisposition for speech perception and expression, may then begin to take over language functions.

Prizant's (1983; Prizant & Rydell, 1984) research on the development of autistic children's language is compatible with the notion of a shift from right to left hemisphere specialization for speech processing. He has argued that autistic children's early language, which is almost entirely echolalic, is the result of an overreliance on holistic rather than analytic processing modes. Prizant has further observed that, as the autistic child's functional usage of echolalic speech becomes more complex, spontaneous, creative speech similar in form to that of normal young children begins to emerge. These two language systems continue to coexist until eventually the spontaneous, creative speech predominates, except during periods of stress. These observations are compatible with a shift in the direction of hemispheric processing of language with development. Clearly, the test of such a theory would depend on a longitudinal study. Also, it is likely that if such a developmental course were documented, it would apply only to a subgroup of autistic children, since the heterogeneity of underlying dysfunction may result in a number of possible patterns of adaption with development.

THE POSSIBLE ROLE OF ABNORMAL HEMISPHERIC SPECIALIZATION IN THE AFFECTIVE AND SOCIAL DEFICITS OF AUTISTIC CHILDREN

As mentioned above, current research suggests that both hemispheres are critically involved in the regulation of affect and social behavior. I now would like to elaborate on some of the current theories regarding the hemispheric basis of emotion, particularly as they may be relevant to our understanding of autism. Although most of these ideas are speculative and based on indirect evidence, they do yield testable hypotheses for future research.

On the basis of data from several different experimental paradigms, including lateralized eye movements (Ahern & Schwartz, 1979), dichotic listening (Reuter-Lorenz & Davidson, 1981), and asymmetrical brain activity (Davidson & Fox, 1982; Davidson, Schwartz, Saron, Bennet, & Goleman, 1979), investigators have reported differential involvement of the hemispheres in the perception and expression of positive and negative emotions. When hemispheric asymmetries are found, the left hemisphere appears to be specialized for the processing of positive affective stimuli while the corresponding regions of the right hemisphere are specialized for the processing of negative affective stimuli. This finding has now been documented for 10-month-old infants (Davidson & Fox, 1982), suggesting that this may be an early functional characteristic of the hemispheres. Clinical data, as reported above, also support the notion of differential involvement of the hemispheres in emotion. For example, pathological laughter is more often associated with right hemisphere damage whereas catastrophic crying and depression are associated with left hemisphere damage (Benson, 1973; Gainotti, 1972).

Recently, Fox and Davidson (1984) have proposed a developmental model of the hemispheric substrates of affect. Similar to Trevarthen (1984), they are suggesting that positive and negative emotions reflect the underlying behavioral dimension of approach and withdrawal, upon which these affective subsystems have evolved. Furthermore, they propose that, in infancy, the early emerging emotions, such as happiness and distress, are each under unilateral hemispheric control. As the functional capacity of the commissural system develops, more complex emotional responses involving coactivation of the hemispheres, as well as inhibition and regulation of right hemisphere-mediated emotions through left hemisphere control, occur. In particular, Fox and Davidson suggest that the ability to inhibit and regulate distress involves left hemisphere inhibition of negative affective responses that are predominantly under right hemisphere control.

This model of the hemispheric basis of affective development has some interesting implications for understanding autism. The most basic social characteristic of young autistic children is that of withdrawal. Approach, as expressed in behavior such as the desire for affiliation with the caretaker and interest in people and surroundings, is characteristically missing in the autistic child. Given Fox and Davidson's model, it is possible that the autistic child's withdrawn behavior reflects impoverished development of the left hemisphere. Also, if regulation of distress reactions depends on left hemisphere inhibition of right hemisphere affective processes, it is possible that the severe and uncontrollable distress exhibited by many young autistic children results from inadequate left hemisphere control. Clearly, these ideas are based only on indirect empirical support. However, they do lead to several testable hypotheses regarding the hemispheric basis of affective and social deficits in autism.

The autistic child's social and affective impairments may also be related to the early failure to imitate others and use gesture for communication. The notion that motor imitation and the use of gesture are left-hemisphere-mediated functions rests on substantial clinical (DeRenzi et al., 1966; Duffy et al., 1975; Kimura & Archibald, 1974; Mateer & Kimura, 1977) and some experimental (Dawson et al., 1985) data. The ability to imitate facial expressions (Field, Woodson, Greenberg, & Cohen, 1982) and facial postures (Meltzoff & Moore, 1977) has been demonstrated in young infants, which suggests that this is an early functional characteristic of the human nervous system. This early form of imitation may be a precursor of later, more sophisticated forms of imitative skills. Thus, the autistic child's failure to imitate may reflect a neurologically based impairment in social functioning that exists from birth.

The role of imitation in early social development has been documented by observations of young infants and their caretakers (Papousek & Papousek, 1977). Imitation is one of the first means of shared communication (Uzgiris, 1981); it is also one of the primary mechanisms by which infants learn to play social games and use gestures, and learn to use a variety of complex facial expressions. Thus, the autistic child's impairment in motor imitation is likely to have severe consequences for social development. In a study of 4- to 6-year-old autistic children, Dawson and Adams (1984) found that the level of motor imitation skill was significantly related to the degree of social responsiveness shown during free play.

Given the left hemisphere's possible role in imitative and gestural behavior, and in the affective processes that are required for forming basic affiliations with others (Sroufe, 1979), it is very possible that inadequate left hemisphere functioning accounts, at least in part, for the autistic child's impaired social development.

CONCLUSION

To date, no particular type or locus of brain dysfunction has been found to be either uniquely or universally associated with autism. It is most likely that autism can arise from a variety of neurological impairments. What is consistent across cases of autism, then, may be, not the specific locus of neurological dysfunction, but rather the specific brain *systems* that are effected. Any type of dysfunction, whether cortical or subcortical, that interferes from early life with the ability to meaningfully process the social environment, in both verbal and nonverbal modalities, may result in a form of autism. The extent and type of dysfunction may influence the degree of autism and eventual developmental outcome, and therefore be a useful prognostic indicator. Thus, some investigation of the relationship between specific types of neurological impairment and the degree of social, language, and other behavioral impairments in autistic children would be useful. I am suggesting a model of autism that emphasizes the role of abnormal left hemisphere development. The cause of abnormal hemispheric specialization and function may be varied, possibly involving brainstem or thalamic regions. Regardless of the cause, abnormal hemisphere development may play an important role in producing the primary symptoms of autism. Its role may be central—that is, abnormal hemisphere development may account for the major symptoms of autism. Or its effects may be additive, with the impairments arising from other related brain regions. Moreover, individual variation in this regard is expected.

A model of two-way interaction between the brain and experience needs to be considered in understanding any developmental disorder. In the case of autism, it is probable that the child's deficiencies in processing social and language stimuli will adversely affect brain development. In general, very little is known about the effects of having a developmental disability on the developing brain. It is likely that when language acquisition begins at an age much later than is normal, many of our assumptions regarding brain development may not apply. For example, certain aspects of brain functioning, such as left hemisphere speech specialization, that normally may be established in infancy may not be present until later childhood or even late adolescence in the developmentally disabled child. The degree to which "normality" can be expected to be achieved may differ according to the type and degree of dysfunction and the age of onset of various functions, such as language.

A more dynamic conception of autism will be useful in understanding the complex neurological and behavioral findings with autistic individuals. In particular, we need to keep in mind that, like normal persons, autistic individuals will differ significantly in their symptoms and neurological characteristics with development. No longer is it acceptable to group together (statistically or conceptually) autistic persons of a wide range of ages and abilities in order to study "autism." Instead, a careful consideration of developmental level may allow for a meaningful interpretation of the heterogeneity of both behavioral and neurological findings across individuals and across studies.

Finally, both neuropsychological and autism research previously have tended to focus on language and cognition and have underemphasized affective and social behavior. Both areas of research have recently shifted this emphasis. It is very likely that the growth of these two complementary fields of study will allow new insights into the nature of autism.

ACKNOWLEDGMENTS

I wish to thank Larry Galpert for his suggestions and critical reading of earlier drafts of this chapter. Much of the research reported in this chapter was supported by NIMH grant MH36612 awarded to Geraldine Dawson.

REFERENCES

Ahern, G. L., & Schwartz, G. E. (1979). Differential lateralization for positive versus negative emotion. *Neuropsychologia, 17*, 693–698.

Arnold, G., & Schwartz, S. (1983). Hemispheric lateralization of language in autistic and aphasic children. *Journal of Autism and Developmental Disorders, 13*, 129–139.

Bakker, D. J., Hoefkens, M., & VanderVlugt, H. (1979). Hemispheric specialization in children as reflected in the longitudinal development of ear asymmetry. *Cortex, 15*, 619–625.

Baltaxe, C. A., & Simmons, J. Q. (1975). Language in childhood psychosis: A review. *Journal of Speech and Hearing Disorders, 30*, 439–458.

Bartak, L., Rutter, M., & Cox, A. (1975). A comparative study of infantile autism and specific developmental language disorders: The children. *British Journal of Psychiatry, 126*, 127–145.

Bates, E. (1979). *The emergences of symbols.* New York: Academic Press.

Benson, D. F. (1973). Psychiatric aspects of aphasia. *British Journal of Psychiatry, 123*, 555–566.

Best, C. T., Hoffman, H., & Glanville, B. B. (1982). Development of right ear asymmetries for speech and music. *Perception and Psychophysics, 31*, 75–85.

Butler, S. R., & Glass, A. (1974). Asymmetries in the electroencephalogram associated with cerebral dominance. *Electroencephalography and Clinical Neurophysiology, 36*, 481–491.

Crowell, P., Jones, R., Kapuniai, L., & Nakagawa, J. (1973). Unilateral cortical activity in newborn humans. An early index of cerebral dominance. *Science, 180*, 205–208.

Curcio, G. (1978). Sensorimotor functioning and communication in mute autistic children. *Journal of Autism and Childhood Schizophrenia, 8*, 281–292.

Davidson, R. J., & Fox, N. A. (1982). Asymmetrical brain activity discriminates between positive and negative affective stimuli in human infants. *Science, 218*, 1235–1237.

Davidson, R. J., Schwartz, G. E., Saron, C., Bennett, J., & Goleman, D. J. (1979). Frontal versus parietal EEG asymmetry during positive and negative affect. *Psychophysiology, 16*, 202–203.

Dawson, G. (1983). Lateralized brain dysfunction in autism: Evidence from the Halstead–Reitan Neuropsychological Battery. *Journal of Autism and Developmental Disorders, 13*, 269–286.

Dawson, G., & Adams, A. (1984). Imitation and social responsiveness in autistic children. *Journal of Abnormal Child Psychology, 12*, 209–225.

Dawson, G., & Galpert, L. (1986). A developmental model for facilitating the social behavior of autistic children. In E. Schopler & G. Mesibov (Eds.), *Social behavior in autism.* New York: Plenum Press.

Dawson, G., Finley, C., Phillips, S., & Galpert, L. (1986). Hemispheric specialization and the language abilities of autistic children. *Child Development, 57*, 1440–1453.

Dawson, G., Warrenburg, S., & Fuller, P. (1982). Cerebral lateralization in individuals diagnosed as autistic in early childhood. *Brain and Language, 15*, 353–368.

Dawson, G., Warrenburg, S., & Fuller, P. (1983). Hemisphere functioning and motor imitation in autistic persons. *Brain and Cognition, 2*, 346–354.

Dawson, G., Warrenburg, S., & Fuller, P. (1985). Left hemisphere specialization for facial and manual imitation. *Psychophysiology, 22*, 237–245.

DeMyer, M. K., Alpern, G. D., Barton, S., DeMyer, W. E., Churchill, D. W., Hingtgen, J. N., Bryson, C. Q., Pontius, W., & Kimberlin, C. (1972). Imitation in autistic, early schizophrenic, and nonpsychotic subnormal children. *Journal of Autism and Childhood Schizophrenia, 2*, 264–287.

DeRenzi, E., Pieczuro, A., & Vignolo, L. A. (1966). Oral apraxia and aphasia. *Cortex, 2*, 50–73.

Doyle, J., Galin, D., & Ornstein, R. E. (1974). Lateral specialization of cognitive mode: EEG frequency analysis. *Psychophysiology, 11*, 567–578.

Duffy, R., Duffy, J., & Pearson, K. (1975). Pantomime recognition in aphasics. *Journal of Speech and Hearing Research, 18*, 115–132.

Entus, A. K. (1977). Hemispheric asymmetry in processing of dichotically presented speech and non-speech sounds by infants. In S. Segalowitz & F. A. Gruber (Eds.), *Language development and neurological theory*. New York: Academic Press.

Field, T. M., Woodson, R., Greenberg, R., & Cohen, D. (1982). Discrimination and imitation of facial expression by neonates. *Science, 218*, 179–181.

Fein, D., Humes, M., Kaplan, E., Lucci, D., & Waterhouse, L. (1984). The question of left hemisphere dysfunction in autism. *Psychological Bulletin, 95*, 258–281.

Fein, D., Skoff, B., & Mirsky, A. F. (1981). Clinical correlates of brain dysfunction in autistic children, *Journal of Autism and Developmental Disorders, 11*, 303–315.

Flaney, R. C., & Balling, J. D. (1979). Developmental changes in hemispheric specialization for tactile spatial ability. *Developmenal Psychology, 15*, 364–372.

Foldi, N., Cicone, M., & Gardner, H. (1983). Pragmatic aspects of communication in brain-damaged patients. In S. J. Segalowitz (Ed.), *Language functions and brain organization* (pp. 51–86). New York: Academic Press.

Fox, N. A., & Davidson, R. J. (1984). Hemispheric substrates of affect: A developmental model. In N. A. Fox & R. J. Davidson (Eds.), *The psychobiology of affective development* (pp. 353–381). Hillsdale, NJ: Erlbaum.

Fromkin, V. A., Krashem, S., Curtiss, S., Rigler, D., & Ringler, M. (1974). The development of language in Genie: A case of language acquisition beyond the "critical period." *Brain and Language, 1*, 81–107.

Gainotti, G. (1972). Emotional behavior and hemispheric side of the lesion. *Cortex, 8*, 41–52.

Glanville, B. B., Best, C. T., & Levinson, R. (1977). A cardiac measure of cerebral asymmetries in infant auditory perception. *Developmental Psychology, 13*, 54–59.

Hammes, J., & Langdell, T. (1981). Precursors of symbol formation and childhood autism. *Journal of Autism and Developmental Disorders, 11*, 331–346.

Hiscock, M., & Kinsbourne, M. (1978). Ontogeny of cerebral dominance: Evidence from time-sharing asymmetry in children. *Developmental Psychology, 14*, 321–329.

Homes, O. R., & Pan-Hysen, L. (1971). Depression and cerebral dominance. A study of bilateral intracartotid amytal in eleven depressed patients. *Psychiatria Neurologia Neurochirurgia, 74*, 259–270.

Hynd, G. W., & Obrzut, J. E. (1977). Effects of grade level and sex on the magnitude of the dichotic ear advantage. *Neuropsychologia, 15*, 689–692.

Kimura, D., & Archibald, Y. (1974). Motor functions of the left hemisphere. *Brain, 97*, 337–350.

Lansdell, H. (1962). Laterality of verbal intelligence in the brain. *Science, 135*, 922–923.

Lansdell, H. (1969). Verbal and nonverbal factors in right hemisphere speech. *Journal of Comparative Physiological Psychology, 69*, 734–738.

Lenneberg, E. H. (1967). *Biological foundations of language*. New York: Wiley.

Mateer, C., & Kimura, D. (1977). Impairment of nonverbal oral movement in aphasia. *Brain and Language, 4*, 262–272.

Meltzoff, A. N., & Moore, M. K. (1977). Imitation of facial and manual gestures by human neonates. *Science, 198*, 75–78.

Milner, B. (1974). Hemispheric specialization: Scope and limits. In F. O. Schmitt & F. G. Worden (Eds.), *The neurosciences. Third study program*. Cambridge, MA.: MIT Press.

Molfese, D. L., Freeman, R. B., & Palermo, D. S. (1975). The ontogeny of brain lateralization for speech and non-speech stimuli. *Brain and Language, 2*, 356–368.

Molfese, D. L., & Molfese, U. J. (1979). Hemisphere and stimulus differences as reflected in the cortical responses of newborn infants to speech stimuli. *Developmental Psychology, 15*, 505–511.

Molfese, D. L., & Molfese, U. J. (1980). Cortical responses of preterm infants to phonetic and nonphonetic speech stimuli. *Developmental Psychology, 16*, 574–581.

Nava, P. L., & Butler, S. R. (1977). Development of cerebral dominance motivated by asymmetries in the alpha rhythm. *Electroencephalography and Clinical Neurophysiology, 43*, 582.

Ornitz, E. (1983). Neuroanatomical basis of early infantile autism. *International Journal of Neuroscience, 19*, 85–124.

Ornitz, E. M., & Walter, D. D. (1975). The effect of sound pressure waveform on human brainstem auditory evoked responses. *Brain Research, 92*, 490–498.

Papousek, H., & Papousek, M. (1977). Mothering and cognitive headstart: Psychobiological considerations. In H. R. Schaffer (Ed.), *Studies in mother-infant interaction* (pp. 63–85). New York: Academic Press.

Perrin, L., Rosadini, G., & Rossi, G. F. (1961). Determination of side of cerebral dominance with amobarbital. *Archives of Neurology, 4*, 173–179.

Piaget, J. (1962). *Play, dreams and imitation in childhood*. New York: Norton.

Prior, M. R., & Bradshaw, J. L. (1979). Hemisphere functions in autistic children. *Cortex, 15*, 73–81.

Prizant, B. M. (1983). Language acquisition and communicative behavior in autism: Toward an understanding of the whole of it. *Journal of Speech and Hearing Disorders, 48*, 296–307.

Prizant, B., & Rydell, P. J. (1984). Analysis of functions of delayed echolalia in autistic children. *Journal of Speech and Hearing Research, 27*, 183–192.

Ricks, D. M., & Wing, L. (1975). Language, communication, and the use of symbols in normal and autistic children. *Journal of Autism and Childhood Schizophrenia, 5*, 191–221.

Rosenblum, S. M., Arick, J. R., Krug, D. A., Stubbs, E. G., Young, N. B., & Pelson, R. D. (1980). Auditory brainstem evoked responses in autistic children. *Journal of Autism and Developmental Disorders, 10*, 215–225.

Rosenblum, D. R., & Dorman, M. F. (1978). Hemispheric specialization for speech perception in language deficient kindergarten children. *Brain and Language, 6*, 378–389.

Rutter, M. (1974). The development of infantile autism. *Psychological Medicine, 4*, 147–163.

Shucard, J. L., Shucard, D. W., Cummins, K. R., & Campos, J. J. (1981). Auditory evoked potentials and sex-related differences in brain development. *Brain and Language, 13*, 91–102.

Sommers, R. K., & Taylor, M. L. (1972). Cerebral speech dominance in language-disordered and normal children. *Cortex, 8*, 224–332.

Springer, S., & Eisenson, J. (1977). Hemispheric specialization for speech in language-disordered children. *Neuropsychologia, 15*, 287–293.

Reuter-Lorenz, P., & Davidson, R. J. (1981). Differential contributions of the two cerebral hemispheres to the perception of happy and sad faces. *Neuropsychologia, 19*, 609–613.

Sroufe, L. A. (1979). Socioemotional development. In J. Osofsky (Ed.), *Handbook of infant development*. New York: Wiley.

Tanguay, P. E. (1976). Clinical and electrophysiological research. In E. R. Ritvo (Ed.), *Autism: Diagnosis, current research and management*. New York: Spectrum.

Tanguay, P. E., Edwards, R. M., Buchwald, J., Schwafel, J., & Allen, V. (1982). Auditory brainstem evoked responses in autistic children. *Archives of General Psychiatry, 39*, 174–180.

Terzian, H. (1964). Behavioral and EEG effects of intracarotid sodium amytal inject. *Acta Neurochirurgica, 12*, 230–239.

Trevarthen, C. (1977). Descriptive analyses of infant communicative behavior. In H. R. Schaffer (Ed.), *Studies in mother–infant interaction* (pp. 227–270). New York: Academic Press.

Trevarthen, C. (1984). Hemispheric specialization. In *Handbook of physiology: Nervous system III* (pp. 1129–1190). Bethesda, Maryland: American Physiological Society.

Uzgiris, I. C. (1981). Experience in the social content. In R. L. Schiefelbusch & D. D. Bricker (Eds.), *Early language: Acquisition and intervention* (pp. 139–168). Baltimore: University Park Press.

Wetherby, A. M., Koegel, R. L., & Mendel, M. (1981). Central auditory nervous system dysfunction in echolalic autistic individuals. *Journal of Speech and Hearing Research, 24,* 420–429.

Wing, L. (1981). Language, social and cognitive impairments in autism and severe mental retardation. *Journal of Autism and Developmental Disorders, 11,* 31–44.

Witelson, S. F. (1977). Early hemisphere specialization and inter hemispheric plasticity: An empirical and theoretical review. In S. J. Segalowitz & F. A. Gruber (Eds.), *Language development and neurological theory* (pp. 213–289) New York: Academic Press.

Witelson, S. F., & Rabinovitch, M. S. (1972). Hemispheric speech lateralization in children with auditory-linguistic deficits. *Cortex, 8,* 412–426.

Brain Lesions in Autism

G. ROBERT DeLONG and MARGARET L. BAUMAN

INTRODUCTION

In this chapter we will review the available data on brain lesions in infantile autism. These encompass clinical and neuroradiological data, as well as neuropathological (autopsy) studies. The pneumoencephalogram and, more recently, the computerized tomographic (CT) scan have contributed to an understanding of brain lesions in autism, and the relevant studies will be reviewed. In addition, we will review a recent careful neuropathological study of the brain of an autistic man, which has provided evidence of a focal brain lesion in autism. Finally, we will discuss possible correlations between the brain lesions found by anatomical techniques and the neurobehavioral dysfunction found in autism.

THE SIGNIFICANCE OF BRAIN LESIONS: NEUROLOGICAL VERSUS NONNEUROLOGICAL AUTISM

Autism is defined as a behavioral syndrome, which may have several different etiologies. Sometimes the etiology is completely obscure; in other cases autism may occur in the context of known brain disease, such as congenital rubella (Chess, Korn, & Fernandez, 1971) or destructive brain lesions (Hauser, DeLong, & Rosman, 1975). Thus, observers speak of neurological and nonneurological autism—i.e., cases in which neurological or somatic signs are present, and those with no such signs. The autistic syndrome, however, appears to be essentially indistinguishable in both. Garreau, Barthelemy, Sauvage, Leddet, and LeLord (1984) compared the clinical features of autistic syndromes with and without associated neurological problems, and showed that the two were remarkably similar in terms of severity and type of autistic symptoms, IQ, and sex distribution. This study argued that conclusions drawn from autistic subjects with identifiable brain lesions may be generalized to cases without such lesions. It suggested that the same neural systems are dysfunctional in both types of autism, even though the etiology may differ. This suggestion spurs the hope

G. ROBERT DeLONG and MARGARET L. BAUMAN • Pediatric Neurology Unit, Massachusetts General Hospital, Boston, Massachusetts 02114.

that study of those cases of autism that show neuropathological lesions may shed light on the pathophysiological processes underlying autism in general.

CLINICAL STUDIES

Knobloch and Pasamanick (1975) carried out an early investigation to determine the relationship of the autistic behavioral constellation to perinatal complications and organic brain disease. They identified 64 children with the symptom complex of autism, of whom 14 had phenylketonuria. The remaining 50 children were evaluated at a mean age of 18 months (a fact that complicates interpretation of the study, since autistic manifestations may not be fully developed, and may be difficult to assess, at such a young age). The authors found, at the time of initial examination, that all 50 showed evidence of organic disease of the nervous system. There was a high incidence of antecedent complications of pregnancy and the neonatal period (21% had seizures, strabismus, and "cerebral palsy" or other major specific neurological disorder—meningitis with secondary hydrocephalus, encephalitis, hypoglycemia, craniostenosis, congenital rubella, congenital hypothyroidism, hypsarrhythmia, and others). These specific disorders closely matched those found in an abnormal comparison group without autism.

Only 20% of the autism patients had initial developmental quotients above 75. The autistic symptoms were qualitatively the same whether the child had mental deficiency or normal intelligence, or whether the process had been present from birth or appeared after a definite cerebral insult, such as encephalitis or seizures. The autistic children differed from the abnormal comparison children only by virtue of having the autistic symptom complex in addition to their other central nervous system abnormalities.

Thirty-nine of these children were followed up at a median age of 7 years. The autistic behavior had disappeared in three-fourths of the patients; it tended to persist in those with the lowest developmental quotients at the time of initial examination, and in those who had been over 3 years of age at initial evaluation.

Knobloch and Pasamanick (1975) concluded that infantile autism is a description of a complex of behavioral symptoms associated with organic disease of the brain of varied etiologies. They called attention to the high incidence of associated mental retardation, language disorders, and convulsive disorders. They observed that most children eventually lose their autistic behavior and establish social interactions; however, they remain as mentally defective as before, or more so.

The authors argued that their sample of autistic children with organic brain disease was essentially comparable to the groups described by Rutter, Greenfield, and Lockyer (1967) and by Kanner (1943), except that the latter were drawn from psychiatric services and were older at initial evaluation. They point out that children with overt neurological abnormalities are unlikely to be referred to psychiatric clinics, and that those initially diagnosed at an older age are more likely to have persistence of their autistic symptoms. The authors point out that their sample and that of Rutter et al. (1967), drawn from a psychiatric clinic, had comparable incidences of mental deficiency, grand mal seizures, central communication disorders and other distortions of language behavior, and similar global clinical outcomes; they suggest that Kanner's (1943) population was not in fact very different, since outcome results were similar.

Other studies of autism have shown a high incidence of encephalopathy. A survey in Western Australia of 25 autistic children (Gubbay, Lobascher, & Kingerlee, 1970), all of whom were retarded, found that 21 (84%) showed evidence of encephalopathy and 13 (56%)

had unequivocal evidence of organic brain disease. In this study, 20 to 30% had abnormal electroencephalograms characterized by focal slowing, spiking, or paroxysmal spike-wave discharges. Others have reported abnormal EEGs in 60 to 80% of autistic children (Creak & Pampiglione, 1969; White, DeMyer, & DeMyer, 1964). Forty-two percent of one group had clinical seizures at the time of the study (Schain & Yannet, 1960).

In summary, clinical study of a broad range of children with autism reveals that many have clearly identifiable organic disease of the brain.

EPIDEMIOLOGICAL FACTORS ASSOCIATED WITH ENCEPHALOPATHY

The role of perinatal complications in causation of autism was investigated by Deykin and MacMahon (1980) in an epidemiological study of 145 autistic children and 330 matched unaffected siblings. Autistic children were significantly more likely than their siblings to have at least one prenatal complication and to have experienced labor and delivery complications. Neonatal complications, including medical interventions in the first year of life, were also significantly more common for the autistic children (in each category, $p < .05$). The authors note that the highest risk ratios were observed for events that involved very small proportions of propositi and siblings, and the complications that carried the highest risk of autism represented various kinds of pathologic processes with no apparent unifying feature. The authors suggest that various types of physical damage may produce autistic symptomatology. Their data suggest, however, that the perinatal complications they studied could account for only a small proportion of autism.

In a related study (Deykin & MacMahon, 1979), the same authors evaluated a number of infectious agents as possible factors in the etiology of autism. The data showed that only two agents, prenatal rubella and prenatal influenza, were significantly more frequent in autistic children than in their siblings. The authors estimated that, at most, only 5% of autism could be attributable to these prenatal infections.

In discussions of brain lesions and autism, congenital rubella holds a special place. Chess et al. (1971) thoroughly evaluated the psychiatric disorders of children with congenital rubella in New York, following the 1964 epidemic. Their sample consisted of 243 children with proven congenital rubella evaluated at 2 to 4 years of age. Of these, 10 were classified as autistic and an additional 8 showed a "partial syndrome of autism." Thus the prevalence rate of autism in this sample of rubella children was betwen 100 and 200 times greater than in the general population. These children also had varying degrees of mental retardation; only 1 of the 10 autistic children, and 1 of the 8 with the partial syndrome of autism, were intellectually normal. Only 1 of the latter had additional symptoms of cerebral dysfunction.

In another detailed investigation of the neurological aftermath of congenital rubella (Desmond et al., 1967), 8 of 64 children surviving at 18 months were characterized as autistic.

NEURORADIOLOGICAL STUDIES

Although congenital encephalopathy is recognized in a high proportion of autistic children, how the encephalopathy produces autism remains unclear. Is it because specific localized brain lesions produce discrete functional deficits? We will focus on the neuroanatomical and neuropathological data pertinent to this question.

Both pneumoencephalography and computerized tomographic scanning have been utilized to study autistic children. The results, while not definitive, have provided useful information.

Pneumoencephalography

Several authors (Aarkrog, 1968; Dalby, 1975; Hauser *et al.*, 1975; Melchior, Dyggve, & Gylstorff, 1965; Schonfelder, 1964) have published the results of pneumoencephalographic (PEG) examinations in autistic children; in most cases measurements have been limited to (a) the Evans ratio (i.e., the span of the anterior horns/the internal transverse diameter of the skull), (b) the width of the third ventricle, and (c) the presence or absence of widened cortical sulci. These were useful parameters to study because normal values had been established (Jacobsen & Melchior, 1967; Melchior, 1961) and abnormalities in these measurements had been shown to correlate with the degree of mental retardation (Melchior, 1961; Melchior *et al.*, 1965; Nielsen, Petersen, Thygesen, & Willanger, 1966a, 1966b) and with the age at onset of seizure disorders (Skatvedt, Eek, & Gardborg, 1959) in childhood. Unfortunately, other potentially useful PEG observations (including note of asymmetries, and measurements of the temporal horns) went for the most part unrecorded. Melchior *et al.* (1965), using the above criteria, found mildly abnormal PEGs in the majority of 27 children diagnosed as autistic. The deviations from normal were mild when compared with nonautistic retarded children of similar intelligence. Boesen and Aarkrog (1967) reported 13 abnormal PEGs out of 33 cases of infantile psychosis studied. PEGs were reviewed from a total of 117 children with a wide variety of psychiatric syndromes, and it was reported that "in the material there are cases of local particularly severe dilatations, e.g., in the temporal region and a smaller number of asymmetrical dilatations. Specific psychiatric clinical pictures corresponding to these locations were not observed." Aarkrog (1968) later expanded this study to include 46 children with infantile autism or "borderline" autism and found that 25 (54%) had abnormalities by PEG. In addition, Schonfelder (1964) reported PEG findings on 2 children with early infantile autism, both from the same family. Atrophy, seen as pathological ventricular dilatation, was generalized in one case and limited to the left hemisphere in the other. Dalby (1975) presented pneumoencephalographic findings in a large group of children characterized by developmental language retardation. Forty of 87 (46%) of these children had dilatation of the left temporal horn, which in 26 (30%) was limited solely to the left temporal horn. A control group of children with petit mal showed only 15% with dilatation of the left temporal horn. Dalby's group was not characterized behaviorally except for language retardation, but in personal communication he has noted that many of them had more extensive behavioral abnormalities.

Hauser *et al.* (1975) described the pneumoencephalographic findings in 17 children with clinical features of the infantile autism syndrome. They paid particular attention to the temporal horns of the lateral ventricles, which were not described in some early pneumoencephalographic studies, and which are poorly evaluated by the CT scan (Damasio, Maurer, Damasio, & Chui, 1980).

Seventeen cases were selected retrospectively from a group of 105 children referred for neurological evaluation of retarded language development and/or infantile autism. The sole criterion for selection was the presence of a pneumoencephalogram as part of the diagnostic study. Identifiable metabolic disorders were absent in all cases. None of the children were blind or deaf. Somatic abnormalities were present in only 2 cases, 1 dolichocephalic and 1 with synostosis of the coronal suture, surgically repaired.

Fifteen of the 17 cases satisfied at least five of the criteria set forth by Creak (1963) for the diagnosis of infantile autism. Sixteen satisfied the two criteria most central to the diagnosis, that is, failure of normal development of communicative language and gross and sustained impairment in emotional relationships.

The primary language disorder could be characterized as a failure to develop expressive speech. Comprehension of spoken language, although also delayed for age, was somewhat less deficient in 14 cases. Five children had failed to develop any speech, 4 were using single words only (range of vocabulary 1 to 50 words), and the remaining 8 had developed four- or five-word sentences. In the last group, acquisition of sentences was accompanied by hyperlalia and echolalia in 5 cases and was used as a form of self-amusement in addition to communication. Although these children were fluent, words were poorly articulated, improperly accented, and often used with incorrect pronouns. Regression was present in only 3 cases. One lost all expressive language following a prolonged episode of status epilepticus; another used only one word at a time, losing a previously spoken word with each new acquisition; and a third had subsequently lost the six or seven words spoken at 15 months. With only three exceptions, the entire group was able to understand and respond appropriately to simple commands. Thirteen could point to common objects and/or parts of the body when requested to do so. Thus, the language disorder observed in these children was interpreted as both receptive and expressive in nature. The expressive deficit predominated in most cases.

All the cases exhibited, during some stage in their development, profound disturbances in relationships with people. Twelve were frankly autistic, refusing to be held, establishing no eye contact, and usually described by family as in a world of their own. Five others could be classified as symbiotic, ignoring all people except for one or two close family members, with whom they were overaffectionate and demanding of attention. These two groups were not separable by other clinical criteria and hence were considered together.

Six children had head circumferences greater than the 97th percentile for age. Five had definite focal findings on examination, including an upgoing right plantar response; slight hyperreflexia in the left arm; neglect of the right visual field; duplication of knee-jerks, ankle clonus, and bilateral adductor spasticity; and bilateral ankle clonus with a left upgoing plantar response.

Of the 17 children, 8 were left-handed and 3 had failed to establish preferred handedness when last seen.

EEGs demonstrated unequivocal paroxysmal activity in eight cases, with spiking in the right temporal area (3), in the left temporal area (1), bitemporally (2), generalized (1), or suggestive of atypical petit mal. Four other cases had probable abnormal EEGs due to excessive slow activity (3) or fast activity for age (1). Only five EEGs were considered to be entirely normal.

Psychological testing was performed on 12 of 17 cases. The other 5 cases, although uncooperative and therefore not tested, would have been expected to perform only on a moderately to severely retarded level. Five cases had normal intelligence as tested by nonverbal means. Two cases were mildly retarded. The remaining 10 cases were significantly retarded in nonverbal and verbal skills.

The most consistent abnormality found in the laboratory investigations was in the pneumoencephalograms. Fifteen cases demonstrated some enlargement of the left lateral ventricle (with respect to the right) and, particularly, enlargement of the left temporal horn (in one case the temporal horns were not visualized). The widening of the temporal horn seemed to vary independently of the overall left ventricular enlargement; the increased width of the temporal horn reflected primarily flattening and atrophy of the hippocampal contours that form the medial wall of the horn, bulging prominently into the ventricle.

In all our cases cited as abnormal, the left coronal cleft was both (a) 4 mm or greater in width, and (b) at least 2 mm wider than its counterpart on the right. The single exception to this was one patient for whom only (a) was true.

In all cases except 2, in which only the temporal horn was involved, the entire left ventricle, but particularly the left temporal horn, was enlarged. Five of these 15 patients had, in addition, some dilatation of the right ventricular system, of either the lateral ventricle or the temporal horn, or both. In these cases of bitemporal horn enlargement, the widening was greater on the left in all cases except 1. Other abnormalities observed by PEG included cortical atrophy in 3 patients, gross central atrophy (lateral ventricular span of 40 mm or greater) in 3, atrophy at the level of the third ventricle (anterior width 7 mm or greater) in 2, widening of the aqueduct (caliber wider than 3 mm) in 2, and increased height of the fourth ventricle (beyond 20 mm) in 3.

In summary, the PEGs demonstrated enlargement of the left ventricular system and especially of the left temporal horns in 13 cases and isolated widening of the left temporal horn in 2 others. These were isolated findings in 5 cases and in the 10 others were associated with a variety of other findings. The 2 patients with no temporal horn enlargement (1 with a normal PEG and 1 with left hemispheral central atrophy) each had prominent electroencephalographic abnormalities focused on the temporal lobe: One had constant left temporal bursts of sharp and slow wave activity, and the other had slow wave phase reversals bitemporally. Thus, all of our patients had either PEG or EEG evidence implicating the temporal lobe, either on the left side or bilaterally.

Computerized Tomography (CT) Scan

Damasio *et al.* (1980) described CT scan findings in 17 patients with autistic behavior that they considered representative of autism as seen in clinical practice. Their cases included both "symptomatic" autism (an autistic syndrome appearing in the setting of identifiable neurologic disease) and idiopathic childhood autism. The extent of recognizable neurologic dysfunction was noteworthy: Two patients had craniostenosis, 2 had sequelae of meningitis (including massive communicating hydrocephalus in 1) and 4 others had a history of seizures. Nine of the 13 in whom an electroencephalogram was reported had major paroxysmal abnormalities; in 2 of these the focus was right temporal, in 3 the focus was localized to left temporal, and the others had generalized discharges. Nearly all of the patients had neuromotor abnormalities, primarily dystonia (8), Babinski responses (2), or clonus, clumsiness, cogwheeling, or unilateral emotional facial paresis; these observations are quite apart from the stereotyped and repetitive movements, flapping, posturing, and motor perseveration that were common to virtually all. Thus, this sample had ample evidence of neurological abnormality. Given this fact, it is perhaps surprising that the CT scan abnormalities were not more marked. Three patients' scans had localizable lesions (2 in frontal lobe and 1 with massive communicating hydrocephalus), 5 had clear evidence of bilateral ventricular enlargement, and 50% were normal or had "soft" abnormalities (right ventricle larger than left, or one lateral ventricle excessively larger than the other). The authors were not able to make any comment about the temporal horns; they acknowledged that the CT scan often fails to show discrete or moderate enlargement of the temporal horns, even if such enlargement is visible in air studies. In addition, they did not find significant differences from normal in petalia (prominence of frontal or occipital poles on one side) and thus did not confirm the findings reported by Hier, Lemay, and Rosenberger (1979).

This CT study adds to the body of data indicating that there are frequent abnormalities of brain parenchymal configuration in cases of autism, in most cases presumably representing the residue of destructive disease. These changes usually are not massive and are not sharply localized, at least as seen by CT scan. The PEG may delineate such changes more precisely, especially in the temporal horns, but is unlikely to be utilized for future studies.

CASES WITH DISCRETE MEDIAL TEMPORAL LOBE LESIONS

We have encountered several special cases that illustrate particularly well a correlation between a discrete brain lesion and autism or an autisticlike syndrome. These will be described.

Bilateral Anterior Temporal Lobe Cavitations

A 4-year-old boy evaluated because of mental deficiency, developmental disorder, and autisticlike behavior was found by computed tomography to have remarkable encephaloclastic atrophic changes limited to the inferior and medial portions of both temporal lobes. The remainder of the brain, including the upper and lateral portions of the temporal lobes, was normal. Because the CT scan was so striking, it is worth presenting the clinical picture in detail.

He was the product of a pregnancy complicated by a maternal seizure early in pregnancy, and by emotional difficulties. Delivery was uncomplicated at term. At 16 days he began having apneic spells treated with phenobarbital, but had no definite seizures. Motor development was slightly delayed, with walking at 15 months. Head circumference was at 2nd percentile, although height and weight were average.

On behavioral evaluation at age 4, he was hyperactive, aggressive, and self-abusive. He pulled away and stiffened when held. He had no eye contact until after 1 week of special reinforcement with food reward. He displayed constant rocking, head banging, hitting, and picking at his ears when agitated. At another time he was described as constantly moving around the room, spitting, slapping other people in the room, hitting his head against the wall, and banging the side of his head with his arms. He had no speech but made thick growling noises and cried loudly when restrained. He would lead his teacher by the hand, reposition the teacher's hand, and point to a favorite reinforcer; these were the limits of his communicative efforts. He explored toys by mouthing them and then threw them across the room. He was not attentive to any object for more than a few seconds. He was not responsive to social interaction and showed little interest in toys or in persons. He was restless and distractible. Formal psychometric assessment yielded an IQ of 38 on the Cattell Infant Behavior Test and an LQ of 22 on the Verbal Language Development Scale.

There were no seizures. EEG at age 2 was normal. EEG at age 4 showed a bilateral posterior temporal delta slow and sharp focus, more prominent on the left.

This child affords an example of the clinical syndrome, consonant with low-functioning autism, resulting in early childhood from bilateral medial temporal lesions. The case makes the argument that the bilateral medial temporal lobe syndrome in early childhood, and low-functioning infantile autism, are indistinguishable. To our knowledge the medial temporal lobe syndrome has never been described as such in young children (Geschwind, 1972). Nor have Korsakoff psychosis or the Kluver-Bucy syndrome been described in the young child—presumably because the characteristic features of those syndromes are overwhelmed in the young child by the massive behavior disorder and failure of communication and learning.

Encephalitis Affecting Medial Temporal Lobe

DeLong, Bean, and Brown (1981) reported three cases in which children demonstrated a full-blown autistic syndrome in the course of an acute encephalopathic illness. In two cases, encephalitis was presumed but not proved. In the third, herpes simplex infection was verified, and an extensive left temporal lobe lesion was verified by computerized tomographic (CT) scan.

The salient clinical neurologic features were limited to sociobehavioral and language abnormalities. By contrast, motor, sensory, reflex, convulsive, or vegetative abnormalities were absent or inconspicuous. The main abnormalities in behavior were failure of social responsiveness despite preserved conscious alertness, failure to recognize persons, loss of communicative language and of all interpersonal communication, perseveration, inappropriate emotional expressions (including uncontrollable aggressiveness or blank apathy), restless hyperactivity, constriction of interest, and absence of purposive or motivated actions. At various times repetitive movements, toe walking, echolalia, obsessive fascination with objects, inappropriate rote stereotyped utterances, hyperexploratory behavior with fleeting attention span, masturbation, and perseverative speech were observed. Finally, the three children showed a distinctive language and communicative deficit, which has not been described except in relation to autism (Bartak, Rutter, & Cox, 1975) and which is clearly differentiated from receptive or global aphasia. In these cases, the abnormalities were acquired and not developmental, but they clearly fit the critical clinical features of the childhood autism syndrome.

In the third case, extensive damage to the left temporal lobe and insula was seen by CT scan, with much more restricted involvement of the right insular region and right temporal lobe. The CT scan gave no evidence of medial or basal frontal lobe disease. This case allowed the suggestion that a major portion of the neurobehavioral syndrome was the consequence of acute extensive temporal lobe lesions, predominantly in the left lobe. Clinically, she had severe impairment of language function. She uttered rote phrases with perseveration, without evident communicative intent, but without defects of articulation. These features contrasted with the better preservation of visuospatial skills (e.g., the ability to copy a three-dimensional cube). These findings indicated that left hemispheral language-related functions were severely impaired, with sparing of right hemispheral visuospatial functions. This correlates with the CT finding. Other striking features, including her lack of social interaction, lack of sustained attention, and aggressive and impulsive behavior, may be correlated with temporal lobe disease.

In the other two cases, though the clinical syndromes were quite similar, CT scans were normal and anatomic localization could not be defined. Electroencephalograms showed bilateral diffuse slowing in both, but one patient had slow wave bursts of greater amplitude in the temporal regions, and the second at one point had paroxysmal spiking localized to the right midtemporal region. These findings suggest that the temporal lobes may have been major foci of disease.

In these cases, the behavioral syndrome was acquired at a clearly definable time, in the context of an acute encephalopathic illness, and was reversible. The third case alone provides data regarding the possible anatomic substrate for this behavioral syndrome complex, supporting in general the idea advanced by Hauser *et al.* (1975) and by DeLong (1978) that extensive medial temporal disease in children, perhaps particularly on the left side, produces a syndrome having many of the characteristic features of the autistic syndrome. Damasio and Maurer (1978) have advanced a similar interpretation, implicating mesolimbic structures, including mesial frontal and temporal lobes.

NEUROANATOMIC STUDIES

In April 1984, using the technique of gapless whole brain serial section, Bauman and Kemper reported selected anatomic abnormalities in the brain of a 29-year-old well-documented autistic man, studied in comparison with an identically processed age- and sex-matched control (Bauman & Kemper, 1985). Both cerebra were well developed and showed no gross lesions, abnormalities of gyral configuration, myelination, or gliosis. No recognizable differences were noted in multiple cerebral cytoarchitectonic areas. However, cell packing density (the number of neuronal nucleoli per 0.001 mm^3) in the brain of the autistic patient was increased bilaterally by 27 to 58% in all areas of the hippocampus, subiculum, and entorhinal cortex (area 28). In addition, in the autistic brain, a clear zone deep to the superficial cell layer in the entorhinal cortex was noted that was not present in the control. This clear zone is generally referred to as a lamina dissecans; it initially appears during the second trimester of fetal life (Filimonov, 1949/1965) and is normally no longer evident by 15 months of age (Conel, 1967).

Increased cell packing density was also noted in the mammillary body, the only abnormality noted in the hypothalamus, where the number of cells was increased by 66%, the most marked increase in any area of the brain. Additional abnormalities were found in the septal area but were confined to the vertical limb of the nucleus of the diagonal band of Broca and the medial septal nucleus. In the former, there was a decrease in the total number of neurons without change in cell packing density. In the latter, the cell packing density was increased by 54%, with a strong reduction in nerve cell size.

Additional abnormalities were seen in selected areas of amygdaloid complex. Cell packing density was increased in the central, medial, and cortical nuclei by 40%, 28%, and 35% respectively, and cell size was reduced. The basolateral complex showed little or no change.

Abnormalities were also seen in the cerebellum and in the cerebellar circuits in the autistic brain. Atrophy of the neocerebellar cortex was present with a marked loss of Purkinje cells and, to a lesser extent, of granule cells. The anterior lobe of the cerebellum and the vermis showed no abnormality. The fastigial, globose, and emboliform nuclei contained small pale neurons that were markedly reduced in number, while the dentate nucleus appeared to be comparable to that of the control brain. The only remaining abnormality in the brainstem was a widening of the upper portion of the fourth ventricle with corresponding thinning and elongation of the superior cerebellar peduncle.

The abnormalities in the forebrain of this autistic patient could disrupt the function of the circuitry of the hippocampal-subicular complex, the amygdala, limbic and sensory association neocortical areas directly related to them, and the relationship of these areas to the reticulate core of the brain.

Given the anatomic abnormalities noted in the cerebellum of this autistic patient, Bauman, LeMay, Bauman, and Rosenberger (1985) reviewed a series of CT scan studies on 19 autistic individuals, ages 3 years to 21 years, in comparison to a comparable number of age-matched controls, with particular attention to the posterior fossa. Measurements of the fourth ventricular width, the greatest internal diameter of the posterior fossa, and the fourth ventricular ratio were made. Sixteen of the 19 autistic individuals demonstrated a fourth ventricular width and fourth ventricular ratio that was significantly larger than that seen in the controls. Further, atrophy of the cerebellar vermis and hemispheres was noted in several cases.

While the significance of these findings is as yet unclear, these observations suggest that further attention to the posterior fossa structures in autistic individuals is warranted. Cerebellar atrophy has been reported by CT scan in chronic schizophrenia (Heath, Franklin, & Shraberg, 1979) and has been more recently noted in three additional autistic patients by Jafken and Van den Berghe (1984). Further, Ritvo et al. have observed Purkinje cell loss in the cerebellum of four autistic patients on neuropathological investigation (personal communication, July 13, 1985). Thus, there appears to be mounting evidence to support the involvement of the cerebellum and cerebellar circuits in some autistic individuals. Given the technical difficulties of viewing the posterior fossa with CT scan, however, MRI studies may be of greater value in studying this portion of the brain in vivo.

DISCUSSION

The studies described above lead to two conclusions: (1) A high proportion of cases of infantile autism are associated with recognizable neurological disease of the child. As investigators look more carefully at autistic children, using more sophisticated techniques to identify brain damage and dysfunction, the proportion of children in which neurological disorder is identified becomes higher. (2) In autistic children there is no clear difference between the autistic symptomatology of the pure or idiopathic autistic child and the neurological or symptomatic autistic. The meaningful distinctions are in the degree of associated retardation, and of other features of encephalopathy.

What lessons can be learned from the observations on brain lesions in autism? First, anatomic abnormalities are common in brains of autistic patients, as seen by PEG and CT scan, but appear to have little specificity. Those abnormalities that have been most frequent are enlargement of the ventricles, especially the lateral ventricles. The findings suggest central atrophy rather than cortical atrophy; that is, there has not been evidence of atrophy involving the cerebral cortex. The enlargement of ventricles, as seen in these patients, does not suggest hydrocephalus. It is generally modest in degree. In addition to the bodies of the lateral ventricles, it often affects the temporal horns, the contours indicating flattening and atrophy of the hippocampal formation. The lesions tend to be more prominent in the left hemisphere. Other lesions, if seen, involve mild atrophic changes in brainstem and cerebellum. These changes are most suggestive of an encephaloclastic insult to developing brain either prenatally or perinatally. They are not in themselves indicative of any specific etiology.

Secondly, isolated cases have shown anatomic lesions that can suggest specific clinical-anatomical correlations. In the case of herpes simplex (DeLong et al., 1981) with evidence of extensive disease of left temporal lobe, the clinical syndrome was of acute onset in a previously normal 11-year-old child; thus it was not autism in a strict sense. However, the clinical features were essentially identical to those of autism, and they give strong support to the concept that disease of the temporal lobe—in this case primarily on the left side, but possibly with a bilateral contribution—may produce a syndrome similar to autism. A second case (the unpublished case of a boy with autism who has large bilateral symmetrical cavitated lesions of anterior temporal lobes) reinforces the same point: Prominent disease of the temporal lobe in the young child—bilateral in this case—may be associated with the clinical picture of autism.

The most elegant example of a correlation between medial temporal lobe disease and the autistic syndrome is the case reported by Bauman and Kemper (1985), which showed apparent arrest of tissue development in the hippocampus, subiculum, entorhinal cortex, amygdala, septum, and mammillary bodies, in contrast to normal development of the neo-cortex. The behavioral significance of this circuitry has been demonstrated in experiments in which lesions in these regions produce prominent effects on motivation, emotion, memory, and learning, many of which resemble behaviors seen in childhood autism.

Behavioral abnormalities similar to those seen in autism were first described by Kluver and Bucy in 1939 following bilateral ablation of the temporal lobe in monkeys. These included purposeless hyperactivity, severe impairment in social interaction, hyperexploratory behavior, and the inability to recognize or remember the significance of visually or manually examined objects. These behaviors have also been noted following similar neurosurgical lesions in man (Terzian & Delle-Ore, 1955). Further, bilateral ablations of the hippocampus in animals have resulted in stereotypic motor behavior and hyperactivity (Kimble, 1963), and a disordered response to novel stimuli (Roberts, Dember, & Brodwick, 1962). Bilateral amygdalectomy in monkeys has resulted in loss of fear of normally aversive stimuli, compulsive indiscriminate examination of objects, withdrawal from previously rewarding social interactions, and reduced ability to attach meaning to a specific situation based on past experience, with resultant incapacity to adapt behavior to new environmental requirements (Mishkin & Aggleton, 1981). Further, lesions of the medial, central, and cortical nuclei of the amygdala were more effective in suppressing the effects of familiarization than laterally placed lesions (Vergnes, 1981).

Of further interest to the clinical picture of autism are the studies of Thompson (1981), in which bilateral amygdaloidectomies were performed on infant monkeys. Although the surgically treated animals initially appeared to be behaviorally similar to controls, they developed poor social interaction by the age of 8 months, and hyperactivity by age 3 years. Thus, these monkeys appeared to "grow into" their symptoms, a series of events that could be linked to the early clinical features seen in some autistic children.

In addition to altered behavior, the medial temporal forebrain areas that have been affected in autistic patients have also been implicated in disturbances of memory function. Severe loss of recognition and associative visual memory was produced in monkeys by Mishkin (1978) with bilateral ablations of both hippocampus and amygdala, and by Mahut, Zola-Morgan, and Moss (1982) following bilateral hippocampal lesions. This memory impairment was more profound following combined lesions than that noted with removal of either structure alone (Mishkin, 1978). More recently, Murray and Mishkin (1983) have also noted a profound loss in tactile memory in monkeys with combined lesions of the hippocampus and amygdala. These authors therefore concluded that bilateral combined lesions of the hippocampus and amygdala result in a severe memory deficit that was at least bimodal and comparable to the global anterograde amnesia seen following medial temporal lobe surgery or pathology in humans. Further support for the role of the amygdala and hippocampus in autistic behavior is provided by Mishkin and Bachevalier (personal communication, June 25, 1984). These investigators have noted that bilateral ablation of the hippocampus and amygdala in neonatal monkeys results in striking autisticlike behavior. These considerations suggest that memory function should receive careful and quantitative study in autism (Boucher & Warrington, 1976).

An important point is suggested by the neuroimaging data and by other experience: There is no indication that autism is associated with lesions of the cerebral neocortex (exclusive of temporal lobe). On the contrary, even extensive hemispheral neocortical lesions are not associated with autism. This observation is of particular interest because it suggests that autism probably cannot be explained by any combination of deficits of cognitive functions mediated by the neocortex.

The question of hemispheral lateralization in autism has been addressed but not definitively answered by neuroimaging studies. Hauser *et al.* (1975) found a preponderance of lesions in the left medial temporal lobe, though some cases clearly had bilateral involvement. DeLong (1978) suggested that low-functioning autism might be associated with bilateral medial temporal lobe disease, while unilateral disease might permit higher function.

Finally, the clinical–anatomical correlations in autism must break new ground; new concepts on both sides will be necessary to develop cogent correlations. The neuropathological substrates of perseveration, stereotypy, echolalia, asociality, and pragmatic language disorders are not known independently; when learned, they will most likely be learned from the study of autism. The conjunction of anatomical and functional-clinical observations reinforce each other, especially the powerful correspondence between medial temporal lobe lesions in pathologic and radiological studies, and clinical and neuropsychological evidence of medial temporal lobe dysfunction. Working out the exact relationships between autistic symptoms and brain lesions should provide a rich chapter in neuropsychology.

ACKNOWLEDGMENTS

We gratefully acknowledge support by grants from the Jessie B. Cox Charitable Trust and the Charles and Sara Goldberg Charitable Trust.

REFERENCES

Aarkrog, R. (1968). Organic factors in infantile psychoses and borderline psychoses. Retrospective study of 46 cases subjected to pneumoencephalography. *Danish Medical Bulletin, 15,* 283–288.

Bartak, L., Rutter, M., & Cox, A. (1975). A comparative study of infantile autism and specific developmental receptive language disorders: I. The children. *British Journal of Psychiatry, 126,* 127–145.

Bauman, M. L., & Kemper, T. L. (1985). Histoanatomic observations of the brain in early infantile autism. *Neurology, 35,* 866–874.

Bauman, M. L., LeMay, M., Bauman, R. A., & Rosenberger, P. B. (1985). Computerized tomographic (C.T.) observations of the posterior fossa in early infantile autism. *Neurology, 35,* 247.

Boesen, V., & Aarkrog, T. (1967). Pneumoencephalography of patients in a child psychiatry department. *Danish Medical Bulletin, 14,* 210–218.

Boucher, J., & Warrington, E. K. (1976). Memory deficits in early infantile autism: Some similarities to the amnesic syndrome. *British Journal of Psychiatry, 67,* 73–87.

Chess, S., Korn, S. J., & Fernandez, P. B. (1971). *Psychiatric disorders of children with congenital rubella.* New York: Brunner/Mazel.

Conel, J. L. (1967). *The postnatal development of the human cerebral cortex.* Cambridge: Harvard University Press.

Creak, M. (1963). Schizophrenic syndrome in childhood: Progress report of a working party. *Cerebral Palsy Bulletin, 3,* 501–503.

Creak, M., & Pampiglione, G. (1969). Clinical and EEG studies on a group of 35 psychotic children. *Developmental Medicine and Child Neurology, 11*, 218–227.

Dalby, M. (1975). Air studies of speech-retarded children: Evidence of early lateralization of language function. Abstract, First International Congress of Child Neurology, Toronto.

Damasio, A. R., & Maurer, R. G. (1978). A neurological model for childhood autism. *Archives of Neurology, 35*, 777–786.

Damasio, H., Maurer, R. G., Damasio, A. R., & Chui, H. C. (1980). Computerized tomographic scan findings in patients with autistic behavior. *Archives of Neurology, 37*, 504–510.

DeLong, G. R. (1978). A neuropsychologic interpretation of infantile autism. In M. Rutter & E. Schopler (Eds.), *Autism* (pp. 207–218). New York: Plenum Press.

DeLong, G. R., Bean, S. C., & Brown, F. R. (1981). Acquired reversible autistic syndrome in acute encephalopathic illness in children. *Archives of Neurology, 38*, 191–194.

Desmond, M. M., Wilson, G. S., Melnick, J. L., Singer, D. B., Zion, T. E., Rudolph, A. J., Pineda, R. G., Ziai, M. H., & Blattner, R. J. (1967). Congenital rubella encephalitis. *Journal of Pediatrics, 71*, 311–331.

Deykin, E. Y., & MacMahon, B. (1979). Viral exposure and autism. *American Journal of Epidemiology, 109*, 628–638.

Deykin, E. Y., & MacMahon, B. (1980). Pregnancy, delivery, and neonatal complications among autistic children. *American Journal of Diseases in Children, 134*, 860–864.

Filimonov, I. N. (1965). Comparative anatomy of the cerebral cortex of mammalians. (V. Dukoff, Trans.). Washington, DC: Joint Publication Research Service. (Original translation published 1949.)

Garreau, B., Barthelemy, C., Sauvage, D., Leddet, I., & LeLord, G. (1984). A comparison of autistic syndromes with and without associated neurological problems. *Journal of Autism and Developmental Disorders, 14*, 105–111.

Geschwind, N. (1972). Disorders of higher cortical function in children. *Clinical Proceedings: Children's Hospital National Medical Center* (Washington, DC), *28*, 261–272.

Gubbay, S. S., Lobascher, M., & Kingerlee, P. (1970). A neurologic appraisal of autistic children: Results of a Western Australian survey. *Developmental Medicine and Child Neurology, 12*, 422–429.

Hauser, S. L., DeLong, G. R., & Rosman, N. P. (1975). Pneumographic findings in the infantile autism syndrome: A correlation with temporal lobe disease. *Brain, 98*, 667–688.

Heath, R. G., Franklin, D. E., & Shraberg, D. (1979). Gross pathology of the cerebellum in patients diagnosed and treated as functional psychiatric disorders. *Journal of Nervous and Mental Disease, 167*, 585–592.

Hier, D., Lemay, M., & Rosenberger, P. (1979). Autism and unfavorable left–right asymmetries of the brain. *Journal of Autism and Developmental Disorders, 9*, 153–159.

Jacobsen, H. H., & Melchior, J. C. (1967). On pneumoencephalographic measuring methods in children. *American Journal of Roentgenography, 101*, 188–194.

Jafken, J., & Van den Berghe, G. (1984). An infantile autistic syndrome characterized by the presence of succinylpurines in body fluids. *Lancet, 2*, 1058–1061.

Kanner, L. (1943). Autistic disturbances of affective contact. *Nervous Child, 2*, 217–250.

Kimble, D. P. (1963). The effects of bilateral hippocampal lesions in rats. *Journal of Comparative Physiological Psychology, 56*, 273–283.

Kluver, H., & Bucy, P. (1939). Preliminary analysis of functions of the temporal lobes in monkeys. *Archives of Neurology and Psychiatry, 42*, 979–1000.

Knobloch, H., & Pasamanick, B. (1975). Some etiologic and prognostic factors in early infantile autism and psychosis. *Pediatrics, 55*, 182–191.

Mahut, H., Zola-Morgan, S., & Moss, M. (1982). Hippocampal resections impair associative learning and recognition memory in the monkey. *Journal of Neuroscience, 2*, 1214–1229.

Melchior, J. C. (1961). Pneumoencephalography in atrophic brain lesions in infancy and childhood. *Acta Paediatrica (Stockholm), Supplement, 128*, 1–320.

Melchior, J.C., Dyggve, H. V., & Gylstorff, H. (1965). Pneumoencephalographic examination of 207 mentally retarded patients. *Danish Medical Bulletin, 12*, 38–42.

Mishkin, M. (1978). Memory in monkeys severely impaired by combined but not by separate removal of amygdala and hippocampus. *Nature, 273*, 297–298.

Mishkin, M., & Aggleton, J. P. (1981). Multiple functional contributors of the amygdala in the monkey from the amygdaloid complex. In Y. Ben-Ari (Ed.), *The amygdaloid complex, INSERM Symposium No. 20.* New York: Elsevier North-Holland Biomedical Press.

Murray, E., & Mishkin, M. (1983). Severe tactual memory deficits in monkeys after combined removal of the amygdala and hippocampus. *Brain Research, 270*, 340–344.

Nielsen, R., Petersen, O., Thygesen, P., & Willanger, R. (1966a). Encephalographic ventricular atrophy. Relationships between size of ventricular system and intellectual impairment. *Acta Radiologica: Diagnosis (Stockholm), 4*, 240–256.

Nielsen, R., Petersen, O., Thygesen, P., & Willanger, R. (1966b). Encephalographic cortical atrophy. Relationships to ventricular atrophy and intellectual impairment. *Acta Radiologica: Diagnosis (Stockholm), 4*, 437–448.

Roberts, W. W., Dember, W. N., & Brodwick, M. (1962). Alteration and exploration in rats with hippocampal lesions. *Journal of Comparative Psychiatry, 55*, 695–700.

Rutter, M., Greenfield, G., & Lockyer, L. (1967). A five to fifteen year study of infantile psychosis: II. Social and behavioral outcome. *British Journal of Psychiatry, 113*, 1183.

Schain, R. G., & Yannet, H. (1960). Infantile autism. *Journal of Pediatrics, 57*, 560–576.

Schonfelder, T. (1964). Uber fruhkindliche Antriebsstorungen [Early childhood autism]. *Acta Paedopsychiatrica, 31*, 112–129.

Skatvedt, M., Eek, S., & Gardborg, O. (1959). Epilepsy in children: A clinical and roentgenological study. *Acta Paediatrica (Stockholm), Supplement, 48*, 99–100.

Terzian, H., & Delle-Ore, G. (1955). Syndrome of Kluver and Bucy reproduced in man by bilateral removal of the temporal lobes. *Neurology, 3*, 373–380.

Thompson, E. I. (1981). Long-term behavioral development of rhesus monkeys after amygdalectomy in infancy. In Y. Ben-Ari (Ed.), *The amygdaloid complex. INSERM Symposium No. 20.* New York: Elsevier North-Holland Biomedical Press.

Vergnes, M. (1981). Effect of prior familiarization with mice on elicitation of mouse killing in rats: Role of the amygdala. In Y. Ben-Ari (Ed.), *The amygdaloid complex. INSERM Symposium No. 20.* New York: Elsevier North-Holland Biomedical Press.

White, P. T., DeMyer, W., & DeMyer, M. (1964). EEG abnormalities in early childhood schizophrenia: A double-blind study of psychiatrically-disturbed and normal children during promazine sedation. *American Journal of Psychiatry, 120*, 950–958.

IV

Neurochemical, Biochemical, and Nutritional Issues

14

Neurochemical Hypotheses of Childhood Psychoses

GLEN R. ELLIOTT and ROLAND D. CIARANELLO

INTRODUCTION

Childhood psychoses are a diverse group of poorly understood disorders that first may become manifest from birth through adolescence. Often, they incapacitate those afflicted for life. Concepts about the etiolgies of childhood psychoses have evolved a great deal over the past decade, and a chapter exploring possible roles of brain neuroregulators no longer requires the justification it once did. Even so, the title of this chapter is somewhat misleading, because as yet no specific hypotheses implicate an abnormality in a single neuroregulatory system as the underlying mechanism for childhood psychoses. Rather, as described in the following pages, investigators have been accumulating data on (1) how disruptions in certain aspects of normal development and metabolism can result in psychotic syndromes in childhood and (2) whether the activity of some known neuroregulators are altered in children with psychoses. Such research provides fundamental building blocks for clarifying the causes of these devastating disorders.

One important factor that has hampered efforts to elucidate the role of brain neuroregulators in childhood psychoses is the heterogeneity of the disorders themselves. Among disorders now lumped together under this term are infantile autism, childhood-onset pervasive developmental disorder, reactive psychosis, and schizophrenia; their interrelationships remain largely unexplored. For example, infantile autism once was thought to be an early form of schizophrenia (Bender, 1971), yet other research strongly suggests that they are unrelated syndromes (Ornitz & Ritvo, 1976; Rutter, 1972). Also, the major signs and symptoms of infantile autism and childhood-onset pervasive developmental disorder are quite similar, and distinguishing between them often hinges on a judgment of whether problems developed before or after the age of 30 months (American Psychiatric Association, 1980; Elliott & Ciaranello, 1986). Other methods of identifying subtypes of childhood psychoses may yield more homogeneous groups that could be of use to researchers and clinicians alike (Siegel, Anders, Ciaranello, Bienenstock, & Kraemer, 1986).

GLEN R. ELLIOTT and ROLAND D. CIARANELLO • Division of Child Psychiatry and Child Development, Department of Psychiatry and Behavioral Sciences, Stanford University School of Medicine, Stanford, California 94305.

Even with a relatively specific diagnosis such as infantile autism, the manifestation of the syndrome can differ markedly among individuals, and a number of quite different etiologies may result in the types of symptoms now identified as autism. Differences also may arise as a result of developmental influences (Bender & Freedman, 1952; Cain, 1969). For instance, an autistic child who has acquired speech may display an array of cognitive abilities and deficits that simply are inaccessible to a prelingual child. Such developmental differences also may help explain the observation that children with schizophrenia are less likely to have delusions than are adults with this disorder. Furthermore, no pathognomonic signs or symptoms of childhood psychoses have been identified. Many of the behaviors can occur transiently in children who are developing normally, especially early in life, and also may be part of other childhood disorders, including mental retardation and certain types of epilepsy.

Another major impediment to research on the roles of neuroregulators in childhood psychoses is the lack of acceptable tools for studying them. The brain is so well protected that investigators have few methods with which to monitor neuroregulatory activity in adult volunteers—and fewer still for studying children (cf. Barchas, Akil, Elliott, Holman, & Watson, 1978; Elliott & Barchas, 1986). To date, most research on neuroregulators in children with psychoses has used measures of neuroregulators or their metabolites in blood or, less often, in cerebrospinal fluid (CSF). Such measures may be poor indicators of what is happening to neuroregulator activity in small brain regions of interest. Nonetheless, children with psychosis—and their parents—who participate in this type of research should be commended for their invaluable contributions to a slowly emerging base of fundamental knowledge about severe childhood disorders.

This chapter reviews the progress that has been made toward clarifying the biochemistry of childhood psychoses. We focus primarily on autism because it is the most uniquely associated with childhood and has by far the largest body of research. However, relevant findings on schizophrenia in childhood are also cited. The next section describes some of the evidence that supports the conclusion that these disorders are the result of damage to the central nervous system. Following that is a brief summary of research on specific neuroregulators, including serotonin and the catecholamines. Fortunately, as described in the last section, several new research methodologies on the horizon promise to make studies of brain function in children both more practical and more informative.

EVIDENCE OF CENTRAL NERVOUS SYSTEM ABNORMALITIES

Initial suggestions that autism results from an insult to the brain were supported indirectly by studies of prevalence and more directly by findings about risk factors for the syndrome. That evidence has been augmented with postmortem findings of neuropathology and X-ray computed tomography (CT) studies of brain neuroanatomy and with noninvasive studies of brain electrophysiology and cognitive functioning.

Prevalence Studies

From 1 to 5 of every 10,000 members of the general population have autism, with a male-to-female ratio of about 4 to 1 (Lotter, 1966; Treffert, 1970). Autism can be found throughout the world in a wide range of races and cultures. Among siblings of children with autism, the prevalence is 2%—much higher than expected by mere chance (Folstein & Rutter, 1978; Ritvo, Spence, et al., 1985). This increased risk is consistent with a relatively mild genetic influence, although it also could be reflect nongenetic environmental factors. The risk appears to be somewhat specific for autism: The prevalence of schizophrenia in these families is not increased (Hanson & Gottesman, 1983). More strongly supportive of a genetic contribution is research on children with autism who have an identical (monozygotic) twin; both twins are autistic about half the time (Folstein & Rutter, 1978; Ritvo, Freeman, Mason-Brothers, Mo, & Ritvo, 1985). More recently, some researchers have identified a phenomenon called the fragile X syndrome, which refers to a peculiar constriction of the distal end of the long arm of the X chromosome under certain *in vitro* conditions. Studies suggest that 5 to 15% of individuals with autism have the fragile X syndrome (Blomquist et al., 1984; Watson et al., 1984) and that, conversely, a large percentage of people with the fragile X syndrome have some autisticlike features (Levitas, Hagerman, Braden, Rimland, & McBogg, 1983).

All of these findings combine to intrigue neuroscientists who are seeking a biochemical explanation of autism, because genetic influences must be expressed through a change in protein production or function. The proteins of interest might be involved at many levels (Ciaranello, Vandenberg, & Anders, 1982). For example, they might affect the delicate and incompletely understood process of neurogenesis early in development. Or, they might alter cellular metabolism, intracellular transport mechanisms, neuronal regulatory mechanisms, or some other critical element of normal brain function. Even though the exact level of abnormality still is far from clear, the overall impression of a defect in the central nervous system is compelling.

Risk Factor Studies

A risk factor is a condition or circumstance the presence of which changes the likelihood of an individual having a specified outcome. Having an autistic sibling or a fragile X chromosome appear to be two risk factors for autism, and a number of others also have been identified, including pre- and perinatal injury, certain neurological and metabolic disorders, and some viral infections (reviewed in Ciaranello et al., 1982). As is true for a positive family history, the great majority of children with such risk factors are not autistic, and no one has found evidence that forges a clear causal link between any condition and the development of autism. In fact, for some risk factors, a still unsuspected process may be responsible both for the risk factor and the autism. Suppose, for instance, that an unknown genetic trait increases the risk both of having a difficult delivery and of being autistic. Children with that trait will contribute to an observed correlation between birth injuries and autism, even though the former does not cause the latter. Even so, information about risk factors is useful because it can help to identify groups of individuals who may need special attention and care as they develop.

Certain types of disruptions of very early development appear to increase the risk for autism. The strongest known risk factor is exposure to rubella virus *in utero*; 8 to 10% of such children subsequently develop symptoms of autism, in addition to a number of physical problems such as blindness and hearing difficulties (Chess, Korn, & Fernandez, 1971; Desmond, Montgomery, Melnick, Cochran, & Verniaud, 1969). Other viral risk factors include *in utero* toxoplasmosis and congenital neurosyphilis (Ornitz & Ritvo, 1976; Rutter, 1974). Also of interest is the observation that phenylketonuria is a risk factor for autism

(Ornitz & Ritvo, 1976). This well-studied genetic disease results from a deficiency of the liver enzyme that converts phenylalanine to tyrosine, the precursor for the whole family of catecholamine neuroregulators.

The identified risk factors for autism seem to have in common the potential disruption of normal central nervous system development, often early in the process. Again, this supports the concept of a biochemical mechanism, but the available data should not be extended too far. Too many questions remain unanswered. Why do 90% of children exposed to rubella fail to become autistic? How similar are the autistic symptoms of children with known risk factors such as rubella exposure or phenylketonuria to each other and to those of children with idiopathic autism? Are the syndromes identical, or are these groups of children distinct subtypes? Until researchers have answers to these and other questions, the risk factors serve primarily to emphasize that biochemical factors can be of key importance at least in some children with autism and to suggest some possible directions for research into its causes.

Neuropathological Studies

Kanner (1943) described the first autistic children only a little over 30 years ago, and most of them still are living, so it is not too surprising that few studies of brain neuropathology are available. However, a few children and young adults with autism have died from unrelated causes under circumstances that permitted studies of the brain. For example, Williams, Hauser, Purpura, DeLong, and Swisher (1980) described postmortem brain studies of four children with mental retardation and autistic symptoms, one of whom was known to have phenylketonuria. They found no evidence of specific abnormalities. A more recent study of a 29-year-old with a well-documented history of autism reported major cellular and structural changes in the amygdala, cerebellum, and hippocampus (Bauman & Kemper, 1985). Clearly, more extensive studies are needed.

The advent of CT scans has made feasible the study of certain aspects of brain anatomy in living human beings. This technology has been applied to autism, but with inconclusive results. Several groups have published results on reasonable, though small, sample sizes (Campbell *et al.*, 1982; Rapoport & Ismond, 1982; Rosenbloom *et al.*, 1984). A few subjects had clear evidence of frank pathology, including one case of hydrocephalus, several of frontal lobe tissue defects, and several with ventricular enlargement, but most subjects had no abnormalities or only nonspecific minor changes. Some researchers have suggested that a disproportionate number of subjects with autism have enlarged right cortical hemispheres, consistent with a relatively dysfunctional left hemisphere (Hier, LeMay, & Rosenberger, 1979); however, others have questioned these findings (Tsai, Jacoby, Stewart, & Beisler, 1982). Still other investigators have implicated subcortical structures (Damasio & Maurer, 1978; Damasio, Maurer, Damasio, & Chui, 1980).

At least to date, this approach has been of limited help in identifying gross brain pathology in individuals with autism. However, few subjects have been studied, and the sophistication of available methods leaves much to be desired. CT can provide quite good anatomical detail under optimal conditions, but the technique cannot be used to detect microscopic abnormalities or changes in brain function. As described in the last section of this chapter, several emerging technologies may offer valuable new tools for acquiring better data.

Studies of Functional Changes

The exact nature of the cognitive deficits of autism remain far from clear. A surfeit of abnormalities have been described, ranging from defects in sensory reception and acquisition through problems with storage and retrieval to difficulties with processing and integration (cf. Litrownik & McInnis, 1982; Ornitz, 1969, 1983; Rimland, 1964). Unfortunately, no consistent findings have emerged to shed light on the underlying pathology of autism. This type of research may be quite sensitive to the problem of multiple forms of the syndrome, and investigators ultimately may discover that a number of dissimilar deficits can lead to a similar clinical picture.

Measures of global electroencephalographic (EEG) activity in children with autism have yielded inconsistent results of uncertain significance. It is not surprising that EEGs are abnormal in a significant proportion of those with autism, given that one-fourth develop grand mal or psychomotor seizures by adolescence (Rutter, Greenfeld, & Lockyer, 1967). Yet no specific pattern has emerged (DeMyer et al., 1973; Kolvin et al, 1971; White, 1974). Studies do suggest that subjects with autism have normal sleep cycles and normal amounts of REM sleep, although the rapid eye movements themselves may be decreased (Tanguay, Ornitz, Forsythe, & Ritvo, 1976).

Electrophysiological studies of autism also have been disappointing, perhaps for the same reasons. Several investigators have described abnormalities in brainstem regulation of auditory, vestibular, and cardiovascular processes (Fein, Skoff, & Mirsky, 1981; Kootz, Marinelli, & Cohen, 1982; Ornitz & Ritvo, 1976; Palkovitz & Wiesenfeld, 1980; Tanguay & Edwards, 1982). These findings are interesting, but their direct relevance to the causes of autism is unknown (cf. Litrownik & McInnis, 1982; Todd & Ciaranello, 1985). For example, vestibular function seems to be disturbed, as evidenced both by a suppression of vestibular nystagmus during waking states (Pollack & Krieger, 1958; Ritvo et al., 1969) and by a failure of vestibular stimulation to affect rapid eye movements during sleep (Ornitz, Forsythe, & de la Pena, 1973). Investigators also have reported prolonged delays in sensory processing, as assessed by transmission times for auditory and visual signals (Fein et al., 1981; LeLord, Laffont, Jusseaume, & Stephant, 1973; Rosenblum et al., 1980) and by the contingent negative variation (CNV) wave form (Small, DeMyer, & Milstein, 1971). Interpretation of changes in physiological parameters that are modulated by cognitive state is especially difficult, because autistic children seldom cooperate with such studies in normal ways, and possible effects of higher cortical functions cannot be ruled out.

Once again, the available evidence points toward abnormalities of brain function in children with autism. However, the nature of the defect or defects and its etiological role in autism, if any, remain unsettled. As with most research efforts in this field, success may require much more careful attention to heterogeneities within the sample populations.

EVIDENCE OF ABNORMALITIES IN BRAIN NEUROREGULATORS

The body of literature on neuroregulators in autism remains relatively small. It focuses mainly on possible changes in the activity of those neuroregulators on which so much of useful psychiatric research has centered until recently—serotonin, dopamine, and norepinephrine. As noted earlier, much of the work has been exploratory, rather than hypothesis-generated, because no one has yet formulated a specific hypothesis that adequately explains the multiple signs and symptoms of autism on the basis of a defect in a single neuroregulatory system.

. One major obstacle to studying autism is the lack of an animal model. A few tentative steps have been made. For example, investigators have considered the possibility that animal stereotypies associated with increased activity of certain brain dopamine systems might be related to the stereotyped behaviors that occur in many children with autism (Young, Kavanagh, Anderson, Shaywitz, & Cohen, 1982). Also of possible interest is a hyperactivity syndrome that seems to be modulated by increased serotonergic activity; this syndrome includes both a general hyperactivity and symmetrical body movements such as forepaw padding and vertical head jerks (Grahame-Smith, 1971; Holman, Seagraves, Elliott, & Barchas, 1976).

Good animal models are of crucial importance because the most sensitive and specific techniques for studying neuroregulators typically require direct sampling and destruction of brain tissues or fluids or the administration of potentially toxic metabolitic inhibitors or radioactive labels (cf. Elliott & Barchas, 1986). As noted earlier, few of these methods are appropriate for studies in human beings, especially children. However, until the syndrome itself is better understood and animal analogues are discovered, clinical studies will continue to provide the most useful data about the biochemistry of autism, despite their obvious limitations.

Serotonin

Interest in serotonin and autism developed with the discovery in the mid-1950s that some individuals with autism have elevated blood serotonin concentrations (hyperserotonemia) (Schain & Freedman, 1961). That report and many others have demonstrated that about one-third of children with autism (Hanley, Stahl, & Freedman, 1977; Ritvo et al., 1970; Takahashi, Kanai, & Miyamoto, 1976) and about half of children who are nonautistic but severely retarded (Hanley et al., 1977; Pare, Sandler, & Stacey, 1960; Partington, Tu, & Wong, 1973) have hyperserotonemia, compared with appropriate age- and sex-matched normal controls.

Efforts to elucidate the mechanism and importance of hyperserotonemia in autism have had little success. Most blood serotonin is contained in the platelets, which have an active serotonin uptake mechanism, and elevated blood serotonin appears to be a result of increased concentrations of serotonin per platelet (Ritvo, Freeman, Geller, & Yuwiler, 1983). However, the cause for that increase has yet to be established. Also, no consistent correlations have been uncovered yet between blood serotonin and any autistic behaviors or symptoms (Hanley et al., 1977; Young et al., 1982).

Interest in serotonin was stimulated further by a report that fenfluramine, an anorexigenic agent that lowers both peripheral and central serotonin, produced marked clinical improvement in 3 children with autism and hyperserotonemia (Geller, Ritvo, Freeman, & Yuwiler, 1982). The same investigators tested 14 children with autism, some of whom had normal blood serotonin concentrations. Observed improvements in this group were reported to include more appropriate motor, social, and sensory behavior in a naturalistic observational setting, better general adaptive functioning, and increased verbal IQ in some higher-functioning subjects (Ritvo et al., 1983, 1984).

We were among 22 institutions that participated in a multicenter study designed to test this preliminary finding more rigorously in a double-blind, crossover design. We enrolled

12 subjects into our study, of whom 10 completed the entire protocol. None of our subjects showed significant clinical improvement, although 2 of the children who had frequent motor stereotypies did have somewhat decreased movements (Siegel, Elliott, Friedman, & Ciaranello, 1986). Our experience generally reflects that of the multicenter trial, in which a total of 175 children took part. Although a few children reportedly had dramatic improvements, the overwhelming majority did not (Ho, Lockitch, Eaves, & Jacobson, 1986).

As part of our study, we drew blood for serotonin on each of 10 monthly visits and obtained two spinal taps on all 10 of the subjects who completed the study, once on placebo and once on fenfluramine. Several interesting results emerged (Elliott, Siegel, Faull, & Ciaranello, 1986). Patients had two baseline visits and then two 4-week drug periods on either placebo or fenfluramine. From baseline to placebo, average serotonin concentrations declined by 21%, with a further decrease from placebo to drug of 50%. The change from placebo to drug, which occurred in every patient, reflected the expected action of fenfluramine. However, the drop from baseline to placebo was unexpected and raises important questions about the sensitivity of blood serotonin to stressful situations. Perhaps "hyperserotonemia" is actually some form of transient response to new settings. This possibility requires further study.

One of the reasons for being interested in blood serotonin is the belief that it may at least partially reflect what is happening to serotonergic systems in the brain. We examined the association between blood serotonin and CSF concentrations of 5-hydroxindoleacetic acid (5-HIAA), the major serotonin metabolite. We found no correlation between the two either on or off fenfluramine. We did find that fenfluramine produced an average 50% decrease in blood serotonin and an average 25% decrease in CSF 5-HIAA. Every single subject had decreases in both while on the drug, but again there was no correlation between these changes. Of course, static measures of a single concentration of either blood serotonin or CSF 5-HIAA may yield little information about the dynamics of the system in the brain, where important changes may be occurring. Still, our findings do raise concerns about the meaning of measures of blood serotonin and suggest the need for a better understanding of what measurable substances best reflect central serotonergic activity.

Several groups have obtained CSF samples from individuals with autism and compared their CSF 5-HIAA concentrations with those of nonautistic controls. Getting adequate controls for such studies is quite difficult, because no one wants to subject a healthy child to that procedure. Typically, controls are recruited from among cancer or neurology patients who had spinal taps as part of their work-up but proved to have no physical disease. Most researchers have assumed that elevated blood serotonin is reflective of increased central serotonergic activity. Yet Cohen and colleagues (Cohen, Caparulo, Shaywitz, & Bowers, 1977; Cohen, Shaywitz, Johnson, & Bowers, 1974) reported that 5-HIAA turnover was decreased in subjects with autism and suggested that central serotonergic activity might be decreased, rather than increased. Their study entailed the use of probenecid, a drug that blocks the active transport of 5-HIAA and other acid metabolites out of the CSF; thus, increases in 5-HIAA after probenecid should correlate with the rate at which new 5-HIAA is entering the CSF. Unfortunately, at least at doses that can be used clinically, the transport blockade is only partial and can be affected by a large number of uncontrollable variables, so interpretation of the results is difficult (Faull, Kraemer, Barchas, & Berger, 1981).

Gillberg, Svennerholm, and Hamiton-Hellberg (1983) reported on CSF results from 22 subjects—13 with autism and 9 with other forms of psychosis, comparing them with 22 sex- and age-matched controls who had undergone neurological evaluations but were of normal intelligence and had no known neurological handicap. This study differs from that just cited because probenicid was not used, so 5-HIAA concentrations are static, rather than reflective of turnover. CSF 5-HIAA concentrations were 122 and 108 nmoles/liter, respectively, for children with autism and their controls, and 132 and 92, respectively, for children with other forms of psychosis and their controls; none of the differences between any of these values reached statistical significance. They also found no correlation between IQ and CSF 5-HIAA concentrations in either group of psychoses.

Another recent finding suggests a quite different mechanism by which the serotonergic system might play a role in autism. Todd and Ciaranello (1984) reported that some children with autism have what appear to be circulating antibodies against specific serotonin receptors. For several children, the antiserotonin receptor activity has been found in both blood and CSF. If confirmed, the existence of such antibodies raises a variety of intriguing questions. When do the antibodies form, and what stimulates their production? Are they specific to autism, or do they occur in other forms of severe mental disorders in children or adults? What is their effect on serotonergic activity—is postsynaptic activity increased, decreased, or unchanged—and how does that affect serotonin turnover? Do the antibodies make changes that produce any of the symptoms of autism? Is the immune system more generally involved in autism?

Even if the antiserotonin-receptor antibodies prove not to be important to the etiology or symptomatology of autism, they call attention to the value of looking beyond static measures of serotonin and 5-HIAA. Also useful are studies of the enzymes involved in the synthesis and degradation of serotonin and of the receptors that mediate serotonin's postsynaptic effects.

Dopamine

Dopamine plays a central role in current hypotheses about schizophrenia and especially about the actions of antipsychotic drugs, so it is not surprising that its activity also should be of interest in childhood psychoses. However, the principal underpinning of the dopamine hypothesis of schizophrenia is the clinical efficacy of dopamine receptor blockers as antipsychotics. As for adults, antipsychotics help control such target symptoms as hallucinations and thought disorders in children and adolescents with schizophrenia, although many clinicians believe the drugs are less effective with this group (Campbell, 1977; Ciaranello & Anders, 1977). In contrast, they have not been found to affect the core signs and symptoms of autism or childhood-onset pervasive developmental disorder; rather, they provide symptomatic relief of certain common behaviors such as hyperactivity, stereotyped behaviors, self-mutilation, and aggressive outbursts (Campbell, 1975; Ciaranello & Anders, 1977).

Homovanillic acid (HVA) is the major dopamine metabolite in the CSF. Using the probenicid method described earlier, Cohen and his colleagues (Cohen & Young, 1977; Cohen et al, 1977; Young et al., 1982) have found elevated concentrations of HVA in the CSF of autistic children, compared with controls. Looking at steady-state, rather than post-probenecid concentrations, Gillberg et al. (1983) also found elevated HVA in 18 of their 22 psychotic subjects. HVA concentrations for subjects with autism and with other forms of childhood psychosis were 451 and 445 nmoles/liter, compared with values of 304 and 270 nmoles/liter for their respective controls. As with 5-HIAA and blood serotonin, HVA concentrations have not been shown to correlate with any autistic behaviors or symptoms.

Cohen *et al.* (1977; Young *et al.*, 1982) proposed that elevated HVA was a secondary effect of lowered central 5-HIAA activity. However, Faull, King, Berger, and Barchas (1984) demonstrated that in adults HVA and 5-HIAA concentrations are closely coupled. We found a high correlation ($r = 0.74$) between HVA and 5-HIAA in the CSF samples of our autistic subjects (Elliott *et al.*, 1986), and calculation from the data reported by Gillberg *et al.* (1983) shows a similar level of correlation for their subjects. This raises serious questions about whether serotonergic and dopaminergic systems are opposing one another.

Norepinephrine

Central noradrenergic systems have been implicated in a wide range of normal and abnormal behaviors and brain functions, but little evidence links them with autism. Plasma norepinephrine has been reported to be elevated in subjects with autism (Lake, Zeigler, & Murphy, 1977). However, urinary excretion of norepinephrine and of 3-methoxy-4-hydroxyphenylethylene glycol (MHPG)—its major brain metabolite—is decreased in subjects with autism, compared with normal controls (Young *et al.*, 1982). Studies suggest no differences in CSF MHPG between individuals with autism and controls (Gillberg *et al.*, 1983; Young *et al.*, 1982).

The enzymes involved in the norepinephrine's synthesis and catabolism offer another approach to studying its possible role in autism. Dopamine-beta-hydroxylase (DBH), the rate-limiting enzyme for norepinephrine synthesis, can be detected in blood. Investigators who have compared blood DBH activities of children with autism with those of normal controls have reported decreases (Lake *et al.*, 1977), increases (Coleman *et al.*, 1974), and no change (Young, Kyprie, Ross, & Cohen, 1975). The meaning of blood DBH activity is unclear, however; normal human beings exhibit wide ranges of activity without evident effect. Two metabolic enzymes, catechol-O-methyl transferase (COMT) and monoamine oxidase (MAO), theoretically might change norepinephrine activity by increasing or decreasing metabolism. Altered COMT activity might also affect dopamine metabolism, and MAO metabolizes both dopamine and serotonin. A study of COMT activity in cultured fibroblasts and in red blood cells revealed no differences between children with autism and controls (Giller *et al.*, 1980). MAO activity also appears to be normal (Boullin, Bhagavan, O'Brien, & Youdim, 1976; Lake *et al.*, 1977; Young *et al.*, 1982).

Other Neuroregulators

A phenomenal expansion has occurred over the past decade in the number of recognized brain neuroregulators (Elliott & Barchas, 1986). Consideration of how those substances might be involved in the etiology of autism has proceeded more slowly. Many of these compounds are peptides, and the development of specific and sensitive assay methods for clinical use still challenges some of the best analytic chemists. Most researchers use radioimmunoassays, relying on antibodies that have been raised specifically against the peptide neuroregulator of interest (Barchas, Evans, Elliott, & Berger, 1985). However, many artifacts can arise—for example, unrecognized competition from unsuspected structural analogues or nonspecific interference from substances present in unpurified or partly purified samples. Especially as reports first begin to appear, readers should look carefully at the strength of the evidence that investigators are measuring what they want to study.

The opioid peptides have been the first of the newly discovered brain neuroregulators for which a role in autism has been suggested. Members of this complex family of interrelated substances, named for the opiatelike physiological actions that many of its members possess, appear to have many functions in the brain beyond the pain systems in which they first were discovered (cf. Barchas *et al.*, 1985). For example, Panskepp and Bishop (1981) have proposed that some opioids may moderate certain aspects of play behavior in animals and that such actions could be relevant to the marked absence of play and other socially interactive behaviors in children with autism. One study has reported that, compared with controls or with children with schizophrenia, subjects with autism have relatively low concentrations of an endorphinlike substance in the blood (Weizman *et al.*, 1984). The actual identity of this substance has yet to be ascertained, however, and researchers have yet to establish the relevance of such a circulating compound to opioid activity in the brain.

Other neuroregulators also might be of importance. For example, gamma-aminobutyric acid (GABA) is thought to be the major inhibitory neuroregulator in the brain; it certainly could play a role in autism. The functions of many of the newer neuropeptide neuroregulators still are largely unknown, and they too might be crucial for an understanding of the autistic syndrome. To date, however, no studies are available about these substances. In many instances, such research must await improvements in sampling and analytical methods that will enable investigators to study the compounds in living human beings.

FUTURE DIRECTIONS FOR RESEARCH

The key role of sound neurochemical techniques for studying some of the major mental disorders of childhood and adolescence seems to have been firmly established, and some intriguing findings are emerging. Still, an enormous amount remains to be done before a clear connection can be drawn between any specific abnormalities in brain function and the clinical signs and symptoms of syndromes such as autism and other childhood psychoses. Fortunately, several developments within the neurosciences promise to provide powerful, noninvasive methods of studying aspects of brain function in human beings that are both safer and far more informative than existing techniques. It seems appropriate to conclude this review with a brief description of some of these exciting advances.

Over the next 5 years a wedding of computers and EEG systems should greatly enhance the ability of researchers to extract information from measurements of brain electrical activity. With available systems, it already is possible to create topographic reconstructions of either spontaneous or evoked electrical activity across the entire brain surface (Duffy, 1982; Morihisa, 1984). Such maps can help investigators detect even relatively subtle aspects of brain activity, such as foci of activity and asymmetries from one part of the brain to another. This approach should be invaluable in refining research on brain electrophysiology that was described earlier.

A second useful technology, positron emission tomography (PET), is the first practicable way to study some aspects of brain metabolism *in vivo* in animals and in human beings. Already in use in research on mental disorders in adults, it promises to enable researchers to look not only at gross measures of brain biochemical activity but at other key elements of the brain. Initially, investigators took advantage of a glucose analogue, 2-fluoro-2-deoxyglucose, which is taken up into neurons but not metabolized. Because neurons use glucose for energy, the pattern of uptake of this substance should reflect the relative metabolic activity of different brain regions. With [^{18}F] as a label, it is possible to acquire sequential pictures of brain sections as a function of mental disorder or of specific mental tasks (cf. Buchsbaum *et al.*, 1984). Perhaps of even greater ultimate importance for psychiatric research, PET also is proving useful for mapping and quantitation of labeled compounds that have a high affinity for specific neuroregulator receptors (Frost *et al.*, 1984; Inoue *et al.*, 1985; Wong *et al.*, 1984). Eventually, it may even be possible to study such aspects of receptor function as synthesis, turnover, activity, and ligand interactions in living human beings.

Application of PET to the study of childhood mental disorders has been slow because of issues about the possible risks of exposure to the radioactive elements used to label substances of interest. In one recent study, Rumsey, Duara, Grady, Rapoport, Margolin, Rapoport, and Cutler (1985) reported that, compared with controls, subjects with autism had substantially elevated utilization of glucose throughout many parts of the brain, including the frontal lobes, the cingulate gyrus and hippocampus, and midbrain regions of the caudate and lenticular nuclei. As more data are gathered about the real magnitude of the risks and as improved techniques help to minimize them, PET clearly should become increasingly important for researchers studying the childhood psychoses. This technology may be the only way to explore the functional status of serotonergic, dopaminergic, and opioid systems in the brains of children with severe psychoses.

Another exciting technology is magnetic resonance (MR). MR uses the innate magnetic properties of hydrogen and phosphorus to provide a completely new window into the brain (Elliott, 1986; Foster, 1984). MR imaging is rapidly displacing X-ray CT scans as the method of choice of obtaining detailed anatomical information about the brain. MR imaging requires no ionizing radiation and has no other known hazards. Also, bone has almost no MR signal, so that the skull does not interfere with the imaging as it does with CT. Furthermore, MR signals are affected by a large number of factors, including the molecules that contain the hydrogen or phosphorus atoms, the presence of paramagnetic substances such as oxygen, and blood flow. Proper utilization of these and other influences makes possible an unparalleled discrimination between even quite similar tissues and also means that the signals provide information about more than just anatomy. At least in a limited sense, images can be created that reflect physiological state.

Another application of MR is further into the future but of even greater potential value for child psychiatric research. Because substances each have characteristic electronic, and hence magnetic, environments, MR can be used as an *in vivo* spectrometer to distinguish among a large array of physiologically important compounds. Researchers already are using this technique to study such phosphorus-containing compounds as ATP, phosphocreatinine, and inorganic phosphate (Prichard, 1983), and MR eventually should enable investigators to use hydrogen spectra to monitor changes in such major brain neuroregulators as GABA and other amino acids (cf. Elliott, 1986). The rapidity with which this technology will become available still remains unclear. Many technical obstacles remain to be overcome. For example, use of MR spectroscopy in human beings requires the development of hollow-core magnets of sufficient internal diameter to admit a human head and shoulders and of high enough field strength and homogeneity to make feasible the identification of the very small differences in MR signals that molecular electronic effects induce.

An improved understanding of basic immunological mechanisms also may suggest mechanisms underlying some childhood psychoses. For example, the report of antiserotonin receptor antibodies in some children with autism (Todd & Ciaranello, 1984) mentioned earlier is only one of a number indications over the years of a connection between autism and immune dysfunction (Fowle, 1968; Stubbs, 1977; Stubbs, Crawford, Burger, & Vandenbark, 1977; Weizman, Weizman, Szekely, Wijsenbeek, & Livni, 1982). The strength and nature or the connection remain tenuous, but it does suggest another avenue along which researchers can seek to identify genetic and early developmental factors that increase the risk of autism (Ciaranello *et al.*, 1982).

Modern molecular biology also will be of use in understanding the neuropathology of infantile autism. Already in use in developmental neurobiology, recombinant DNA techniques have helped identify protein factors that guide, modulate, and direct neuronal growth and development. Because it is likely that aberrant central nervous system development is the primary defect of autism, identification of the factors controlling brain development is an essential priority for basic research in this field. The use of restriction fragment length polymorphisms also may be a valuable for identifying genetic defects in autistic individuals. These techniques already have helped investigators to identify the gene involved in Huntington chorea. Applied to monozygotic twins concordant for autism, they also might provide insight into the genetic basis of that form of autism that occurs in multiple members of the same family. The identification, isolation, and characterization of the genes controlling the expression of neurotrophic factors offers much hope for new understanding of autism in the near future.

Although improved technologies will be invaluable, more is needed in the effort to elucidate the underlying brain mechanisms in childhood psychosis. The burgeoning constellation of neuroregulators makes efforts to link a single neuroregulator to a given disorder seem naive, at best. Conceptual advances also are required to incorporate the increasingly complex interactions among neuroregulators that basic neuroscientists and electrophysiologists continue to identify. Such conceptual frameworks can, in turn, mold research strategies that make optimal use both of methods for observing how behavior and brain function interact and of ways to monitor key aspects of brain electrical and biochemical activity. Only such combined approaches show any true promise of unlocking the mysteries that are the childhood psychoses.

REFERENCES

American Psychiatric Association. (1980). *Diagnostic and statistical manual of mental disorders (3rd ed.).* Washington, DC: Author.

Barchas, J. D., Akil, H., Elliott, G. R., Holman, R. B., & Watson, S. J. (1978). Behavioral neurochemistry: Neuroregulators and behavioral states. *Science, 200,* 964–973.

Barchas, J. D., Evans, C., Elliott, G. R., & Berger, P. A. (1985). Peptide neuroregulators: The opioid system as a model. *Yale Journal of Biology and Medicine, 58,* 579–596.

Bauman, M. I., & Kemper, T. L. (1985). Histoanatomic observations of the brain in early infantile autism. *Neurology, 35,* 866–873.

Bender, L. (1971). Alpha and omega of childhood schizophrenia. *Journal of Autism and Childhood Schizophrenia, 1,* 115–118.

Bender, L., & Freedman, A. M. (1952). A study of the first three years in the maturation of schizophrenic children. *Quarterly Journal of Child Behavior, 4,* 245–272.

Blomquist, H. K., Bohman, M., Edvinsson, S. O., Gillberg, C., Gustavson, K. H., Holmgren, G., & Wahlstrom, J. (1984). Frequency of the fragile X syndrome in infantile autism—A Swedish multicenter study. *Clinical Genetics, 27,* 113–117.

Boullin, D. J., Bhagavan, H. N., O'Brien, R. A., & Youdim, M. B. H. (1976). Platelet monoamine oxidase in children with infantile autism. In M. Coleman (Ed.), *The autistic syndromes.* Amersterdam: North-Holland.

Buchsaum, M. S., Cappelletti, J., Ball, R., Hazlett, E., King, A. C., Johnson, J., Wu, J., & Delisi, L. E. (1984). Positron emission tomographic image measurement in schizophrenia and affective disorder. *Annals of Neurology, (Supplement), 15*, S157–S165.

Cain, A. C. (1969). Special "isolated" abilities in severely psychotic young children. *Psychiatry, 32*, 137–149.

Campbell, M. (1975). Pharmacotherapy in early infantile autism. *Biological Psychiatry, 10*, 339–423.

Campbell, M. (1977). Treatment of childhood and adolescent schizophrenia. In J. M. Weiner (Ed.), *Psychopharmacology in childhood and adolescence* (pp. 101–118). New York: Basic Books.

Campbell, M., Rosenbloom, S., Perry, R., George, A., Kricheff, I., Anderson, L., Small, A., & Jennings, S. (1982). Computerized axial tomography in young autistic children. *American Journal of Psychiatry, 139*, 510–512.

Chess, S., Korn, S. J., & Fernandez, P. B. (1971). *Psychiatric disorders of children with congenital rubella.* New York: Brunner/Mazel.

Ciaranello, R. D., & Anders, T. F. (1977). Drug treatment of childhood psychotic disorders. In J. D. Barchas, P. A. Berger, R. D. Ciaranello, & G. R. Elliott (Eds.), *Psychopharmacology: From theory to practice* (pp. 436–447). New York: Oxford University Press.

Ciaranello, R. D., Vandenberg, S. R., & Anders, T. F. (1982). Intrinsic and extrinsic determinants of neuronal development: Relation to infantile autism. *Journal of Autism and Developmental Disorders, 12*, 115–146.

Cohen, D. J., Caparulo, B. K., Shaywitz, B. A., & Bowers, M. B. (1977). Dopamine and serotonin metabolism in neuropsychiatrically disturbed children. *Archives of General Psychiatry, 34*, 545–550.

Cohen, D. J., Shaywitz, B. A., Johnson, W. T., & Bowers, M. (1974). Biogenic amines in autistic and atypical children. *Archives of General Psychiatry, 31*, 845–853.

Cohen, D. J., & Young, J. G. (1977). Neurochemistry and child psychiatry. *Journal of the American Academy of Child Psychiatry, 16*, 353–411.

Coleman, M., Campbell, M., Freedman, L. S., Roffman, M., Ebstein, R. P., & Goldstein, M. (1974). Serum dopamine-beta-hydroxylase levels in Down's syndrome. *Clinical Genetics, 5*, 312–315.

Damasio, A. R., & Maurer, R. G. (1978). A neurological model of childhood autism. *Archives of Neurology, 35*, 777–785.

Damasio, H., Maurer, R. G., Damasio, A. R., & Chui, H. C. (1980). Computerized tomographic scan findings in patients with autistic behavior. *Archives of Neurology, 37*, 504–510.

Desmond, M. M., Montgomery, J. R., Melnick, J. L., Cochran, G. G., & Verniaud, W. (1969). Congenital rubella encephalitis. *American Journal of Diseases of Children, 118*, 30–31.

DeMyer, M. K., Barton, S., DeMyer, W. E., Norton, J. A., Allen, J., & Steel, R. (1973). Prognosis in autism: A follow-up study. *Journal of Autism and Childhood Schizophrenia, 3*, 199–246.

Duffy, F. H. (1982). Topographic display of evoked potentials: clinical applications of brain electrical activity mapping (BEAM). *Annals of the New York Academy of Sciences, 388*, 183–196.

Elliott, G. R. (1986). Magnetic resonance and *in vivo* studies of the human brain. In P. A. Berger & H. K. H. Brodie (Eds.), *The American handbook of psychiatry* (Vol. 8), (pp. 249–262). New York: Basic Books.

Elliott, G. R., & Barchas, J. D. (1986). Behavioral neurochemistry: The study of brain and behavior. In P. A. Berger & H. K. H. Brodie (Eds.), *The American handbook of psychiatry* (Vol. 8), (pp. 34–63). New York: Basic Books.

Elliott, G. R., & Ciaranello, R. D. (1986). Biological aspects of and drug treatments for selected childhood mental disorders. In P. A. Berger & H. K. H. Brodie (Eds.), *The American handbook of psychiatry* (Vol. 8), (pp. 620–650). New York: Basic Books.

Elliott, G. R., Siegel, B., Faull, K. F., & Ciaranello, R. D. (1986). *A double-blind clinical trial of fenfluramine on children with autism. II. Biochemical findings in cerebrospinal fluid and blood.* Manuscript in preparation.

Faull, K. F., King, R. J., Berger, P. A., & Barchas, J. D. (1984). Systems theory as a tool for integrating functional interactions among biogenic amines. In E. Usdin (Ed.), *Catecholamines:*

Neuropharmacology and central nervous system—Therapeutic aspects (pp. 143–152). New York: Alan R. Liss.

Faull, K. F., Kraemer, H. C., Barchas, J. D., & Berger, P. A. Clinical application of the probenecid test for measurement of monoamine turnover in the CNS. *Biological Psychiatry, 16*, 879–899.

Fein, D., Skoff, B., & Mirsky, A. F. (1981). Clinical correlates of brainstem dysfunction in autistic children. *Journal of Autism and Developmental Disorders, 11*, 303–315.

Folstein, S., & Rutter, M. (1978). A twin study of individuals with infantile autism. In M. Rutter & E. Schopler (Eds.), *Autism: A reappraisal of concepts and treatment* (pp. 219–242). New York: Plenum Press.

Foster, M. A. (1984). *Magnetic resonance in medicine and biology*. Oxford: Pergamon Press.

Fowle, A. M. (1968). A typical leukocyte pattern of schizophrenic children. *Archives of General Psychiatry, 18*, 666–680.

Frost, J. J., Wagner, H. N., Dannals, R. F., Ravert, H. T., Links, J. M., Wilson, A. A., Burns, H. D., Wong, D. F., McPherson, R. W., Rosenbaum, A. E., Kuhar, M. J., & Snyder, S. H. (1984). Imaging opiate receptors in the human brain by positron tomograph. *Journal of Computer Assisted Tomography, 9*, 231–236.

Geller, E., Ritvo, E., Freeman, B. J., & Yuwiler, A. (1982). Preliminary observations on the effect of fenfluramine on blood serotonin and symptoms in three autistic boys. *New England Journal of Medicine, 307*, 165–169.

Gillberg, C., Svennerholm, L., & Hamilton-Hellberg, C. (1983). Childhood psychosis and monoamine metabolites in spinal fluid. *Journal of Autism and Developmental Disorders, 13*, 383–396.

Giller, E. L., Jr., Young, J. G., Breakefield, X. O., Carbonari, C., Braverman, M., & Cohen, D. J. (1980). Monoamine oxidase and catechol-O-methyltransferase activities in cultured fibroblasts and blood cells from children with autism and the Gilles de la Tourette syndrome. *Psychological Research, 2*, 187–197.

Grahame-Smith, D. G. (1971). Studies in vivo on the relationship between brain tryptophan, brain 5-HT synthesis and hyperactivity in rats treated with a monoamine oxidase inhibitor and L-tryptophan. *Journal of Neurochemistry, 18*, 1053–1066.

Hanley, H. G., Stahl, S. M., & Freedman, D. X. (1977). Hyperserotonemia and amine metabolism in autistic and retarded children. *Archives of General Psychiatry, 34*, 521–531.

Hanson, D. R., & Gottesman, I. I. (1983). The genetics of childhood psychoses. In L. Wing & J. K. Wing (Eds.), *Handbook of psychiatry* (Vol. 3, pp. 222–232). Cambridge: Cambridge University Press.

Hier, D. B., LeMay, M. & Rosenberger, P. B. (1979). Autism and unfavorable left–right asymmetries of the brain. *Journal of Autism and Developmental Disorders, 9*, 153–159.

Ho, H. H., Lockitch, G. Eaves, L., & Jacobson, B. (1986). Blood serotonin concentrations and fenfluramine therapy in autistic children. *Journal of Pediatrics, 108*, 465–469.

Holman, R. B., Seagraves, E., Elliott, G. R., & Barchas, J. D. (1976). Stereotyped hyperactivity in rats treated with tranylcypromine and specific inhibitors of 5-HT reuptake. *Behavioral Biology, 16*, 507–514.

Inoue, Y., Wagner, H. N., Wong, D. F., Links, J. M., Frost, J. J., Dannals, R. F., Rosenbaum, A. E., Takeda, K., DiChiro, G., & Huhar, M. J. (1984). Atlas of dopamine receptor images (PET) of the human brain. *Journal of Computer Assisted Tomography, 9*, 129–140.

Kanner, L. (1943). Autistic disturbances of affective contact. *Nervous Child, 2*, 217–250.

Kolvin, I., Ounsted, C., Humphrey, M., Richardson, L., Garside, R., Kidd, J., & Roth, M. (1971). Six studies in the childhood psychoses. *British Journal of Psychiatry, 118*, 381–419.

Kootz, J. P., Marinelli, B., & Cohen, D. J. (1982). Modulation of response to environmental stimuli in autistic children. *Journal of Autism and Developmental Disorders, 12*, 185–193.

Lake, C. R., Zeigler, M. G., & Murphy, D. L. (1977). Increased norepinephrine levels and decreased DBH in primary autism. *Archives of General Psychiatry, 35*, 553–556.

Lelord, G., Laffont, P., Jusseaume, P., & Stephant, J. L. (1973). Comparative study of conditioning of averaged evoked responses by coupling sound and light in normal and autistic children. *Psychophysiology, 10*, 415–425.

Levitas, A., Hagerman, R. J., Braden, M., Rimland, B., & McBogg, P. (1983). *Journal of Developmental and Behavioral Pediatrics, 4*, 151–158.

Litrownik, A. J., & McInnis, E. T. (1982). Cognitive and perceptual deficits in autistic children: A model of information processing, critical review, and suggestions for the future. In J. J. Steffen & P. Karoly (Eds.), *Autism and severe psychopathology* (pp. 103–155). Lexington, MA: Lexington Books.

Lotter, V. (1966). Epidemiology of autistic conditions in young children. I. Prevalence. *Social Psychiatry, 1*, 124–137.

Morihisa, J. M. (1984). *Brain imaging in psychiatry.* Washington, DC: American Psychiatric Press.

Ornitz, E. M. (1969). Disorders of perception common to early infantile autism and schizophrenia. *Comprehensive Psychiatry, 10*, 259–274.

Ornitz, E. M. (1983). The functional neuroanatomy of infantile autism. *International Journal of Neuroscience, 19*, 85–124.

Ornitz, E. M., Forsythe, A. M., & de la Pena, A. (1973). The effect of vestibular and auditory stimulation on the rapid eye movements of REM sleep in autistic children. *Archives of General Psychiatry, 29*, 786–791.

Ornitz, E. M., & Ritvo, E. R. (1976). The syndrome of autism: A critical review. *American Journal of Psychiatry, 133*, 609–621.

Palkovitz, R. J., & Wiesenfeld, A. R. (1980). Differential autonomic responses of autistic and normal children. *Journal of Autism and Developmental Disorders, 10*, 347–360.

Panksepp, J., & Bishop, P. (1981). An autoradiographic map of 3H-diphrenophrine binding in rat brain: Effects of social interaction. *Brain Research Bulletin, 7*, 405–410.

Pare, C. M. B., Sandler, M., & Stacey, R. S. (1960). 5-Hydroxyindoles in mental deficiency. *Journal of Neurology, Neurosurgery and Psychiatry, 23*, 341–346.

Partington, M., Tu, J., & Wong, C. (1973). Blood serotonin levels in severe mental retardation. *Developmental Medicine and Child Neurology, 15*, 616–627.

Pollack, M., & Krieger, H. P. (1958). Oculomotor and postural patterns in schizophrenic children. *Archives of Neurology and Psychiatry, 79*, 720–726.

Prichard, J. W. (1983). Cerebral metabolic studies in vivo by 31P NMR. *Proceedings of the National Academy of Sciences (USA), 80*, 2748–2751.

Rapoport, J. L., & Ismond, D. R. (1982). Biological research in child psychiatry. *Journal of American Academy of Child Psychiatry, 21*, 543–548.

Rimland, B. (1964). *Infantile autism.* New York: Appleton-Century-Crofts.

Ritvo, E. R., Freeman, B. J., Geller, E., & Yuwiler, A. (1983). Effects of fenfluramine on 14 autistic outpatients. *Journal of the American Academy of Child Psychiatry, 22*, 549–558.

Ritvo, E. R., Freeman, B. J., Mason-Brothers, A., Mo, A., & Ritvo, A. M. (1985). Concordance for the syndrome of autism in 40 pairs of afflicted twins. *American Journal of Psychiatry, 142*, 74–78.

Ritvo, E. R., Freeman, B. J., Yuwiler, A., Geller, E., Yokota, A., Schroth, P. & Novak, P. (1984). Study of fenfluramine in outpatients with the syndrome of autism. *Journal of Pediatrics, 105*, 823–828.

Ritvo, E. R., Ornitz, E. M., Eviatar, A., Markham, C. H., Brown, M. B., & Mason, A. (1969). Decreased post-rotary nystagmus in early infantile autism. *Neurology, 19*, 653–658.

Ritvo, E. R., Spence, M. A., Freeman, B. J., Mason-Brothers, A., Mo, A., & Marazita, M. L. (1985). Evidence for an autosomal recessive type of autism in 46 multiple incidence families. *American Journal of Psychiatry, 142*, 187–192.

Ritvo, E. R., Yuwiler, A., Geller, E., Ornitz, E. M., Saeger, K., & Plotkin, S. (1970). Increased blood serotonin and platelets in early infantile autism. *Archives of General Psychiatry, 23*, 566–572.

Rosenbloom, S., Campbell, M., George, A. E., Kricheff, I. I., Taleporas, E., Anderson, L., Reuben, R. N., & Korein, J. (1984). High resolution CT scanning in infantile autism: A quantitative approach. *Journal of the American Academy of Child Psychiatry, 23*, 72–77.

Rosenblum, S. M., Arick, J. R., Krug, D. A., Stubbs, E. G., Young, N. B., & Pelson, R. O. (1980). Auditory brainstem evoked responses in autistic children. *Journal of Autism and Developmental Disorders, 10,* 215–225.

Rumsey, J. M., Duara, R., Grady, C., Rapoport, J. L., Margolin, R. A., Rapoport, S. I., & Cutler, N. R. (1985). Brain metabolism in autism. Resting cerebral glucose utilization, rates as measured with positron emission tomography. *Archives of General Psychiatry, 42,* 448–455.

Rutter, M. (1972). Childhood schizophrenia reconsidered. *Journal of Autism and Childhood Schizophrenia, 2,* 315–337.

Rutter, M. (1974). The development of infantile autism. *Psychological Medicine, 4,* 147–163.

Rutter, M., Greenfeld, D., & Lockyer, L. (1967). A five to fifteen year follow-up study of infantile psychosis. II. Social and behavioral outcome. *British Journal of Psychiatry, 113,* 1183–1200.

Schain, R. J., & Freedman, D. X. (1961). Studies on 5-hydroxyindole metabolism in autistic and other mentally retarded children. *Journal of Pediatrics, 58,* 315–329.

Siegel, B., Anders, T. F., Ciaranello, R. D., Bienenstock, B., & Kraemer, H. C. (1986). Empirically derived subclassification of the autistic syndrome. *Journal of Autism and Developmental Disorders, 16,* 275–293.

Siegel, B., Elliott, G. R., Friedman, S., & Ciaranello, R. D. (1986). *A double-blind clinical trial of fenfluramine on children with autism. I. Behavioral characteristics and treatment response.* Manuscript in preparation.

Small, J. G., DeMyer, M. K., & Milstein, V. (1971). CNV responses of autistic and normal children. *Journal of Autism and Childhood Schizophrenia, 1,* 215–231.

Stubbs, E. G. (1977). Autistic children exhibit undetectable hemagglutination-inhibition antibody titers despite previous rubella vaccination. *Journal of Autism and Childhood Schizophrenia, 6,* 269–274.

Stubbs, E. G., Crawford, M. L., Burger, D. R., & Vandenbark, A. A. (1977). Depressed lymphocyte responsiveness in autistic children. *Journal of Autism and Childhood Schizophrenia, 7,* 49–55.

Takahashi, S. Kanai, H., & Miyamoto, Y. (1976). Reassessment of elevated serotonin levels in blood platelets in early infantile autism. *Journal of Autism and Childhood Schizophrenia, 6,* 317–326.

Tanguay, P. E., & Edwards, R. M. (1982). Electrophysiological studies of autism: The whisper of the bang. *Journal of Autism and Developmental Disorders, 12,* 117–184.

Tanguay, P. E., Ornitz, E. M., Forsythe, A. B., & Ritvo, E. R. (1976). Rapid eye movement (REM) activity in normal and autistic children during REM sleep. *Journal of Autism and Childhood Schizophrenia, 6,* 275–288.

Todd, R. D., & Ciaranello, R. D. (1984). Demonstration of inter- and intraspecies differences in serotonin binding sites by antibodies from an autistic child. *Proceedings of the National Academy of Sciences (USA), 82,* 612–616.

Todd, R. D., & Ciaranello, R. D. (1985). Infantile autism and the childhood psychoses. In P. J. Vinken, G. W. Bruyn, & H. L. Klawans (Eds.), *Handbook of clinical neurology,* (Vol. 2, pp. 189–197). New York: Elsevier.

Treffert, D. A. (1970). Epidemiology of infantile autism. *Archives of General Psychiatry, 22,* 431–4382.

Tsai, L., Jacoby, C. G., Stewart, M. A., & Beisler, J. M. (1982). Unfavorable left–right asymmetries of the brain and autism: A question of methodology. *British Journal of Psychiatry, 140,* 312–319.

Watson, M. S., Leckman, J. F., Annex, B., Breg, W. R., Boles, D., Volkmer, F. R., Cohen, D. J., & Carter, C. (1984). Fragile X in a survey of 75 autistic males. *New England Journal of Medicine, 310,* 1462.

Weizman, R., Weizman, A., Tyano, S., Szekely, G., Weissman, B. A., & Sarne, Y. (1984). Humoral-endorphin blood levels in autistic, schizophrenic and healthy subjects. *Psychopharmacology, 82,* 368–370.

Weizman, A., Weizman, R., Szekely, G. A., Wijsenbeek, H., & Livni, E. (1982). Abnormal immune response to brain tissue antigen in the syndrome of autism. *American Journal of Psychiatry, 139,* 1462–1465.

White, L. (1974). Organic factors and psychophysiology in childhood schizophrenia. *Psychological Bulletin, 81*, 238–255.

Williams, R. S., Hauser, S. L., Purpura, D., DeLong, R., & Swisher, C. N. (1980). Autism and mental retardation: Neuropathologic studies performed in four retarded persons with autistic behavior. *Archives of Neurology, 37*, 749–753.

Wong, D. F., Wagner, H. N., Dannals, R. F., Links, J. M., Frost, J. J., Ravest, H. T., Wilson, A. A., Rosenbaum, A. E., Gjedde, A., Douglass, K. H., Petronis, J. D., Folstein, M. F., Toung, J. K. T., Burns, H. D., & Kuhar, M. J. (1984). Effects of age on dopamine and serotonin receptors measured by positron tomography in the living human brain. *Science, 226*, 1393–1396.

Young, J. G., Kavanagh, M. E., Anderson, G. M., Shaywitz, B. A., & Cohen, D. J. (1982). Clinical neurochemistry of autism and associated disorders. *Journal of Autism and Developmental Disorders, 12*, 147–165.

Young, J. G., Kyprie, R. M., Ross, N. T., & Cohen, D. J. (1975). Serum dopamine-beta-hydroxylase activity: Clinical applications in child psychiatry. *Journal of Autism and Developmental Disorders, 5*, 83–98.

15

Neurotransmitter Research in Autism

ARTHUR YUWILER and DANIEL X. FREEDMAN

GENERAL INTRODUCTION

The irritants used by some organisms to discourage predators have been adapted by nature as a chemical nudge by which one cell can communicate with its neighbor. A nervous system is merely a group of long skinny cells interconnected and communicating with each other by the release of, and response to, such irritants, which are then termed *neurotransmitters*. Neurotransmitters are the communication links between nerve cells and are involved in all behaviors. This is not to say that transmitters or even the brain need be involved in the etiology of the disorders that produce abnormal behaviors. Phenylketonuria is a genetic disease of the liver, and its effect on the brain is secondary to a blockage of amino acid transport into developing brain as a result of disturbed liver metabolism. Whatever the nature of the initiating problem, however, the abnormal behavior involves abnormal neural communication in the form either of inappropriate linkages between neurons or of abnormalities in transmitter metabolism or function. Most transmitter research assumes the latter and consists of a search for dysfunction. This search is especially complicated for the neurochemist because the involved neurons are in the brain and the human brain is, and should be, inviolate. The result is an indirect hunt for traces of the neural activity of dreams, thoughts, and feelings in urine, blood, cerebrospinal fluid, and other available tissues. The general problem, then, is to examine sufficiently large populations with tests capable of identifying pathophysiologically or causally relevant neurotransmitter mechanism in autistic behavior in the hope of identifying either a common abnormality or subgroups with related transmitter dysfunctions. Specific practical problems exist both in finding appropriate tests and in obtaining large and homogeneous populations for testing.

Available tests mostly involve measurements of the concentrations of transmitters, their precursors, or products in peripheral tissues; of the concentrations of compounds whose production or release is controlled by the brain; and of the activities of enzymes or metabolic processes in peripheral tissues analogous to those in the brain. Methods for making such

ARTHUR YUWILER • Neurobiochemistry Research, Veterans Administration, Los Angeles, California 90073; and Department of Psychiatry, University of California at Los Angeles, Los Angeles, California 90024. DANIEL X. FREEDMAN • Department of Psychiatry, University of California at Los Angeles, Los Angeles, California 90024.

measures are constantly being refined and the array of possibly relevant measures enlarged. Further, our fundamental knowledge of the origin, disposition, and function of transmitters is still evolving. It is increasingly clear, however, that concentrations of transmitters, their precursors, or their breakdown products in peripheral tissues alone do not directly or reliably predict brain transmitter status. In order to provide better measures of transmitter function applicable to clinical populations, much more work is needed determining the extent to which the brain signals the periphery by nervous and hormonal mechanisms and in identifying the complex of peripheral compartments involved in the metabolism and utilization of transmitters. In brief, "upstairs–downstairs" relationships still need to be clarified and better tests devised. Nonetheless, enough is now known of the basic physiology of transmitters and sufficient data have been developed in studies on autistic behavior to yield some picture of the current biological status of the syndrome and permit some speculation on what might logically be done to further our understanding of transmitter malfunction in this puzzling disorder.

Nor is the problem of population resolved. Often, too few subjects are studied with any one test to permit generalizing the results beyond the sample. Further, very few studies have been replicated. Additionally, as in other areas of study on autistic behavior, populations are seldom described in sufficient detail to assure investigators they are studying the same disease. This uncertainty about the relationship between diagnosis and etiology also bears heavily on research strategy. A diagnosis of autistic behavior involves identification of features codified in the DMS-III (299.0) and/or by the National Society for Children and Adults with Autism (NSAC). While this provides a diagnosis, it does not necessarily identify a common cause. Indeed, the association of autistic behavior with diseases such as maternal rubella (Chess, 1971), histidinemia (Kotsopoulos & Kutty, 1979), phenylketonuria (Friedman, 1969), mucopolysaccharidoses (Knoblock & Pasamanick, 1975), aberrant purine metabolism (Becker, Paivio, Bakay, Adams, & Nyhan, 1980; Coleman, Landgrebe, & Landgrebe 1976; Nyhan, James, Tebert, Sweetman, & Nelson, 1969), fragile X syndrome (Brown et al., 1982; Folstein, Chapter 5; Gillberg, 1983), neurofibromatosis (Gillberg & Forsell, 1984), and abnormalities in carbohydrate metabolism (Coleman & Blass 1985) suggests that autistic behavior has multiple etiologies. However, if autistic behavior does not have a single etiology, then any neurotransmitter disorder found in all with autistic behavior also does not relate to etiology. Rather, at best, the biochemical abnormality is linked to some common final pathway of the separate etiologies leading to symptom expression or, at worst, it may reflect symptoms or treatment. That is, if "autistic behavior," like "mental retardation," is a cover name for a cluster of etiologically distinct diseases, a better strategy than searching for a biochemical abnormality common to all those with the syndrome might be to search for the mechanisms for any abnormalities common to a subpopulation, even if this strategy risks detailing the medically trivial. Most of the studies to be reported here have tacitly assumed a single etiology for autistic behavior and have compared those with such behavior with other populations.

TRANSMITTERS

Introduction

Currently some dozen and a half small molecules and 50 or so peptides may serve as neurotransmitters; new ones are proposed daily. Of these, the transmitters dopamine, norepinephrine, and serotonin have been at the focus of research on transmitter abnormalities in mental disease both because their chemical structures permit easy detection and quantification and because they modulate fundamental behaviors such as sleep, mood, motor control, and arousal, which are often disturbed in psychiatric and neurological diseases. These transmitters (collectively termed *monoamines*) have a wide distribution in the brain but they are made by highly localized cells that together make up only a small fraction of the neurons in the brain. Moreover, each monoaminergic system is organized into anatomical and functional subsystems with independent actions, and each interacts with, is affected by, and is interconnected to other transmitter systems. Serotoninergic terminals synapse on some dopamine cell bodies (Dray, Gonye, Oakley, & Tanner, 1976), noradrenergic terminals on some serotoninergic cell bodies (Baraban & Aghajanian, 1981), dopaminergic terminals on some noradrenergic cell bodies (Simon, LeMoal, Stinus, & Calas, 1979), and opiate receptors occur on terminals of serotoninergic neurons (Parenti, Tirone, Olgiati, & Groppetti, 1983), and so on. Hence, a disturbance in one transmitter system is likely to affect the activity of other transmitter systems and an abnormality in one does not preclude linked abnormalities in others as well. Another layer of complexity is added by the fact that several transmitters may coexist in some nerve terminals. Substance P coexists with serotonin in about 25% of the serotoninergic neurons of the Raphe nuclei (Chan-Palay, Jonsson, & Palay, 1978), enkephalins may coexist with adrenergic and cholinergic transmitters (Klein, Wilson, Dzielak, Yang, & Viveros, 1982), and dopamine sometimes coexists with cholecystokinin (Hokfelt *et al.*, 1980). Thus, even if an aberrant transmitter system is identified there may still be ambiguity as to which transmitter need be manipulated to treat the symptoms. The literature survey that follows is grouped according to transmitter for the sake of convenience in presentation and should not be taken to imply single transmitter etiologies of this syndrome.

Serotonin

Serotonin is the trivial name for 5-hydroxytryptamine (5-HT), which is made from the essential amino acid tryptophan. It is formed in a two-step reaction. The first involves the addition of an atom of molecular oxygen to the tryptophan nucleus to produce the compound 5-hydroxytryptophan (5-HTP). This is the rate-limiting step in serotonin formation, and the rate is sensitive both to the amount and activity of the enzyme tryptophan hydroxylase, that carries out the reaction and to the amount of substrate, tryptophan, available to it. In the second step, 5-hydroxytryptophan is converted to 5-hydroxytryptamine by the enzyme aromatic amino acid decarboxylase. Serotonin is degraded by the action of still another enzyme, monoamine oxidase, to an intermediate that, in most tissues, is further oxidized to the end product 5-hydroxyindoleacetic acid (5-HIAA) and, in some, is reduced to the alcohol 5-hydroxytryptophol (5-HIOH).

Data from three sources have been taken as evidence for serotoninergic involvement in autistic behavior: elevated blood serotonin concentration, antiserotonin antibodies, and, to a lesser extent, behavioral response to pharmacological agents affecting the serotonin system.

Tissue Levels

Elevated blood serotonin among children showing autistic behavior was first reported by Schain and Freedman 91961) and confirmed by investigators throughout the world (Campbell, Friedman, De Vito, Greenspan, & Collins, 1984; Douay, Debray-Ritzen, & Kamoun, 1980; Goldstein, Mahanad, Lee, & Coleman, 1976; Hanley, Stahl, & Freedman, 1977;

Ritvo, *et al.*, 1970; Takahashi, Kanai, & Miyamoto, 1976; Yuwiler, Ritvo, Bald, Kipper, & Koper, 1971; Yuwiler *et al.*, 1975). To date it is the only confirmed biological abnormality in this syndrome. This observation raises a number of questions.

A first question concerns incidence. Only about 30% of children with autistic behaviors have elevated blood serotonin, and a similar incidence is found among those with mental retardation [exclusive of those with phenylketonuria, who instead have low blood (Pare, Sandler, & Stacey, 1960; Partington, Tu, & Wong, 1973; Schain & Freedman, 1961) and brain serotonin (McKean, 1972) or those with Down syndrome]. High blood serotonin concentrations are also found among patients with some intestinal tumors (Pernow & Waldenstrom, 1954; Sjoerdsma, Weissbach, & Udenfriend 1956), nontroptical sprue (Pimparker, Senesky, & Kakser, 1961), bipolar manic-depressive illness (Sarai & Kayano, 1968), and some chronic schizophrenics (Freedman, Belendiuk, Belendiuk, & Crayton, 1981), in the latter of whom it may be associated with enlargement of brain ventricles (De Lisi, Neckers, Weinberger, & Wyatt, 1981). Fifteen percent of children with autistic behavior are also reported to have enlarged ventricles (Gillberg & Svendsen, 1983; Hauser, DeLong, & Rosman, 1975) or other geometric brain abnormalities (Damasio, Maurer, Damasio, & Chui, 1980; Gillberg & Svendsen 1983; Hier, LeMay, & rosenberg, 1979), but how many of these also have high blood serotonin is not known. Elevated blood serotonin was also noted (Belendiuk, Belendiuk, & Freedman, 1980; Belendiuk, Belendiuk, Freedman, & Antel, 1981; Irwin, Belendiuk, McCloskey, & Freedman, 1981) in other disorders like attention deficit disorder with normal IQ, Huntington disease, amyotrophic lateral sclerosis, and lower neuron motor disease. People with Type A personalities also appear to have slightly higher blood serotonin concentrations than others (Marsden & McGuire 1984).

A second question is whether blood serotonin concentration is related to a specific clinical feature, and the answer is not settled but seems to be no. Although blood serotonin concentrations can vary widely among individuals, consistency within an individual is high and persistent. Levels in some children with the autistic syndrome remained unchanged through puberty and into young adulthood despite hospitalization and institutionalization. Whether it would change with clinical remission is not known (Hanley *et al.*, 1977; Yuwiler, Ritvo, Freeman, Yarborough, & Santat, 1984). Interestingly, among some monkeys blood serotonin seems to be state-dependent. In these animals the dominant male has twice the blood serotonin concentration of subordinates (McGuire, Raleigh, & Brammer, 1982; Steklis & Raleigh, 1984) so long as he remains leader and in contact with the group. Isolation or overthrow leads to a fall in blood serotonin concentration (Raleigh, McGuire, Brammer, & Yuwiler, 1984). Perhaps blood serotonin in humans is also subject to social influences and it is only the social buffering provided by the multiple hierarchical positions humans hold in different social contexts (employee, parent, spouse, child, citizen) that prevents this from being seen.

Since elevated blood serotonin is neither found among all autistic people nor unique to them, the remaining critical question is whether the *mechanism* for the elevated serotonin of those with autistic behaviors is unique (Hanley *et al.*, 1977; Yuwiler *et al.*, 1975). The question is important because it is uniqueness of mechanism that determines clinical utility. Blood glucose is a clinically useful measure, even though abnormal concentrations occur in many conditions, only because in each instance it occurs by a unique mechanism. In one group it is due to insulin deficiency, in another to a lack of insulin receptors, and in yet another to increased formation of glucose. And in each instance, mechanism points the way for possible therapy and at possible etiology. A similar pattern may be the case for increased blood serotonin. For example, in motor neuron disease, blood serotonin concentration correlates with severity and relates to another biochemical measure (monoamine oxidase activity) (Belendiuk, Belendiuk, Freedman, & Antel, 1981), but these relationships are not seen among those with autistic behaviors. Similarly, the number of serotonin-producing cells increase in some intestinal cancers, leading to increased blood serotonin, but there is no evidence to suggest that this is the mechanism for the increased serotonin associated in any other case of hyperserotoninemia.

Despite its potential importance, however, very few studies are explicitly directed at uncovering the mechanism for hyperserotoninemia among those with the syndrome of child-hood autism. Rather, most examine for population differences, and relationships to hyper-serotoninemia must be indirectly inferred on the assumption of a higher incidence among those with autism than among controls.

Because all the serotonin in blood is normally contained within platelets (DeMet, Halaris, & Bhatarakamul 1978), information on serotonin metabolism, platelet physiology, and such things as platelet distribution in various organs (Shulman, Watkins, Itscoitz, & Students, 1969) or rates of platelet travel through regions of serotonin formation are relevant. The search for mechanism could be narrowed by a definitive answer to the question of whether hyperserotoninemia among those with childhood autism is the result of more platelets, more serotonin per platelet, or both. Calculations from existing data suggest that the answer is more serotonin per platelet (Boullin, Coleman, O'Brien, & Rimland 1971; Douay et al., 1980; Hanley et al., 1977; Ritvo et al., 1970; Takahashi et al., 1976; Yuwiler et al., 1971, 1975) rather than more platelets, although some studies report modestly increased platelet numbers as well (Boullin, Coleman, & O'Brien, 1970; Ritvo et al., 1970). Presumably the children with high blood serotonin are responsible for this difference. If so, then the mech-anism for their hyperserotoninema likely involves serotonin metabolism or serotonin uptake, release, or storage in platelets. Direct measures of the serotonin content of platelets from children with high and normal blood serotonin concentration are needed to confirm these calculations, however.

Data relevant to serotonin metabolism consist of measures of the concentrations of the serotonin catabolite 5-hydroxindoleacetic acid, and the serotonin precursor tryptophan, and of the activity of the enzyme monoamine oxidase, which degrades serotonin. The results, in toto, are ambiguous.

Some tenuous support for increased serotonin synthesis comes from indications of increased urinary 5-HIAA excretion by a small number of children with autistic behavior both under basal conditions and after tryptophan loading (Hanley et al., 1977; Schain & Freedman, 1961). However, as the authors note, 24-hour collections were precluded because of incontinence, and despite normalizing the values to the indirect measure of muscle mass, creatinine, the findings must be regarded as tentative. This is doubly so because 5-HIAA excretion is volume-dependent, and it was later discovered that some caretakers encouraged the children to drink water heavily so as to increase urinary volume. An elevation in urinary tryptamine was also found by Hanley et al. (1977), which could indicate a greater flux of peripheral tryptophan or might itself be an artifact of volume-dependent excretion. Normal urinary 5-HIAA was found in hyperserotoninemic children without the syndrome of autism (Irwin, Belendiuk, McClosky, & Freedman, 1981) and among hyperserotoninemic children with retardation (Partington et al., 1973). Clearly, more information is needed.

Equally ambiguous are measurements of the concentration of the serotonin precursor tryptophan. This essential amino acid is largely bound to albumin in the blood, and the small unbound fraction has been considered by some to be the most relevant measure for serotonin synthesis. Total blood tryptophan is reported to be normal (Douay et al., 1980; Hoshino et al., 1984). In one study free tryptophan also appeared to be normal for the group, but (Hoshino et al., 1979) two markedly aggressive and hyperactive children with autism had high concentrations of both serotonin and free tryptophan. The same investigators (Hoshino et al., 1984) in a later study found elevated free tryptophan that correlated positively with activity and clinical status and negatively with developmental quotient. The blood serotonin of the children with autism was also elevated but did not correlate with free tryptophan; this is not surprising since platelets have an 8- to 10-day half-life and their serotonin content largely reflects past accumulations, whereas free tryptophan concentrations portend future synthesis. Compatible with elevated free tryptophan is the report that autistic people have increased serum fatty acid concentrations (DeMyer, Schwier, Bryson, Solow, & Roeske, 1971) since free fatty acids can displace tryptophan from its albumin binding sites and thereby increase the free tryptophan without affecting the total.

There is no evidence for decreased serotonin breakdown among children with autistic symptoms. Dietary tryptophan increased their excretion of 5-HIAA by at least as much as it did controls (Hanley et al., 1977; Schain & Freedman, 1961; Shaw, Lucas, & Rabinovitch, 1959), and increased serotonin breakdown within platelets is unlikely. Monoamine oxidase is located on the outer membrane of the mitochondria while most platelet serotonin is sequestered in vesicles. Further, serotonin is not a good substrate for the form of monoamine oxidase (MAO B) in platelets. Finally, MAO B activity in platelets (Boullin, Bhagavan, Coleman, O'Brien, & Youdim, 1975; Cohen, Young, & Roth, 1977; Young, Cohen, & Roth, 1978) and in cultured skin fibroblasts from children with autism (Giller et al., 1980) does not differ from controls.

Existing platelet studies are no more definitive and are largely limited to measures of serotonin uptake, efflux, and storage. Serotonin enters platelets by active uptake and passive diffusion. One study using short incubation times and low serotonin concentrations appropriate to measure initial uptake rate reported 50% greater uptake by platelets from four children with autistic symptoms than that from six hospitalized psychotic controls (Rotman, Caplan, & Szekely, 1980). Three studies using experimental conditions measuring active and passive serotonin accumulation produced conflicting results. In one (Sankar, Cates, Broer, & Sankar 1963), platelets from children with autism accumulated significantly less serotonin than platelets from controls; in two attempted replications (Lucas, Warner, & Gottlieb, 1971; Yuwiler et al., 1975), groups did not differ, and in yet another (Boullin et al., 1970), platelets from those with autism accumulated more serotonin. These differences likely result from differences in diagnostic criteria and experimental procedures.

Serotonin uptake into platelets reflects turnover at each uptake site and the number of sites. Imipramine is a serotonin reuptake inhibitor that binds to a regulatory site proximal to the serotonin uptake site. Controls and children with autism did not differ in either the number of binding sites or their affinity for imipramine (Anderson, Minderaa, van Benthem, Volkmar, & Cohen, 1984). Specific attention was not given to whether hyperserotoninemic and normoserotonemics differ on these measures.

The rate of repletion of platelet serotonin after impairment of serotonin binding by reserpine treatment seemed the same for both four hyperserotoninemic autistic subjects and four controls (Hanley et al., 1977), although final serotonin concentrations were higher for the autistic subjects.

Platelets tightly sequester serotonin but some release (efflux) does occur. Measurements of efflux have produced mixed results. Early studies indicated that platelets from children with high "E-2 scores" (Rimland, 1979) had increased serotonin efflux that could even predict the range of the E-2 score (Boullin et al., 1970, 1971). Results could not be replicated in later studies on populations defined by E-2 score (Boullin, 1978), by clinical criteria (Yuwiler *et al.*, 1975), or by both (Boullin *et al.*, 1982). Efflux is measured by procedures involving separation steps that could segregate or injure platelets, and it seems likely that the procedures producing the initial promising results were sensitive to factors, other than efflux, on which populations differ. Platelet size or platelet fragility are among the possibilities and reexamination for such factors may be worthwhile.

Finally, there is the question of whether blood serotonin levels in children with autism has any relationship to brain serotonin. Certainly there is no reason why the two must be related. Serotonin in brain is made in nerve cells, where it acts as a neurotransmitter. Serotonin in blood is made by specialized cells in the intestine (Bertaccini, 1960), is carried in blood in platelets, and serves to decrease blood loss after injury. Neither can contribute to the concentration of the other, and examples can be cited in which they change quite independently. On the other hand, serotonin in brain and in the periphery are formed and metabolized in the same way, both are affected in the same manner by precursors and a number of drugs, and the platelet and the neurons have very similar systems for serotonin uptake, transport, and storage. Further, there are instances, such as phenylketonuria, where both change in roughly the same degree.

Measures of brain serotonin content, metabolism, and/or receptors would help answer the question but these have yet to be obtained. However, 5-HIAA in the cerebrospinal fluid (CSF) has been studied and to the extent that measures of CSF metabolites reflect the status of their parent transmitters, brain serotonin is normal in patients with autism. It is not clear if it is also normal in hyperserotoninemics with childhood autism. The qualification is important, however. CSF samples are taken from the lumbar region below the end of the spinal cord. 5-HIAA from brain contributes to this pool, since there is an appreciable cerebral-cadal concentration gradient, but so does 5-HIAA from the cord (Garelis, Young, Lal, & Sourkes, 1974), and it takes about 6 hours for material to travel from the brain to the lumbar region so that brain contributions to lumbar 5-HIAA are diluted and delayed (Pletscher, Bartholini, & Tissor, 1967). To further complicate matters, CSF is seldom taken from normal children and comparisons are usually between various patient populations.

The 5-HIAA content of cerebrospinal fluid has been determined under basal conditions and after administration of the drug probenecid, which competitively inhibits transport of acidic catabolites from brain. The rate of accumulation of these acidic catabolites provides a measure of the turnover of their precursors.

Basal CSF 5-HIAA concentration was found to be the same for 13 children with autism and 13 sex-matched nonpsychotic children with neurological symptoms but without detectable disease (Gillberg, Svennerholm, & Hamilton-Hellberg, 1983). Similarly, 5-HIAA accumulation after probenecid did not differentiate children (Cohen, Caparulo, Shaywitz and Bowers, 1977; Cohen, Shaywitz, Johnson, & Bowers, 1984; Leckman *et al.*, 1980; Winsberg, Sverd, Castells, Hurwic, & Perel, 1980). However, probenecid blockade was not complete in many of these studies, as evidenced by correlations between probenecid and catabolite concentrations, precluding valid turnover estimates and conclusions on the gross status of brain serotonin.

Immunology

Immunological evidence for a role for serotonin in autism comes from the discovery, in a hyperserotoninemic autistic girl, of circulating and CSF antibodies against human cortical 5HT 1A serotonin receptors (Todd & Ciaranello, 1985). Serotonin receptors are classified by binding properties, and 5HT 1A receptors are those with nanomolar affinities for serotonin and spiperone and micromolar affinity for ketanserine. Although actual data were presented on only a single subject, antibodies against serotonin receptors were reportedly also detected in half of 13 autistic subjects surveyed but not in 13 controls (Todd & Ciaranello, 1985).

A possibly related finding is that of a cell-mediated immune response to human myelin basic protein in 13 of 17 autistic subjects but not in 17 controls (Weizman, Weizman, Szekely, Wijsenbeek, & Livni, 1982). Myelin basic protein contains a serotonin binding site associated with the peptide sequence Arg Phe Ser Trp (Root-Bernstein & Westall, 1983). It is conceivable that this sequence also occurs in the 5HT 1A receptor site and that antibodies directed to one would appear directed to both.

Presumably a receptor antibody would target receptors for destruction and diminish postsynaptic stimulation. Such is the case for the autoimmune disease myasthenia gravis, in which antibodies are directed against cholinergic receptors. This disease is treated with cholinesterase inhibitors to increase intrasynaptic acetylcholine concentration and more effectively stimulate the diminishing number of receptor sites. By analogy, increasing intrasynaptic serotonin around 5HT 1A sites or stimulating serotonin receptors with agonists should be therapeutic, while serotonin antagonists or treatments diminishing intrasynaptic serotonin should be deleterious.

How such autoimmunity would affect blood serotonin is not clear. Blockade of some receptors in the central nervous system results in compensatory increases of transmitter metabolism in the presynaptic neurone, but blood serotonin is made in the gut and stored in the platelet and there is no known feedback in this system. On the other hand, hyperserotoninemia might contribute to the genesis of the autoimmunity. It has been suggested that serotonin binding to fragments of myelin basic protein (or 5HT 1A receptor) released during normal turnover might protect the protein against catabolism long enough for immunological processing (Westall & Root-Bernstein, 1983). Presumably concomitant disease or metabolic damage would also be required to expose the peptide fragment to immunologically competent cells, and, as noted in the introduction, pre- and neonatal disease is commonly found in autism. Clearly this is an area likely to be vigorously pursued.

Pharmacology

Pharmacological studies also provide some, albeit mixed, support for serotoninergic involvement in autism, although interpretation is confounded by problems of drug specificity. A total of seven relevant compounds have been used. Because of inadequate detail or questions of diagnosis, early studies on responses of psychotic and autistic children to LSD (Bender, Cobrinik, Faretra, & Sankar, 1966) and to reserpine (Hanley et al., 1977) will not be reviewed here except to say that the former, at doses likely to increase brain serotonin concentration but decrease transynaptic release, appeared to have some therapeutic effects while the latter, which lowers brain amines generally, had none.

Two of the five remaining compounds, 5HTP and imipramine, should increase serotoninergic transmission but both also can affect catecholaminergic systems. 5-hydroxytryptophan is the immediate precursor to serotonin and circumvents the rate-limiting step of tryptophan hydroxylation. However, it can be taken into catecholaminergic neurons as well and be decarboxylated there by ubiquitous amino acid decarboxylase to a false transmitter. Administration to a total of five children with autism in two studies (Sverd, Kupietz, Winsberg, Hurwic, & Becker, 1978; Zarcone et al., 1973) did not improve symptomatology and may even have worsened it. The tricyclic antidepressant imipramine blocks serotonin reuptake into tissues (Axelrod & Inscoe, 1963), thereby increasing its intrasynaptic concentration.

However, it is rapidly demethylated *in vivo* to the rather specific norepinephrine reuptake inhibitor desmethylimipramine. This compound had mixed clinical effects on 10 autistic and schizophrenic children. Some initial transient improvement of apathy, hypoactivity, irritability, and withdrawal was noted, but at the end of the treatment period, while two subjects improved, five had increased psychotic symptoms, behavioral disorganization, blunted affect, sedation, both hyper- and hypoactivity, irritability, and insomnia (Campbell, Fish, Shapiro, & Floyd, 1971). Studies with more specific serotonin reuptake inhibitors may now be in order.

Neither compound, then, improved, and both may even have worsened, autistic behaviors. While these findings are compatible with the view that increasing serotoninergic stimulation is deleterious, the data are too few, the changes too small, and the drug action too uncertain to be more than merely suggestive.

The drugs methylsergide, dopa and fenfluramine all diminish serotonin concentration or serotoninergic transmission by different mechanisms. Methylsergide, a serotonin receptor blocker with limited effectiveness in brain, reportedly temporarily brightened affect, increased eye contact, and enhanced alertness and responsivity of schizophrenic and autistic children. However, this was shortly followed by irritability and disorganized activity (Fish, Campbell, Shapiro, & Floyd, 1969b).

Dopa is the immediate precursor to dopamine, and this is the basis for its wide clinical use in Parkinsonism to replace the dopamine lost by the death of dopaminergic neurons. As an incidental feature, dopa interferes with serotonin by the same mechanism as 5HTP interferes with dopamine metabolism (Ng, Chase, Colburn, & Kopin, 1970). Two studies on a total of 16 children with autism examined the therapeutic response to dopa (3,4-dihydroxyphenylalanine) on autistic behaviors. In one study (Ritvo *et al.*, 1971) urinary 5-HIAA and blood 5HT of 4 children were reduced by dopa, although postdrug blood serotonin concentrations were still higher than those of controls. Treatment did not alter global assessments of perception, motility, relatedness, or language beyond normal variance. A second larger study employed a crossover comparison of dopa with placebo and L-amphetamine. Only 2 of the 12 subjects had initially elevated blood serotonin concentrations, and effects of dopa on blood serotonin were inconsistent—half increasing and half declining. Behavioral changes were equally inconsistent, with half of the children showing some improvement and half worsening. None of the changes met statistical criteria and behavioral and serotonin responses were wholly unrelated (Campbell *et al.*, 1976). Neither study included a peripheral decarboxylase inhibitor to prevent tissue conversion of dopa, which can pass the blood brain barrier, to dopamine, which cannot; the dose delivered to the brain is therefore uncertain, as are the relative contributions of serotonin and catecholamines to the results.

Somewhat stronger pharmacological evidence for serotoninergic involvement in autism comes from studies with fenfluramine. Widely used as an anorectic, fenfluramine reduces brain and blood serotonin and brain and CSF 5-HIAA (Duhault & Boulanger, 1977; Duhault & Verdavainne, 1967; Raleigh *et al.*, 1984), inhibits serotonin reuptake (Costa, Groppetti, & Revuelta, 1971; Garattini *et al.*, 1979), increases serotonin release (Costa *et al.*, 1971), inhibits tryptophan hydroxylase activity (Sanders-Bush, Bushing, & Sulser, 1975), and decreases serotonin turnover (Fuller & Perry, 1983). These actions probably occur at the nerve terminal.

Fenfluramine reportedly improved motor behavior, socialization, and even intellectual performance of about 30% of children with autism (August, Raz, & Baird, 1984; August *et al.*, 1984; Geller, Ritvo, Freeman, & Yuwiler, 1982; Klykylo, Feldis, O'Grady, Ross, & Halloran, 1985; Ritvo, Freeman, Geller, & Yuwiler, 1983; Ritvo *et al.*, 1984; Ritvo, Freeman, Yuwiler, Geller, Schroth, Yokota, Mason-Brothers, August, Klykylo, Leventhal, Lewis, Piggot, Realmuto, Stubbs, & Umansky, 1986; Campbell, Deutsch, Perry, Wolsky, & Palij,

1986). An equal percentage failed to respond. The major effect appears to be to enhance the ability to attend, and improvement generally follows the sequence of decreased stereotypic motor behaviors, sequential changes in personality, attentional and performance components of the syndrome, and finally, in some few cases, performance on standard IQ tests. Symptoms reappear in the same order after discontinuation of drug, stereotypic behavior reappearing first and performance deteriorating last.

Although much more information is needed on the nature and extent of drug effectiveness and persistence, as well as on such clinical issues as dosage, dosage interval, and especially long-term safety, it seems likely that the effects of the drug on responders involves the serontoninergic system. It is of some interest, however, that response tends to be inversely related to basal serotonin blood level (Ritvo et al., 1986) or, since the fixed dosage used halves serotonin concentration, to postdrug serotonin concentration. Whether this means that hyperserotoninemics require a higher dose or are more refractory to the drug is unclear. Further, although fenfluramine clearly decreases serotonin concentrations and turnover, some data suggest that it may also increase postsynaptic stimulation (Dumbrille-Ross & Tang, 1983; Samanin, Mennini, Ferraris, Bendotti, & Borsini, 1980). That is, more information is needed on its acute and chronic effects on the systems under serotoninergic control. There is even some question as to the compound responsible for therapeutic actions. Fenfluramine in clinical use is a racemic mixture of d and l isomers that are both converted to active metabolites. All differ in their pharmacological properties, and their relative contributions to behavioral change are yet to be sorted out (Borroni, Ceci, Garattini, & Mennini, 1983; Caccia et al., 1981; Mennini, Garattini, & Caccia, 1985). Finally, as indicated in the introduction, neurotransmitter systems are interactive, and although brain serotonin but not brain catecholamines are affected by low doses of fenfluramine, higher doses of acutely administered drug increases the dopamine metabolite homovanillic acid in the striatum (Jori & Bernardi, 1969) but not dopamine, perhaps by blocking postsynaptic dopamine receptors (Garattini, Buczko, Jori, & Samanin, 1975). Acute administration at relatively high doses also increases striatal and hippocampal acetylcholine (Samanin, Quattrone, Peri, Ladinsky, & Consolo, 1978) and noncompetitively inhibits both GABA and glutamate uptake into synaptosomes while stimulating glutamic acid decarboxylase and inhibiting GABA transaminase (Kouyoumdjian, Gonnart, & Balin, 1979). The drug also acts on the autonomic nervous system to lower circulating norepinephrine and dopamine-B-hydroxylase (De la Vega, Slater, Ziegler, Lake, & Murphy, 1977; Leventhal, Schaffer, & Freedman, 1985). The importance of any of these to fenfluramine's clinical actions remains to be determined.

Catecholamines

The catecholamines, dopamine and norepinephrine, share with serotonin the dubious honor of being implicated in a variety of neurological and psychiatric diseases as well as in normal behaviors. They also closely resemble serotonin in metabolism. Catecholamines are made from the essential amino acid tyrosine to which is added an atom of molecular oxygen by the rate-limiting enzyme tyrosine hydroxylase. The product 3,4-dihydroxyphenylalanine or dopa is decarboxylated to 3,4-dihydroxyphenethylamine or dopamine (DPM), which is taken into storage vesicles to be released upon nerve stimulation. In dopaminergic neurons synthesis stops here. In noradrenergic neurons the vesicles contain another enzyme, dopamine-beta-hydroxylase, which hydroxylates the side chain to form norepinephrine. Some of the dopamine-beta-hydroxylase is also released with norepinephrine when the nerve discharges (Weinshilboum, Raymond, Elveback, & Weidman, 1973).

As with serotonin, the side chain of the catecholamines undergoes oxidation by mono-amine oxidase (MAO) to finally yield the corresponding acids or alcohols. Monoamine oxidase is located within the cell. In addition, another enzyme, catechol-O-metyltransferase (COMT), located outside the cell, adds a methyl (CH_3) group to the ring hydroxyl at position 3. The combined action of these two enzymes produce a series of oxidized, meth-ylated, and both oxidized and methylated compounds, the more relevant of which will be discussed in context below. Because oxidation is carried out intracellularly and methylation extracellularly, unmethylated oxidation products are considered to represent intracellular turnover while methylated compounds are thought to reflect transmitter released into the synaptic space and recaptured. The former is likely true; the latter is more complicated since oxidized, inactive, metabolites can also be released and methylated.

Dopamine

Tissue Levels. The most popular current theory of the etiology of schizophrenia is the hyperdopaminergic theory, which derives largely from the fact that most antipsychotics interfere with some aspect of dopaminergic transmission. The status of the dopamine system in autism therefore is of obvious interest. The major product of the combined action of MAO and COMT on dopamine is 3-methoxy-4-hydroxy phenylacetic acid or homovanillic acid (HVA). The contribution of brain dopamine to the HVA in blood and urine is estimated as between 30 and 60% (Maas, Hattok, Greene, & Landis, 1980), most of the remainder coming from the adrenal and the gut. Autistic children diagnosed according to the parental inventory (Rimland, 1979) are reported to have an elevated ratio of urinary HVA to urinary creatinine roughly proportional with severity (Garreau et al., 1980). Whether these subjects showed adrenal activation is unknown. Nor is it known whether variations in urinary creatinine might contribute to this relationship. Although commonly used as an indicator of muscle mass, urinary creatinine is influenced by clinical state (Yuwiler, 1969) and symptom severity. Vitamin B6 and magnesium loading is reported to improve clinical status (Rimland, Callaway, & Dreyfus, 1978) and reduce elevated urinary HVA to normal (Lelord et al., 1978; Martineau, Garreau, Barthelemy, Callaway, & Lelord, 1981). This somewhat paradoxical finding sug-gests that B6 and Mg probably do not act by increasing enzymatic efficiency since the only pyridoxal phosphate-metal-requiring enzyme in dopamine biosynthesis is aromatic amino acid decarboxylase. While not the rate-limiting enzyme in this pathway, these agents should, if anything, increase decarboxylase activity, dopamine synthesis, and HVA formation. These findings need to be verified on subjects diagnosed by parental inventory and by clinical criteria since the two populations may differ.

Present data suggest that lumbar HVA derives mainly from the brain since there is a steep HVA concentration along the cord (Garelis et al., 1974), concentrations increase above and decrease below any block in the spinal arachnoid space (Gerelis & Sourkes 1973; Young, Lal, Martin, Ford, & Sourkes, 1973), and HVA does not appear to enter CSF from blood (Bartholini, Pletscher, & Tissot 1966). As might be expected, the number of studies on CSF from children with autism is small. Only one study measured basal CSF concentrations and found that mean HVA concentrations for 13 drug-free autistic children were higher than for matched controls (451 nmoles/L vs. 304). One child had a particularly high concentration (894) (Gillberg et al., 1983). In the same study, 9 children with other psychoses also had high values (445) as compared to matched controls (270). Clearly this study warrants attempted replication to verify an association with childhood autism specifically or disturbed children more generally.

Unfortunately, lesser differences have been reported in studies measuring CSF concentrations after probenecid blockade of HVA transport from the brain. Thus, 9 autistic subjects had lower HVA concentrations than 11 atypical children (141 vs. 175 ng/ml) in one study (Cohen et al., 1974) but were not different from various nonautistic populations in two others—205 for autistic subjects, 231 for nonautistic subjects, 196 for contrast subjects (Cohen, Caparulo, et al., 1977), 192 for autistic subjects, and 191 for other subjects (Leckman et al., 1980). The problems associated with probenecid studies have been alluded to already and may serve to obscure, rather than clarify, the status of the dopamine system in autism.

Pharmacology. The increased urinary and, perhaps, CSF HVA provides some support for a dopaminergic role in at least the symptom expression of autism. Additional support can be taken from the fact that amphetamine, which can act as an indirect dopamine agonist, exacerbates the preexisting stereotypic motor behavior of the autistic subject (Campbell et al., 1976) while neuroleptics, which have dopamine blocking properties, have some therapeutic efficacy (Campbell et al., 1976; Cohen et al., 1980; Fish et al., 1969a). The therapeutic effects of antipsychotics will be discussed in detail elsewhere in this series and will not be detailed here. In general, however, their effects in reducing the frequency of stereotyped behaviors and hyperactivity could be taken to further support a role for dopamine in the motor disturbances in autism.

Norepinephrine

Tissue Levels. Plasma norephinephrine concentrations of subjects with childhood autism have been reported to be elevated whether subjects were sampled when supine or erect (Lake, Ziegler, & Murphy, 1977), and hyperserotoninemic children with autism had strikingly higher levels of norepinephrine than siblings or stressed or tranquil controls (Leventhal, Schaffer, & Freedman, 1985). This suggests enhanced discharge of the sympathetic nervous system, which is compatible with reports that children with autism have higher mean blood flow and lower vascular resistance (Cohen & Johnson, 1977). Such increased sympathetic discharge could result from psychogenic fear and anxiety or from physiological processes like defective norepinephrine reuptake or sympathetic control. A single blood measure, however, is a single instantaneous glimpse of metabolic traffic between tissues; a momentary glimpse of variables such as blood catecholamines and cardiovascular status, which are responsive to the moment's environmental stimuli and to circadian changes, is insufficient to establish a mean level of sympathetic arousal. This is evidenced by results on dopamine-beta-hydroxylase (DBH) activity in autism. As indicated in the introduction, DBH is stored together with norepinephrine in the storage vesicles in the nerve terminal and is partly released with it upon sympathetic stimulation. Because the enzyme has a longer half-life in blood than circulating catecholamines, its activity has been used as an index of chronic, but not acute, changes in sympathetic tone. Accordingly, elevated DBH might parallel chronically elevated sympathetic tone. Its status in autistic children, however, is uncertain, being reported as above normal (Freedman, Roffman, & Goldstein, 1973), the same as that of children with organic psychosis but lower than that of childhood schizophrenics (Belmaker, Hattab, & Ebstein, 1978), and lower than normal (Goldstein et al., 1976; Lake et al., 1977). Since the enzyme is under considerable genetic control, a study comparing the DBH of relatives of children with autism and especially of members of families with multiple incidence would provide interesting information on genetic contributions to the conflicting findings.

Both of the catecholamine-degrading enzymes are found in peripheral tissues and have been measured. As previously discussed, MAO activity in platelets and fibroblasts from children with autism appears normal. So too does COMT activity in red cells and fibroblasts (O'Brien, Semenuk, Coleman, & Spector, 1976; Walker, Danielson, & Levitt, 1976). Schizophrenic children, however, seemed to have lower COMT activity than children with or without psychosis or autistic symptoms (Walker *et al.*, 1976). This difference, if confirmed, may be relevant to the continuing debate over the relationship between autism and childhood schizophrenia. Again it should be stressed that these results do not preclude population difference in the activities of these enzymes in the brain.

The final product of norepinephrine oxidation in the brain and the periphery differs, providing possible distinction between the two in body fluids. In the brain, norepinephrine is largely converted to the alcohol 3,4-dihydroxyphenylglycol, which when methylated by COMT becomes 3-methoxy-4-hydroxyphenylglycol (MHPG). In peripheral tissue it is largely changed to the acid 3,4-dihydroxymandelic acid, which is converted by COMT to 3-methyl-4-hydroxymandelic acid or, more commonly, vanillymandelic acid (VMA).

Increased sympathetic tone among children with autism might be expected to be evident in concentrations of VMA. This has not been directly measured, but it is interesting that Hanley *et al.* (1977) found that autistic children had markedly greater VMA in urines obtained after tryptophan loading than did mildly retarded children. Unfortunately, baseline measures were not made but it seems unlikely that this difference was due to the tryptophan loading itself.

While MHPG largely derives from brain, the magnitude of the contribution is not yet settled. About 60% of total body MHPG was originally thought to derive from brain on the basis of the MHPG content of blood in vessels entering and leaving the brain (Maas, Hattox, Greene, & Landis, 1980). This has been revised downward to account for the relatively easy exchange of MHPG between CSF, blood, and urine (Chase, Gordon, & Ng, 1973; Kopin, Gordon, Jimerson, & Polinksy, 1983) and the discovery that much of the MHPG from brain is converted to VMA (Blombery, Kopin, Gordon, Markey, & Ebert, 1980).

In contrast to the reported elevated blood norepinephrine in children with autism (Lake *et al.*, 1977), blood MHPG concentration is either less than (Young, Cohen, Caparulo, Brown, & Maas, 1979) or the same as that of controls (Young, *et al.*, 1981). Similarly, urinary and CSF MHPG concentrations are also indistinguishable from those of controls (Gillberg *et al.*, 1983; Young *et al.*, 1981).

Pharmacology. Relevant pharmacological studies are limited to the use of tricyclic antidepressants, many of which are norepinephrine reuptake inhibitors, and amphetamines and dopa, which affect dopamine as well as norepinephrine. In general, tricyclic antidepressants have not proven to be particularly efficacious (Kurtis, 1966), while amphetamines or methylphenidate appear to worsen symptoms (Campbell *et al.*, 1972). The effects of dopa have been discussed already.

In sum, there is currently no data indicative of a major noradrenergic abnormality in autism.

Neuropeptides

The clinical significance of the neuropeptides is the object of much investigation, but only a few studies on opioid peptides have been directed to autism. This large complex family of compounds derives largely from three precursor polypeptides, proenkephalin A, proenkephalin B, and proopiomelanocortin, which are cleaved by specific peptidases in specific tissues to give, respectively, the methionine and leucine enkephalins, the dynorphins, and polypeptides like beta-endorphin, ACTH, and MSH. These show different anatomical distributions and have somewhat different properties. On the basis of similarities in responses to pain and social contacts, first Kalat (Kalat, 1978) and then Panksepp (1979) suggested that autistic children might suffer from chronic or intermittent hyperactivity of enkephalin and/or endorphin system. Support for this is reviewed in Chapter 19. In one study an opiate receptor assay was used to examine for opiate peptides in two factions of CSF; I, rich in dynorphins and II, rich in enkephalins (Gillberg, Terenius, & Lönnerholm, 1985). CSF from 20 autistic, 4 psychotic nonautistic, and a comparison group of 8 children initially suspected of having neurological symptoms were examined. Groups did not statistically differ in mean CSF concentrations of Fraction I peptides (derived largely from proenkephalin B), although one-third of the autistic subjects had values well outside the range for the comparison group. Similarly, these subjects did not differ from the comparison group in the concentration of Fraction II peptides, although half had values well outside the normal range. Concentrations of Fraction I and Fraction II did not correlate, demonstrating the heterogeneity of response of the opiate systems, but values for Fraction II were reportedly high in subjects with decreased pain sensitivity. This, together with the large variance among autistic and psychotic subjects, would be compatible with etiological heterogeneity.

More information on the exact composition of Fractions I and II are needed in order to evaluate if the results support the hypothesis of opioid hyperactivity in autism or whether they help define an etiological subgroup.

In seeming contrast to possible increased enkephalin levels in the CSF of autistic and psychotic children, blood levels of humoral endorphin H, an opioid peptide having a bell-shaped dose response to naloxone blockade, was about half as great in 4 unmedicated autistic subjects, and 4 schizophrenic subjects as in 11 healthy controls. In contrast, 6 medicated autistic subjects and 8 medicated schizophrenic subjects had blood levels equal to that of controls (Weizman et al., 1984). This suggests that endorphin H concentration either is related to the behaviors controlled by these drugs or is directly affected by drug. In addition, the similar endorphin H concentrations of untreated autistic and schizophrenic subjects suggests that concentration reflects some feature common to these populations; it seems unlikely to be directly related to etiology.

Only 8% of autistic children are reported to show "normal" chromatographic patterns of urinary peptides and protein-associated peptide complexes. The remainder showed one of four abnormal patterns. Three of these patterns were common to the children who were autistic, psychotic or mentally retarded, had minimal brain function, or had attention deficit disorder. Twelve percent of the autistic subjects showed a relatively distinctive pattern of excretion (Gillberg, Trygstad, & Foss, 1982). It remains to be determined whether these peptides have any relationship to peripheral levels of opioid peptides or whether they mirror diet, drug, or activity level.

CONCLUSION

What, then, is one to make of all this? First, it is clear that current data are insufficient to draw any conclusions regarding the status of brain transmitter systems in autism. Many of the variables studied may alter for reasons unrelated to these systems, and most studies neither have been replicated nor involve enough subjects to permit a compelling conclusion.

Seldom have a full array of relevant variables been studied on the same populations (Freedman *et al.*, 1981), so that the bulk of the literature is a hodgepodge of disparate findings on disparate populations. Further, the paucity of subjects has hindered serious attempts to examine for etiologically distinct subpopulations. It can be expected that progress on the etiology of autism (and other diseases of low incidence) will remain slow until logistical procedures develop for sharing populations and tissues and for rapid independent replication of promising preliminary results. At present, reports that autistic subjects differ from controls in platelet serotonin uptake, free blood tryptophan, urinary HVA-creatinine ratio, circulating antibodies to 5HT 1A receptors or myelin basic protein, and perhaps in basal CSF HVA and endorphin H concentrations all need replication, and more work is needed on establishing the mechanism for hyperserotoninemia in autism. Further, new procedures now permit investigations into the status of a host of transmitters other than the monoamines. In addition, there have been recent advances in noninvasive imaging techniques that may contribute to information on the status of transmitter systems in autism. Especially promising are magnetic and positron emission tomography, although at the moment the former is largely limited to examining protons and the latter virtually requires an adjacent cyclotron. Finally, brain banks have facilitated biochemical studies on postmortem brain. We do not yet have sufficient information to infer quantitative or qualitative variations in skills and aptitudes from altered regional concentrations of transmitters and their metabolites, enzymic activities, or receptor densities and properties. However, major disruptions in transmitter systems, as occurs, for example, in Parkinsonism, are detectable even over the statistical noise contributed by variations in agonal state, drug, time, storage, and dissection techniques.

While progress has been slow, the identification of autism is only 40 years old and only 20 years have elapsed since the first biochemical studies on the syndrome. Neurochemical and behavioral understanding of the fundamental properties of the brain is growing at an exponential rate, and there is much hope for the future.

REFERENCES

Anderson, G. M., Minderaa, R. B., van Benthem, P-P, G., Volkmar, F. R., & Cohen, D. J. (1984). Platelet imipramine binding in autistic subjects. *Psychiatry Research, 11,* 133–141.

August, G. J., Raz, N., & Baird, T. D. (1985). Brief report: Effects of fenfluramine on behavioral, cognitive, and affective disturbances in autistic children. *Journal of Autism and Developmental Disorders, 15,* 97–107.

August, G. J., Raz, N., Papanicolaou, A. C., Baird, T. D., Hirsh, S. L., & Hsu, L. L. (1984). Fenfluramine treatment in infantile autism. *Journal of Nervous and Mental Disease, 172,* 604–612.

Axelrod, J., & Iscoe, J. K. (1963). The uptake and binding of circulating serotonin and the effects of drugs. *Journal of Pharmacology and Experimental Therapeutics, 141,* 161–165.

Baraban, J. H., & Aghajanian, G. K. (1981). Noradrenergic innervation of serotoninergic neurones in the dorsal raphe. Demonstration by electronmicroscopic autoradiography. *Brain Research, 204,* 1–11.

Bartholini, G., Pletscher, A., & Tissot, R. (1966). On the origin of homovanillic acid in the cerebrospinal fluid. *Experientia (Basel), 22,* 609–610.

Becker, M. A., Paivio, K. O., Bakay, B., Adams, W. B., & Nyhan, W. L. (1980). Variant human phosphoriboxylpyrophosphate synthetase altered in regulatory and catalytic functions. *Journal of Clinical Investigation, 65,* 109–120.

Belmaker, R. H., Hattab, J., & Ebstein, R. P. (1978). Plasma dopamine-beta hydroxylase in childhood psychosis. *Journal of Autism and Childhood Schizophrenia, 8,* 293–298.

Belendiuk, K., Belendiuk, G. W., and Freedman, D. X. (1980). Blood monoamine metabolites in Huntington's disease. *AMA Archives of General Psychiatry, 37,* 325–332.

Belendiuk, K., Belendiuk, G. W., Freedman, D. X., & Antel, J. P. (1981). Neurotransmitter abnormalities in patients with motor neuron disease. *Archives of Neurology, 38,* 415–417.

Bender, L., Cobrinik, L., Faretra, G., & Sankar, D. V. S. (1966). The treatment of childhood schizophrenia with LSD and UML. In M. Rinkel (Ed.), *Biological treatment of mental illness.* New York: C. Page.

Bertaccini, G. (1960). Tissue serotonin and urinary 5-HIAA after partial or total removal of the gastrointestinal tract in the rat. *Journal of Physiology, 153,* 239–243.

Blombery, P. A., Kopin, I. J., Gordon, E. K., Markey, S. P., & Ebert, M. H. (1980). Conversion of MHPG to vanillymandelic acid. *AMA Archives of General Psychiatry, 37,* 1095–1098.

Borroni, E., Ceci, A., Garattini, S., & Mennini, T. (1983). Differences between d-fenfluramine and d-norfenfluramine in serotonin presynaptic mechanisms. *Journal of Neurochemistry, 40,* 891–893.

Boullin, D. J. (1978). Biochemical indication of central serotonin function. In D. J. Boullin (Ed.), *Serotonin and mental abnormalities.* New York: Wiley.

Boullin, D. J., Bhagavan, H. N., Coleman, M., O'Brien, R. A., & Youdim, M. B. (1975). Platelet monoamine oxidase activity and hematocrit in children with infantile autism. *Medical Biology, 53,* 210–213.

Boullin, D. J., Coleman, M., & O'Brien, R. A. (1970). Abnormalities in platelet 5-hydroxytryptamine efflux in patients with infantile autism. *Nature, 226,* 371–372.

Boullin, D. J., Coleman, M., O'Brien, R. A., & Rimland, B. (1971). Laboratory predictions of infantile autism based on 5-hydroxytryptamine efflux from blood platelets and their correlation with the Rimland E2 score. *Journal of Autism and Childhood Schizophrenia, 1,* 63–71.

Boullin, D., Freeman, B. J., Geller, E., Ritvo, E., Rutter, M., & Yuwiler, A. (1982). Toward the resolution of conflicting findings. *Journal of Autism and Developmental Disorders, 12,* 97–98.

Brown, W. T., Jenkins, E. C., Friedman, E., Brooks, J., Wisniewski, K., Raguthu, S., & French, J. (1982). Autism associated with fragile-X syndrome. *Journal of Autism and Developmental Disorders, 12,* 303–308.

Caccia, S., Dagnino, G., Garattini, S., Guiso, G., Madonna, R., & Zanini, M. G. (1981). Kinetics of fenfluramine isomers in the rat. *European Journal of Drug Metabolism and Pharmacokinetics, 6,* 297–301.

Campbell, M., Deutsch, S. I., Perry, R., Wolsky, B. B., & Palij, M. (1986). Short term efficacy and safety of fenfluramine in hospitalized preschool-age autistic children: An open study. *Psychopharmacology Bulletin, 22,* 141–147.

Campbell, M., Fish, B., David, R., Shapiro, T., Collins, P., & Koh, C. (1972). Response to triiodothyronine and dextroamphetamine: A study of preschool schizophrenic children. *Journal of Autism and Childhood Schizophrenia, 2,* 343–358.

Campbell, M., Fish, B., Shapiro, T., & Floyd, A., Jr. (1971). Imipramine in preschool autistic and schizophrenic children. *Journal of Autism and Childhood Schizophrenia, 1,* 267–282.

Campbell, M., Friedman, E., DeVito, E., Greenspan, L., & Collins, P. J. (1974). Blood serotonin in psychotic and brain-damaged children. *Journal of Autism and Childhood Schizophrenia, 4,* 33–41.

Campbell, M., Small, A. M., Collins, P. J., Friedman, E., Davyd, R., & Genieser, N. B. (1976). Levodopa and levoamphetamine: A crossover study in schizophrenic children. *Current Therapeutic Research, 18,* 70–86.

Chan-Palay, V., Jonsson, G., & Palay, S. L. (1978). Serotonin and substance P coexist in neurones of the rat central nervous system. *Proceedings of the National Academy of Sciences, USA, 75,* 1582–1586.

Chase, T. N., Gordon, E. K., & Ng, L. K. Y. (1973). Norepinephrine metabolism in the central nervous system of man: Studies using 3-methoxy-4-hydroxyphenylethylene glycol levels in cerebrospinal fluid. *Journal of Neurochemistry, 21,* 581–587.

Chess, S. (1971). Autism in children with congenital rubella. *Journal of Autism and Childhood Schizophrenia, 1,* 33–47.

Cohen, D. J., Caparulo, B. K., Shaywitz, B. A., & Bowers, M. B., Jr. (1977). Dopamine and serotonin metabolism in neuropsychiatrically disturbed children, CSF homovanillic acid and 5-hydroxyindoleacetic acid. *AMA Archives of General Psychiatry, 34*, 545–556.

Cohen, D. J., & Johnson, W. T. (1977). Cardiovascular correlates of attention in normal and psychiatrically disturbed children. *AMA Archives of General Psychiatry, 34*, 561–567.

Cohen, D. J., Shaywitz, B. A., Johnson, W. T., & Bowers, M. (1974). Biogenic amines in autistic and atypical children: Cerebrospinal fluid measures of homovanillic acid and 5-hydroxyindoleacetic acid. *AMA Archives of General Psychiatry, 31*, 845–853.

Cohen, D. J., Young, J. G., & Roth, J. A. (1977). Platelet monoamine oxidase in early childhood autism. *AMA Archives of General Psychiatry, 34*, 534–537.

Cohen, I. L., Campbell, M., Posner, D., Small, A. M., Triebel, D., & Anderson, L. T. (1980). Behavioral effects of haloperidol in young autistic children. *Journal of the American Academy of Child Psychiatry, 19*, 665–677.

Coleman, M., & Blass, J. P. (1985). Autism and lactic acidosis. *Journal of Autism and Developmental Disorders, 15*, 1–8.

Coleman, M., Landgrebe, M. A., & Landgrebe, A. R. (1976). Purine autism. Hyperuricosuria in autistic children; does this identify a subgroup of autism? In M. Coleman (Ed.), *The autistic syndromes*. Amsterdam: North-Holland.

Costa, E., Groppeti, A., & Revuelta, A. (1971). Action of fenfluramine on monoamine stores in rat tissue. *British Journal of Pharmacology and Chemotherapy, 41*, 57–63.

Damasio, H., Maurer, R. G., Damasio, A. R., & Chui, H. C. (1980). Computerized tomographic scan findings in patients with autistic behavior. *Archives of Neurology, 37*, 504–510.

De la Vega, C. E., Slater, S., Ziegler, M. G., Lake, C. R., & Murphy, D. L. (1979). Reductions in plasma norepinephrine during fenfluramine treatment. *Clinical Pharmacology and Therapy, 21*, 216–221.

De Lisi, L. E., Neckers, L. M., Weinberger, D. R., & Wyatt, R. J. (1981). Increased whole blood serotonin concentrations in chronic schizophrenic patients. *AMA Archives of General Psychiatry, 38*, 647–650.

DeMet, E. M., Halaris, A. E., & Bhatarakamul, S. (1978). Indoleamine compartmentation in human blood. *Clinica Chimica Acta, 89*, 285–292.

DeMyer, M. K., Schwier, H., Bryson, C. Q., Solow, E. B., & Roeske, N. (1971). Free fatty acid response to insulin and glucose stimulation in schizophrenic, autistic, and emotionally disturbed children. *Journal of Autism and Childhood Schizophrenia, 1*, 436–452.

Douay, O., Debray-Ritzen, P., & Kamoun, P. (1980). Serotonine et tryptophane sanguin dans l'autisme. *Annales de Biologie Clinique, 38*, 243.

Dray, A., Gonye, T. J., Oakley, N. R., & Tanner, T. (1976). Evidence for the existence of a raphe projection to the substantia nigra in the rat. *Brain Research, 113*, 45–57.

Duhault, J., & Boulanger, M. (1977). Fenfluramine long-term administration and brain serotonin. *European Journal of Pharmacology, 43*, 203.

Duhault, J., & Verdavainne, C. (1967). Modification du taux de serotoinine cerebrale chez le rat par les trifluoro ethyl-phenyl-2-ethylaminopropane (fenfluramine). *Archives of International Pharmacodynamics and Therapy, 170*, 276.

Dumbrille-Ross, A., & Tang, S. W. (1983). Manipulations of synaptic serotonin: Discrepancy of effects on serotonin S1 and S2 binding sites. *Life Sciences, 32*, 2677–2684.

Fish, B., Campbell, M., Shapiro, T., & Floyd, A., Jr. (1969a). Comparison of trifluperidol, trifluoperazine and chlorpromazine in preschool schizophrenic children: The value of less sedative antipsychotic agents. *Current Therapeutic Research, 11*, 589–595.

Fish, B., Campbell, M., Shapiro, T., & Floyd, A., Jr. (1969b). Schizophrenic children treated with methylsergide (Sansert). *Diseases of the Nervous System, 30*, 534–540.

Freedman, D. X., Belendiuk, K., Belendiuk, G. W., & Crayton, J. W. (1981). Blood tryptophan metabolism in chronic schizophrenics. *AMA Archives of General Psychiatry, 38*, 655–659.

Freedman, L. S., Roffman, M., & Goldstein, M. (1973). In E. Usdin & S. Snyder (Eds.), *Frontiers in catecholamine research*. Elmsford, New York: Pergamon Press.

Friedman, E. (1969). The "autistic syndrome" and phenylketonuria. *Schizophrenia, 1,* 249–261.

Fuller, R. W., & Perry, K. W. (1983). Decreased accumulation of brain 5-hydroxytryptophan after decarboxylase inhibition in rats treated with fenfluramine, norfenfluramine or p-chlorphenylalanine. *Journal of Pharmacy and Pharmacology, 35,* 0597–0598.

Garattini, S., Buczko, W., Jori, A., & Samanin, R. (1975). The mechanism of action of fenfluramine. *Postgraduate Medical Journal, 51,* (Supplement 1), 27.

Garattini, S., Caccia, S., Mennini, T., Samanin, R., Consolo, S., & Ladinsky, H. (1979). Biochemical pharmacology of the anorectic drug fenfluramine: A review. *Current Medical Research Opinion, 6* (Supplement 1), 15–270.

Garelis, E., & Sourkes, T. L. (1973). Sites of origin in the central nervous system of monoamine metabolites in human cerebrospinal fluid. *Journal of Neurology, Neurosurgery and Psychiatry, 4,* 625–629.

Garelis, E., Young, S. N., Lal, S., & Sourkes, T. L. (1974). Monoamine metabolites in lumbar CSF: The question of their origin in relation to clinical studies. *Brain Research, 79,* 1–8.

Garreau, B., Barthelemy, C., Domenech, J., Sauvage, D., Muh, J. P., Lelord, G., & Callaway, E. (1980). Troubles du metabolisme de la dopamine chez des infants ayant un comportement autistique. Resultats des examens clinique et des dosages urinaires de l'acide homovanilique (AHV). *Acta Psychiatrica Belgica, 80,* 249–265.

Geller, E., Ritvo, E. R., Freeman, B. J., & Yuwiler, A. (1982). Preliminary observations on the effect of fenfluramine on blood serotonin and symptoms in three autistic boys. *New England Journal of Medicine, 307,* 165–169.

Gillberg, C. (1983). Identical triplets with infantile autism and the fragile-X-syndrome. *British Journal of Psychiatry, 143,* 256–260.

Gillberg, C., & Forsell, C. (1984). Childhood psychosis and neurofibromatosis—More than a coincidence? *Journal of Autism and Developmental Disorders, 14,* 1–8.

Gillberg, C., & Svendsen, P. (1983). Childhood psychosis and computed tomographic brain scan findings. *Journal of Autism and Developmental Disorders, 13,* 19–32.

Gillberg, C., Svennerholm, L., & Hamilton-Hellberg, C. (1983). Childhood psychosis and monoamine metabolites in spinal fluid. *Journal of Autism and Developmental Disorders, 13,* 383–396.

Gillberg, C., Terenius, L., & Lönnerholm, G. (1985). Endorphin activity in childhood psychosis. Spinal levels in 24 cases. *AMA Archives of General Psychiatry, 42,* 780–783.

Gillberg, C., Trygstad, O., & Foss, I. (1982). Childhood psychosis and urinary excretion of peptides and protein-associated peptide complexes. *Journal of Autism and Developmental Disorders, 12,* 229–241

Giller, E. L., Jr., Young, G., Breakefield, X. O., Carbonari, C., Braverman, M., & Cohen, T. J. (1980). Monoamine oxidase and catechol-O-methyltransferase activities in cultured fibroblasts and blood cells from children with autism and Gilles de la Tourette syndrome. *Psychiatric Research, 2,* 187–197.

Goldstein, M., Mahanad, D., Lee, J., & Coleman, M. (1976). Dopamine-beta hydroxylase and endogenous total 5-hydroxyindole levels in autistic patients and controls. In M. Coleman (Ed.), *The autistic syndromes.* Amsterdam: North-Holland.

Hanley, H. G., Stahl, S. M., & Freedman, D. X. (1977). Hyperserotonemia and amine metabolites in autistic and retarded children. *Archives of General Psychiatry, 34,* 521–531.

Hauser, S., DeLong, G., & Rosman, N. (1975). Pneumographic findings in the infantile autism syndrome: A correlation with temporal lobe disease. *Brain, 98,* 667–688.

Hier, D. E., LeMay, M., & Rosenberg, P. B. (1979). Autism and unfavorable left-right asymmetries of the brain. *Journal of Autism and Developmental Disorders, 9,* 153–159.

Hokfelt, T., Renfeld, J. F., Skirboll, L., Ivemark, B., Goldstein, M., & Markey, K. (1980). Evidence for the coexistence of dopamine and CCK in meso-limbic neurones. *Nature, 285,* 476–478.

Hoshino, Y., Kumashiro, H., Kaneko, M., Numata, Y., Honda, K., Yashima, Y., Tachibana, R., & Watanabe, M. (1979). Serum serotonin, free tryptophan and plasma cyclic AMP levels in autistic children with special reference to hyperkinesia. *Fukushima Journal of Medical Science, 26,* 79–91.

Hoshino, Y., Yamamoto, T., Kaneko, M., Tachibana, R., Watanabe, M., Ono, Y., & Kumashiro, H. (1984). Blood serotonin and free tryptophan concentration in autistic children. *Neuropsychobiology, 11*, 22–27.

Irwin, M., Belendiuk, K., McCloskey, K., and Freedman, D. X. (1981). Tryptophan metabolism in children with attentional deficit disorder. *American Journal of Psychiatry, 138*, 1082–1085.

Jori, A., & Bernardi, D. (1969). The effects of amphetamine and amphetamine-like drugs on homovanillic acid concentration in the brain. *Journal of Pharmacy and Pharmacology, 21*, 694.

Kalat, J. W. (1978). Letter to the editor: Speculations on similarities between autism and opiate addiction. *Journal of Autism and Childhood Schizophrenia, 8*, 477–479.

Klein, R. L., Wilson, S. P., Dzielak, D. J., Yang, W. H., & Viveros, D. H. (1982). Opioid peptides and noradrenaline co-exist in large dense-cored vesicles from sympathetic nerve. *Neuroscience, 7*, 2255–2256.

Klykylo, W. M., Feldis, D., O'Grady, D., Ross, D. L., & Halloran, C. (1985). Brief report: Clinical effects of fenfluramine in ten autistic children. *Journal of Autism and Developmental Disorders, 15*, 425–436.

Knoblock, H., & Pasamanick, B. (1975). Some etiological and prognostic factors in early infantile autism and psychosis. *Pediatrics, 55*, 182–191.

Kopin, I. J., Gordon, E. K., Jimerson, D. C., & Polinsky, R. J. (1983). Relation between plasma and cerebrospinal fluid levels of 3-methoxy-4-hydroxyphenylglycol. *Science, 219*, 73–75.

Kotsopoulos, S., & Kutty, K. M. (1979). Histidinemia and infantile autism. *Journal of Autism and Developmental Disorders, 9*, 55–60.

Kouyoumdjian, J. C., Gonnart, P., & Balin, M. F. (1979). Effect of fenfluramine administration on synaptosomal uptake of some neurotransmitters and on synaptosomal enzymes which metabolise GABA. *Naunyn-Schmiedebergs Archiv für Pharmacologie, 309*, 7–11.

Kurtis, L. B. (1966). Clinical study of the response to nortriptyline on autistic children. *International Journal of Neuropsychiatry, 2*, 552–563.

Lake, C. R., Ziegler, M. G., & Murphy, D. L. (1977). Increased norepinephrine levels and decreased dopamine-beta-hydroxylase activity in primary autism. *AMA Archives of General Psychiatry, 34*, 553–556.

Leckman, J. F., Cohen, D. J., Shaywitz, B. A., Caparulo, B. K., Heninger, G. R., & Bowers, M. B., Jr. (1980). CSF monoamine metabolites in child and adult psychiatric patients. *AMA Archives of General Psychiatry, 37*, 677–681.

Lelord, G., Callaway, E., Muh, J. P., Arlot, J. C., Sauvage, D., Garreau, B., & Domenechi, J. (1978). Modification in urinary homovanillic acid after ingestion of vitamin B6: Functional study in autistic children. *Revue Neurologique, 134*, 797–801.

Leventhal, B. L., Schaffer, M., & Freedman, D. X. (1985). [Blood catecholamines in childhood diseases.] Unpublished raw data.

Lucas, A. R., Warner, K., & Gottlieb, J. S. (1971). Biological studies in childhood schizophrenia. *Biological Psychiatry, 38*, 39–48.

Maas, J. W., Hattox, S. E., Greene, N. M., & Landis, D. H. (1980). Estimate of dopamine and serotonin synthesis by the awake human brain. *Journal of Neurochemistry, 34*, 1547–1549.

Marsden, D., & McGuire, M. T. (1984). Whole blood serotonin and the Type A behavior pattern. *Psychosomatic Medicine, 46*, 546–548.

Martineau, J., Garreau, B., Barthelemy, C., Callaway, E., & Lelord, G. (1981). Effects of vitamin B6 on averaged evoked potentials in infantile autism. *Biological Psychiatry, 16*, 627–641.

McGuire, M. T., Raleigh, M. J., & Brammer, G. L. (1982). Sociopharmacology. *Annual Review of Pharmacology and Toxicology, 22*, 643–661.

McKean, C. N. (1972). The effects of high phenylalanine concentrations on serotonin and catecholamine metabolism in the human brain. *Brain Research, 42*, 469–476.

Mennini, T., Garattini, S., & Caccia, S. (1985). Anorectic effect of fenfluramine isomers and metabolites: Relationship between brain levels and in vitro potencies on serotoninergic mechanisms. *Psychopharmacology, 85*, 111–114.

Ng, K. Y., Chase, T. N., Colburn, R. W., & Kopin, I. J. (1970). L-dopa-induced release of cerebral monoamines. *Science, 170,* 76–77.

Nyhan, W. L., James, J. A., Tebert, A. J., Sweetman, L., & Nelson, L. G. (1969). A new disorder of purine metabolism with behavioral manifestations. *Journal of Pediatrics, 74,* 20.

O'Brien, R. A., Semenuk, G., Coleman, M., & Spector S. (1976). Cathechol-O-methyltransferase in erythrocytes of children with autism. *Journal of Clinical and Experimental Pharmacology and Physiology, 3,* 9–14.

Panksepp, J. (1979). A neurochemical theory of autism. *Trends in Neuroscience, 2,* 174–177.

Pare, C. M. B., Sandler, M., & Stacey, R. S. (1960). The relationship between decreased 5-hydroxyindole metabolism and mental defect in phenylketonuria. *Archives of Disease in Childhood, 34,* 422–425.

Parenti, M., Tirone, F., Olgiati, V. R., & Groppetti, A. (1983). Presence of opiate receptors on striatal serotoninergic nerve terminals. *Brain Research, 280,* 317–322.

Partington, M. W., Tu, J. B., & Wong, C. Y. (1973). Blood serotonin levels in severe mental retardation. *Developmental Medicine and Child Neurology, 15,* 616–627.

Pernow, B., & Waldenstrom, J. (1954). Paroxysmal flushing and other symptoms caused by 5-hydroxytryptamine and histamine in patients with malignant tumors. *Lancet, 2,* 951.

Pimparker, B. P., Senesky, D., & Kakser, M. H. (1961). Blood serotonin in non-tropical sprue. *Gastroenterology, 40,* 504–506.

Pletscher, A., Bartholini, G., & Tissor, R. (1967). Metabolic fate of L-(14C) dopa in cerebrospinal fluid and blood plasma of humans. *Brain Research, 4,* 106–109.

Raleigh, M. J., McGuire, M. T., Brammer, G. L., & Yuwiler, A. (1984). Social and environmental influences on blood serotonin concentrations in monkeys. *AMA Archives of General Psychiatry, 41,* 405–410.

Rimland, B. (1979). Institute for child behavior research form E-2. In D. J. Boullin (Ed.), *Serotonin and mental abnormalities.* New York: Wiley.

Rimland, B., Callaway, E., & Dreyfus, P. (1978). The effects of high doses of vitamine B6 on autistic children: A double blind crossover study. *American Journal of Psychiatry, 135,* 472–475.

Ritvo, E. R., Freeman, B. J., Geller, E., & Yuwiler, A. (1983). Effect of fenfluramine on 14 outpatients with the syndrome of autism. *Journal of the American Academy of Child Psychiatry, 6,* 549–558.

Ritvo, E. R., Freeman, B. J., Yuwiler, A., Geller, E., Schroth, P., Yokota, A., Mason-Brothers, A., August, G. J., Klykylo, W., Leventhal, B., Lewis, K., Piggot, L., Realmuto, G., Stubbs, E. G., & Umansky, R. (1986). Fenfluramine treatment of autism: UCLA collaborative study of 81 patients at nine medical centers. *Psychopharmacology Bulletin, 22,* 133–140.

Ritvo, E. R., Freeman, B. J., Yuwiler, A., Geller, E., Yokota, A., Schroth, P., & Novak, P. (1984). Study of fenfluramine in outpatients with the syndrome of autism. *Journal of Pediatrics, 105,* 823–828.

Ritvo, E. R., Yuwiler, A., Geller, E., Kales, A., Rashkis, S., Schicor, A., Plotkin, S., Axelrod, R., & Howard, C. (1971). Effects of L-dopa in autism. *Journal of Autism and Childhood Schizophrenia, 2,* 190–205.

Ritvo, E. R., Yuwiler, A., Geller, E., Ornitz, E., Saeger, K., & Plotkin, S. (1970). Increased blood serotonin and platelets in early infantile autism. *AMA Archives of General Psychiatry, 23,* 566–572.

Root-Bernstein, R. S., & Westall, F. C. (1983). Serotonin binding sites I. Structures of sites on myeline basic protein, LHRH, MSH, ACTH, interferon, serum albumin, ovalbumin and red pigment concentrating hormone. *Brain Research Bulletin, 12,* 425–436.

Rotman, A., Caplan, R., & Szekely, G. A. (1980). Platelet uptake of serotonin in psychotic children. *Psychopharmacology, 67,* 245–248.

Samanin, R., Mennini, T., Ferraris, A., Bendotti, C., & Borsini, F. (1980). Hypo- and hypersensitivity of central serotonin receptors: (3H) serotonin binding and functional studies in the rat. *Brain Research, 189,* 449–457.

Samanin, R., Quattrone, A., Peri, G., Ladinsky, H., & Consolo, S. (1978). Evidence for an interaction between serotoninergic and cholinergic neurones in the corpus striatum and hippocampus of the rat brain. *Brain Research, 151,* 73–82.

Sanders-Bush, E., Bushing, J. A., & Sulser, F. (1975). Long term effects of chloramphetamine and related drugs on central serotoninergic mechanisms. *Journal of Pharmacology and Experimental Therapeutics, 192*, 33–41.

Sankar, D. V. S., Cates, N., Broer, H. B., & Sankar, D. B. (1963). Biochemical parameters of childhood schizophrenia (autism) and growth. *Recent Advances in Biological Psychiatry, 5*, 76–83.

Sarai, K., & Kayano, M. (1968). The level and diurnal rhythm of serotonin in manic-depressive patients. *Folia Psychiatrica et Neurologica Japonica, 22*, 138–140.

Schain, R. J., & Freedman, D. X. (1961). Studies on 5-hydroxyindole metabolism in autistic and other mentally retarded children. *Journal of Pediatrics, 58*, 315–318.

Shaw, C., Lucas, J., & Rabinovitch, R. (1959). Metabolic studies in childhood schizophrenia. Effects of tryptophan loading on indole excretion. *AMA Archives of General Psychiatry, 1*, 366–370.

Shulman, N. R., Watkins, S. P., Jr., Itscoitz, S. B., & Students, A. B. (1969). Evidence that the spleen retains the youngest and hemostatically most effective platelets. *Transactions of the American Association of Physiology, 81*, 302–313.

Simon, H., LeMoal, M., Stinus, L., & Calas, A. (1979). Anatomical relationships between the ventral mesencephalic tegmentum-A10 region and the locus coeruleus as demonstrated by antegrade and retrograde tracing techniques. *Journal of Neural Transmission, 44*, 77–86.

Sjoerdsma, A., Weissbach, H., & Udenfriend, S. (1956). A clinical, physiological and biochemical study of patients with malignant carcinoid (argentoffinoma). *American Journal of Medicine, 20*, 520.

Steklis, H. D., Raleigh, M. J., Kling, A. S., & Tachiki, K. (1986). Biochemical and hormonal correlates of dominance and social behavior in male groups of squirrel monkeys (*Saimiri sciureus*). *American Journal of Primatology, 11*, 133–146.

Sverd, J., Kupietz, S. S., Winsberg, B. G., Hurwic, M. J., & Becker, M. A. (1978). Effects of 5-hydroxytryptophan in autistic children. *Journal of Autism and Childhood Schizophrenia, 8*, 1971–1980.

Takahashi, S., Kanai, H., & Miyamoto, Y. (1976). Reassessment of elevated serotonin levels in blood platelets in early infantile autism. *Journal of Autism and Childhood Schizophrenia, 6*, 317–326.

Todd, R. D., & Ciaranello, R. D. (1985). Demonstration of inter- and intraspecies differences in serotonin binding sites by antibodies from an autistic child. *Proceedings of the National Academy of Sciences (USA), 82*, 612–616.

Walker, H. A., Danielson, E., & Levitt, M. (1976). Catechol-O-methyltransferase activity in psychotic children. *Journal of Autism and Childhood Schizophrenia, 6*, 263–268.

Weinshilboum, R. M., Raymond, F. A., Elveback, L. R., & Weidman, W. H. (1973). Dopamine beta hydroxylase activity in serum. In E. Usdin & S. Snyder (Eds.), *Frontiers in catecholamine research*. New York: Pergamon Press.

Weizman, A., Weizman, R., Szekely, G. A., Wijsenbeek, H., & Livni, E. (1982). Abnormal immune response to brain tissue antigen in the syndrome of autism. *American Journal of Psychiatry, 139*, 1462–1465.

Weizman, R., Weizman, A., Tyano, S., Szekely, G., Weissman, B. A., & Sarne, Y. (1984). Humoral-endorphin blood levels in autistic, schizophrenic and healthy subjects. *Psychopharmacology, 82*, 368–370.

Westall, F. C., & Root-Bernstein, R. S. (1983). Suggested connection between autism, serotonin, and myelin basic protein. *American Journal of Psychiatry, 140*, 1260.

Winsberg, B. G., Sverd, J., Castells, S., Hurwic, M., & Perel, J. M. (1980). Estimation of monoamine and cyclic-AMP turnover and aminoacid concentrations of spinal fluid in autistic children. *Neuropediatrics, 11*, 250–255.

Young, J. G., Cohen, D. J., Caparulo, B. K., Brown, S. L., & Maas, J. W. (1979). Decreased 24-hour urinary MHPG in childhood autism. *American Journal of Psychiatry, 136*, 1055–1057.

Young, J. G., Cohen, D. J., Kavanagh, M. E., Landis, H. D., Shaywitz, B. A., & Maas, J. W. (1981). Cerebrospinal fluid, plasma, and urinary MHPG in children. *Life Sciences, 28*, 2837–2845.

Young, J. G., Cohen, D. J., & Roth, J. A. (1978). Association between platelet MAO and hematocrit in childhood autism. *Life Sciences, 23,* 797–806.

Young, S. N., Lal, S., Martin, J. B., Ford, R. M., & Sourkes, T. L. (1973). 5-hydroxyindole acetic acid, homovanillic acid, and tryptophan levels in the CSF above and below a complete block of CSF flow. *Psychiatria Neurologia Neurochirurgia* (Amsterdam), *76,* 439–444.

Yuwiler, A. (1969). Basal biochemical measures and their possible influence on biochemical tests for schizophrenia. In D. V. Siva-Sankar (Ed.), *Schizophrenia: Current concepts and research.* Hicksville, NY: PJD Press.

Yuwiler, A., Ritvo, E., Freeman, E. J., Yarborough, E., & Sanat, U. (1984). [Stability of blood serotonin in autistic children.] Unpublished raw data.

Yuwiler, A., Ritvo, E., Bald, D., Kipper, D., & Koper, A. (1971). Examination of circadian rhythmicity of blood serotonin and platelets in autistic and non-autistic children. *Journal of Autism and Childhood Schizophrenia, 1,* 421–435.

Yuwiler, A., Ritvo, E., Geller, E., Glousman, P., Schneiderman, G., & Matsuno, D. (1975). Uptake and efflux of serotonin from platelets of autistic and nonautistic children. *Journal of Autism and Childhood Schizophrenia, 5,* 83–98.

Zarcone, V., Kales, A., Scharf, M., Tan, T-L., Simmons, J. Q., & Dement, W. C. (1973). Repeated oral ingestion of 5-hydroxytryptophan. *AMA Archives of General Psychiatry, 28,* 843–846.

16

A Neurophysiological View of Autism

ERIC COURCHESNE

INTRODUCTION

Attentional Orientation

Parents, teachers, clinicians, and researchers consistently observe that people with autism do not seem to pay attention to their environment in a normal fashion, and do not, as a rule, respond to stimuli that would be surprising and attention-getting to normal people.

People with autism may sometimes seem, for example, completely oblivious to even novel, unexpected sounds and may not give any overt indication that they were surprised or startled (giving an orienting response), or that they were curious about the source (focusing their attention on the event). At other times, they may seem intensely attentive to something to the total exclusion of everything else, and they may become intensely upset by even small changes from a regular, expected pattern of stimulation.

Autistic people seem, therefore, to be able to attend and to orient, but it is not clear how these mechanisms function differently from those of normal individuals. In other words, their *attentional orientation* to the world clearly differs from normal, but at present there exists no adequate framework for predicting their attentional orientations. Moreover, no adequate model exists for explaining how neural dysfunction creates this difference developmentally each and every day of the child's life.

Although Rimland (1964) suggested that autism may involve some sort of disordered functioning of the reticular formation, it has remained an important research question as to whether these defects are characterized by increased and/or decreased sensitivity and attention to novel stimulation (Gold & Gold, 1975; James & Barry, 1980; Kootz & Cohen, 1981; Rutter, 1979). There is sometimes clinical evidence of more dysfunction with auditory stimulus processing than with visual (e.g., Hoffman & Prior, 1982). Since detecting, paying attention to, and learning about new and significant information is an essential requirement

ERIC COURCHESNE • Neurosciences Department, School of Medicine, University of California at San Diego, La Jolla, California 92093; and Neuropsychology Research Laboratory, Children's Hospital Research Center, San Diego, California 92123.

for normal development, a defect in attentional orientation to new and significant information could have devastating consequences.

Finally, since autistic infants and children sometimes seem oblivious to sounds, natural questions would be whether abnormal hearing is the cause for the failure to attentionally orient to the auditory world.

Conceptual Orientation

Normal people maintain not only an attentional orientation to the sources of information but also a *conceptual orientation* to the pattern and the significance of specific information that is useful, expected, or important to us coming from this source.

In our normal everyday living, we keep up-to-date ideas about what has been happening and what is happening, so that we can better anticipate future events. Also, among our ideas, we hold some to be more important than others. Input which disconfirms our ideas of what is important causes us to alter them.

Broadly speaking, our conceptual orientation, or ideas, have many facets, among which are the following four. First, we form a general concept of the overall ongoing context, such as the global probability of certain events that are taking place. Second, we "automatically" keep account of the most recent patterns of stimulation (see Johnson & Donchin, 1982) to form an idea of the local context. Third, we keep track of specific information that we know will aid us in accomplishing our goals. Fourth, we tag certain ideas as more important than others, and we treat input relating to such ideas accordingly. Whenever input does not coincide with one of these four facets, we alter our concepts.

People with autism seem to have deficits in conceptual orientation as well as in attentional orientation. They have remarkable difficulties in altering their ideas about the world, as well as attending to the world. I am reminded of one subject who drives a car. He was able to find his way to Children's Hospital the first time but parked his car at the opposite end of the hospital from our laboratory. Although he knew, after the first visit, that we were located at the other end of the hospital, he still insisted on parking his car in the same place, walking to the same entrance, and waiting for us in the same way he did on the first visit.

It sometimes seems that even when autistic people are intensely attentive to a stimulus input, they still have difficulty altering their ideas about it in the face of changing environmental information. It is as if they make cognitive representations of fragments or chunks of information that, once made, exist independently of the environmental context; these representations persist despite changes in the context, which, in normal people, would require changes in the original representation.

Autistic individuals are also notoriously indifferent to how important an incoming piece of information may be. They often do not seem to make distinctions between pieces of information of different values.

A Question

What, in autism, is the nervous system doing with information? Invocations of disordered reticular formation, abnormal hearing, abnormal levels of serotonin, abnormal hippocampi, abnormal frontal cortex, and similar factors do not explain why autistic individuals process visual information better than they do auditory; why autistic persons (especially nonretarded ones) have such idiosyncratic and diverse "islands of skill or knowledge" such as the ability to do rapid multicolumn multiplication, or the ability to recall precisely types of bicycles, types of street lamps, and TV program schedules; why even very high-functioning nonretarded autistic people have great difficulty with social and auditory language information but not with highly complex visual information, such as reading; why many terribly disturbed autistic infants and children eventually develop so many remarkable skills; why autistic children may seek the same information or perform the same action over and over—yet with no two children doing, saying, or seeking exactly the same things; and so on.

The combination of recording the neural activity of autistic people and of measuring their behavior may provide important answers. After all, if one wants to know what the nervous system in autism is doing with information, why not record this activity?

Currently, the best way to do this is to record a person's neural responses to specific pieces of information delivered to him or her. This technique is called ERP recording. ERP refers to the "event-related potential" of the brain in direct response to information. ERP recordings pick up a great deal of neural activity, but not all the responses to a particular piece of information. ERPs provide a good sample of neural activity from sensory, cognitive, and motor levels of the nervous system.

As with all technical approaches to studying the brain, ERP recording makes certain requirements of the scientist if it is to be used properly. The following two sections provide information about ERPs so that the reader and the non-ERP scientist may better appreciate these requirements and may better discern useful from not-so-useful research reports on ERPs.

AN INTRODUCTION TO ERPS

Description of Recording and Basic Terms

ERPs in humans are recorded, in nonsurgical settings, by placing EEG electrodes on the surface of the scalp and sending the electrical potentials detected by the electrodes through electrical amplifiers to an electrical data storage device such as a computer. The ERPs recorded in this way represent a sample of the activity of the brain.

ERPs are distinguished from EEG in that the brain activity represented by the ERP is evoked by a specified event. That is, the ERP is time-locked to a specified event. The exact time of occurrence of this event must be known. The event may be physical, such as a musical chord or a picture, or psychological, such as the decision that something that was supposed to happen did not, or that something novel happened. The moment of this psychological event may be inferred from a button press by the subject, for example.

Also, the brain activity evoked by the specified event generates an electrical field of some magnitude and duration. The metal electrode on the scalp represents a body in this field and, therefore, is at some electrical potential relative to the part of the brain generating the field.

Thus, a particular recorded potential of the ERP has several characteristics: It occurs at some time or latency after an event; latency is measured in milliseconds (ms) after the occurrence of the event. It has a magnitude or amplitude, which is measured in micro-volts (μV) or millionths of a volt. It has a duration, which is how long the potential lasts

in ms. Finally, it has a spatial distribution, which refers to the fact that some scalp electrode sites may be at a position of greater potential (amplitude in μV) than other electrode
sites.

Description of an ERP "Record"

A particular event evokes a volley of activities in numerous parts of the brain at
numerous times following it. An auditory stimulus, for example, evokes activity detectable
by scalp electrodes at a latency of less than 2 ms (0.002 s). Activity in response to this
stimulus may be recorded from that early latency to as late as 1200 ms (1.2 s). The amplitude
of the potentials recorded can range from 0.3 μV (0.3 millionths of a volt) to perhaps 80 μV.

Each electrode is capable of detecting a number of potentials. These may be early or
late in latency, large or small in amplitude. An ERP record from a single scalp electrode,
therefore, is a series of potentials, each with its own latency, amplitude, duration, and spatial
distribution (Figure 1). For example, a single auditory stimulus may evoke more than 20
different potentials, each generated by a different neural system.

Such discrete potentials are called components. Each has a characteristic latency range
and a characteristic spatial distribution. "Characteristic spatial distribution" refers to the idea
that for each component, there are scalp electrode sites where it tends to be largest in
amplitude, and other sites where it tends to be smaller or absent. Each component is assumed
to be associated with discrete processes or functional states of the brain.

In one ERP record, it is certain that many components overlap to a lesser or greater
degree in time and spatial distribution. This overlapping sometimes presents difficulties in
identifying and measuring individual components.

In sum, a single ERP record consists of a series of components that are generated by
neural systems involved in sensory, cognitive, and motor processes. Although a record is a
series of components, a sequential activation or "domino effect" model is not applicable.
The occurrence, amplitude, latency, etc., of each component is not necessarily dependent
upon preceding components (that is, upon the neural activity that generates those preceding
components).

An Illustration of an ERP Record

Figure 1 shows an idealized illustration of one ERP record. It shows the electrical
potentials evoked in the brain, as detected by scalp electrodes, by a single auditory stimulus—
in this case, a 70-dB nHL click—from time 0 (stimulus onset) to 1 s after the onset.

In an ERP record, the first five (known) components occur in the first 10 ms after the
auditory stimulus. They are called Waves I, II, III, IV, and V. They represent activity of
the auditory nerve and auditory braimstem structures. Possible structures involved include
the ventral cochlear nucleus, superior olive, and lateral lemniscus (Scherg & Von Cramon,
1985).

These early sensory components are followed by other sensory components, including
Na and Pa. These occur from 18 to 40 ms after the stimulus. Na and Pa are "middle latency"
components. Current evidence suggests that Na and Pa may be produced by thalamic structures and auditory cortex. They are absent or too small to be reliably detected during early

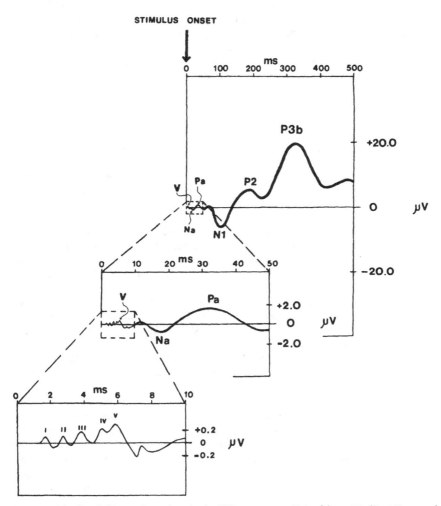

Figure 1. Idealized illustration of a single ERP response elicited by a 70-dB nHL sound—a click. The ERP is a continuous series of components occurring at various latencies after stimulus onset and having various amplitudes and durations. Shorter latency components—Waves I, II, III, IV, and V, and Na and Pa—are classic examples of *exogenous* components. The longer latency component P3b is a classic example of an *endogenous* component.

childhood, and they do not evidence the reliable adult pattern until preadolescence (Kraus, Smith, Reed, Stein, & Cartee, 1985).

.   Middle laTency components are followed by long-latency components, such as N1 and P2. These occur from 70 to 200 ms after the stimulus. Strictly speaking, they fall into a gray zone because they do not seem to represent purely sensory or purely cognitive functions.

Lastly, we have shown P3b, which can occur any time between 280 and 900 ms after the stimulus. P3b was the first component to be recognized as representing purely cognitive functions. P3b matures gradually from early childhood through adolescence (Figure 2).

Types of Components

In an ERP record, components may be divided into two general classes: exogenous and endogenous.

Exogenous Components. Exogenous components occur within the first 200 ms after a stimulus. Waves I, II, III, IV, and V shown in Figure 1 illustrate prototypical examples of exogenous components; these five components will be a focus of discussion later in this chapter.

These components are associated with sensory processes. They vary as a function of physical stimulus parameters such as light intensity or tonal frequency. They may be thought of as "obligatory" responses because stimulation external to the nervous system is the necessary and sufficient condition for them to be evoked—without external stimulation, they do not occur.

Endogenous Components. Endogenous components occur from as early as 30 ms to as late as more than a second after a stimulus. These components are associated with cognitive processes. They vary as a function of the tasks assigned to the subject; the subject's intentions about his own performance of the assigned tasks; the subject's subjective understanding, assessment of, and experience with the stimuli presented and the tasks assigned; the subject's subjective assessment of the importance of the stimuli and tasks; and the subject's experience, abilities, and knowledge.

In contrast to exogenous components, endogenous components are nonobligatory responses to stimuli. This can be shown in two ways. First, endogenous components may be elicited whether a stimulus is present or absent, provided the presence or omission of the stimulus means the same thing to the subject (Figure 3). Second, even very different stimuli (e.g., tones, words, auditory or visual stimuli) can elicit the very same endogenous response, provided they mean the same thing to the subject (Figure 3). Figure 3 illustrates prototypical examples of endogenous components: Nc and P3b; these components will be a focus of discussion later in this chapter.

Advantages of ERPs

ERPs can be obtained from infants, children, and adults in a completely noninvasive fashion. A subject may be tested repeatedly without any side effects. Normative data may be obtained easily from large numbers of subjects. With the exception of EEG, there is no other direct measure of human neural activity that is noninvasive.

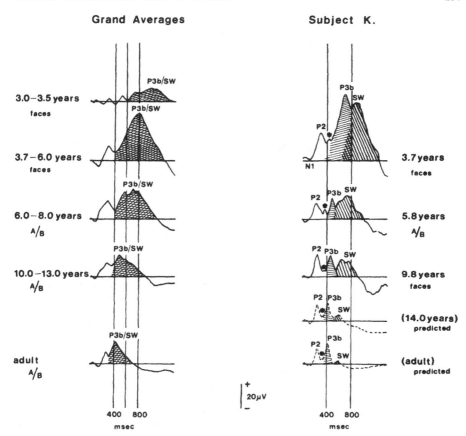

Figure 2. ERPs to targets at Pz. Lefthand panel shows the maturation of P3b (P3b/SW complex) from early childhood to adulthood. P3b (P3b/SW complex) evoked by target stimuli in subjects of different ages. These target stimuli were randomly intermixed with nontarget, background stimuli. P3b (P3b/SW complex) shaded; 3- to 3.5-year-olds (3 subjects) and 3.7- to 6.0-year-olds (6 subjects) are from Courchesne, Ganz, and Norcia (1986), in which target stimuli were human faces; 6- to 8-year-olds (16 subjects), 10- to 13-year olds (16 subjects), and 24- to 36-year-olds (12 subjects) are from Courchesne (1978), in which the target stimulus was the letter A.

Righthand panel shows the maturation of P3b (P3b/SW complex) in one subject. ERPs from subject K. recorded at 3.7, 5.8, and 9.8 years; dashed lined ERPs are predicted.

All ERPs from the Pz scalp electrode site. (From Courchesne, Ganz, & Norcia, 1986.)

Summary Points about Interpretation of ERPs

In order to interpret a particular component evoked by an event, it must be considered in the context of theory, experimental manipulations, subject variables (e.g., age), subject behavior and performance, and in relation to other components (see further discussion in Courchesne & Yeung-Courchesne, in press).

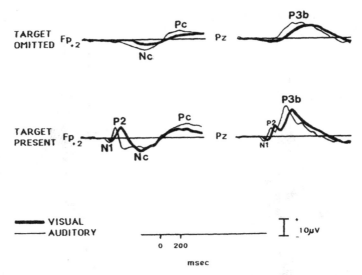

Figure 3. ERPs elicited from two types of target events. Normal subjects were presented a series of stimuli occurring once every 1.05 sec. In some series, "standard" stimuli were brief tones, and in others, standard stimuli were brief flashes of a colored slide on a screen. Occasionally one of these standard stimuli was omitted. Normal subjects were asked to detect these occasional omissions, termed *target omitted*. We recorded the ERP response to omitted targets. The top half of the figure shows three of the "endogenous components" elicited by omissions—P3b, which is largest at Pz (over parietal cortex), and Nc and Pc, which are largest at Fp$_{+2}$ (over frontal cortex halfway between Fp$_2$ and F8).

In a second experiment, we also presented the same standard auditory and visual stimuli, but now the target to be detected by normal subjects was an occasional replacement of a standard by a different stimulus (a different tone or colored slide), termed *target present*. The bottom half of the figure shows the same three endogenous components. In addition, now visual and auditory N1 and P2 components can be seen; they are "exogenous components" and must be elicited by a physical stimulus (they cannot be elicited by an omitted event).

These points are equally true of all other direct and indirect measures of neural activity, whether they be electrical, chemical, or otherwise, because neuroscience has not yet discovered how information is encoded in the brain. Without this knowledge, all measures of brain activity can be logically considered only as signs or correlates of information processing. Similarly, measures of neuroanatomy can also be considered only as correlates of neural functioning, because it is not known, for any human cognitive system, how information is encoded in neuroanatomical structures.

ERP RESEARCH REQUIREMENTS AND STUDIES OF AUTISM

In recent years, there have been changes in the criteria by which ERP studies are judged to have met basic research standards (Courchesne & Yeung-Courchesne, in press; Donchin *et al.*, 1977; Rosler, 1983). ERP studies of autism are best when they (1) reveal abnormality in components associated with processes implicated by theory or clinical observation, (2) reveal normality in other components associated with other processes not implicated, (3) provide corroborative performance and behavioral measures, (4) control for general attentiveness and cooperation, (5) take into account subject factors such as ability level, presence of pathology, and age, and (6) follow generally accepted technical procedures in ERP recording.

As more is known about conditions necessary to obtain reliable and interpretable ERP data, this field of science has come to recognize the limitations of past designs.

The literature on ERPs in autism, particularly on endogenous components, is not extensive. Few ERP studies achieve current criteria. Not surprisingly, these tend to be the most recent studies. Older studies often did not include controls for, and measurements of, performance and behavior; did not control for attentiveness and cooperation; did not group children according to age and abilities; and did not incorporate various technically required procedures.

While the data from these pioneering studies are difficult to interpret, the efforts have nonetheless been valuable to us by pointing out the need for better design and technical procedures. Since the older literature has been reviewed by James and Barry (1982), we will review only recent work whose methodology meets current requirements for research on ERPs, as mentioned above.

The only studies of endogenous components that meet criteria are studies of people with autism who were cooperative and capable of performing tasks per the instructions of researchers (Courchesne, Kilman, Galambos, & Lincoln, 1984; Courchesne, Lincoln, Kilman, & Galambos, 1985; Courchesne, Lincoln, Yeung-Courchesne, Elmasian, & Grillon, 1986; Dawson, Finley, Phillips, & Galpert, 1986; Novick, Kurtzberg, & Vaugahn, 1979; Novick, Vaughan, Kurtzberg, & Simson, 1980). In Novick *et al.* (1979, 1980) these autistic individuals were adolescents; in Courchesne *et al.* (1984, Courchesne, Lincoln, *et al.*, 1985, 1986) they were adolescents and young adults; and in Dawson *et al.* (1986) they were children and adolescents. Since it has been the goal of our laboratory to use endogenous components to elucidate the neural functioning in autism, the majority of studies discussed below come from our research effort.

ERP STUDIES IN AUTISM

Short-Latency ERP Components

Brainstem Auditory Components: 1 to 10 ms Poststimulus

Background Information. At least five ERP components are known to be generated by neural structures in the brainstem auditory sensory pathways; they are Waves I, II, III, IV, and V (see Figure 1) (Achor & Starr, 1980a, 1980b; Picton, Stapells, & Campbell, 1981; Robinson & Rudge, 1982a, 1982b). Each component reflects a different step in auditory sensory processing. These five components are evoked by click stimuli and reflect some of the rapid neural activity which takes place during the first 8 ms following the onset of the click.

The recording of these components gives an objective measure of normal versus disordered functioning in some of these structures. Such recordings are an important tool in neurology and audiology. Middle ear and cochlear pathologies and brainstem pathologies (tumors, demyelinating diseases) may create abnormalities in these auditory components (Chiappa, 1983; Galambos & Hecox 1978; Picton & Smith 1978; Starr & Achor, 1975; Starr & Hamilton, 1976; Starr, Sohmer, & Celesia, 1978; Stockard, Stockard, & Sharbough, 1977).

The most clinically reliable measures of these brainstem ERPs are (a) the latency of a component, especially wave V, and (b) the interpeak interval (time interval) between the peaks of waves I, III, and V (Galambos & Hecox, 1978; Starr et al., 1978; Stockard, Stockard, & Sharbough, 1978). This review will emphasize findings involving the clinically reliable and useful measures of brainstem auditory ERPs.

ERP Findings in Autism. The question has arisen over the years as to whether people with autism hear normally. Another question has been whether abnormal hearing is causally implicated in the development of autism. To answer these questions, a number of researchers have recently studied brainstem auditory ERPs (Courchesne, Courchesne, Hicks, & Lincoln, 1985; Gillberg, Rosenhall, & Johansson, 1983; Novick et al., 1980; Rumsey, Grimes, Pikus, Duara, & Ismond, 1984; Skoff, Mirsky, & Turner, 1980; Tanguay, Edwards, Buchwald, Schwafel, & Allen, 1982; Taylor, Rosenblatt, & Linschoten, 1982).

The first question is a straightforward clinical one: Do some people with autism have abnormal hearing? The answer is yes; ERP and audiological studies suggest that between 20 and 40% of autistic people may not have normal hearing (e.g., Gillbert et al., 1983; Rumsey et al., 1984; Taylor et al., 1982).

The second question requires an experimental perspective and careful experimental design: In order for autism to be present, must there be abnormal functioning of auditory brainstem pathways? The answer is no (Courchesne, Courchesne, et al., 1985).

In order to make this determination, one must rule out confounding secondary pathologies—i.e., other neurological syndromes such as tuberous sclerosis and audiological disorders such as otitis media (see Rutter, 1979). One must also account for age, gender, body temperature at the time of ERP recording, potentially confounding muscle artifact in the ERP data, and reliability of the ERP data. One must thoroughly evaluate auditory functioning by systematically studying stimulus parameters that have a functional relationship with these auditory brainstem components. This requires systematically varying neurophysiologically relevant parameters such as stimulus intensity, stimulus rate, and ear of stimulus delivery.

Of all the auditory brainstem ERP studies, only two incorporated most of these methodological points (Rumsey et al., 1984; Tanguay et al., 1982) and only one incorporated all of them (Courchesne, Courchesne, et al., 1985). All three studies found no evidence to support the idea that auditory brainstem systems must be abnormal for autism to develop.

Tanguay et al. (1982) incorporated all of the above methodological points except the ruling out of confounding secondary neurological syndromes (not stated in their paper), and taking body temperature into account. Rumsey et al. (1984) incorporated all but temperature and systematic variation of stimulus rate and intensity. Both studies used retarded and nonretarded autistic subjects. Tanguay et al. and Rumsey et al. did not find the relatively high incidence of abnormality in auditory brainstem responses, which have been reported by other studies that have not incorporated most of these methodological points.

In the most recent auditory brainstem study of autism, we (Courchesne, Courchesne, et al., 1985) incorporated all of the above points. We compared ERPs from 14 autistic subjects to the ERPs from 14 carefully matched normal controls. We also compared the ERPs from these autistic subjects to ERP clinical norms with a data base of more than 100 subjects. We found that all of these autistic subjects had clinically and neurophysiologically

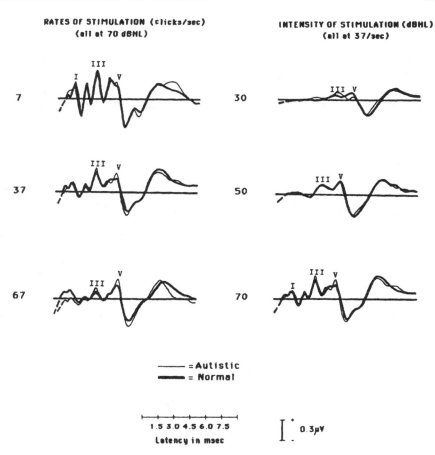

Figure 4. Functioning of brainstem auditory sensory pathways (ERPs to click stimulation). Figure shows similarity in brainstem auditory sensory ERPs between normal and autistic subjects. ERP responses to rarefaction clicks are monaurally delivered to left and right ears (each trace is the average response from both the left and right ears). Also shown are the ERP responses to clicks presented at three different rates and at three different stimulus intensities. The thick tracings are the averages of ERP responses from 14 normals. Superimposed onto these are thin tracings representing the averages of ERP responses from 14 autistic subjects. (From Courchesne, Courchesne, et al., 1985).

normal auditory brainstem ERP components. Figure 4 shows the auditory brainstem ERP responses of our normal and autistic subjects under a variety of sensory stimulation conditions. This figure shows how very similar the ERP responses were in these two subject groups.

Thus, the ERP data from the three most carefully designed studies show that the development of autism occurs despite normal functioning of pathways that generate brainstem auditory ERPs. Research must look elsewhere for the neural systems that must be disordered for autism to develop.

Other Sensory Components: 10 to 120 ms Poststimulus

Background Information. In the human ERP, there are a number of soma-tosensory, visual, and auditory components that reflect sensory processing systems besides the auditory brainstem components (Goff, Allison, & Vaughan, 1978; Spehlmann, 1985; Starr et al., 1978). Somatosensory components represent neural activity in the spinal cord, medial lemniscus, thalamus and/or thalamocortical radiations, and somatosensory cortex. Visual components represent activity in the retina and visual cortex. It remains an unsettled question as to whether any auditory components (e.g., Na and Pa) represent thalamic or auditory cortex activity.

ERP Findings in Autism. Disappointingly, there have not been studies of these components in autistic subjects, with the exception of N1 (see next section for comments). Such studies would be most valuable if they followed the general guidelines used by the recent ERP research on auditory brainstem components, as discussed in the preceding section (e.g., Courchesne, Courchesne, et al., 1985; Rumsey et al., 1984; Tanguay et al., 1982): (a) the study of autism unconfounded by secondary neurological syndromes, (b) stringent quality control of ERP data, (c) systematic variation of stimulus parameters, (d) ERP meas-urement using clinically reliable and useful procedures, (e) recording of later cognitive components in the same subjects for comparison and correlation and (f) the use of properly matched control groups and clinical norms where feasible.

From the standpoint of discerning where the nervous system begins to behave abnor-mally, it would be very helpful to know whether these other sensory ERP responses are normal in autism.

Long-Latency ERP Components

Auditory and Visual N1 and P2: 70 to 270 ms Poststimulus

Background Information. The N1 and P2 components, as detected by scalp electrodes, occur with maximal amplitudes over the central and frontal cortical areas. They are evoked by auditory, visual, and somatosensory stimuli (Figures 1 and 3). They are usually considered to be exogenous components, because their amplitudes and latencies are affected by the physical parameters of eliciting stimuli such as stimulus intensity, tonal frequency, and spatial frequency. Auditory and visual N1 occur ca 100 and 130 ms, respectively, after stimulus onset. Auditory and visual P2 occur ca 200 and 230 ms, respectively, after stimulus onset (Figures 1 and 3).

It is quite possible that these components are generated by cortical neural activity. Currently, research is attempting to establish whether they are generated by the primary and secondary sensory cortex of each sensory modality or if they are generated by polymodal association cortex where sensory integration may occur. The complex question of their neural generators is discussed elsewhere (Wood et al., 1984; Woods, Clayworth, Knight, Simpson, & Naesser, in press).

N1 and P2 responses to phonemes are slow to mature. Up to 2 years of age, the N1 and P2 responses to phonemes are markedly different from those of adults (Kurtzberg 1985; Kurtzberg, Stone, & Vaughan & 1986). They change gradually and do not achieve the adult form until after 8 to 10 years of age (Courchesne, in press).

It is becoming apparent that these components reflect more than sensory-specific information. For instance, N1 responses to stimulation in one sensory modality may be significantly reduced in amplitude by prior stimulation in another sensory modality. This sort of intermodality interaction tends to favor the idea that these components are dependent upon polymodal association cortex where sensory integration takes place.

Also, when a particular stimulus is repeatedly presented (for instance, at intervals 0.5 or 1.0 s), the amplitude of the N1 response to each repetition becomes smaller and smaller, eventually reaching a stable size after 4 to 6 repetitions (Woods & Elmasian, 1986). Yet, while N1 becomes smaller and smaller, subjects continue to perceive each repetition of the stimulus as being unchanged in intensity, tonal frequency, hue, etc.

The fact that N1 amplitude decreases with stimulus repetition suggests that N1 may, in some fashion, be associated with short-term habituation mechanisms. Moreover, if some characteristic of the repeated stimulus is changed, this changed stimulus elicits a larger response than the "habituated" one (Woods & Elmasian, 1986). The more change given the repeated stimulus, the larger the recovered response. Such short-term habituation and recovery of response to a change in stimulation, along with other evidence, has led some researchers to suggest that N1 may be associated with short-term memory or perhaps modulation of polymodal association cortex.

Although N1 may be associated with short-term habituation and memory, it does not appear to be associated with mechanisms available for conscious awareness and use. This may be inferred from N1 studies of people who are functionally deaf as a result of having suffered from some neurological disorder. Despite not consciously hearing auditory stimuli, such a person nevertheless produces N1 responses that show normal short-term habituation, recovery, and specificity of responsiveness dishabituation (Woods, Knight, & Neville, 1984).

In summary, then, central to the characteristic physiologies of N1 and P2 are (a) their reductions in amplitudes with stimulus repetition, (b) their amplitude covariation with the rate of stimulus delivery (the faster the rate, the smaller the amplitude response), and (c) their recovery of response amplitude when there is a change in a repeated stimulus (the more change, the bigger the recovery).

It is known that N1 and P2 are overlapped by another component, which is termed *Nd*. Nd has been associated with attentional mechanisms. In normal subjects, Nd occurs between ca 70 and 250 ms after an attended auditory stimulus. It has not been studied in autism. When one simply measures the amplitude at the peak of the N1 component, this amplitude measure is a composite of N1 and Nd. How much of the amplitude is due to N1 and how much to Nd must be determined by certain procedures beyond the scope of this chapter. The interested reader is referred to Hansen and Hillyard (1980, 1983) and Hillyard and Kutas (1983).

ERP Findings in Autism. There have been no systematic studies of N1 and P2 in autism: No auditory, visual, or somatosensory studies have been done on intensity effects, rate of stimulation effects, intersensory modality effects, and so on. The studies that are available usually did not control for potentially confounding effects of attention on N1 and P2 measures. Ideally, studies of N1 and P2 might start by systematically varying stimulus parameters in one sensory modality while actively and fully engaging the attention of subjects in a task in a different sensory modality. With attention directed to a different sensory modality, and the attention quantified, the N1 and P2 responses can then be measured free of overlapping attentional components.

Some studies have recorded N1 and P2 without objectively quantifying the degree and direction of attention to the eliciting stimuli. The results of such studies cannot be interpreted, because ERP differences between normals and controls could be due to differences between the subject groups in attentiveness, rather than to differences in exogenous, sensory-related processes.

The few studies that have taken measures to ensure that attentional demands were comparable between autistic subjects and control groups have not reported a consistent pattern of results on N1 and P2 (e.g., Courchesne *et al.*, 1984; Courchesne, Lincoln, *et al.*, 1985; Dawson *et al.*, 1986; Novick *et al.*, 1980).

Because of this inconsistent pattern of results and the lack of proper systematic studies, no conclusions about N1 and P2 in autism can be made at this time.

Several studies have found that the auditory N1 and P2 components tend to be smaller in autistic subjects as compared to normals (Courchesne *et al.*, 1984; Courchesne, Lincoln, *et al.*, 1985; Dawson *et al.*, 1986; Novick *et al.*, 1980) (e.g., see Figure 5). However, not in all cases was this tendency statistically significant.

For example, in an initial report, we (Courchesne *et al.*, 1984) found our autistic subjects to have insignificantly smaller auditory N1 and P2 responses, but in a second report in which more subjects were used, we (Courchesne, Lincoln, *et al.*, 1985) found the auditory N1 to be significantly smaller. In both reports, we presented subjects with complex stimuli (e.g., the sound *me*). Novick *et al.* (1980) and Dawson *et al.* (1986) reported P2 to be significantly smaller in their autistic subjects, but not N1 (Figure 5 from Dawson *et al.*). However, as shown in Figure 5, N1 was noticeably, though statistically insignificantly, smaller in the autistic subjects of Dawson *et al.* (1986).

It is possible that the Nd component associated with selective attention (see section below on Nc and Attention) may account for these different results. As noted above, it is known that N1 is overlapped by the Nd component. Changes in the amplitude or timing of this attentional Nd component can alter the amplitude measures of N1. None of the studies to date were designed to allow independent measurement of these two overlapping components.

It is known that Nd is larger with easier discrimination tasks than with more difficult ones. Perhaps the discrimination tasks used by Novick *et al.* (1980) and Dawson *et al.* (1986) were equally easy for their autistic and normal subjects, while the word discrimination task of Courchesne, Lincoln, *et al.* (1985) was more difficult for the autistic subjects than for the normal ones. Such differences in task difficulty could create differences in the amplitude of Nd, which overlaps N1 and may confound measurement of it.

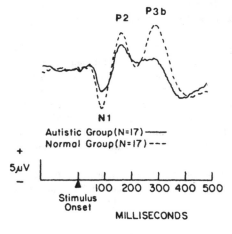

Figure 5. ERPs elicited by the target sound "da." This target was intermixed with nontarget, background sounds, which were brief clicks. Subjects raised a hand to indicate whenever they heard the "da" sound. ERP traces from the Cz (over central cortex) scalp electrode site. (Adapted from Dawson *et al.*, 1986.)

In sum, conventional measures of auditory N1 are composed of N1 itself in addition to some amount of an early auditory attentional component that overlaps N1 in time. These conventional measures of a "composite" N1 (e.g., N1 + Nd) suggest that the composite may be smaller in autism in response to auditory stimuli. It is an open question as to whether the smaller auditory "composite" N1 results from a smaller N1 component, or from a smaller, overlapping attentional Nd component. A definitive answer to this question will be important in developing theories of autism, since each component is associated with functions relevant to the disorder—auditory memory and attention.

We (Courchesne, Lincoln, *et al.*, 1985) also recorded visual N1 responses in a design analogous to our auditory one; the same subjects participated in both. Autistic and normal subjects had similar N1 amplitudes at Cz, which is over central cortex. However, preliminary data in our laboratory suggest that the visual N1 at Oz, which is over primary visual cortex, *might* be smaller in autistic than in normal subjects. Again, since the design had not anticipated allowing N1 to be measured separately from early attentional components, their contribution to the N1 measure is uncertain.

A/Pcz/300, a Frontocentral P3, and Orienting to Novelty: 250 to 450 ms Poststimulus

Background Information. Several ERP components have been found to be associated with the detection of novel, surprising stimuli. There is evidence that one component, A/Pcz/300, may be associated with an auditory mechanism that makes rapid detections of such stimuli.* This component is largest at scalp electrode sites situated midway between superior parietal and frontal cortical areas. It occurs at 300 ms after the onset of an unexpected, surprising sound in normal children and adults (Courchesne, 1983). It is small in patients with prefrontal lobe lesions, and does not habituate in these patients as it does in normal individuals (Knight, 1984).

Another component, the frontocentral P3, may be associated with an analogous visual mechanism. It occurs at 380–450 ms after an unexpected event and habituates rapidly in normal people (Courchesne, 1978b; Courchesne, Hillyard, & Galambos, 1975; Kok, 1983, personal communication). Unlike the auditory A/Pcz/300 component, this component is not readily seen in the waveforms of children and preadolescents. Future research will be required to determine whether this component is a late developmental phenomenon, or if it exists during childhood but is obscured in children's waveforms, which tend to have very large Nc components that occur at the same latency as the frontocentral P3. It also remains to be experimentally determined whether the frontocentral P3 and A/Pcz/300 are analogous physiologically.

ERP Findings in Autism. If individuals with autism were hypersensitive to novel stimuli, these two components would then be predicted to be as large as, or larger than, normal, and they would not be expected to habituate. On the other hand, if individuals with autism misperceive novel stimuli as *non*novel and insignificant, these two ERP components would be predicted to be no different from responses to expected, nonnovel stimuli.

To investigate these possibilities, we presented a monotonous, repetitive series of stimuli ("standard" stimuli) to autistic and normal subjects; occasionally, a surprising, novel

---

*A/Pcz/300 refers to the following: A = the auditory modality, P = positive in polarity, cz = largest amplitudes found at electrode site cz (over central cortical areas), and 300 = mean latency is 300 msec.

stimulus was inserted into this series (Courchesne *et al.*, 1984; Courchesne, Lincoln, *et al.*, 1985). We presented visual and auditory conditions separately. Subjects were not told that the novel stimuli would be presented. We recorded the A/Pcz/300 component evoked by auditory stimuli and the frontocentral P3 evoked by visual stimuli.

To control for attention, general arousal, and cooperation, subjects were required to press a button whenever they detected a specific "target" stimulus (auditory condition: the sound *you*; visual: the letter *A*).

This Sokolovian-type orienting paradigm (Berlyne, 1960; Bernstein, 1979; Luria & Homskaya, 1970; Sokolov, 1958, 1960, 1963) was identical to one that we have used to chart the normal development of these two ERP components. In these studies, we collected data from 113 normal 4- to 44-year-olds (Courchesne, 1977, 1978a, 1983). Thus, we were able to compare the ERPs from our autistic subjects to this extensive normative data base as well as to age-matched controls. In this way, we had the opportunity to consider the question of maturational delay in neurophysiological systems associated with the detection of novel, surprising stimuli.

To reiterate, the auditory A/Pcz/300 component and the visual frontocentral P3 are associated with the subject's detection of novelty; both components are higher in amplitude to novel stimuli than to monotonous background stimuli in normal subjects from 4 to 44 years. The question was, will this also be true for autistic subjects?

The auditory and visual ERPs of autistic subjects indicated that they *do* detect and perceive novelty when it occurs. This is evidenced by the finding that the auditory component A/Pcz/300 and the visual frontocentral P3 responded with higher amplitudes to novel than

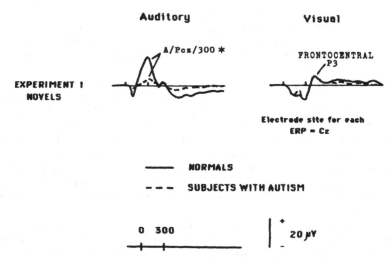

Figure 6. Orientation to surprising new information. Figure shows differences in auditory A/Pcz/300 amplitudes between normal and autistic subjects. ERPs elicited by novel stimuli showing the A/Pcz/300 and frontocentral P3 components at Cz electrode site (central midline site). The thick tracings are the averages of ERP responses from 10 normals. Superimposed onto these are dashed tracings representing the averages of ERP responses from 9 autistic subjects. * = Significant differences (Adapted from Courchesne *et al.*, 1984; Courchesne, Lincoln, *et al.*, 1985.)

to the monotonous "standard" stimuli, as is the normal pattern (see Figure 6). Nonetheless, several important differences were found between autistic and normal subjects.

The first major finding was that the averaged auditory A/Pcz/300 component was still much smaller in autistic than in normal subjects (see Figure 6), but the visual frontocentral P3 was similar in size in both subject groups.

The abnormal A/Pcz/300 response may be a sign of mechanisms abnormally inhibiting the reticular formation, limbic structures, or prefrontal cortex (Groves & Lynch, 1972; Luria & Homskaya, 1970; O'Keefe, 1976; Ranck, 1973; Sokolov, 1963; Vinogradova, 1970). Adults who have sustained lesions of the prefrontal cortex also have smaller A/Pcz/300 responses to auditory novelty (Knight, 1984). The coincidence of these results may be a useful clue about the neural disorder in autism.

Because autistic and normal subjects were almost equally accurate in giving a behavioral response to the targets—which were randomly mixed with the presentation of the novels and standards—the abnormal A/Pcz/300 responses cannot be easily accounted for by differences between autistic and normal subjects in general arousal, cooperation, or task difficulty.

There was a second major finding. The fact that the *averaged* A/Pcz/300 amplitude was smaller in autism still left open the question of whether every novel sound elicited a diminished amplitude. To find an answer to this question, we recently reexamined the data from several subjects. We looked at the A/Pcz/300 amplitude to the very first novel trial and to each of the following five novel trials. We found that autistic subjects usually have normal amplitude A/Pcz/300 responses to the very first novel stimulus. However, after this first trial, each of the following responses is usually very much smaller, and the wave shape changes radically from trial to trial (Figure 7).

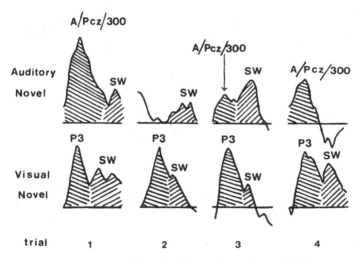

Figure 7. Subject R., a 15-year-old male. Figure shows large initial response to auditory novel, but extreme variability to subsequent auditory novels. In contrast, large and consistent response to visual novels is shown. Single trial ERP responses from one autistic subject elicited by the first four auditory and visual novel stimuli showing A/Pcz/300 and frontocentral P3 components at Cz electrode site (over central cortex). (Adapted from Courchesne, Lincoln, et al., 1985.)

This evidence suggests that the neural generators involved in detecting novelty have the capacity for normal functioning, and, occasionally, they do respond normally. *Most importantly, however, this evidence raises the possibility that the operation of this apparently otherwise normal neural system is usually abnormally interfered with or hindered by some other system.* Thus, our autistic subjects had a limited or diminished opportunity to respond to auditory novelty compared with visual novelty, and compared with normal subjects. This evidence and the conclusion it leads to are especially relevant to the theory of autism presented in the last section of this chapter.

On the basis of the normative data from the 113 4- to 44-year-olds, this abnormal A/Pcz/300 response in autistic subjects is not consistent with maturational delay. Rather, the abnormal response is indicative of a diminished capacity relative to normal persons of all ages, even 4-year-olds—this despite the high level of functioning of these autistic subjects.

These are the only published studies of novelty and ERPs in autism.

P3b, Concept Modification, and Attention to Event Importance: 300 to 900 ms Poststimulus

Background Information.   The P3b component is associated with concept modification and attention to event importance (Courchesne, 1978b; Donchin, 1981; Donchin *et al.*, 1984; Donchin, Ritter, & McCallum, 1978; Paul & Sutton, 1972; Sutton & Ruchkin, 1984). It is the grandfather of all cognitive components and was discovered by Sutton, Braren, Zubin, and John (1965, 1967). It has a positive polarity, occurs 300–900 ms after an event, and is largest at electrode sites situated over parietal cortex. It is the most thoroughly studied of all cognitive components. It behaves in a highly predictable manner under certain circumstances. For example, when an infrequent event (a target) is unpredictably inserted into a repetitive sequence of another event (standard), and subjects are asked to respond to the target, a large P3b is evoked every time a normal subject detects this important target event. The event can even be an omission of a stimulus from a repetitive sequence of standards. The P3b response is similar whether visual, auditory, or somatosensory modalities are used.

P3b appears to be a component affected by multiple factors. It is associated with all of the *four* facets of conceptual orientation to the ongoing environment (i.e., our ideas about what is happening). (1) It is sensitive to global event probabilities: It is larger to improbable events than to highly likely ones. (2) Its amplitude varies with the sequential pattern of eliciting events; for instance, an event that has been alternating with another event will produce a smaller P3b than if it occurs after a string of the other event. (3) It is larger when subjects do not know when the eliciting event will occur than when they are told in advance exactly when it will occur, even if the global probability is the same in each case. (4) Finally, it is larger to events with more value or importance, such as monetary value, subjective interest, or task-relevance (target stimuli to which subjects must respond).

There are numerous studies showing each of these effects. Selective citing of a few would neglect others. Please refer to any one of several excellent reviews (Donchin *et al.*, 1978, 1984; Pritchard, 1981; Rosler, 1983; Sutton & Ruchkin, 1984).

ERP Findings in Autism.   Of the four facets of conceptual orientation that affect P3b, all studies of autism to date have tested only the fourth: attention to stimulus value or importance (Courchesne *et al.*, 1984; Courchesne, Lincoln, *et al.*, 1985, 1986; Dawson *et al.*, 1986; Novick *et al.*, 1979, 1980).

In our research on stimulus importance, we studied the P3b component in three different experiments (Courchesne *et al.*, 1984; Courchesne, Lincoln, *et al.*, 1985, 1986) (Figure 8). In each experiment, (a) we used the basic outline of the highly predictable and reliable type of design for eliciting P3b, described above in the background information of P3b, (b) we used analogous auditory and visual sequences, (c) targets occurred unpredictably, and (d) targets occurred with a 0.10 probability.

One of our experiments was the one in which we used novel events, described on pages 299–300 in the preceding subsection "A/Pcz/300, a Frontocentral P3, and Orienting to Novelty." The visual target was the letter *A*, and the auditory was the word *you.*

In our second experiment, the visual target was a brief flash of a slide of one color (e.g., red) and the standard was a brief flash of a slide of another color (e.g., blue). The auditory target in this experiment was one brief tone (e.g., 1000 Hz) and the standard stimulus was another brief tone (e.g., 2000 Hz). The auditory portion of this experiment was analogous to Novick *et al.* (1980) and Dawson *et al.* (1986).

In our third experiment, the visual target was the omission (target/omit) of one of the regularly and repetitively presented (1/s) brief flashes of a slide of one color, and the auditory target was the omission (target/omit) of one of the regularly and repetitively presented (1/s) brief tones. This third experiment was similar to the Novick *et al.* (1979) study of three autistic adolescents.

In the experiments of Novick *et al.* (1980) and Dawson *et al.* (1986) and in each of our own, subjects were asked to respond whenever they detected a designated target (e.g., the letter *A*, a tone, or a target/omit). In Novick *et al.* (1980) and in our experiments, the response required was a button press that allowed these researchers to evaluate reaction time as well as accuracy of task performance. Finally, in our experiments, we also examined each subject's answers to questions about each condition after the condition was completed.

In these ways, the general behavioral attentiveness, cooperation, and understanding of the task demands of the autistic subjects could be assessed. In Novick *et al.* (1980), although autistic subjects were less accurate than normal subjects, the median and interquartile ranges of reaction time of the autistic subjects did not differ from normal subjects. In Dawson *et al.* (1986), many autistic subjects were less accurate than normal ones. However, in their study, the accuracy of 10 autistic subjects was similar to normal subjects; they compared the ERPs of these autistic subjects (as well as those who were less accurate) to the ERPs of normal subjects.

In our experiments, there were no differences between autistic and normal groups in general behavioral attentiveness, cooperation, and understanding of the tasks. Accuracy to targets was similar in the autistic and normal subject groups in all three of our experiments. Reaction times were similar in both groups in our second and third experiments described just above, but they were somewhat longer in the autistic group in our first set of experiments (Courchesne *et al.*, 1984; Courchesne, Lincoln, *et al.*, 1985, 1986).

P3b elicited by auditory targets in autistic subjects was significantly smaller than normal in the experiments of Novick *et al.* (1979, 1980) and Dawson *et al.* (1986), and in all three of our experiments (see Figures 5 and 8). In contrast, we found that, in autistic subjects, P3b elicited by visual targets (e.g., the letter *A* or target/omit) was insignificantly different from normal (Figure 8), although it was sometimes slightly (but insignificantly) smaller than normal (Courchesne, Lincoln, *et al.*, 1985; Courchesne, Lincoln, *et al.*, 1986).

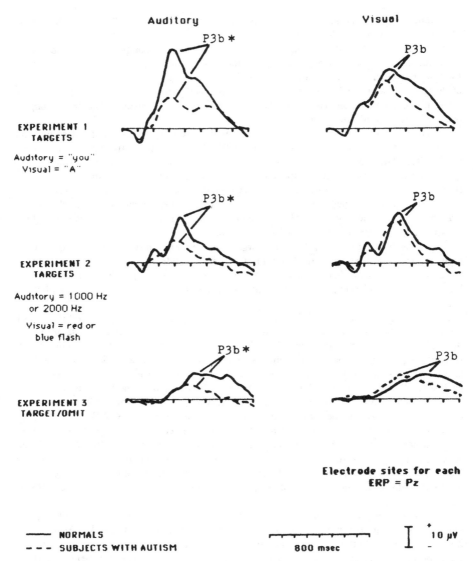

Figure 8. Concept modification and concept updating. Figure shows differences in auditory and visual P3b amplitudes between normal and autistic subjects. ERPs elicited by different types of targets showing the P3b component at the Pz electrode site (over parietal cortex) in Experiments 1, 2, and 3, described in this subsection. The thick tracings are the averages of ERP responses from normal subjects. Superimposed onto these are dashed tracings representing the averages of ERP responses from autistic subjects. ERPs from normal and autistic subjects represent averages of 8 to 10 people, depending on the experiment. * = Significant differences between subject groups. (Adapted from Courchesne et al., 1984; Courchesne, Lincoln, et al., 1985; and Courchesne, Lincoln, et al., 1986.)

Further research is needed to establish whether there are any special information-processing conditions or any subgroups of autistic people wherein visual P3b does significantly differ from normal.

In all three of our experiments (Figure 8), the auditory P3b was only about 50% of the P3b amplitude obtained from normal subjects. In contrast, the visual P3b was about 75% or more of the P3b amplitude obtained from normal subjects. Thus, we have found that the auditory P3b amplitude in our autistic subjects was much more reduced than was the visual P3b. We did not find any subjects for whom the auditory P3b was substantially larger than the visual P3b.

Since P3b to an omitted event is triggered by an internal decision and not by actual sensory stimulation, the smaller P3b to auditory target/omits leaves little doubt that autism involves a cognitive deficit independent of low-level sensory processing.

Also, since the autistic group performed with accuracy and speed equal to those of the normal group in both auditory and visual tasks, there is no evidence of disordered perception and recognition memory. That is, our autistic subjects were able to learn and remember the exact target event (word, letter, color, tone, omitted event) as well as normal subjects. Moreover, because the smaller auditory P3b was found in such a variety of experiments from several laboratories, it cannot be due to stimulus complexity, the use of verbal stimuli, the complexity of the stimulus context, or subtle methodological procedures.

Because P3b in response to an omitted auditory event was smaller, the implicated cognitive deficit could be related to the *use* of auditory memory, rather than to the initial storage of auditory memory. In terms of suggestions about the functional significance of P3b (Courchesne, 1978b; Donchin, 1981; Donchin *et al.*, 1978), the results suggest the hypothesis that autistic subjects may differ from normal subjects in the use of contextual information to optimally *modify* their auditory memory. In other words, once autistic subjects generate a template of the auditory target event, they might not modify it but, rather, only compare it in a fixed, mechanical way to what is happening in the environment.

P3b could prove to be a window to this information-processing problem. This hypothesis predicts that they would not use probability, cuing, or salience information in the same way, or to the same degree, as normal individuals. Future experiments should investigate these possibilities, as well as investigate the other three facets of conceptualization associated with P3b mentioned in the background section above.

We wanted to know whether the smaller *averaged* P3b responses meant that autistic people have a constant diminished capacity to use contextual information to modify memory. We reexamined the P3b responses elicited by auditory targets in some subjects (as we did with our A/Pcz/300 data to novels; see above subsection "A/Pcz/300, a Frontocentral P3, and Orienting to Novelty").

We found that most of the single trial responses of P3b to auditory targets are small. Interestingly, however, they are occasionally of normal amplitude. Task performance remained relatively constant throughout the trials despite these variations in P3b amplitude. This evidence shows that systems that generate P3b are capable of normal responding, and raises the possibility that they may usually be abnormally *prevented* from responding. This suggestion implies that, because of abnormal neural interference of some sort, our autistic subjects usually had a diminished opportunity to engage mechanisms used for modifying memory on the basis of contextual information. However, this interference may occasionally be overridden.

This evidence and conclusion are especially relevant to the theory of autism presented in the last section of this chapter.

Nc and Attention: 200 to 900 ms Poststimulus

Background Information. There are numerous theories of attention, many of which feature no less than two central mechanisms. One is a mechanism for the voluntary selection of what is to be attended; another is a mechanism that compares these attentional choices with input from the environment. When a match occurs, it is treated differently from the way it is treated when the comparison results in no match.

At least two ERP components are associated with these attentional mechanisms in the brain. One component has been termed *Nd* or the *modality-specific processing negativity*. It was introduced in the previous section in the context of N1 findings in autism. It has been extensively studied in normal adults, but not in autistic people. It occurs between ca 70 and 250 ms after an attended stimulus. In Naatanen's view (1982), it is associated with a comparison process that identifies a sensory event as matching the short-term memory of events that are being attended, or sought.

Another component appears between ca 200 and 900 ms after an attended stimulus. Naatanen (1982) has termed this the *frontal component of the processing negativity,* to indicate that its location is more prominent at scalp electrode sites over frontal cortex (e.g., Fz and Fpz). This component is similar in many ways to Nc, which was first described in children (Courchesne, 1977, 1978a) but was later also found in infants (Courchesne, Ganz, & Norcia, 1981; Karrer & Ackles, in press; Kurtzberg, 1985). Nc should probably be termed *Ni*, because we now know that it first appears in infants (Ackles & Karrer, 1985; Courchesne *et al.,* 1981; Karrer & Ackles, in press; Kurtzberg, 1985); indeed, it may be the first cognitive ERP component to appear in the human ERP waveform.

These terms—*frontal component of the processing negativity* and *Nc*—have been used to describe phenomena that share similar waveforms, latencies, scalp distributions, and the propensity to be larger in response to perceptually more easily distinguished or more deviating stimulation (e.g., data from Courchesne, 1977, 1978a, 1983; Courchesne *et al.,* 1981; Hansen & Hillyard, 1980, 1983; Naatanen, 1982; Naatanen, Gaillard, & Varey, 1981). Courchesne (1978a) and Courchesne *et al.* (1981) proposed that Nc is associated with the "further processing of attention-getting events." This proposal is suggestive of Naatenen's (1982) later proposal that the frontal component of the processing negativity is associated with "further processing" and selective directing of internal attention to each sensory event that matches the memory of events to be attended. The relationship between Nc and "the frontal component of the processing negativity" remains to be established.

Nc may be a sign of a mechanism for voluntary control and focusing of internal attention on important information that has just occurred. In this model, Nc occurs to stimuli that subjects must pay attention to because of the experimenter's instructions or to stimuli that are subjectively attention-getting for the subjects (e.g., surprising, interesting events) (Courchesne, 1978a; Courchesne *et al.,* 1981; Karrer & Ackles, in press). In the normal population, this component may occur at all ages from infancy to adulthood (Courchesne, 1977, 1978a, 1983; Courchesne *et al.,* 1981), and in auditory and visual modalities (see reviews of Nc by Courchesne, 1983, and Courchesne, Elmasian, & Yeung-Courchesne, 1986).

It is noteworthy that there are differences and parallels between Nc and P3b (Courchesne, Elmasian, & Yeung-Courchesne, 1986). Both are elicited by significant, surprising information. Thus, they occur in each stimulus trial as parts of the same ERP record in adolescents and young adults. Also, they begin to appear 200 to 350 ms after stimulus onset in adolescents and young adults. However, Nc and P3b have different spatial distributions: Nc is largest at scalp sites over frontal cortex, while P3b is largest over parietal cortex. They also differ in duration: Nc may last many hundreds of ms, while P3b ends much sooner, often lasting only 150 to 250 ms. Also, Nc appears in infancy, but P3b is not reliably seen until about 3 years of age.

ERP Findings in Autism. We have recorded Nc in each of three recent experiments (Courchesne, Lincoln, *et al.*, 1985, 1986), described in the preceding section. Each had analogous auditory and visual tasks and stimulus sequences. In each experiment, we randomly inserted a target event into a sequence of stimuli, and we instructed subjects to press a button to each target event. The targets were the sound *you* and the letter *A* in Experiment 1, a tone (e.g., 1000 Hz) or a color slide (e.g., red) in Experiment 2, and the *omission* of a tone or a color slide from a regularly, repetitively presented sequence (e.g., all 1000 Hz tones or all red slides) in Experiment 3.

The use of an omitted event allowed us to measure Nc uncontaminated by overlapping sensory ERP components. In Experiment 1, which used the *you* and *A* stimuli as targets, we also inserted unexpected, novel stimuli: bizarre, complex sounds or color patterns. (ERPs to these novel stimuli were discussed in the subsection entitled "A/Pcz/300, a Frontocentral P3, and Orienting to Novelty: 250 to 450 ms Poststimulus.")

One of the most striking findings in our experiments is that the Nc seems to be consistently very much smaller (less negative in potential) in the autistic group. In fact, rather than a negative potential where Nc should have been, autistic subjects often had a slightly *positive* potential—exactly the opposite of normal subjects. These findings in the autistic subjects were significant for all visual targets and visual novels. These findings were also significant for auditory target/present and target/omit events and showed a tendency to be significant for auditory novels (overlapping sensory components may have obscured a statistically significant effect). These Nc differences are depicted in Figure 9.

In terms of the model of Nc presented above (Courchesne, 1978a; Courchesne *et al.*, 1981), it could be tentatively suggested that the smaller Nc negative amplitude and often positive potential where Nc should have been indicate that nonretarded autistic people have a diminished or altered capacity for selectively channeling information for further internal attention and processing.

There also appears to be a subtle, but very interesting, effect in the data in Figure 9. Only the longest-lasting, most extremely deviant stimuli produced Nc responses in the autistic subjects—the wild, clanging, ringing novel sounds; the bright, colorful novels; and the word *you*, which, perhaps fortuitously, was pronounced with special emphasis.

In contrast, all target and novel stimuli produced substantial Nc responses in the normal subjects, even the complete omission of a stimulus. This latter effect may be significant. Despite detecting such stimulus omissions and short-lasting simple target stimuli such as a 1000-Hz tone as accurately and rapidly as normal subjects, the autistic subjects evidenced very little Nc. Single trial analysis on several autistic subjects showed that Nc was small on every trial.

The evidence suggests that the Nc generator can be engaged, but the stimulation must be much more extreme than is true for normal people. That is, whether information is auditory or visual, it must be much more extreme (or perhaps of special, idiosyncratic significance to the subject) to gain access to mechanisms for voluntary control and focusing of internal attention in people with autism as compared to normal individuals. This is relevant to the discussion in the next section.

The fact that Nc is clearly seen in normal people in response to auditory and visual target/omits is noteworthy. This is solid evidence that this component is purely endogenous; that is, its occurrence is triggered entirely by internal cognitive activity, not by the sensory stimulation *per se*. This puts it in the special class of endogenous/cognitive components along with P3b.

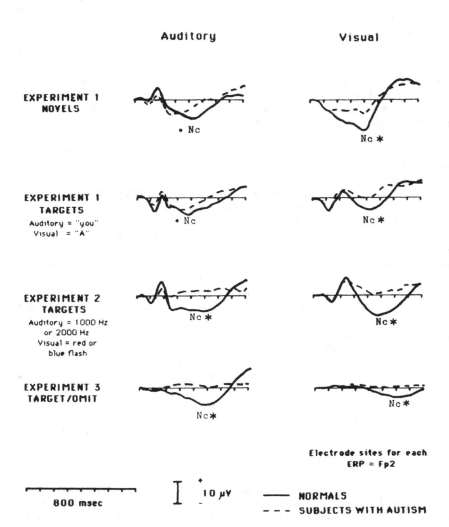

Figure 9. Attention. Figure shows differences in Nc between normal and autistic subjects.
ERP responses showing the Nc component at Fp_{+2} electrode site (over right frontal cortex
halfway between Fp_2 and F8) in the three experiments which are described in the preceding
subsection. ERPs were elicited by novels and different types of targets. The thick tracings
are the averages of ERP responses from normal subjects. Superimposed onto these are
dashed tracings representing the averages of ERP responses from autistic subjects. ERPs
from normal and autistic subjects represent averages of 8 to 10 people, depending on the
experiment. * = Significant differences; • = tendency to be different. (Adapted from Courchesne et al., 1984; Courchesne, Lincoln, et al., 1985; and Courchesne, Lincoln, et al.,
1986.)

Special notice should be given to the fact that the attention-related component Nc is one of the first endogenous ERP components to appear during development (Courchesne *et al.*, 1981; Karrer & Ackles, in press; Kurtzberg, 1985). It can be found in newborns. One wonders whether this component reflects some facet of neurophysiological mechanisms fundamental to normal cognitive development.

Since Nc is present even in normal newborns, its abnormality in our autistic subjects is particularly curious. Is it possible that, from the very onset of postnatal development, these abnormalities in Nc have existed in our autistic subjects? If so, might the type of Nc abnormality we observed be a sign of abnormal functioning of neurophysiological mechanisms that are essential to the development of a normal attentional orientation to the environment? Our present rudimentary knowledge about Nc makes these questions highly speculative; much research is needed.

In the previous section, we also discussed suggestive evidence that another attention component, the auditory Nd, may have been smaller in our autistic subjects. We concluded that the evidence was suggestive only because our designs did not allow separate, direct measures of this Nd component and the overlapping N1 component.

More specific conclusions about Nd must await systematic studies of attention and ERPs in autism. There are no other studies of Nc in autism.

Some Ideas about the Neurogenerators of Nc. What neurophysiological system might be responsible for Nc? Two possibilities come to mind: acetylcholine systems, and the reticular-thalamic-cortical "activating" system. Arousal, reticular stimulation, behaviorally important stimuli, and novel stimuli increase the release of acetylcholine in cortex and also trigger the reticular-thalamic-cortical activating system. The consequences of these two physiological responses is the selective enhancement of the responsiveness of thalamic and cortical neurons. The specific nature of the triggering stimulation presumably determines exactly which thalamic and cortical neural activity is selectively enhanced. The precise relationship between these two physiological responses to significant environmental information has yet to be established; the increased release of acetylcholine at cortex may, in fact, be part of the reticular-thalamic-cortical activating response (see Hobson & Steriade, 1986, for further discussion).

As regards acetylcholine systems, neurons in nucleus basalis (a subcortical nucleus) send axons to the cortex, where they release the neurotransmitter acetylcholine, and the cortex also has its own "intrinsic" acetylcholine system (Cuello & Sofroniew, 1984; Hedreen, Struble, Whitehouse, & Price, 1984). This transmitter is received by muscarinic receptors on certain cortical neurons. When this happens, these neurons become more easily excited by subsequent stimulation (Brown, 1983). This facilitated state may last many seconds. Stimuli that have significance for the organism may trigger acetylcholine systems. The facilitated state could establish a condition by which information occurring across several seconds may be temporally tagged and integrated. Degeneration of the nucleus basalis system in Alzheimer patients may be a contributing factor in their memory disorder; however, it is not clear whether the disorder involves muscarinic receptors (Arendt, Bigl, Arendt, & Tennstedt, 1983; Price *et al.*, 1982; Terry & Katzman, 1983).

A number of characteristics of Nc are consistent with the physioanatomical and maturational characteristics of acetylcholine systems affecting cortex: Nc—latency of several hundred milliseconds, long duration, negative polarity, largest over central-frontal cortex, appears in newborns, elicited by novel and significant stimuli (Courchesne, 1977, 1983, this subsection; Karrer & Ackles, in press; Kurtzberg, 1985; Kurtzberg, Stone, & Vaughan, 1986). Acetylcholine systems—latency of several hundred milliseconds, long duration, effect of action would be negative polarity potential over cortex, largest over central frontal areas, early maturation of function, increases in acetylcholine release with novel and arousing situations (Brown, 1983; Cuello & Sofroniew, 1984; Hobson & Steriade, 1986; Price, 1985, personal communication; Johnston, 1985, personal communication).

As regards the reticular-thalamic-cortical activating system, this system is necessary for normal attention and awareness (see germinal article by Moruzzi & Magoun, 1949; Hobson & Steriade, 1986). Carpenter (1976, p. 593) writes, "It seems generally accepted that the [reticular-thalamic-cortical] projection system regulates the local and general excitability of the cortex, and, therefore, the state of consciousness and awareness." Sensory stimulation may activate and arouse by triggering portions of the reticular formation in the brainstem. Reticular cells then excite intralaminar cells in the thalamus that, in turn, excite cortex (e.g., Hobson & Steriade, 1986; Steriade & Glenn, 1982). This excitatory input to cortex could produce a negative potential on the surface of the cortex, followed by a positive one generated by secondary excitatory input to a deep layer of cortex where association fibers leave to provide information to other cortical areas. Nc, and the positive potential Pc that follows it, are elicited by the same sorts of stimuli (novel, important, or specifically attended stimuli) that would be expected to excite this reticular-thalamic-cortical activating system. Lesions in this system in man may produce deactivation, lethargy, and loss of awareness (Castaigne, Buge, Escourolle, & Masson, 1962; Facon, Steriade, & Wertheim, 1958). In the two patients described by Castaigne et al. (1962) and Facon et al. (1958), intense stimulation or loud interactions were necessary to maintain awareness.

ERP FINDINGS: SUMMARY AND CONCLUDING REMARKS

Although relatively few ERP studies of autism have been published that meet contemporary methodology standards, a number of interesting and consistent findings have emerged. These studies are important beginnings in the effort to find and characterize the physiological as well as psychological points at which information processing in autism goes awry.

Several recent studies have found no evidence to support the idea that auditory brainstem systems must be abnormal for autism to develop (Figure 4). Thus, the earliest stages of auditory sensory processing do not seem crucial to this disorder. The neural systems crucial to the development of autism must be sought elsewhere. "Elsewhere" includes not only hippocampus, thalamus, dopaminergic and serotonergic systems, cerebellum, and cortex, but also brainstem systems other than those auditory ones that are responsible for generating auditory brainstem ERPs.

Although these very early stages of auditory sensory processing have been thoroughly studied, this has not been true of later stages in auditory sensory processing, somatosensory processing, and visual sensory processing. ERP studies of these other sensory stages and modalities are necessary if we are to establish where and how information processing goes awry. Is sensory input distorted at some stage? Is it attenuated? Is it normal in some modalities but not in others? Knowing the answers to these questions will facilitate the interpretation of ERP findings on endogenous components associated with attention, orienting, and memory. In designing studies of exogenous, sensory components, experimenters must eliminate all potentially confounding effects of attention-related ERP components. These attention-related components may occur during the same time zones as do exogenous, sensory components.

Beyond studies of exogenous components associated with sensory processing stages, a number of studies have found important and consistent abnormalities in endogenous components associated with attention, orienting, and memory.

1. First, autistic people may have a reduced capacity, on the average, to attach appropriate levels of importance to auditory information. The magnitude of this reduction appears to be much more for auditory than for visual information; future research needs to explore and explain this modality effect. The evidence is that autistic people have, on the average, smaller auditory P3b and A/Pcz/300 responses when they are confronted with significant information, whether target or novel sounds (Figures 5, 6, and 8). Of the six ERP experiments reviewed here, all found smaller auditory P3b to targets—a consistent and apparently robust finding.

Important, however, is the additional fact that, while these responses were smaller most of the time, sometimes a single response would be normal—for example, the response to the very first novel sound (Figure 7). This suggests that, in autism, the generators of the auditory P3b component and the auditory A/Pcz/300 component may not be abnormal, but, instead, they seem to be affected by whatever neural systems *are* malfunctioning in autism. The study of these endogenous components appears to be a good starting place for the search for this malfunction.

2. Second, the conditions resulting in abnormal responses do not seem to involve a simple verbal/nonverbal dimension. Since P3b to an omitted event is triggered by internal decisions and not by actual sensory stimulation, the smaller auditory P3b to omitted events indicates considerable independence of the abnormal responses from the precise physical quality or details of stimuli. Moreover, the abnormally small auditory P3b responses have been elicited in tasks demanding processing of spoken words, phonemes, and tones, as well as omitted auditory events.

3. Third, the small and often absent Nc responses to both auditory and visual stimuli suggests that autistic people may not alter or increase internal attention even when they detect significant information. It is as though they register the stimulus event but do not react—categorization without consequence.

The autistic versus normal group differences just mentioned cannot be due to malfunctioning of processes at sensory, perceptual, recognition memory, or categorization levels. First, in our experiments, the autistic subjects were able to perform the auditory target detection tasks (tones and omissions) as accurately and rapidly as did normal subjects, and they were able to recall information about the stimulus sequences (types of stimuli, descriptions of individual novel sounds) after the experiments were over. The use of several measures of task performance and the high level of performance actually found permit the conclusion that task involvement, arousal, attentiveness, cooperation, and ability to understand the task demands cannot account for the subject group differences.

Is it possible that one source of neurophysiological malfunctioning is responsible for these smaller endogenous ERP responses in autism (i.e., P3b, Nc, A/Pcz/300)? Perhaps the clue we are looking for exists in the finding that the *first* auditory novel stimulus did succeed in eliciting a large normal response in several autistic subjects (Figure 7), but subsequent stimuli generally did not. Interestingly, the largest Nc responses were also to the most extreme events (Figure 9)—the wild, clanging, ringing novel sounds and the bright, colorful novel pictures. Is it possible that for a stimulus to gain "full" access to the processing pathways, much more attention-getting stimulation might be required? Just such extreme stimulation is apparently necessary to alert people who have disorders of attention and awareness after lesions of the reticular-thalamic-cortical activating system (Castaigne *et al.*, 1962; Facon *et al.*, 1958). Perhaps the critical malfunctioning in autism involves this system or, judging from the ERP data, involves a neural system that *interferes* with the normal functioning of this activating system.

A CONJECTURE ABOUT THE PATHOPHYSIOLOGY OF AUTISM

Summary

We propose that autism is due to physioanatomical sources of abnormal neural activity analogous to, but not necessarily the same as, epilepsy. The active process interferes with otherwise normal neural systems. The interference prevents the normal functioning of neural systems responsible for attention and awareness (cholinergic and reticular-thalamic-cortical activating systems) and, consequently, prevents normal memory, language, and social functioning. Interference may include (a) random excitation of attentional systems, (b) excitation of only a greatly narrowed neural channel within attentional systems, and (c) inhibition of portions of attentional systems. Again analogous to epilepsy, the activity of the abnormal physioanatomical source would be expected to fluctuate, and this, in turn, should cause fluctuations in the amount and possibly the type of interference with attentional systems. During moments of diminished interference, the whole nervous system is free to function normally and should acquire knowledge whenever this happens. The more severe the interference (whether random excitation, highly narrowed excitation, or inhibition) and the longer the periods of interference, the more impaired the person's memory, language, and social functioning should be.

The time of onset of this proposed abnormal neural activity may be critical. Onset during fetal development would be especially debilitating. Lesions that are sustained before neural pathways are normally established will allow abnormal neural pathways to be established (Schneider, 1979). Such aberrant connections will create abnormal neural activity which will have persistent interfering effects not easily overcome by maturation, experience, or training (Gramsbergen & Ijkema-Paassen, 1985). Abnormally active processes created directly and indirectly by such early lesions should be more debilitating to cognitive and social development than similar ones that occur after substantial knowledge has been acquired. That is, people who sustain similar lesions by way of neurological disorders or trauma during childhood or later in life would not be expected to exhibit the autism syndrome. The physioanatomical source of the abnormal neural activity could be one of several neural systems that have the potential for disrupting or distorting the functioning of attention and awareness mechanisms. Neuroanatomical studies have verified that autism is not the result of massive or widespread abnormalities (Prior, Tress, Hoffman, & Boldt, 1984) but, instead, may be the result of subtle abnormalities involving several neural structures such as the amygdala, hippocampus, and cerebellum (Bauman, 1986, personal communication; Bauman & Kemper, 1985; Williams, Hauser, Purpura, DeLong, & Swisher, 1980). Neurochemistry studies implicate serotonergic and dopaminergic systems (see Chapters 14 and 15), although noradrenergic and acetylcholine systems would also be likely candidates.

Further Discussion

Suppose that most of the nervous system responsible for sensation, perception, memory, recognition, categorization, speech, language, and emotion was normal. Suppose, too, that from the earliest days of life, some neural abnormality existed, and it was an *active* neural influence—neurons acting in a way and at a site that is not normal (e.g., excitatory neurons functioning in the absence of normal inhibitory controls).

Unlike the results of a lesion that eliminates functioning altogether, or produces constantly impaired functioning, an active neural process would produce fluctuations in function across time. At times when these abnormal neurons have diminished activity, functioning of the rest of the nervous system might be near normal; at times of heightened amounts of abnormal activity, functioning of the rest of the nervous system might be distorted, disrupted, or prevented altogether.

Three general types of interference can be considered. First, abnormal activity could randomly excite subgroups of cells within attentional systems. For instance, subgroups of cells within the intralaminar thalamic nucleus (part of the RAS, or reticular activating system) are known to excite different areas of cortex (Steriade & Glenn, 1982); this may also be true of subgroups of cells in the nucleus basalis whose input to cortex, as mentioned earlier, may facilitate the temporal integration of important information. Random excitation of subgroups of cells within attentional systems could activate cortex and behavior in a haphazard fashion. In addition to disorganizing behavior, if haphazard excitations of disparate areas of cortex co-occurred, anomalous corticocortical associations might be established. Second, abnormal activity might affect only limited subgroups of cells within attentional systems. Such limited influence could result, for example, in frequent or persistent excitation of only limited areas of cortex to the exclusion of others—effectively "locking in" very narrow channels of cortical activation, attention, and behavior (which might be manifested as highly restricted activities and interests). Third, abnormal activity may inhibit subgroups of cells within attentional systems; other subgroups, however, would be free to function in response to environmental input. Such inhibition might be associated with deactivation of affected cortical areas. Behavioral attention might then become dominated by whichever cortical areas remained unaffected.

In our conjecture about the pathophysiology of autism, each of these three states of interference is the consequence of abnormal neural activity in a hypothetical physioanatomical source (e.g., analogous to an epileptic site); each state may be expected to fluctuate as a result of fluctuations in the activity of the abnormal neural source. Fluctuations in the abnormal physioanatomical source should lead not only to different degrees of interference, but might also lead to fluctuations in the state of interference which is manifested (i.e., fluctuations from a state of random kaleidoscope-like excitation of numerous cortical areas to a state of "locked in" excitation of few cortical areas). Fluctuations might also include large enough reductions in the abnormal activity such that the state of interference disappears, freeing attention systems to function more normally. Depending on what elements control the amount of activity of these abnormally acting neurons, the fluctuations and their various consequences might be evident across seconds, minutes, hours, or days.

This sort of neural abnormality is not uncommon in humans and animals. An example in humans is epilepsy. In some cases, the abnormal neural activity is infrequent and does not produce widespread disruption of the nervous system. Such people may lead quite normal and very productive intellectual and emotional lives. In other cases, the abnormal neural interference is so frequent and so widespread in its influence that it can reduce an otherwise potentially normal person to the level of severe intellectual, emotional, and social incapacity. The earlier the epilepsy begins, the greater the jeopardy is to the acquisition of general knowledge, language, and social ability.

Training and experience do not prevent or get around such active, fluctuating abnormal actions of epileptic neurons. Knowledge is acquired during times of diminished activity of such interfering neurons. Note that, in our supposition, the nervous system is largely normal otherwise. The more time free from the interfering neural activity, the more normal the person will be. With such abnormal neural activity, it can be expected that various internal conditions—oxygen levels, hormonal levels, nutrients available—and various external conditions—flashing lights, loud sounds—will be able to affect the activity of these interfering neurons.

Might autism be a disorder analogous to this sort of neurophysiological dysfunction? Specifically, if interfering neural activity did exist in neural systems implicated in the ERP studies cited above, could the disruption in early development account for autism? As a reminder, current ERP findings (on A/Pcz/300, P3b, Nc) implicate neural systems involved in attention and awareness: systems necessary for consciously tagging and remembering information as important. We suggested above that Nc, which appears even in the newborn, might be associated with such neural systems, systems essential to normal cognitive development. The Nc abnormality in autism, therefore, raises the question of whether a fundamental disturbance exists in mechanisms of attention and awareness during development. We also stated above that massive interference of these mechanisms in adults produces dramatic reductions in awareness, the absolute level of which, however, does fluctuate; loud stimuli, for instance, could greatly increase attention and awareness for brief moments (Castaigne et al., 1962; Facon et al., 1958).

Descriptions of this type of interference are reminiscent of the self-description of an autistic young man recently published by Volkmar and Cohen (1985), "I was living in a world of daydreaming. . . . One thing I loved that not even the Fear could stop was Airplaines. I saw an air show the planes—f4s—were loud. I was allway(s) Impressed by Airplaines. . . . [I] had and still have mental blocks and great difficulty paying attention." Coincidentally, a young autistic man in our studies also said that he "daydreams"; he said, "It is almost like I'm asleep. . . . One time [when this young man was an adolescent] a math teacher yelled at me and told me I was tuned out and I was looking at the lights and I was doing this." He then moved his hand closer and further from his nose. During this episode of "tuning out," this young man said he had no recollection of anything—either thoughts or things from the outside world. He said, "I'm aware this [tuning out] happens because I suddenly see the whole room again and I knew that that is where I have always been [before tuning out]. One time [while tuned out], I thought I heard someone say 'small world after all'; then my teacher yelled at me . . . and startled me . . . and asked what music the class was talking about." This young man answered, "Small world after all," and his teacher said that was right!

If interference of attention and awareness essential for properly tagging information for later remembrance and use was occurring in an infant, he or she would have a fragmented, haphazard, and narrowed representation of the external world. Interference might only *attenuate*, not completely block, normal sensory information passing through thalamus to cortex. During moments of diminished interference, the infant's nervous system would be free to more normally absorb sights and sounds. So, as the hypothesized interference fluctuates, the autistic person's knowledge of the world would be made up of disconnected fragments of information. The fragments would have no context or temporal continuity for the child. What fragments do enter conscious memory would be, in large measure, initially due to chance, as the interference randomly fluctuates, activating and deactivating patches of cortex in a kaleidoscopic fashion; randomly "locks in" or narrows the focus of activation to a few patches of cortex; or is briefly overridden by loud or strong stimulation. Perhaps this accounts for the observation of tremendous variability in the knowledge acquired by autistic people.

I am reminded of the self-report of one of the adult nonretarded autistic subjects in our studies. He stated that one of his earliest memories was when he was 5 years old and noticed for the first time that a man had something around his mouth, which he was told was a beard. He said he had not been aware before this that men had beards. Apparently for years after that, beards served as powerful stimuli, such that whenever he encountered beards, he became alert, but utterly focused on the beard itself. He excitedly went on to say that 2 years later, he suddenly discovered that men also have sideburns. His fascination with beards remains to this day, more than a decade later. Such moments of highly focused awareness brought him fragments of information that became his knowledge base of the world. Just as the sound of your name being called while you are drowsy may rouse you to consciousness, so too, it seems, do such fragments of consciously remembered information serve as powerful stimuli for the autistic child.

So, for one autistic child, then, a random, chance fluctuation brought him a world of beards, and, perhaps for another autistic child, a world of airplanes. These children then build on what they know and become specialists in especially narrow channels of knowledge—beards, airplanes, bicycles, numbers, helicopters. Information not within these narrow channels of knowledge might not be any more intelligible to them than a foreign language—information without a knowledge base for comprehending it.

A fragment of knowledge about objects in a room or a sequence of movements by the child itself would be usable knowledge. Objects have constant values; the lamp by the bed does not change from moment to moment. The child can throw the light switch time and again and the same thing happens.

On the other hand, haphazard fragments of social and language information may be more confusing than useful. A fragment of a sentence, or the expression, posture, and dress of mother, for example, offer little useful information in the variable, complex, and temporally dependent world of language and social interactions. A spoken phrase or a brief facial expression make little sense without a context of actions, words, people, and events. Imagine a symphony you have never heard before being played on your radio, but the transmission is so faulty that you only occasionally hear a few bars. If the social world were imagined to be like a symphony, with complex and temporally dependent interactions of players, how socially handicapped would a person be if he experienced only occasional snippets?

Emotional states such as pain, satiety, or hunger build up through automatic functions of the nervous system. As with other strong stimulation, we can presume that these emotional states may reach a level at which they may override the interference of attention and awareness systems. However, when such emotional states are triggered, and as they are building up, the neural activity interfering with awareness would preclude the autistic child's making the normal link between the triggering events and the emotional state. More anomalous, however, would be the result of momentary fluctuations in the abnormal interference during emotional states. A momentary decrease in interference (perhaps due to strong internal emotional stimulation analogous to strong, loud external stimulation) could allow a fragment of information to be consciously processed and linked with the emotional state. The environmental information attended to and linked up could be anything—a chance glance at a toy helicopter, or a spoken phrase. The anomalous result would be an environmental event emotionally tagged, but devoid of context or consequence.

Just like a normal child, the autistic child will use the information he or she has acquired. The child will perform the actions known, speak the words known, and respond to stimulation according to remembrances. Occurrences such as these might be seen as ritualistic, echolalic, and anomalous responses to the environment.

From the above comments, it may already be seen that we suggest that fluctuations in the interference may come about in several ways. Strong emotional states, intense stimulation, stimuli that, by chance, have become linked with special emotion and importance (e.g., beards) may each override, for periods of time, the abnormally interfering activity and take control. Perhaps, with increasing maturity of cortex and with increasing amounts of fragments of knowledge that have been strongly emotionally and consciously tagged, behavior and thought become organized around, oriented towards, and controlled by such fragments of emotionally charged knowledge.

More than one neural system could play such a devastating role in interfering with normal attention and awareness mechanisms at reticular, thalamic, and cortical levels. It is possible that, while all cases of autism result from this speculated general sort of abnormal neurophysiology, different subgroups of autism might be the consequence of different neural systems that are disrupting these mechanisms to different degrees and at different levels (reticular, thalamic, or cortical). Alternatively, perhaps only one crucial and especially vulnerable neural system is responsible. Differences in intelligence and level of functioning would then be due to two factors: (1) the severity and duration of the abnormal activity— for instance, severe interference for long periods of time versus mild levels for short periods of time; and (2) the presence of additional lesions.

What neural systems are reasonable candidates? Normal activation of attention and awareness involves precisely timed sequences of excitation and inhibition of numerous neural systems at reticular, thalamic, and cortical levels. The serotonergic, dopaminergic, noradrenergic, and cholinergic neurotransmitter systems either play a role in this activation or are connected in such a way as to have potential for disrupting activation (see review by Hobson & Steriade, 1986). Chapters 14 and 15 discuss the evidence of abnormality in several of these systems.

Neuroanatomical studies of autism have provided few and somewhat perplexing clues about candidate neural systems. Some CT scan studies have found that the neuroanatomy of nonretarded autistic people is not distinctively different from normal at the gross morphological level, although examination of the cerebellum has seldom been specifically mentioned (e.g., Prior et al., 1984). When abnormalities have been found, they have most frequently been in the hippocampus and the cerebellum of retarded autistic people (Bauman, 1986, personal communication; Bauman & Kemper, 1985; Hauser, DeLong, & Rosman, 1975; Jaeken & VandenBerghe, 1984; Williams et al., 1980). The hippocampus plays a critical role in memory making, and the cerebellum in modulation of motion and perhaps also in certain facets of memory (Leaton & Supple, 1986; McCormick & Thompson, 1984; see review of recent research on memory and the cerebellum, Gellman & Miles, 1985).

The hippocampus and cerebellum are two of the brain structures most sensitive to damage from hypoxia. Severe prenatal or perinatal damage to the hippocampus would, very likely, lead to lasting memory problems. Also, the hippocampus is especially susceptible to becoming epileptic. The hippocampus has a significant, although indirect, influence over the reticular-thalamic-cortical activating system and reciprocal interactions with nucleus basalis cholinergic system.

These facts seem to make the hippocampus an attractive candidate for the source of abnormality in autism.

Yet damage and epilepsy cannot easily account for certain important facts. Hippocampal epilepsy is not typical of autism, in general, and is relatively unusual in nonretarded autistic individuals, in particular. Damage to hippocampus would produce consistent memory deficits, not fluctuations in the capacity to create new memory across seconds, minutes, and hours, as seen in nonretarded autistic individuals. Also, hippocampal damage cannot readily explain how it can be that nonretarded individuals can remember all manner of details about such things as types of streetlamps, bicycles, days and dates, the sequence and time of programs on one TV station, and the exact words and intonations of a phrase from a raucous TV commercial. The same individual may turn around and not remember anything at all about an experimenter with whom they have just spent 1 to 2 hours.

It is easy to see how hippocampal damage could lead to mental retardation in autism or in any other disorder, but it remains to be seen how it can explain the remarkable variety and variability of memory in autism. Nonetheless, hippocampal malfunctioning cannot be ruled out as a potential contributor to autistic symptomatology, particularly in mentally retarded autistic people.

On the face of it, damage to the cerebellum seems unlikely to be a candidate for a source of abnormal neural activity causing autism. Yet the recent neuropathology findings of Bauman and Kemper (1985) do have some interesting features. The cerebellar pathology they reported was loss of Purkinje neurons and significant neuronal loss in several deep nuclei of the cerebellum. The neuronal loss in their single case of autism might have occurred very early in fetal development before final neural connections were in place (see comments below). Purkinje neurons control the activity of these deep cerebellar nuclei. One of these nuclei, the dentate nucleus, was not damaged in the case reported by Bauman and Kemper (1985).

This may have had three consequences. First, Purkinje cells and deep cerebellar nuclei (dentate and interpositus) may play an important role in associative learning, and disorder in their functioning due to Purkinje cell loss could have affected such learning (Gellman & Miles, 1985). Second, the activity of the neurons of the dentate nucleus would no longer have been controlled (the Purkinje neurons having been lost). Third, the dentate nucleus might have made abnormal connections with other neural systems; that is, it might have made axonal connections to brainstem, thalamus, and limbic system left vacated by its neighboring degenerated nuclei. Aberrant neural connections have been described in rodents following damage to dentate nucleus, as well as other parts of the nervous system (e.g., Gramsbergen and Ijkema-Paassen, 1985; Schneider, 1979). Aberrant neural connections are thought to produce long-lasting physiological and behavioral abnormalities, abnormalities difficult if not impossible to overcome (see discussions by Gramsbergen and Ijkema-Paassen, 1984; Schneider, 1979). To understand the pathophysiology of autism, it is essential to consider the possibility of such aberrant neural connections whenever there is a report of neuronal loss, whether in cerebellum or anywhere else.

What are the connections of the deep cerebellar nuclei, and the dentate nuclei in particular (Carpenter, 1976; Gilman, Bloedel, & Lechtenberg, 1981; Gramsbergen & Ijkema-Paassen, 1985; Hendry, Jones, & Graham, 1979; Miller & Strominger, 1977; Nieuwenhuys, Voogd, & van Huijzen, 1981)? The dentate nuclei, as well as other deep cerebellar nuclei, can be expected to make direct connections with several levels of the reticular-thalamic-cortical activating system. They include nucleus reticularis gigantocellularis, nucleus reticularis pontis caudalis, nucleus reticularis pontis oralis, reticulotegmental nuclei, mesencephalic reticular formation, nucleus centralis lateralis thalamus, nucleus paracentralis thalamus, possibly nucleus ventralis medialis thalamus, and possibly nucleus reticularis thalamus. They also make direct connections to thalamic nuclei that represent a major point of confluence of cortical, cerebellar, and basal gangliar initiation and fine control of motor actions. They include nucleus ventralis anterioralis thalamus and nucleus ventralis lateralis thalamus. They also make direct connections to portions of the serotonergic neurotransmitter system—namely, nucleus raphe magnus and nucleus raphe pontis. Abnormal levels of serotonin are sometimes reported in autism (see Chapters 14 and 15).

The neural projections of the dentate nuclei constitute an excitatory system reaching out to, and potentially significantly affecting, the normal functioning of several levels of the systems which mediate attention and awareness, intentional motor behavior, and emotional behavior. Moreover, the major control over this excitatory system are the cerebellar Purkinje neurons, and, according to a recent neuropathology report, there is a loss of these Purkinje neurons in a postmortem single case study of a severely retarded autistic individual (Bauman & Kemper, 1985). Recently, we tested the idea that the cerebellum might be abnormal in some cases of autism. We wanted concrete *in vivo* evidence from a classic (Kanner syndrome) case uncomplicated by mental retardation, epilepsy, or a history of drug use or neurological disease. In the first such autistic person we tested, we found *in vivo* MRI (magnetic resonance imaging) evidence of a macroscopic maldevelopment of the cerebellum in a person with classic (Kanner syndrome) autism; the dentate nuclei appeared normal (Courchesne, Hesselink, Jernigan, & Yeung-Courchesne, in press). This cerebellar maldevelopment could be accounted for by massive Purkinje cell loss during fetal development, but, of course, such a possibility cannot be proven with *in vivo* MRI technology.

The deep cerebellar nuclei, including the dentate nuclei, are known to provide excitatory input to thalamus and potentially also to the reticular formation. The consequence could be either excitation of thalamic output, inhibition, or an oscillation between the two states. Which it is has yet to be fully established by scientists. In either case, if these nuclei, including dentate, were not normally regulated (e.g., by Purkinje cells), they could be capable of producing abnormally patterned bursts of activity. Such ongoing abnormal activity would have an aberrant relationship to events in the external world. The harmful consequences to the normal functioning of attention and awareness systems and to systems mediating intentional motor behavior could be substantial.

Although the neuropathology of the cerebellum provides an interesting candidate for our view of the pathophysiology of autism, great caution is in order. Few cases of cerebellar damage in autistic individuals have been reported and they have been predominantly cases of retarded individuals. The cerebellar damage could be a secondary or associated pathology, rather than the pathology (or pathologies) without which autism does not develop. This possibility is especially important to remember when reading reports that do not provide evidence of brain sites other than the cerebellum. Also, the observation that cerebellar damage sustained during fetal development could be a candidate in some autistic individuals does not preclude other sites of pathology from also being responsible for analogous disruptions in other autistic individuals. Lastly, there are degenerative disorders of Purkinje neurons that do not lead to autism. Such disorders are thought to begin usually after local cerebellar circuitry and cerebellar afferent circuitry have been laid down; and many occur after a period of time has passed during which the nervous system has had a chance to begin maturing normally and acquired a broad foundation of knowledge (e.g., middle childhood, adulthood).

Our model of the pathophysiology in autism is a general one (and indeed may have application in understanding order disorders such as schizophrenia): occult abnormal neural activity secondary to neuronal loss and aberrant neural connections interferes with the normal functioning of attentional systems; the interference could take the form of a kaleidoscopic, random pattern of cortical activation and deactivation; of a "locked in," focused activation of relatively few patches of cortex; and of a deactivation of large areas of cortex. The abnormal activity fluctuates, and this creates fluctuations in those states of interference. More generally, the proposed model of pathophysiology includes the idea that disorders of information processing more subtle than autism may involve analogous pathophysiologies.

ACKNOWLEDGMENTS

This research was supported by NIMH grant 1-RO1-MH36840 awarded to E. Courchesne and by NINCDS grant 5-RO1-NS19855 awarded to E. Courchesne. Valuable assistance has also been provided by the San Diego Regional Center for the Developmentally Disabled. Special thanks go to Beverly A. Kilman, whose understanding of autism and whose help were keys given to the author that unlocked doors to his research on autism. Thanks go to Rachel Yeung-Courchesne for helpful comments on the manuscript, to Martha B. Denckla, Magda Campbell, and Anne Petersen for acting as critical catalysts, and to Jeannette Johnson, Jon Rolf, and Wright and Barbara Williamson.

REFERENCES

Achor, L. J., & Starr, A. (1980a). Auditory brain stem responses in the cat: I. Intracranial and extracranial recordings. *Electroencephalography and Clinical Neurophysiology, 48,* 154–173.

Achor, L. J., & Starr, A. (1980b). Auditory brain stem responses in the cat: II. Effects of lesions. *Electroencephalography and Clinical Neurophysiology, 48,* 174–190.

Ackles, P., & Karrer, R. (1985). *Development of late visual event-related potentials and information processing in infants.* Paper presented at the meetings of the Society for Research in Child Development, Toronto.

Arendt, T., Bigl, V., Arendt, A., & Tennstedt, A. (1983). Loss of neurons in the nucleus basalis of meynert in Alzheimer's disease, paralysis agitans and Korsakoff's disease. *Acta Neuropathologica, 61,* 101–108.

Bauman, M., & Kemper, T. L. (1985). Histoanatomic observations of the brain in early infantile autism. *Neurology, 35,* 866–874.

Berlyne, D. D. (1960). *Conflict, arousal and curiosity.* New York: McGraw-Hill.

Bernstein, A. S. (1979). The orienting response as novelty and significance detector: Reply to O'Gorman. *Psychophysiology, 16,* 263–273.

Brown, D. A. (1983). Slow cholinergic excitation—A mechanism for increasing neuronal excitability. *Trends in Neurosciences, 6,* 302–307.

Carpenter, M. B. (1976). *Human neuroanatomy.* Baltimore: Williams and Wilkins.

Castaigne, P., Buge, A., Escourolle, R., & Masson, M. (1962). Ramollissement pedonculaire median, tegmento-thalamique avec ophtalmoplegie et hypersomnie. *Revue Neurologique, 106,* 357–367.

Chiappa, K. H. (1983). *Evoked potentials in clinical medicine.* New York: Raven Press.

Courchesne, E. (1977). Event-related brain potentials: A comparison between children and adults. *Science, 197,* 589–592.

Courchesne, E. (1978a). Neurophysiological correlates of cognitive development: Changes in long-latency event-related potentials from childhood to adulthood. *Electroencephalography and Clinical Neurophysiology, 45,* 468–482.

Courchesne, E. (1978b). Changes in P3 waves with event repetition: Long-term effects on scalp distribution and amplitude. *Electroencephalography and Clinical Neurophysiology, 45,* 754–766.

Courchesne, E. (1979). From infancy to adulthood: The neurophysiological correlates of cognition. In J. E. Desmedt (Ed.), *Cognitive components in cerebral event-related potentials and selective attention: Progress in clinical neurophysiology* (Vol. 6, pp. 224–242). Basel: Karger.

Courchesne, E. (1983). Cognitive components of the event-related brain potential: Changes associated with development. In A. W. K. Gaillard & W. Ritter (Eds.), *Tutorials in ERP research: Endogenous components* (pp. 329–344). Amsterdam: North-Holland.

Courchesne, E. (in press). Chronology of post-natal human brain development: ERP, PET, myelinogenesis and synaptogenesis studies. In J. W. Rohrbaugh, R. Parasuraman, & R. Johnson (Eds.), *Event-related brain potentials: Issues and interdisciplinary vantages.* New York: Oxford Press.

Courchesne, E., Courchesne, R. Y., Hicks, G., & Lincoln, A. J. (1985). Functioning of the brainstem auditory pathway in non-retarded autistic individuals. *Electroencephalography and Clinical Neurophysiology: Evoked Potentials, 61*, 491–501.

Courchesne, E., Elmasian, R., & Yeung-Courchesne, R. (1986). Electrophysiological correlates of cognitive processing: P3b and Nc, basic, clinical, and developmental research. In A. M. Halliday, S. R. Butler, & R. Paul (Eds.), *A textbook of clinical neurophysiology* (pp. 645–676). London: Wiley.

Courchesne, E., Ganz, L., & Norcia, A. (1981). Event-related brain potentials to human faces in infants. *Child Development, 52*, 804–811.

Courchesne, E., Ganz, L., & Norcia, A. M. (1986). *The P3b/SW complex in young children in a face discrimination task.* Manuscript submitted for publication.

Courchesne, E., Hesselink, J. R., Jernigan, T. L., & Yeung-Courchesne, R. (in press). Neuropathology of a non-retarded person with autism: Unusual findings from magnetic resonance imaging. *Archives of Neurology.*

Courchesne, E., Hillyard, S. A., & Galambos, R. (1975). Stimulus novelty, task relevance and the visual evoked potential in man. *Electroencephalography and Clinical Neurophysiology, 39*, 131–143.

Courchesne, E., Kilman, B. A., Galambos, R., & Lincoln, A. J. (1984). Autism: Processing of novel auditory information assessed by event-related brain potentials. *Electroencephalography and Clinical Neurophysiology: Evoked Potentials, 59*, 238–248.

Courchesne, E., Lincoln, A. J., Kilman, B. A., & Galambos, R. (1985). Event-related brain potential correlates of the processing of novel visual and auditory information in autism. *Journal of Autism and Developmental Disorders, 15*, 55–76.

Courchesne, E., Lincoln, A. J., Yeung-Courchesne, R., Elmasian, R., & Grillon, C. (1986). *Pathophysiology in social and language disorders: Autism and receptive developmental dysphasia.* Manuscript in preparation.

Courchesne, E., & Yeung-Courchesne, R. (in press). Event-related brain potentials and developmental psychopathologies. In M. Rutter, H. Tuma, & I. Lann (Eds.), *Assessment and diagnosis in child and adolescent psychopathology.* New York: Guilford Publications.

Cuello, A. C., & Sofroniew, M. V. (1984). The anatomy of the CNS cholinergic neurons. *Trends in Neurosciences, 7*, 74–78.

Dawson, G., Finley, C., Phillips, P., & Galpert, L. (1986). *P300 of the auditory evoked potential and the language abilities of autistic children.* Manuscript in preparation.

Donchin, E. Surprise! . . . Surprise? *Psychophysiology, 18*, 493–513.

Donchin, E., Callaway, E., Cooper, R., Desmedt, J. E., Goff, W. R., Hillyard, S. A., & Sutton, S. (1977). Publication criteria for studies of evoked potentials (EP) in man. In J. E. Desmedt (Ed.), *Progress in clinical neurophysiology* (Vol. 1, pp. 1–11). Basel: Karger.

Donchin, E., Heffly, E., Hillyard, S. A., Loveless, N., Maltzman, I., Ohman, A., Rosler, F., Ruchkin, D., & Siddle, D. (1984). Cognition and event-related potentials: II. The orienting reflex and P300. In R. Karrer, J. Cohen, & P. Tueting (Eds.), *Brain and Information: Event-related potentials. Annals of the New York Academy of Sciences, 425*, 39–57.

Donchin, E., Ritter, W., & McCallum, W. C. (1978). Cognitive psychophysiology: The endogenous components of the ERP. In E. Callaway, P. Tueting, & S. H. Koslow (Eds.), *Event-related brain potentials in man* (pp. 349–411). New York: Academic Press.

Facon, E., Steriade, M., & Wertheim, N. (1958). Hypersomnie prolongée engendrée par des lesions bilaterales du système activateur médial. Le syndrome thrombotique de la bifurcation du tronc basilaire. *Review of Neurology, 106*, 357–367.

Galambos, R., & Hecox, K. E. (1978). Clinical applications of the auditory brain stem response. *Otolaryngological Clinics of North American, 11*, 709–722.

Gellman, R. S., & Miles, F. A. (1985). A new role for the cerebellum in conditioning? *Trends in Neurosciences, 8*, 181–182.

Gillberg, C., Rosenhall, U., & Johansson, E. (1983). Auditory brainstem responses in childhood psychosis. *Journal of Autism and Developmental Disorders, 13*, 181–195.

Gilman, S., Bloedel, J., & Lechtenberg, R. (1981). *Disorders of the cerebellum*. Philadelphia: F. A. Davis Company.

Goff, W. R., Allison, T., & Vaughan, H. G., Jr. (1978). The functional neuroanatomy of event related potentials. In E. Callaway, P. Tueting, & S. H. Koslow (Eds.), *Event-related brain potentials in man* (pp. 1–79). San Francisco: Academic Press.

Gold, M. S., & Gold, J. R. (1975). Autism and attention: Theoretical considerations and a pilot study using set reaction time. *Child Psychiatry and Human Development, 6,* 68–80.

Gramsbergen, A., & Ijkema-Paassen, J. (1985). Cerebellar hemispherectomy at young ages in rats. In J. R. Bloedel, J. Dichgans, & W. Precht (Eds.), *Cerebellar functions* (pp. 164–167). Berlin: Springer-Verlag.

Groves, P. M., & Lynch, G. S. (1972). Mechanisms of habituation in the brain stem. *Psychological Review, 79,* 237–244.

Hansen, J. C., & Hillyard, S. A. (1980). Endogenous brain potentials associated with selective auditory attention. *Electroencephalography and Clinical Neurophysiology, 49,* 277–290.

Hansen, J. C., & Hillyard, S. A. (1983). Selective attention to multidimensional auditory stimuli. *Journal of Experimental Psychology: Human Perception and Performance, 9,* 1–19.

Hauser, S. L., DeLong, G. R., & Rosman, N. P. (1975). Pneumographic findings in the infantile autism syndrome. *Brain, 98,* 667–688.

Hedreen, J. C., Struble, R. G., Whitehouse, P. J., & Price, D. L. (1984). Topography of the magnocellular forebrain system in the human brain. *Journal of Neuropathology and Experimental Neurology, 43,* 1–21.

Hendry, S. H. C., Jones, E. G., & Graham, J. (1979). Thalamic relay nuclei for cerebellar and certain related fiber systems in the cat. *Journal of Comparative Neurology, 185,* 679–714.

Hobson, J. A., & Steriade, M. (1986). The neuronal basis of behavioral state control: Internal systems of the brain. In F. Bloom (Ed.), V. Mountcastle (Series Ed.), *Handbook of physiology: volume on intrinsic regulatory systems of the brain*. Bethesda, Maryland: American Physiological Society Press.

Hoffman, W. L., & Prior, M. R. (1982). Neuropsychological dimensions of autism in children: A test of the hemispheric dysfunction hypothesis. *Journal of Clinical Neuropsychology, 4,* 27–41.

Jaeken, J., & Van den Berghe, G. (1984). An infantile autistic syndrome characterized by the presence of succinylpurines in body fluids. *Lancet, 10,* 1058–1059.

James, A. L., & Barry, R. J. (1980). Respiratory and vascular responses to simple visual stimuli in autistics, retardates and normals. *Psychophysiology, 17,* 541–547.

James, A. L., & Barry, R. J. (1982). A review of psychophysiology in early onset psychosis. *Schizophrenia Bulletin, 6,* 506–525.

Johnson, R. E., Jr., & Donchin, E. (1982). Sequential expectancies and decision making in a changing environment: An electrophysiological approach. *Psychophysiology, 19,* 183–200.

Karrer, R. & Ackles, P. K. (in press). Visual event-related potentials of infants during a modified oddball procedure. *Electroencephalography and Clinical Neurophysiology (Suppl.)*.

Knight, R. (1984). Decreased response to novel stimuli after prefrontal lesions in man. *Electroencephalography and Clinical Neurophysiology, 59,* 9–20.

Kootz, J. P., and Cohen, D. J. (1981). Modulation of sensory intake in autistic children. *Journal of the American Academy of Child Psychiatry, 20,* 692–701.

Kraus, N., Smith, D. I., Reed, N. L., Stein, L. K. and Cartee, C. (1985). Auditory middle latency responses in children: Effects of age and diagnostic category. *Electroencephalography and Clinical Neurophysiology: Evoked Potentials, 62,* 343–351.

Kurtzberg, D. (1985). *Late auditory evoked potentials and speech sound discrimination in newborns*. Paper presented at the meetings of the Society for Research in Child Development, Toronto.

Kurtzberg, D., Stone, C. L., Jr., & Vaughan, H. G., Jr. (1986). Cortical responses to speech sounds in the infant. In R. Q. Cracco & I. Bodis-Wollner (Eds.), *Frontiers of clinical neuroscience: Vol. 3. Evoked potentials* (pp. 513–520). New York: Alan R. Liss.

Leaton, R. N. and Supple, W. F. (1986). Cerebellar vermis:essential for long-term habituation of the acoustic startle response. *Science, 232*, 513–515.

Luria, A. R., & Homskaya, E. D. (1970). Frontal lobes and the regulation of arousal process. In D. I. Mostofsky (Ed.), *Attention: Contemporary theory and analysis* (pp. 303–330). New York: Appleton-Century-Crofts.

McCormick, D. A., & Thompson, R. F. (1984). Cerebellum: Essential involvement in the classically conditioned eyelid response. *Science, 223*, 296–299.

Miller, R. A., & Strominger, N. L. (1977). An experimental study of the efferent connections of the superior cerebellar peduncle in the rhesus monkey. *Brain Research, 133*, 237–250.

Moruzzi, G., & Magoun, H. W. (1949). Brainstem reticular formation and activation of the EEG. *Electroencephalography and Clinical Neurophysiology, 1*, 455–473.

Naatanen, R. (1982). Processing negativity: An evoked-potential reflection of selective attention. *Psychological Bulletin, 92*, 605–640.

Naatanen, R., Gaillard, A. W. K., & Varey, C. A. (1981). Attention effects on auditory EPs as a function of interstimulus interval. *Biological Psychology, 13*, 173–187.

Nieuwenhuys, R., Voogd, J., & van Huijzen, C. (1981). *The human central nervous system*. Berlin: Springer-Verlag.

Novick, B., Kurtzberg, A., & Vaughan, H. G., Jr. (1979). An electrophysiologic indication of defective information storage in childhood autism. *Psychiatry Research, 1*, 101–108.

Novick, B., Vaughan, H. G., Jr., Kurtzberg, D., & Simson, R. (1980). An electrophysiologic indication of auditory processing defects in autism. *Psychiatry Research, 3*, 107–114.

O'Keefe, J. (1976). Place units in the hippocampus of the freely moving rat. *Experimental Neurology, 51*, 78–109.

Paul, D., & Sutton, S. (1972). Evoked potential correlates of response criterion in auditory signal detection. *Science, 177*, 362–364.

Picton, T. W., & Smith, A. D. (1978). The practice of evoked potential audiometry. *Otolaryngological Clinics of North America, 11*, 263–282.

Picton, T. W., Stapells, D., & Campbell, K. B. (1981). Auditory evoked potentials from the human cochlea and brainstem. *Journal of Otolaryngology, 10*, 1–41.

Price, D. L., Whitehouse, P. J., Struble, R. G., Coyle, J. T., Clark, A. W., DeLong, M. R., Cork, L. C., & Hedreen, J. C. (1982). Alzheimer's disease and Down's syndrome. *Annals of the New York Academy of Sciences, 398*, 145–164.

Prior, M. R., Tress, B., Hoffman, W. L., & Boldt, D. (1984). Computed tomographic study of children with classic autism. *Archives of Neurology, 14*, 482–484.

Pritchard, W. S. (1981). Psychophysiology of P300. *Psychological Bulletin, 89*, 506–540.

Ranck, J. B. (1973). Studies on single neurons in dorsal hippocampal formation and septum in unrestrained rats. I. Behavioral correlates and firing repertories. *Experimental Neurology, 4*, 185–200.

Rimland, B. (1964). *Infantile autism*. New York: Appleton-Century-Crofts.

Robinson, K., & Rudge, P. (1982a). Centrally generated auditory potentials. In A. M. Halliday (Ed.), *Evoked potentials in clinical testing* (pp. 345–372). London: Churchill Livingston.

Robinson, K., & Rudge, P. (1982b). The use of auditory potentials in neurology. In A. M. Halliday (Ed.), *Evoked potentials in clinical testing* (pp. 373–392). London: Churchill Livingstone.

Rosler, F. (1983). Endogenous ER"Ps" and cognition: Probes, prospects, and pitfalls in matching pieces of the mind–body puzzle. In A. W. K. Gaillard & W. Ritter (Eds.), *Tutorials in event related potential research: Endogenous components*. Amsterdam: Elsevier/North-Holland.

Rumsey, J. M., Grimes, A. M., Pikus, A. M., Duara, R., & Ismond, D. R. (1984). Auditory brainstem responses in pervasive developmental disorders. *Biological Psychiatry, 19*, 1403–1418.

Rutter, M. (1979). Language, cognition, and autism. In R. Katzman (Ed.), *Congenital and acquired cognitive disorders* (pp. 247–264). New York: Raven Press.

Scherg, M., & Von Cramon, D. (1985). A new interpretation of the generators of BAEP waves I–V: Results of a spatio-temporal dipole model. *Electroencephalography and Clinical Neurophysiology: Evoked Potentials, 62*, 290–299.

Schneider, G. E. (1979). Is it really better to have your brain lesion early? A revision of the "Kennard Principal." *Neuropsychologia, 17*, 557–583.

Skoff, B. F., Mirsky, A. F., & Turner, D. (1980). Prolonged brainstem transmission time in autism. *Psychiatry Research, 2*, 157–166.

Sokolov, E. N. (1958). The orienting reflex, its structure and mechanisms. In L. G. Voronin, A. N. Leontiev, A. R. Luria, E. N. Sokolov, and O. S. Vinogradova (Eds.), *Orienting reflex and exploratory behavior* (pp. 141–151). Moscow: Academy of Pedagogical Sciences of RSFSR.

Sokolov, E. N. (1960). Neuronal models and the orienting reflex. In M. A. B. Brazier (Ed.), *The central nervous system and behavior* (pp. 187–276). New York: Macy Foundation.

Sokolov, E. N. (1963). Higher nervous functions: The orienting reflex. In V. E. Hall, R. R. Sonnenschein, & A. C. Giese (Eds.), *Annual review of physiology* (pp. 545–580). Palo Alto: Annual Reviews.

Spehlmann, R. (1985). *Evoked potential primer: Visual, auditory and somatosensory evoked potentials in clinical diagnosis.* Boston: Butterworth.

Starr, A., & Achor, L. J. (1975). Auditory brain stem responses in neurological disease. *Archives of Neurology, 32*, 761–768.

Starr, A., & Hamilton, A. E. (1976). Correlation between confirmed sites of neurological lesions and abnormalities of far-field auditory brainstem responses. *Electroencephalography and Clinical Neurophysiology, 41*, 595–608.

Starr, A., Sohmer, H., & Celesia, G. G. (1978). Some applications of evoked potentials to patients with neurological and sensory impairment. In E. Callaway, P. Tueting, & S. H. Koslow (Eds.), *Event-related brain potentials in man* (pp. 155–196). San Francisco: Academic Press.

Steriade, M., & Glenn, L. (1982). Neocortical and caudate projections of intralaminar thalamic neurons and their synaptic excitation from midbrain reticular core. *Journal of Neurophysiology, 48*, 352–371.

Stockard, J. J., Stockard, J. E., & Sharbrough, F. W. (1977). Detection and localization of occult lesions with brainstem auditory responses. *Mayo Clinic Proceedings, 52*, 761–669.

Stockard, J. J., Stockard, J. E., & Sharbrough, F. W. (1978). Nonpathologic factors influencing brainstem auditory evoked potentials. *American Journal of EEG Technology, 18*, 177–209.

Sutton, S., Braren, M., Zubin, J., & John, E. R. (1965). Evoked potential correlates of stimulus uncertainty. *Science, 150*, 1187–1188.

Sutton, S., Braren, M., Zubin, J., & John, E. R. (1967). Information delivery and the sensory evoked potential. *Science, 155*, 1436–1439.

Sutton, S., & Ruchkin, D. S. (1984). The late positive complex: Advances and new problems. In R. Karrer, J. Cohen, and P. Tueting (Eds.), *Brain and information: Event-related potentials. Annals of the New York Academy of Sciences, 425*, 1–23.

Tanguay, P., Edwards, R. M., Buchwald, J., Schwafel, J., & Allen, V. (1982). Auditory brainstem evoked responses in autistic children. *Archives of General Psychiatry, 39*, 174–180.

Taylor, M. J., Rosenblatt, B., & Linschoten, L. (1982). Electrophysiological study of the auditory system in autistic children. In A. Rothenberger (Ed.), *Event-related potentials in children* (pp. 379–386). New York: Elsevier Biomedical Press.

Terry, R. D., and Katzman, R. (1983). Senile dementia of the Alzheimer type. *Annals of Neurology, 14*, 497–506.

Vinogradova, O. S. (1970). Registration of information and the limbic system. In G. Horn and R. A. Hinde (Eds.), *Short-term changes in neural activity and behavior*. Cambridge: Cambridge University Press.

Volkmar, F. R., & Cohen, D. J. (1985). The experience of infantile autism: A first-person account by Tony W. *Journal of Autism and Developmental Disorders, 15*, 47–54.

Williams, R. S., Hauser, S. L., Purpura, D. P., DeLong, G. R., & Swisher, C. N. (1980). Autism and mental retardation: Neuropathologic studies performed in four retarded persons with autistic behavior. *Archives of Neurology, 37*, 749–753.

Wood, C. C., McCarthy, G., Squires, N. K., Vaughan, H. G., Jr., Woods, D. L., & McCallum, W. C. (1984). Anatomical and physiological substrates of event-related potentials. In R. Karrer,

J. Cohen, and P. Tueting (Eds.), *Brain and information: Event-related potentials. Annals of the New York Academy of Sciences, 425,* 681–721.

Woods, D. L., & Elmasian, R. (1986). The habituation of event-related potentials to speech sounds and tones. *Electroencephalography and Clinical Neurophysiology, 65,* 447–459.

Woods, D. L., Clayworth, C. C., Knight, R. T., Simpson, G. V., & Naesser, M. A. (in press). Generators of middle and long-latency auditory evoked potentials: Implications from studies of patients with bitemporal lesions. *Electroencephalography and Clinical Neurophysiology.*

Woods, D. L., Knight, R. T., & Neville, H. J. (1984). Bitemporal lesions dissociate auditory potentials and perception. *Electroencephalography and Clinical Neurophysiology, 57,* 208–220.

Woods, D. L., Clayworth, C. C., Knight, R. T., Simpson, G. V., and Naesser, M. A. (in press). Generators of middle and long-latency auditory evoked potentials: Implications from studies of patients with bitemporal lesions. *Electroencephalography and Clinical Neurophysiology.*

Nutrition and Developmental Disabilities
Issues in Chronic Care

DANIEL J. RAITEN

INTRODUCTION

The autistic syndrome has been a frustrating and tragic mystery to both parents and clinicians since it was first identified by Kanner (1943). Much like other topics for research within the now widely accepted medical model of autism/pervasive developmental disabilities (PDD) (Maurer & Damasio, 1982), most research in nutrition can be classified as descriptive or as interventionist. Descriptive studies have attempted to characterize the autistic/PDD population in terms of dietary intake (DeMyer, Ward, & Lintzenich, 1968; Raiten, Massaro, & Zuckerman, 1984; Raiten & Massaro, 1986; Shearer, Larson, Neuschwander, & Gedney, 1982) or nutritional biochemistry (Lis, McLaughlin, McLaughlin, Lis, & Stubbs, 1976; Raiten *et al.*, 1984; Sankar, 1979). The presumption of these studies has been that any differences in analyzed parameters may be related etiologically or are the consequence of behavioral problems that distinguish these disorders. The studies that employ nutritional interventions— e.g., megavitamins—are based on an assumption that pharmacological doses of essential nutrients will ameliorate an underlying biochemical or metabolic anomaly responsible in part for the clinical manifestations of these disorders.

The major impetus behind those studies linking such nutritional factors as vitamins to developmental disorders is the intimate part that nutrition plays in the integrity of the nervous system (Winick, 1979). Specific nutrients, such as the water-soluble "B" vitamins, are important in brain neurochemistry because of their role as coenzymes in the synthesis of neurotransmitters (Dakshinamurti, 1977). Owing to the focus on these associations, however, there has been the tendency to lose sight of nutrition in the broader sense.

Nutrition may be defined as the sum total of the processes involved in the ingestion and utilization of nutrients that are subsequently involved in the growth, repair, and maintenance

DANIEL J. RAITEN • Department of Behavioral Medicine, Children's Hospital, National Medical Center, Washington, DC 20010.

of the body's components and their function. These processes include ingestion, digestion, absorption, metabolism, and functional utilization of nutrients. Furthermore, the acquisition of a balanced diet is influenced by an array of physical, sociocultural, economic, behavioral, genetic, and medical factors (Raiten & Massaro, 1986; Wodarski, 1985). Malnutrition may be a consequence of changes in any of the processes involved in nutrition or those factors affecting it, and may result in either over- or undernutrition. Overnutrition leading to obesity may be the result of decreased activity, psychosocial influences, metabolic changes, overeating, or psychopharmacology. Undernutrition, associated with deficiencies of one or more nutrients, has the following five primary causes outlined by Herbert (1973): (1) inadequate ingestion, (2) inadequate absorption, (3) inadequate utilization, (4) increased excretion, and (5) increased requirement. This fifth cause may be associated with such natural states as pregnancy or other stages in the life cycle, disease states, or genetic differences such as vitamin-dependent inborn errors of metabolism, e.g., B_6 responsive homocysteinuria.

While any of these factors may influence the nutrition of the developmentally disabled child, number 5, increased requirement, has been the major focus of attention because of the publicity and controversy surrounding "megavitamin" or "orthomolecular" treatment (Raiten & Massaro, 1987). It is conceivable that there is a subgroup of autistic children who have a metabolic defect resulting in increased requirements of one or more nutrients. The various theories regarding neurochemical differences among subgroups of autistic/PDD children have been recently reviewed (Anderson & Hoshino, 1986). There are other types of biochemical problems that may characterize subgroups of the autistic population and may also have nutritional implications. Among these are the genetic inborn errors of metabolism, including phenylketonuria (PKU). Although urinary screening tests are mandated in most states for detection of children with such disorders, several authors have found groups of children with autisticlike behavioral disturbances (Friedman, 1969; Lowe, Tanaka, Seashore, Young, & Cohen, 1980). Generally, these types of genetic diseases result from defects in the apoenzyme or protein portion of enzymes involved in key points in metabolic pathways. Treatment of these disorders often requires dietary interventions, such as the restriction of phenylalanine, and supplementation with tyrosine in PKU children. The clinical outcome of the genetic disorders is the direct result of nutritional problems. However, there may be functional changes associated with nutritional anomalies that are unrelated to the primary disorder. Five domains of functional competence that may be compromised by a nutritional deficiency have been identified (National Academy of Sciences, 1977). These areas included cognitive ability, disease response (immunity), reproductive competence, physical activity, and work performance and social/behavioral performance. In a normal population, changes in any of these parameters may be clearly identifiable. In an already compromised group such as autistic or PDD children, however, these types of changes could blend easily into the preexisting symptomology and thereby be attributed to the primary disorder. In these children, the problem becomes one of sensitivity to the possibility of a nutritional problem and taking the steps necessary for its identification.

Within the perspective of Herbert's (1973) basic causes of nutritional deficiency and the processes of nutrition, there are three essential questions that may be asked when considering the possibility of a nutritional problem in a disabled individual. These are as follows: (1) Does the disability/disorder directly interfere with the child's ability to obtain and assimilate an adequate diet? (2) Does the child have modulations in behavior that are related to either food habits or sensitivities? (3) Is there a potential for a iatrogenic effect from the treatment, e.g., effects on growth rate, changes in appetite (obesity), specific drug/nutrient interactions?

The remainder of this paper will review literature in support of the relevence of these questions to the autistic/PDD child.

DIETARY ADEQUACY

Children with developmental disabilities may be either physically compromised or developmentally delayed in those basic skills necessary for the procurement of an adequate diet. Bizarre food habits and specific nutrient deficiencies have been observed across various disorders (Palmer, 1978). It is generally recognized that autistic children have unusual eating habits (Wing, 1979). However, there have been few efforts to document either the incidence of these behaviors or their impact on dietary adequacy. Several investigators have compared the adequacy of dietary intake of autistic children to that of matched controls and found essentially no differences (Raiten *et al.*, 1984; Shearer *et al.*, 1982). In a recent study, several factors that may influence dietary adequacy in groups of autistic/PDD children— e.g., eating habits and behavior, caregivers' attitudes and knowledge—were examined (Raiten & Massaro, 1986). It was found that while there was no difference in the quality of the diet when compared to that of a group of normal children, the autistic subjects did have a higher incidence of unusual eating behaviors as perceived by their primary caregivers. The food habits were clustered into three main categories: those implying adherences to sameness (e.g., rituals), those associated with specific eating behaviors (messy eaters), and those involving specific food preferences (preference for carbohydrate-rich foods). The autistic group had higher percentages in each cluster when compared to the control group. Moreover, there was a higher incidence of food-related idiosyncracies—i.e., food cravings—reported for the autistic children. In 8 out of 21 cases of reported food cravings in the autistic group, the caregivers also reported an association between disturbed behaviors and ingestion of the craved food.

Food idiosyncracies may also be associated with nutrient deficiencies. As is often the case in the general population, special children may have aversions to certain foods or food groups. Shearer *et al.* (1982) reported differences in calcium and riboflavin intake between autistic and control subjects. They attributed these differences to decreased intake of milk and dairy products in the autistic group.

The potential for nutritional deficiency is great in a child who refuses to accept a variety of foods or has specific aversions to foods such as dairy products or foods that require extensive chewing. Although the study of the functional implications of marginal nutrient deficiencies has been virtually ignored, there is ample evidence to show that marginal intakes of specific nutrients such as riboflavin (Sterner & Price, 1973), thiamine (Platt, 1958), pyridoxine (Dakshinamurti, 1977), or iron (Oski, Honig, Helu, & Howanitz, 1983) will result in such nonspecific behavioral changes as depression, anxiety, hyperirritability, appetite changes, or lassitude. It is the caregiver's responsibility to be aware of the possibility of these types of problems developing in a child, and to initiate appropriate steps.

NUTRITION AND BEHAVIOR

Specific food cravings and idiosyncracies have been reported in samples of autistic/ PDD children and linked to nonspecific modulations in behavior (Raiten & Massaro, 1986). Changes in behavior have been associated with eating habits such as missed meals or changes in protein to carbohydrate ratios due to specific food cravings. The scientific basis for theories in the area of nutrition and behavior has been developed by Wurtman and co-workers, who have linked changes in levels of neurotransmitter precursors to alterations in neurotransmitter synthesis (Fernstrom & Wurtman, 1971; Wurtman, Larin, Mostafadour, & Fernstrom, 1974). Examples of precursors include the amino acids: tyrosine, the parent compound for the catecholamines, dopamine and norepinephrine; tryptophan, which is converted to serotonin; and choline, a component of acetylcholine. Most precursors must be supplied through a well-balanced diet. The amount and availability of the major neurotransmitters—e.g., dopamine, norepinephrine, serotonin, or acetylcholine—are therefore inherently linked to the nutritional status of the individual as well as to factors influencing the absorption and transport of precursors, and the biosynthetic machinery required for neurotransmitter production. Figure 1 illustrates the biosynthetic pathways for production of the catecholamines and serotonin, and includes the dietary precursors and coenzymes required.

The intimate association between dietary components and neurotransmitters is undeniable. However, the functional impact of fluctuations in precursor availability has just begun to be examined. Fernstrom (1981) suggested that precursors may be useful for the treatment of selected disease states that may be related to reduced release or availability of neurotransmitters. To date, clinical studies have been inconsistent in demonstrating the therapeutic efficacy of precursor therapy.

Several researchers have continued to examine the effects of precursors or factors affecting their availability (e.g., protein to carbohydrate ratio) on parameters of behavior such as mood and performance (Lieberman, Corkin, Spring, Growdon, & Wurtman, 1983; Spring, Maller, Wurtman, Digman, & Cozolino, 1983). Wurtman and Wurtman (1983) linked the appetite for carbohydrates to brain serotonin metabolism through the control of the availability to the brain of the serotonin precursor tryptophan. It is postulated that this relationship may be responsible for some forms of obesity (Wurtman, 1984). The relationship involving serotonin, obesity, and food cravings may be particularly relevant to the autistic population in light of supporting evidence of a hyperserotonemic group of autistic children (Ritvo et al., 1970) and a recent finding of a possible defect in tryptophan-serotonin metabolism (Hoshino et al., 1984). Researchers have linked changes in levels of serotonin and its precursor to modulations in pain threshold (Seltzer, Marcus, & Stoch, 1981; Spinweber, Ursin, Hilbert, & Hildebrand, 1983), affective disorders (Moller & Larsen, 1984), sleep, and appetite control (Crisp & Stonehill, 1973). Unfortunately, despite the relationship between serotonin and autism and the frequently reported disturbances in sleep and eating habits, there have been no studies linking these phenomena. Clinically, the use of precursors such as tryptophan should be tempered by an awareness of recently recognized pharmacological factors (Hedaya, 1984) and toxicology (Sourkes, 1983).

Other nutritional factors that have received attention include the negative effects of missed meals on cognitive performance in children (Conners & Blouin, 1983; Pollitt, Lewis, Garza, & Shulman, 1983), and the effect of such dietary substances as sugar (Conners &

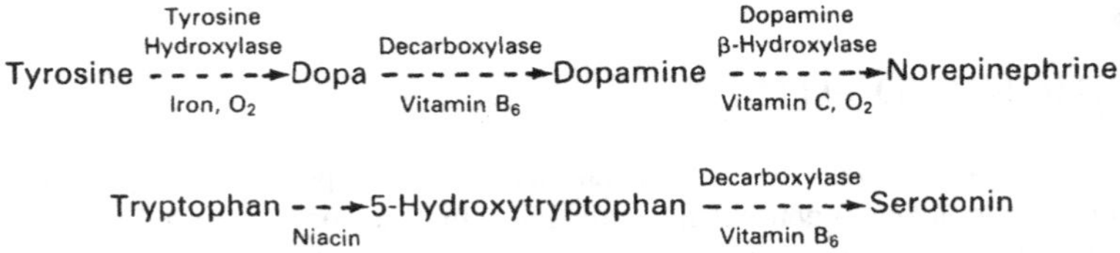

Figure 1. Representation of the role of vitamins in neurochemistry.

Blouin, 1983) and caffeine (Rapoport, Berg, Ismond, Zahn, & Neims, 1984) on behavior and performance. The study of the effects of these types of factors in the autistic/PDD child is complex and requires a multidisciplinary approach similar to the model proposed by Conners & Blouin (1983).

Food Reactions

Changes in behavior associated with food cravings reported by Raiten and Massaro (1986) raised several questions, including the possibility that the behavioral changes may have been secondary to somatic manifestations of food allergy or sensitivities that otherwise had been undetected in nonverbal children who were unable to express their discomfort. Crook (1975) outlined the possible sequence of events leading to behavioral problems associated with food allergies. He listed nervous system symptoms such as headache, fatigue, drowsiness, slowness in thinking, inability to attend to tasks, irritability, and hyperactivity. Many of these symptoms would either go unnoticed or be attributed to the primary disorder in the autistic child. It is not unreasonable to suspect that food allergies or sensitivities may exist in this population with the same frequency as in the general population.

There are many immunological and genetic mechanisms that may be responsible for food intolerances (Goldstein & Heiner, 1970). MacGibbon (1983) added pharmacological and toxicological factors as potential precipitators of adverse effects to food. Presumably food allergies result from immunological reactions to specific foods such as milk, while sensitivities to food additives, as proposed by Feingold (1975), would be caused by toxicological mechanisms. The continuing controversy surrounding the Feingold diet for treatment of hyperactivity is concerned primarily with sensitivity to food additives (Lipton & Mayo, 1983; Thorley, 1983). The research done to date, while marred by methodological flaws and nosological inconsistencies, clearly indicates a subgroup of children who are behaviorally affected by food additives (Trites & Tryphonas, 1983). It is therefore reasonable to expect that there may be atypical children who also have similar sensitivities. Consequently, clinicians should be cognizant of this possibility when taking a detailed history for a given child. Parents and other primary caregivers often are the best sources of insight into problems facing an individual child, and their testimony should be regarded objectively as important clinical data.

The diagnosis of food allergy or sensitivity is complicated and controversial (Fries, 1981), and it is confounded by a variety of diagnostic procedures and questions regarding relative sensitivity (Metcalfe, 1984). Several authors have presented a reasonable diagnostic flow chart for the clinician who relies on a detailed history given by the caregiver (Bock, 1980; Lockey, 1981). For the individual caregiver, awareness of these issues and of the potential for a specific food allergy or sensitivity is essential for initiation of appropriate interventions.

One final phenomenon related to eating idiosyncracies is the incidence of pica, or eating of nonfood items. The higher reported incidence of pica in autistic children (Cohen, Johnson, & Caparulo, 1976; Raiten & Massaro, 1986) may be related to overall developmental delay in these children. Infantile mouthing of objects is a common phenomenon in autistic children. These behaviors may result in exposure to environmental pollutants such as lead. The impact that low-level exposure to lead may have on behavior and cognitive performance remains a major concern and continues to be actively investigated (Bellinger,

Needleman, Bromfield, & Mintz, 1984; Gittelman & Eskenazi, 1983; Needleman, 1983). Nutritionally, there are several factors that may enhance the toxicity of lead, including deficiencies in total calories, calcium, iron, zinc, and phosphorus (Mahaffey, 1983). Moreover, Tandon, Flora, and Singh (1984) suggested that deficiencies in "B complex" vitamins may increase the vulnerability to the neurotoxic effects of lead. Thus, the recommendations made by Cohen, Paul, Anderson, and Harcherik (1982) regarding routine monitoring of autistic/PDD children for lead exposure should be rigorously followed and universally adopted.

PHARMACOLOGY AND NUTRITION

Pharmacology, or the use of substances to ameliorate specific symptomology, is a major issue in the chronic care of autistic/PDD children. While there are many aspects of the effects that drugs produce, one aspect has received minimal clinical attention: the relationship between nutrition and drugs. This is an area that can have profound impact on children and adults in terms of both growth and development, and subsequent response to other treatment modalities. It is this issue, perhaps more than any other, that raises questions about our commitment to, and our definition of, the quality of life of the disabled individual. This section will be divided into two parts. The first part will cover basic concepts concerning the effects of nutrition and its processes on drug delivery, metabolism, and therapeutics. The second part will review issues related to specific drug–nutrient interactions.

Nutrient–Drug Interactions

Both the timing and the composition of meals can affect drug absorption (Hathcock, 1985). In addition, marginal nutrient status can also interfere with the delivery and metabolism of drugs (Campbell, 1977). Hayes and Borzelleca (1985) have reviewed these interactions and suggested that drugs and nutrients undergo similar metabolic processes—i.e., absorption, activation, and excretion. Consequently, if a nutrient interferes with the processing of a drug, there will be a change in the effect of the drug and vice versa. For example, since calcium interferes with the absorption of tetracycline via the formation of insoluble calcium compounds, one can expect a decrease in the therapeutic response to tetracycline and loss of calcium when it is given with a glass of milk. Other factors that may affect drug absorption include meal composition (i.e., high fat versus low fat), the presence or absence of food in the stomach, changes in acidity or alkalinity, or high fiber content, which may adsorb therapeutic agents as well as decrease intestinal transit time, thereby decreasing absorption (Hathcock, 1985). The general nutritional status of any individual will also affect the many components involved in the absorptive process. The morphological integrity of the gastrointestinal tract depends on adequate nutrition. As found in celiac disease, change in gastrointestinal morphology will affect absorption of drugs and nutrients alike. Similarly, malnutrition will influence other aspects of the absorptive process, including carrier mechanisms involved in membrane transport and ultimate passage into the circulation.

Beyond absorption, the metabolic fate of drugs ultimately depends on nutritional factors. The large majority of drugs undergo a series of biotransformations by the mixed function oxidase system (MFO) located primarily in the liver, culminating in either their activation or deactivation. The ultimate goal of this process is to render them more water-soluble, and therefore more easily eliminated. The MFO system is dependent not only on general nutritional status—i.e., protein, fat, and carbohydrates—but also on the availability of specific nutrients such as vitamins (e.g., riboflavin, niacin, thiamine, and folate) and minerals (e.g., iron, zinc, and copper) (Becking, 1976; Bidlack & Smith, 1984; Campbell & Hayes, 1976).

Other factors that have been found to influence drug metabolism are substances found in food that enhance the activity of these systems. For example, there have been reports of substances found in vegetables such as broccoli and cabbage, and others found in charcoal-broiled meats, that increase the activity of the MFO systems (Anderson, Conney, & Kappas, 1982). Caffeine consumption has been linked to decreased therapeutic response to psychotropic medications. This may result from an induction of liver metabolism and/or the formation of insoluble precipitates (Lasswell, Weber, & Wilkins, 1984; Mikkelsen, 1978). As caffeine consumption in the form of coffee, tea, and soft drinks is a common phenomenon, these contingencies may have considerable clinical importance.

Dietary substances that bind drugs in the gastrointestinal tract will prevent absorption and increase excretion. High fat intake may increase the absorption of fat-soluble drugs, while a low-fat meal may have the opposite effect since fat and fat soluble substances must undergo a series of specific steps to allow them to enter the bloodstream. Factors such as dietary fiber that increase the contractions or motility of the gastrointestinal tract will decrease absorption by speeding up the passage and elimination of GI contents.

The majority of information regarding both nutrient–drug and drug–nutrient interactions is based on animal studies. The few clinical studies performed have been with adults. It is clear that nutritional factors have an intimate role in drug metabolism. It is not clear, however, whether developing infants and children are more susceptible to these effects. Sonawane, Coates, Yaffe, and Koldovsky (1983), found that the adult progeny of rats fed deficient diets had changes in drug metabolism. Sonawane and Catz (1981) further reviewed the research on the developmental aspects of the drug–nutrient question and concluded that there may be an increased susceptibility for children to the effects of malnutrition on drug metabolism. In the case of neuroleptics, adults can be expected to respond with the amelioration of major psychiatric symptoms, yet children may respond only with the possible extinctions of selected behaviors—e.g., reduced stereotypies in autistic children (Campbell, Cohen, & Anderson, 1981). Are the differences in response to psychopharmacology between adults and autistic children due to neurological or neurochemical differences or to developmental differences in the metabolism of psychotropic drugs?

Neuroleptic drugs are the most commonly prescribed pharmacological treatment for the autistic/PDD population (Weiner, 1984). Neuroleptics can generally be characterized as lipophilic or fat-soluble, and consequently, their absorption can be facilitated by the presence of fat in the diet. Furthermore, their lipophilic nature allows them to be deposited in adipose or fat tissue. This deposition becomes clinically significant both during drug withdrawal, since storage depots of the drug can be mobilized, and during periods of weight loss (Seeman, 1981). Beyond absorption, most neuroleptics require extensive liver metabolism into metabolites that are predominantly transported bound to plasma proteins. Unfortunately, there have been no clinical studies on the relationship between nutritional factors and neuroleptic therapies. Clearly, there is a multiplicity of factors that can change the response to these medications and may, in part, account for the inter- and intraindividual variabilities seen in the clinical responses to these drugs.

Drug–Nutrient Interactions

The other side of the nutrition–pharmacology relationship is the effect that drugs have on both the processes of nutrition and the availability and viability of specific nutrients. Chronic drug therapy may lead to impairment of liver function, resulting in an alteration in the ability of this organ to enzymatically produce the coenzymatic forms of many vitamins that are essential for carrying out normal metabolic functions both peripherally and in the central nervous system (CNS). Clinical manifestations of a drug-induced nutrient deficiency may appear as a detectable change in circulating metabolites or vitamins, or as neuromotor and behavioral disturbances.

A major class of drugs often used in the autistic population that has been shown to produce a number of adverse effects is the anticonvulsants. Paramount among these effects is the disturbance in normal vitamin D metabolism and function. Normal functioning of vitamin D requires hepatic conversion of the dietary or endogenous provitamin to the 25, hydroxy D3 form. This in turn is converted to the biologically active 1,25 hydroxy D3 form in the kidney. This active form of vitamin D plays a pivotal role in calcium absorption and bone homeostasis. Richens and Rowe (1970) found reduced serum calcium and elevated alkaline phosphatase in individuals maintained on chronic anticonvulsant therapy. Christensen *et al.*, (1981) and Morijiri and Sato (1981) have demonstrated that anticonvulsant therapy results in a reduction in circulating forms of vitamin D in epileptic patients maintained on single and combined regimens. Several reports have shown this impairment to eventually culminate in osteomalacia (Tolman, Jubiz, & Sannella, 1975) and rickets (Morijiri & Sato, 1981) in adult and young individuals, respectively. Although numerous factors have been implicated in the development of these clinical manifestations—i.e., diet, ambulation, and exposure to sunlight—anticonvulsants appear to be the major contributing factor responsible for the observed manifestations.

Chronic anticonvulsant therapy has also been associated with impaired red blood cell synthesis or hemopoiesis. In particular, anticonvulsant drugs have been shown to precipitate megaloblastic anemia, characterized by abnormal red cell maturation and often associated with low serum folic acid (Waxman, Corcino, & Herbert, 1970). Morphological changes in the epithelial lining of the gastrointestinal tract, lip, tongue, and inner surface of the mouth have also been observed in folate deficiency associated with anticonvulsant therapy (Mallek & Nakamoto, 1981). Since folic acid plays a major role in DNA synthesis, it is not surprising that epithelial tissues with such a high rate of turnover, and normal processes involved in red blood cell synthesis, are affected earlier and to a greater extent than other tissues as a result of a drug-induced folate deficiency.

It is important to recognize, however, that prior to the appearance of severe clinical manifestations, a deficiency of folic acid has been associated with various neurological and behavioral symptoms, including mild polyneuropathies, fatigue, hypotonia, depression, and impaired intellectual performance (Botez & Reynolds, 1979). Recent observations depicted the presence of thiamin deficiency in folate-deficient patients (Thomson, Baker, & Leevy, 1976) and microcytic hypochromic anemia (characteristic of pyridoxine deficiency) in a young adolescent patient treated for petit mal seizures (John, 1981). Thus, it is unclear to what extent the observed changes in neurological functions and behavioral symptoms can be attributed solely to a deficiency of folic acid. Recent studies have implicated anticonvulsant therapies in deficiencies of biotin (Krause, Berlit, & Bonjour, 1982), zinc, and vitamin E (Higashi, Ikeda, Matsukura, & Matsuda, 1982). These findings raise the possibility of multiple deficiencies, especially in individuals receiving a marginal diet.

Neuroleptic drugs constitute one of the major classes of drugs prescribed for the amelioration of behavioral anomalies in both children and adults who presumably have not responded to alternative, drug-free therapies. Dependent on the dose and duration, the neuroleptics have been associated with metabolic and physiological side effects that may interfere with the processes of nutrition. These side effects include abdominal pain and distension, and vomiting. A more chronic problem is constipation caused by the anticholinergic effect of neuroleptics (Seeman, 1981). This side effect is often treated with laxatives— e.g., mineral oil or other cathartic drugs—thereby creating another potentially dangerous nutritionally related problem. Laxatives, such as mineral oil, can bind nutrients or prevent their absorption, thereby creating the possibility of nutrient deficiencies (Roe, 1976). In addition, the therapeutic effect of these drugs is decreased transit time in the gut, which can cause decreased nutrient absorption.

A number of other metabolic effects have been associated with chronic neuroleptic therapy related to abnormalities in endocrine status of the individual. Neuroleptics have been shown to stimulate prolactin secretion (Hays & Rubin, 1981), which has been implicated in producing a hyperglycemic-diabetogenic effect, and enhancing fat deposition. Simpson, Pi, and Sramek (1981) have sugested that one of the metabolic consequences of chronic neuroleptic therapy—i.e., weight gain—may be caused by fluid retention, fat redistribution, and altered glucose sensitivity.

Awad (1984) suggested several other possible drug-induced mechanisms that might lead to obesity. Improved mental status, mouth dryness associated with increased consumption of soft drinks, and decreased activity are the most commonly cited possibilities. Another explanation might center around neuroleptic-induced changes in central neurochemistry associated with appetite control. In light of the recent statement issued by the National Institute of Health (NIH) declaring it a disease (Kolath, 1985), obesity must be considered a major issue in the chronic care of autistic/PDD children. Aside from the direct impact that obesity can have, Mallick (1983) pointed out some of the deleterious consequences of weight control and diets on growth, development, and mental functioning of children and adolescents. Furthermore, since autistic adults are at risk for the same chronic disease as the general population, obesity will ultimately affect the length and quality of life of these individuals. There is a need for clinical studies addressing either the mechanisms involved in neuroleptic-induced obesity or potential treatments or management protocols for the autistic/PDD population. Harris and Bloom (1984) demonstrated the feasibility of weight reduction programs for mentally retarded adolescents and adults, but they cautioned that long-term success was correlated with individual IQ, residential status, and perseverence of the primary caregiver. Similar studies could be performed with autistic subjects to assess the relevance of these findings.

The hepatotoxic effects of neuroleptics constitute one of the more serious side effects of prolonged treatments and are often accompanied by jaundice and elevated serum alkaline phosphatase levels. Little information is available regarding the indirect effects of neuroleptics on the metabolic integrity of the liver in terms of its ability to form the necessary coenzymatic forms of many of the water-soluble or B vitamins.

It is important to recognize that results of several recent animal studies have demonstrated possible profound effects of neuroleptic drugs on normal metabolic processes in the CNS. Schatzman, Wise, and Kuo (1981) demonstrated that neuroleptics inhibit protein kinase in rat brain, which is involved in the activation of numerous active compounds, including neurotransmitters. It is conceivable that pyridoxine, which plays an integral role in the biosynthesis of neurotransmitters and requires activation by a similar enzyme (Segalman

& Brown, 1981), may likewise be affected by such a mechanism and, as a result, be required in increased amounts in order to maintain its normal efficacy. A more direct and insidious effect of both neuroleptic drugs and certain antidepressants has been demonstrated by Pinto, Huang, and Rivlin (1981). Prompted by the similar structures of riboflavin and the drugs chlorpromazine, imipramine, and amitriptyline, these workers sought to determine any effects these drugs may have on the conversion of riboflavin to its active coenzyme form. The results indicated that all three drugs inhibited the activation of riboflavin in liver, cerebrum, and cerebellum. An even more dramatic result was seen in a study of long-term administration of chlorpromazine (Pinto et al., 1981). After periods of 3 to 7 weeks "at doses comparable on a weight basis to those used clinically," this study showed that chlorpromazine led to riboflavin deficiency even in animals fed 30 times their recommended daily allowance of B_2. The authors concluded the study by stating that the results "raise the possibility that drug-induced nutritional deficiency may be an unrecognized and undesirable result of antipsychotic drug therapy, particularly when treatment is prolonged."

We must recognize that psychopharmacology has other consequences besides the amelioration of specific symptoms. The potential functional impact of drug- or diet-induced nutrient deficiencies on behavior and cognition have received minimal attention. Future studies should address these issues, while clinicians and caregivers must be vigilant in their recognition and monitoring of those clinical parameters that may indicate a potential problem.

REFERENCES

Anderson, G. M., & Hoshino, Y. (1986). Neurochemical studies of autism. In D. J. Cohen, A. Donnellan, & R. Paul (Eds.), *Handbook of autism and disorders of atypical development*. New York: Wiley.

Anderson, K. E., Conney, A. H., & Kappas, A. (1982). Nutritional influences in chemical biotransformations in humans. *Nutrition Review, 40,* 161–171.

Awad, A. G. (1984). Diet and drug interactions in the treatment of mental illness—A review. *Canadian Journal of Psychiatry, 29,* 609–613.

Becking, G. C. (1976). Trace elements and drug metabolism. *Medical Clinics of North America, 60,* 813.

Bellinger, D., Needleman, H. L., Bromfield, R., & Mintz, M. (1984). A followup study of the academic attainment and classroom behavior of children with elevated dentine lead levels. *Biological Trace Element Research, 6,* 207–223.

Bidlack, W. R., & Smith, C. H. (1984). The effect of nutritional factors on hepatic drug and toxicant metabolism. *Journal of the American Dietetic Association, 84,* 892–898.

Bock, S. A. (1980). Food sensitivity: A critical review and practical approach. *American Journal of Diseases of Children, 134,* 973–982.

Botez, M. I., & Reynolds, E. H. (1979). *Folic acid in neurology, psychiatry, and internal medicine* (p. 534). New York: Raven Press.

Campbell, M., Cohen, T. L., & Anderson, L. T. (1981). Pharmacotherapy for autistic children: A summary of research. *Canadian Journal of Psychiatry, 26,* 265–273.

Campbell, T. C. (1977). Nutrition and drug metabolizing enzymes. *Clinical Pharmacology and Therapeutics, 22,* 699–706.

Campbell, T. C., & Hayes, J. R. (1976). The effect of quantity and quality of dietary protein on drug metabolism. *Proceedings of the Federation of the American Society for Experimental Biology, 35,* 2470–2474.

Christensen, C. K., Lund, B. I., Lund, B. J., Sorensen, O. H., Nielsen, H. E., & Mosekilde, L. (1981). Reduced 1, 25-dihydroxy vitamin D and 24, 25-dihydroxy vitamin D in epileptic patients receiving chronic combined anticonvulsant therapy. *Metabolic Bone Disease and Related Research, 3*, 17.

Cohen, D. J., Johnson, W. T., & Caparulo, B. K. (1976). Pica and elevated blood lead level in autistic and atypical children. *American Journal of Diseases of Children, 130* 47–48.

Cohen, D. J., Paul, R., Anderson, G. M., & Harcherik, D. F. (1982). Blood lead in autistic children. *Lancet, 2,* 94–95.

Conners, C. K., & Blouin, A. G. (1983). Nutritional effects on behavior of children. *Journal of Psychiatric Research, 17,* 193–201.

Crisp, A. M., & Stonehill, E. (1973). Aspects of the relationship between sleep and nutrition: A study of 375 psychiatric outpatients. *British Journal of Psychiatry, 122,* 379–394.

Crook, W. G. (1975). Food allergy—the great masquerader. *Pediatric Clinics of North America, 22,* 227–238.

Dakshinamurti, K. (1977). B vitamins and nervous system function. In R. J. Wurtman & J. J. Wurtman (Eds.), *Nutrition and the Brain* (Vol. 1). New York: Raven Press.

DeMyer, M. K., Ward, S. D., & Lintzenick, J. (1968). Comparison of macronutrients in the diets of psychotic and normal children. *Archives of General Psychiatry, 18,* 584.

Feingold, B. F. (1975). Hyperkinesis and learning disabilities linked to artificial food flavors and colors. *American Journal of Nursing, 75,* 797–803.

Fernstrom, J. D. (1981). Dietary precursors and brain neurotransmitter formation. *Annual Review of Medicine, 32,* 413–425.

Fernstrom, J. D., & Wurtman, R. J. (1971). Brain serotonin content: Physiological dependence on plasma tryptophan levels. *Science, 173,* 149–152.

Friedman, E. (1969). The autistic syndrome and phenylketonuria. *Schizophrenia, 1,* 249–261.

Fries, J. H. (1981). Food allergy—current concerns. *Annals of Allergy, 41,* 260–263.

Gittelman, R., & Eskenazi, B. (1983). Lead and hyperactivity revisited. *Archives of General Psychiatry, 40,* 827–833.

Goldstein, G. B., & Heiner, D. C. (1970). Clinical and immunological perspectives in food sensitivities. *Journal of Allergy, 46,* 270–281.

Harris, M. B., & Bloom, S. R. (1984). A pilot investigation of a behavioral weight control program with mentally retarded adolescents and adults: Effects on weight, fitness, and knowledge of nutritional and behavioral principles. *Rehabilitation Psychology, 29,* 177–182.

Hathcock, J. N. (1985). Metabolic mechanisms of drug–nutrient interactions. *Proceedings of the Federation of the American Society for Experimental Biology, 44,* 124–129.

Hayes, J. R., & Borzelleca, J. F. (1985). Nutrient interaction with drugs and their zenobiotics. *Journal of the American Dietetic Association, 85,* 335–339.

Hays, S. E., & Rubin, R. T. (1981). Differential prolactin responses to Haloperidol and TRH in normal adult men. *Psychoneuroendocrinology, 6,* 45.

Hedaya, R. J. (1984). Pharmacokinetic factors in the clinical use of tryptophan. *Journal of Clinical Psychopharmacology, 4,* 347–348.

Herbert, V. (1973). The five possible causes of all nutrient deficiency: Illustrated by deficiencies of Vitamin B_{12} and folic acid. *American Journal of Clinical Nutrition, 26,* 77–88.

Higashi, A., Ikeda, T., Matsukura, M., & Matsuda, I. (1982). Serum zinc and Vitamin E in handicapped children treated with anticonvulsants. *Developmental Pharmacology and Therapeutics, 5,* 109–113.

Hoshino, Y., Yamamoto, T., Kaneko, M., Tachibana, R., Watanabe, M., Ono, Y., & Kumashiro, H. (1984). Blood serotonin and free tryotophan concentration in autistic children. *Neuropsychobiology, 11,* 22–27.

John, G. (1981). Transient osteosclerosis associated with sodium valproate. *Developmental Medicine and Childhood Neurology, 23,* 234.

Kanner, L. (1943). Autistic disturbances of affective contact. *Nervous Child, 2,* 217–250.

Kolath, G. (1985). Obesity declared a disease. *Science, 227,* 1019–1020.

Krause, K. H., Berlit, P., & Bonjour, J. P. (1982). Impaired biotin status in anticonvulsant therapy. *Annals of Neurology, 12,* 485–486.

Lasswell, W. L., Weber, S. S., & Wilkins, J. M. (1984). In vitro interaction of neuroleptics and tricyclic antidepressants with coffee, tea, and gallotannic acid. *Journal of Pharmaceutical Science, 73,* 1056.

Lieberman, H. R., Corkin, S., Spring, B. J., Growdon, J. H ., & Wurtman, R. J. (1983). Mood, performance, and pain sensitivity: Changes induced by food constituents. *Journal of Psychiatric Research, 17,* 135–145.

Lipton, M. A., & Mayo, J. P. (1983). Diet and hyperkinesis—an update. *Journal of the American Dietetic Association, 83,* 132–134.

Lis, A. W., McLaughlin, D. I., McLaughlin, R. K., Lis, E. W., & Stubbs, E. G. (1976). Profiles of ultraviolet absorbing components of urine from autistic children as obtained by high resolution ion-exchange chromatography. *Clinical Chemistry, 22,* 1528–1532.

Lockey, R. F. (1981). Food allergy: A clinical approach. *Bulletin of the New York Academy of Science, 57,* 595–599.

Lowe, T. L., Tanaka, K., Seashore, M. R., Young, J. G., & Cohen, D. J. (1980). Detection of phenylketonuria in autistic and psychotic children. *Journal of the American Medical Association, 243,* 126–128.

MacGibbon, B. (1983). Adverse reactions to food additives. *Proceedings of the Nutrition Society, 42,* 233–240.

Mahaffey, K. R. (1983). Biotoxicity of lead: Influence of various factors. *Proceedings of the Federation of the American Society for Experimental Biology, 42,* 1730–1734.

Mallek, H. M., & Nakamoto, T. (1981). Dilantin and folic acid status. *Journal of Periodontology, 52,* 255.

Mallick, M. J. (1983). Health hazards of obesity and weight control in children: A review of the literature. *American Journal of Public Health, 73,* 78–82.

Maurer, R. G., & Damasio, A. R. (1982). Childhood autism from the point of view of behavioral neurology. *Journal of Autism and Developmental Disorders, 12,* 195–204.

Metcalfe, D. D. (1984). Diagnostic procedures for immunologically mediated food sensitivity. *Nutrition Reviews, 42,* 92–97.

Mikkelsen, E. J. (1978). Caffeine and schizophrenia. *Journal of Clinical Psychiatry, 39,* 732–735.

Moller, S. E., & Larsen, O. B. (1984). Tryptophan and tyrosine availability: Relation to chemical response to antidepression pharmacotherapy. In E. Usdin, M. Asberg, L. Bertilsson, & F. Sloqvist (Eds.), *Frontiers in biochemical and pharmacological research in depression* (pp. 319–326). New York: Raven Press.

Morijiri, Y., & Sato, T. (1981). Factors causing rickets in institutionalized handicapped children on anticonvulsant therapy. *Archives of Disease in Childhood, 56,* 446.

National Academy of Sciences. (1977). *Report of study team IX, World food and nutrition study.* National Academy of Science, 1977, Washington, DC: Author.

Needleman, H. L. (1983). Lead at low dose and the behavior of children. *Acta Psychiatrica Scandanavica, 67*(Suppl. 303), 26–37.

Oski, F. A., Honig, A. S., Helu, B., & Howanitz, P. (1983). Effect of iron therapy on behavior performance in non-anemic, iron deficient infants. *Pediatrics, 71,* 877–880.

Palmer, S. (1978). Nutrition and developmental disorders: An overview. In S. Palmer & S. Ervall (Eds.), *Pediatric nutrition in developmental disorders* (pp. 21–24). Springfield, IL: Charles C Thomas.

Pinto, J., Huang, Y. P., & Rivlin, R. S. (1981). Inhibition of riboflavin metabolism in rat tissue by chlorpromazine, imipramine, and amitriptyline. *Journal of Clinical Nutrition, 67,* 1500.

Platt. B. S. (1958). Clinical features in endemic beri-beri. *Proceedings of the Federation of the American Society for Experimental Biology, 17,* 8–20.

Pollitt, E., Lewis, N. L., Garza, C., & Shulman, R. J. (1983). Testing and cognitive function. *Journal of Psychiatric Research, 17,* 169–174.

Raiten, D. J., & Massaro, T. F. (1986). Perspectives on the nutritional ecology of autistic children. *Journal of Autism and Developmental Disorders, 16,* 133–143.

Raiten, D. J., & Massaro, T. F. (1987). Nutrition and developmental disabilities: An examination of the orthomolecular hypothesis. In D. J. Cohen, A. Donnellan, & R. Paul (Eds.), *Handbook of autism and disorders of atypical development.* New York: Wiley.

Raiten, D. J., Massaro, T. F., & Zuckerman, C. H. (1984). Vitamin and trace element assessment of autistic and learning disabled children. *Nutrition and Behavior, 2,* 9–17.

Rapoport, J. L., Berg, C. J., Ismond, D. R., Zahn, T. P., & Neims, A. (1984). Behavioral effects of caffeine in children. *Archives of General Psychiatry, 41,* 1073–1079.

Richens, A., & Rowe, D. J. F. (1970). Disturbance of calcium metabolism by anticonvulsant drugs. *British Medical Journal, 4,* 73.

Ritvo, E. R., Yuwiler, A., Geller, E., Ornitz, E. M., Saeger, K., & Plotkin, S. (1970). Increased blood serotonin and platelets in early infantile autism. *Archives of General Psychiatry, 23,* 566–572.

Roe, D. (1976). *Drug induced nutritional deficiencies.* Westport: AVI.

Sankar, D. V. (1979). Plasma levels of folates, riboflavin, Vitamin B_6, and ascorbate in severely disturbed children. *Journal of Autism and Developmental Disorders, 9,* 73.

Schatzman, R. C., Wise, B. C., & Kuo, J. F. (1981). Phospholipid sensitive calcium-dependent protein kinase: Inhibition by antipsychotic drugs. *Biochemical Biophysical Research Communications, 98,* 669.

Seeman, M. V. (1981). Pharmacological features and effects of neuroleptics. *Canadian Medical Association Journal, 125,* 821–826.

Segalman, T. K., & Brown, R. R. (1981). The metabolism of ^{3}H-Pyridoxine in rat liver and brain. *American Journal of Clinical Nutrition, 34,* 1321.

Seltzer, S., Marcus, R., & Stoch, R. (1981). Perspectives in the control of chronic pain by nutritional manipulation. *Pain, 11,* 141–148.

Shearer, T. R., Larson, K., Neuschwander, J., & Gedney, B. (1982). Minerals in the hair and nutrient intake of autistic children. *Journal of Autism and Developmental Disorders, 12,* 25–34.

Simpson, G. M., Pi, E. H., & Sramek, J. J. (1981). Adverse effects of antipsychotic agents. *Drugs, 21,* 138–151.

Sonawane, B. R., & Catz, C. (1981). Nutritional status and drug metabolism during development. In L. F. Soyka & G. P. Redmond (Eds.), *Drug metabolism and the immature human.* New York: Raven Press.

Sonawane, B. R., Coates, P. M., Yaffe, S. J., & Koldovsky, O. (1983). Influence of perinatal nutrition on hepatic drug metabolism in the adult rat. *Developmental Pharmacology and Therapeutics, 6,* 323–332.

Sourkes, T. L. (1983). Toxicology of serotonin precursors. *Advances in Biological Psychiatry, 10,* 160–175.

Spinweber, C. L., Ursin, R., Hilbert, R. P., & Hildebrand, R. L. (1983). L-tryptophan: Effects on daytime sleep latency and waking EEG. *Electroencephalography and Clinical Neurophysiology, 55,* 652–661.

Spring, B., Maller, O., Wurtman, J., Digman, L., & Cozolino, L. (1983). Effects of protein and carbohydrate meals on mood and performance: Interactions with sex and age. *Journal of Psychiatric Research, 17,* 155–167.

Sterner, R. T., & Price, W. R. (1973). Restricted riboflavin: Within subject behavioral effects in humans. *American Journal of Clinical Nutrition, 26,* 150–160.

Tandon, S. K., Flora, S. J. S., & Singh, S. (1984). Influence of vitamin B complex deficiency on lead intoxication in young rats. *Indian Journal of Medical Research, 80,* 444–448.

Thomson, A. D., Baker, H., & Leevy, C. (1976). Folate induced malabsorption of thiamine. *Gastroenterology, 60,* 756.

Thorley, G. (1983). Childhood hyperactivity and food additives. *Developmental Medicine and Childhood Neurology, 25,* 531–534.

Tolman, K. G., Jubiz, W., & Sannella, J. J. (1975). Osteomalacia associated with anticonvulsant drug therapy in mentally retarded children. *Pediatrics, 56,* 45.

Trites, R. L., & Tryphonas, H. (1983). Food additives: The controversy continues. *Topics in Early Childhood Education, 3,* 43–47.

Waxman, S., Corcino, J., & Herbert, V. (1970). Drugs, toxins, and dietary amino acids affecting vitamin B_{12} or folic acid absorption or utilization. *American Journal of Medicine, 48,* 599.

Weiner, J. M. (1984). Psychopharmacology in childhood disorders. *Psychiatric Clinics of North America, 7,* 831–843.

Wing, L. (1979). *Children apart.* Washington, DC: National Society for Autistic Children.

Winick, M. (1979). Malnutrition and mental development. In R. B. Alfin-Slater & D. Kritchesky (Eds.), *Human nutrition* (p. 41). New York: Plenum Press.

Wodarski, L. A. (1985). Nutrition intervention in developmental disabilities: An interdisciplinary approach. *Journal of the American Dietetic Association, 85,* 218–221.

Wurtman, J. J. (1984). The involvement of brain serotonin in excessive carbohydrate snaking by obese carbohydrate cravers. *Journal of the American Dietetic Association, 84,* 1004–1007.

Wurtman, R. J., Larin, F., Mostafadour, S., & Fernstrom, J. D. (1974). Brain catechol synthesis: Control by brain tyrosine concentration. *Science, 185,* 183–184.

Wurtman, J. J., & Wurtman, R. J. (1983). Studies on the appetite for carbohydrates in rats and humans. *Journal of Psychiatric Research, 17,* 213–221.

Medication Issues

18

Overview of Drug Treatment in Autism

MAGDA CAMPBELL, RICHARD PERRY, ARTHUR M. SMALL, and WAYNE H. GREEN

INTRODUCTION

Infantile autism is a pervasive developmental disorder characterized by a failure to develop relatedness, language abnormalities, and cognitive lags and deficits of various degrees. Mental subnormality is an important aspect in the majority of autistic children. The goals of treatment are twofold: first, to decrease the behavioral symptoms and, second, to promote development and to foster skills that are absent or only rudimentary.

There are a variety of behavioral symptoms: "There is no symptom which is pathognomonic of infantile autism and, what is more, single symptoms characteristic of autism occur in a wide variety of other conditions (Rutter, Bartak, & Newman, 1971, p. 148)." Autistic behavior is most obvious during the preschool years (Wing, 1972), and therefore a correct diagnosis is most feasible at this time. It is at this stage of life that an individualized and comprehensive treatment intervention can be expected to yield maximum results. For this reason the Children's Psychopharmacology Unit concentrates its efforts on assessing the efficacy and safety of psychoactive drugs in young autistic children, housed in a therapeutic nursery, in Bellevue Hospital. In the past 25 years, about 270 children, ages 2 to 7 years, have participated in this research. Though the objective of our research was to study various psychoactive drugs in this population of children, we view pharmacotherapy as part of a comprehensive treatment program tailored to meet each child's individual needs.

Most investigators today believe that autism is a biologically determined condition; most probably it is etiologically heterogeneous. Numerous studies were conducted in the past 10 to 15 years in an attempt to identify the causes of infantile autism (for review, see Campbell, Cohen, & Anderson, 1981; Campbell & Green, 1985; Cohen & Young, 1977; De Myer, Hingtgen, & Jackson, 1981; Fish & Ritvo, 1979; Young, Kavanagh, Anderson, Shaywitz, & Cohen, 1982). Up to the present time no biological marker has been found to identify this syndrome, though a variety of biochemical, neuroendocrine, structural, and

MAGDA CAMPBELL, RICHARD PERRY, ARTHUR M. SMALL, and WAYNE H. GREEN • Department of Psychiatry, New York University Medical Center, New York, New York 10016.

Table 1. Clinical Response to Psychoactive Agents and Its Relationship to Relevant Biochemical Findings in Subgroups of Autistic Children

Relevant biochemical findings	Psychoactive drugs	Clinical response	Main side effects	Representative references
I. *Elevated serotonin levels* (Campbell et al., 1975; Ritvo et al., 1970; for review Young et al., 1982)	1. *Serotonin antagonists*			
	a. Methysergide	In general poor: mixture of stimulating, disorganizing, and sedative effects; tolerance developing; improvement in 2 of 9 patients	Excessive sedation, vomiting, insomnia, increased irritability	Fish et al., 1969a
	b. L-dopa	In general some positive response: mainly stimulating effects; improvement in 5 of 12 patients	Vomiting, decreased appetite, increased irritability, motor retardation, increase of stereotypies and stereotypies de novo	Campbell et al., 1976
	c. Fenfluramine	Conflicting findings: mixture of stimulating and tranquilizing effects	Excessive sedation, transient loss of weight, and irritability	August et al., 1985; Campbell et al., 1986; Geller et al., 1982; Leventhal, 1985; Ritvo et al., 1983, 1984
	2. *Serotonin agonists*			
	a. Imipramine (?)	Poor: mixture of stimulating, tranquilizing, and disorganizing effects; 2 of 10 children improved	Worsening of psychotic symptoms, excessive sedation, irritability, insomnia, catatoniclike state, lowering of seizure threshold, transient increase of SGOT and SGPT	Campbell et al., 1971b

b. Lithium (?)	Minimal effect on symptoms except on aggressiveness and explosiveness	Motor retardation, motor excitation, vomiting, polydipsia, polyuria, leukocytosis with lymphocytopenia, decrease of T4, and EKG changes	Campbell, Fish, Korein, et al., 1972
II. Dopaminergic abnormalities: Elevated dopamine levels (Cohen et al., 1974; 1977; for review, Young et al., 1982); alteration of hypothalamic dopamine receptor sensitivity (Deutsch, Campbell, Perry, et al., 1985; Deutsch, Campbell, Sachar, et al.., 1985)			
1. Dopamine antagonists a. Sedative type of neuroleptics: chlorpromazine	In general poor: some decrease of symptoms accompanied by excessive sedation; narrow therapeutic margin	Excessive sedation, motor retardation, irritability, and catatoniclike state	Campbell, Fish, Korein, et al., 1972
b. High potency neuroleptics: thiothixene, molindone, fluphenazine, trifluoperazine, and haloperidol	In general good: marked decrease of symptoms, wide therapeutic margin; with haloperidol, marked decrease of symptoms, enhancement of learning without untoward effects (when administered over a period of 3½ months cumulatively)	Excessive sedation, acute dystonic reaction, Parkinsonian side effects, excessive weight gain, and tardive and withdrawal dyskinesias	Anderson et al., 1984; Campbell, Anderson, Cohen, et al., 1982; Campbell, Anderson, Meier, et al., 1978; Campbell, Anderson, Small, et al., 1982; Campbell et al., 1970, 1971a; Campbell, Grega, et al., 1983; Campbell, Perry, et al., 1983; Engelhard et al., 1973; Faretra et al., 1970; Fish et al., 1966; Perry et al., 1985

(continued)

Table 1. (Continued)

Relevant biochemical findings	Psychoactive drugs	Clinical response	Main side effects	Representative references
	2. *Dopamine agonists* a. D-amphetamine	In general, only slight decrease of hyperactivity and increases of attention span and verbal production accompanied by side effects	Irritability, motor excitability, worsening of stereotypies and stereotypies *de novo*, loss of appetite, excessive sedation	Campbell, Fish, David, *et al.*, 1972; Campbell, Fish, Shapiro, & Floyd, 1972
	b. L-amphetamine	Poor: only decrease in hyperactivity, in 5 of 11 patients	Increase of preexisting stereotypies, and stereotypies *de novo*, decrease of appetite, loss of weight, excessive sedation, and worsening of preexisting symptoms	Campbell *et al.*, 1976
	c. L-dopa	See above	See above	See above
III. *Hypothalamic dysregulation*: abnormal response to TRH (Campbell, Hollander, *et al.*, 1978); elevated triiodothyronine levels (Campbell *et al.*, 1980; Campbell, Green, *et al.*, 1982; Deutsch, Campbell, Perry, *et al.*, 1985; Deutsch, Campbell, Sachar, *et al.*, 1985	Triiodothyronine (T₃)	Decrease of stereotypies and overall improvement at home	Fluctuating blood pressure, tachycardia, and irritability	Campbell, Small, *et al.*, 1978

IV. Abnormalities of endogenous opiate system[b]				
1. Reduction of urinary free catecholamines and MHPG (Young et al., 1978, 1979)	Opiate antagonists: 1. Naloxone[a] 2. Naltrexone[a]	Tranquilizing and stimulating effects: decreases in hyperactivity, impulsivity, stereotypies, and aggressiveness; increases in language production and social behavior	Hypoactivity and "as if dazed"	Campbell, 1985
2. Reducation of H-endorphin in plasma (Weizman et al., 1984); elevated endorphin fraction II levels in cerebrospinal fluid (Gillberg et al., 1985)				
3. Correlation between high endorphin fraction II levels, self-destructiveness, and decreased pain sensibility (Gillberg et al., 1985)				

[a]For a review of literature in normal adults and psychiatric patients, an article by Verebey et al., (1978) is recommended. On the effects of self-injurious behavior, see Bernstein et al. (1984), Davidson et al. (1983), and Sandman et al. (1983).
[b]See Kalat (1978) and Panksepp (1979).

Table 2. Doses[a] of Psychoactive Drugs

| Drug | Therapeutic dose range | |
	mg/day	mg/kg/day
Chlorpromazine	10–200	0.441–2.0
Trifluoperazine	2–20	0.11–0.69
Fluphenazine	2–16	
Haloperidol	0.5–16	0.019–0.217
Thiothixene	1–30	
Molindone	1–40	
Fenfluramine[b]	15–40	1.093–1.787

[a]For children under 12 years of age.
[b]Given twice a day: 8 a.m., and 12:00 noon (or 4:00 p.m.).

genetic influences have been reported, usually only in subgroups of autistic children. There could be several reasons for such failure: small patient samples, diagnostic heterogeneity within samples, wide age range of patients, and lack of adequate or appropriate controls.

Psychopharmacological research in autism attempts to relate behavioral abnormality (symptoms) to underlying biochemical abnormalities, and attempts to correct both with a therapeutically effective psychoactive drug (Campbell *et al.*, 1981). Even though no specific biochemical marker has been found for autism, we will attempt to relate the biochemical and neuroendocrine abnormalities found in subgroups of these children to their responses to various psychoactive drugs, as shown in Table 1; dosages of representative drugs are given in Table 2. Because autistic children are heterogeneous both behaviorally and biochemically, we can only aim for a rational pharmacotherapy. Behavioral, cognitive, and side effect measures were recently reviewed (Campbell & Palij, 1985a, 1985b; Campbell, Green, & Deutsch, 1985) and will be discussed further in other chapters.

HISTORICAL BACKGROUND

Neuroleptics

Fish (1970) began systematic studies of psychoactive drugs in autistic children. She made the observation that autistic children resemble chronic schizophrenic adults in regard to their response to the standard neuroleptic drug chlorpromazine: They get sedated at low doses that yield few, if any, decreases in symptoms (Campbell, Fish, Korein, *et al.*, 1972). This is true not only for hypoactive patients but also for those with hyperactivity and aggressiveness (Campbell, Fish, Korein, *et al.*, 1972). The more potent and less sedative types of neuroleptics, such as trifluoperazine (Fish, Shapiro, & Campbell, 1966), fluphenazine (Engelhardt, Polizos, Waizer, & Hoffman, 1973), thiothixene (Campbell, Fish, Shapiro, & Floyd, 1970; Simeon, Saletu, Saletu, Itil, & Da Silva, 1973; Waizer, Polizos, Hoffman, Englehardt, & Margolis, 1972), and molindone (Campbell, Fish, Shapiro, & Floyd, 1971a) seemed to be therapeutically more effective and to have a wider therapeutic margin. However, none of these studies were placebo-controlled and the sample sizes were small. The only exception was the clinical trial of trifluoperazine, where amphetamine served as a control; it involved 22 subjects, 2 to 6 years of age (Fish *et al.*, 1966). Trifluperidol, a potent butyrophenone, had a combination of excitatory and tranquilizing properties and was more effective than chlorpromazine or trifluoperazine in the same children (Fish, Campbell, Shapiro, & Floyd, 1969b; Campbell, Fish, Shapiro, & Floyd, 1972). However, it had a narrow therapeutic margin and was frequently associated with untoward extrapyramidal effects. Subsequently this drug was withdrawn from investigational use in this country.

Drugs with Stimulating Properties

The disappointing clinical experience with chlorpromazine prompted Fish and associates to search for pharmacologic agents with stimulating effects, and led to trials of methysergide maleate, imipramine hydrochloride, dextroamphetamine, levoamphetamine, triodothyronine (T3), and L-dopa, each involving small samples of children.

Methysergide, administered to 11 children, ages 2 to 5 years, resulted in a mixture of decreases and worsening of symptoms (only the two children with the lowest IQs showed clear improvement, with increases of affective responsiveness, alertness, and goal-directedness) (Fish, Campbell, Shapiro & Floyd, 1969a). Imipramine, in 10 children, ages 2 to 6 years, had stimulating, tranquilizing, and disorganizing properties, with therapeutic effects usually outweighed by untoward effects (Campbell, Fish, Shapiro, & Floyd, 1971b). Only in the most retarded and anergic children (2) did this drug warrant further study. In treatment with dextroamphetamine, the same doses were associated with only slight improvements (decreases in hyperactivity, increases in attention span and language production) and a variety of severe untoward effects, including irritability, motor excitability, worsening of withdrawal and stereotypies, and motor retardation, among others (Campbell, Fish, David, et al., 1972; Campbell, Fish, Shapiro, & Floyd, 1972; Campbell et al., 1973). A trial of T3 was commenced after Sherwin, Flach, and Stokes (1958) reported positive stimulating effects of this hormone in 2 euthyroid autistic children. In a study involving 14 autistic children, 3 to 6 years of age, T3 appeared to have a variety of stimulating effects; however, the study was not well controlled (Campbell, Fish, David, et al., 1972; Campbell et al., 1973). Interestingly, the responders to T3 had significantly higher thyroxine iodine (T4) values than the nonresponders, and 4 had somewhat elevated T4 levels on baseline. In a subsequent carefully designed, double-blind, and placebo-controlled study involving 30 children, ages 2 years 3 months to 7 years 2 months (mean, 4 years 5 months), the superiority of T3 to placebo was reflected only in the decrease of a few symptoms (Campbell, Small, et al., 1978). The subgroup of 4 children who were good responders to T3 could not be differentiated from the remaining children on any variable. Our earlier speculation that T3 deficiency existed in some autistic children and that administration of T3 therefore yielded beneficial behavioral effects was not confirmed in this study: Actually 13 children had somewhat elevated T3 on baseline, though they were clinically euthyroid. As in our previous study, the greater the reduction of symptom severity, the more marked was the reduction of T4 with T3 administration. The behavioral response to T3 seemed to be related to low IQ.

Elevation of baseline T4 and/or T3 values was also found in a larger sample of autistic children (Campbell, Green, Caplan, & David, 1982). We therefore hypothesized that in a subgroup of autistic children a hypothalamic dysfunction may exist associated with thyroid abnormalities. In a pilot study involving 10 young autistic children, all subjects showed deviant responses of T3 and/or TSH to intravenous administration of thyrotropin-releasing hormone (TRH) though individual variability was marked (Campbell, Hollander, Ferris, &

Greene, 1978). The abnormalities were suggestive of hypothalamic dysfunction. Administration of TRH was associated with transient decrease in hyperactivity, and increases in affective responsiveness, spontaneous speech, focusing, and euphoria. However, no thyroid abnormalities were found in two samples of older subjects by Cohen, Young, Lowe, and Harcherik (1980; $N = 58$, mean age 12.5, $SD \pm 5.1$), and by Abbassi, Linscheid, and Coleman (1978; $N = 13$, age range 7 to 21). Levodopa administration was associated with improvement in 5 of 12 children (Campbell et al., 1976). Positive changes were characterized by increased stimulation and included decreases in negativism and increases in play, language, energy, and motor initiation in hypoactive children. However, side effects were also observed and included worsening of stereotypies and stereotypies de novo. Thus, these drugs with stimulating properties, which included dopamine agonists (d-amphetamine, 1-amphetamine, and L-dopa), were not considered very effective therapeutically and had many side effects in this population. It is of interest that, while d-amphetamine (and methylphenidate) administration to hyperactive children with attention deficit disorder may be associated with tics (Denckla, Bemporad, & Mackay, 1976), d- and 1-amphetamine and L-dopa frequently yielded worsening of preexisting stereotypies and stereotypies de novo in autistic patients.

Lithium

Lithium was explored in a sample of 10 children and compared to chlorpromazine. In general, neither of the two drugs was therapeutically effective, and lithium was less so than chlorpromazine (Campbell, Fish, Korein, et al., 1972). Lithium is known to have antiaggressive properties in animals, in adult psychiatric patients, and in children (for review, see Campbell, Fish, Korein, et al., 1972; Campbell, Perry, & Green, 1984). In this study, aggressiveness decreased in only 2 of the 5 aggressive children. However, in 1, a 6-year-old boy, the response to lithium was dramatic; lifelong explosiveness, self-mutilation, head banging, and temper tantrums practically ceased on 600 mg/d of lithium (blood level 0.593–0.760 mEq/1). Lowering of brain serotonin increases aggressiveness in experimental animals. If lithium indeed increases the rate of synthesis of brain serotonin (Perez-Cruet, Tagliamonte, Tagliamonte, & Gessa, 1971), this could explain not only the decrease of aggressiveness in 2 of our patients but also the minimal change of other behavioral symptoms in this sample.

RECENT STUDIES

As noted above, the low-potency, sedative type of neuroleptic, chlorpromazine, was not sufficiently therapeutically effective in our population of autistic children. It had a narrow therapeutic margin and its administration was associated with excessive sedation, which seemed to impair the children's learning and functioning. The high-potency neuroleptics (fluphenazine, trifluoperazine, thiothixene, and molindone) had a wider therapeutic margin and appeared to be more effective in reducing behavioral symptoms (for review, see Campbell et al., 1981). We will discuss here only haloperidol, fenfluramine, and naltrexone in some detail, for the following reasons. Haloperidol has been studied systematically in the past decade in this population, and more is known about its efficacy and safety in autistic children than of any other psychoactive drug. Fenfluramine was chosen because many physicians prescribe it to autistic children; though reports appear to be promising, the efficacy and safety of this drug remains to be demonstrated. Naltrexone, like fenfluramine, is an experimental drug in this population; because of its relative safety in adults and its biochemical properties, it seems an interesting and important drug to study in infantile autism.

Other drugs were covered elsewhere in recent years (Campbell *et al.*, 1981, 1985).

Haloperidol

Haloperidol, a high-potency neuroleptic with strong antidopaminergic properties, was reported to be therapeutically effective in both hospitalized (Faretra, Dooher, & Dowling, 1970) and outpatient autistic children (Englehardt *et al.*, 1973). These observations were based on pilot studies that were not well controlled. However, the encouraging results, which required replication under more stringent conditions, led us to systematic studies of this drug. In two major studies, each involving 40 autistic hyper- and normoactive children, ages 2 to 7 years, we have demonstrated that haloperidol, when its dose is individually regulated for each child, can significantly decrease behavioral symptoms in the absence of untoward effects (Anderson *et al.*, 1984; Campbell, Anderson, *et al.*, 1978). Furthermore, at the same dose levels (0.5 to 4.0 mg/day, or $M = 1.11$ to 1.78 mg/day) the clinical therapeutic changes are associated with facilitation of learning in the laboratory (Anderson *et al.*, 1984; Campbell, Anderson, Cohen, *et al.*, 1982; Campbell, Anderson, Meier, *et al.*, 1978). This is an important finding, because with similar doses (mg/kg/d) haloperidol had adverse effects on cognition in aggressive children diagnosed as conduct-disorder (Platt, Campbell, Green, & Grega, 1984). Haloperidol is a dopamine antagonist; there is some evidence that a subgroup of autistic children show evidence of excess dopaminergic activity, associated with stereotypies, hyperactivity, and low intellectual functioning (Cohen & Young, 1977; Young *et al.*, 1982). Both stereotypies and hyperactivity decreased significantly with administration of haloperidol in our studies. As noted above, dopamine agonists frequently yielded worsening of preexisting stereotypies and stereotypies *de novo* (Campbell, Fish, David, *et al.*, 1972; Campbell, Fish, Shapiro, & Floyd, 1972; Campbell *et al.*, 1973). Not only the short-term but also the long-term efficacy of haloperidol has been demonstrated (Campbell, Anderson, Cohen, *et al.*, 1982; Campbell, Perry, *et al.*, 1983). In a subsample ($N = 15$) of these children, IQs were retested on follow-up; 8 children showed marked increases in intellectual functioning (Die Trill *et al.*, 1984). However, about 22% of the subjects developed drug-related dyskinesias (tardive and withdrawal dyskinesias) on conservative doses of haloperidol (0.5–3.0 mg/d) when studied prospectively (Campbell, Grega, Green, & Bennett, 1983; Campbell, Perry, *et al.*, 1983; Perry *et al.*, 1985). Our review of the literature revealed an absence of prospective studies of drug-related dyskinesias in children (for review, see Campbell, Grega, *et al.*, 1983). On the basis of retrospective studies and reports, the prevalence of drug-related abnormal involuntary movements in children receiving neuroleptics ranges from 8 to 51% (for review see Campbell, Grega, *et al.*, 1983). In our carefully conducted prospective study the prevalence was 22% (Campbell, Grega, *et al.*, 1983, Perry *et al.*, 1985). Reasons for this discrepancy are many (Campbell, Grega, *et al.*, 1983): One is a failure to differentiate drug-related dyskinesias from voluntary (e.g., stereotypies) and other involuntary (e.g., stereotyped movement disorders, and Tourette syndrome) abnormal movements. We have shown that neuroleptic-related movements can represent a change in severity, amplitude, and frequency/or topography of stereotypies in autistic children. Tourett syndrome may also be associated with neuroleptic administration. In young autistic children, it is at times difficult or impossible to differentiate stereotypies involving the mouth, tongue, and jaw from neuroleptic-related dyskinesias. Furthermore, since we have repeatedly demonstrated that haloperidol will significantly reduce stereotypies, it requires careful prospective studies to differentiate the reemergence of suppressed stereotypies upon drug withdrawal from withdrawal dyskinesias. Findings of institutionalized and mentally retarded children and adolescents (Gualtieri, Quade, Hicks, Mayo, & Schroeder, 1984) cannot be extrapolated and applied to young autistic children such as our subjects, who were never in institutions and who had no history of chronic neuroleptic intake prior to enrollment in an anterospective study. In their autistic patients, Polizos and Engelhardt (1980) reported only 2 cases of tardive dyskinesia involving tongue movements and noted that only 20% of the withdrawal dyskinesias were oral (and always mild). However, in our prospective study the orolingual topography was found to be the most common involvement (Campbell, Grega, et al., 1983; Campbell, Perry, et al., 1983; Perry et al., 1985). We also found that continuous versus discontinuous administration of haloperidol had no effect on the development of abnormal involuntary movements, and that a minimum of 3 months' total cumulative exposure to drug is necessary for the development of dyskinesias. Furthermore, up to the present, dyskinesias have been reversible in all patients. In this prospective study of haloperidol (0.5 to 3.0 mg/d), in a subsample ($N = 42$) of children, ages 2 to 7.6 years, after 6 months' maintenance there was a decrement (4.7 points) in mean height percentile (n.s.), and an 8.2-point increase in mean weight percentile ($p < .05$) (Green et al., 1984).

Fenfluramine

Because of the association of tardive and withdrawal dyskinesias with chronic neuroleptic administration, we began to study fenfluramine. This drug has received great publicity since the preliminary observations and report of Geller, Ritvo, Freeman, and Yuwiler (1982) on 3 autistic children, suggesting behavioral improvement associated with increases in IQs. The rationale for treating this population with fenfluramine was as follows: About 30% of autistic children have elevated serotonin levels as compared to normal controls (Campbell et al., 1975; Ritvo et al., 1970). As a group, autistic children with lower IQs and more florid psychoses have higher serotonin levels (Campbell et al., 1975). Serotonergic activity of the brain has been said to affect appetite, sleep, learning, and memory (for review, see Young et al., 1982). Administration of fenfluramine, which has potent antiserotonergic activity in animal brains, was expected to decrease serotonin levels in autistic children, and this, in turn, should result in decreases of behavioral symptoms. Fenfluramine has structural similarities to amphetamine; stimulating effects may be dose-dependent, and it possesses tranquilizing properties. A study of Ritvo, Freeman, Geller, & Yuwiler (1983) involved 14 outpatients, ages 3 to 18 years. Following a 3-month baseline period, all subjects were treated with fenfluramine (1.5 mg/kg/day) over a period of 4 months, followed by 2 months of placebo. Behavioral improvements included decreases of motility disturbances, restlessness, and "sensory symptoms," improvements in sleep pattern, increases in eye contact, socialization, and communicative language. IQ scores rose too. Serotonin levels in blood decreased markedly after 1 month of fenfluramine maintenance. Low baseline serotonin levels were associated with good response to fenfluramine (Ritvo et al., 1984). Side effects were few and minor. However, results of others differed: Behavioral improvement was not associated with increases in IQ for 9 outpatients ages 5 to 13 years (August, Raz, & Baird, 1985), while in 16 subjects, ages 3 to 12 years, significant decreases of serotonin levels were not accompanied by behavioral or cognitive changes while on fenfluramine maintenance (Leventhal,

1985). All three of these studies employed the same design. It should be noted that subjects were not assigned randomly to treatments and that monthly IQ testing could have had a practice effect in the Ritvo *et al.* study (1983, 1984).

We completed an open pilot study of fenfluramine involving 10 inpatients, ages 3 to 5.75 years (mean, 4.15). They were carefully monitored and a variety of assessments were carried out by several raters independently, including videotaping (Campbell, Deutsch, Perry, Wolsky, & Palij, 1986). Our findings, based on 1 to 2 months of fenfluramine maintenance, are as follows: The drug had both stimulating and tranquilizing properties, which were reflected both in therapeutic and in side effects. The most significant changes were increases in relatedness and affective responsiveness, and decreases in insomnia, irritability, aggressiveness directed against self or others, temper tantrums, and hyperactivity. Four of the 10 children showed marked improvement; however, in some, therapeutic effects were transient. Onset of positive changes occurred as early as the second day of drug administration. The therapeutic margin was good: Above optimal doses, drowsiness, uncontrollable irritability, and transient weight loss were rated. We found no laboratory abnormalities associated with fenfluramine administration, and blood pressure, heart rate, and electrocardiogram remained unchanged through the study. No child developed drug-related abnormal movement. Unlike Ritvo *et al.* (1983, 1984), who used a fixed dose schedule (1.5 mg/kg/d of fenfluramine), we found drug treatment more effective if doses were individually regulated in each child, since optimal doses in our study ranged from 1.1 to 1.8 mg/kg/d (mean, 1.4). The therapeutic effects observed during fenfluramine treatment could be attributed to amphetaminelike, or antiserotonergic or antidopaminergic properties of this drug.

Our preliminary findings await replication: We have begun a double-blind and placebo-controlled study of fenfluramine, where children are randomly assigned to treatment conditions. In this clinical trial, we wish to critically assess the effects of fenfluramine on behavioral symptoms and on discrimination learning in an automated laboratory, and finally, its safety. Preliminary analyses of data involving 11 subjects suggest that there are no significant differences between placebo and fenfluramine (Campbell, Small, Palij, Perry, Polonsky, Lukashok, & Anderson, in press).

Naltrexone

We also wished to explore the possible therapeutic effects of naltrexone in severely disturbed autistic children, to establish its effective dosage and dose range, and its safety using an open acute dose trial design.

The rationale to explore naltrexone, a potent and long-lasting opiate antagonist, in infantile autism is as follows: There is some supportive, though inconclusive, evidence that abnormalities in activity or in the level of endogenous opioids exist in some autistic children (Weizman *et al.*, 1984; Young, Cohen, Brown, & Caparulo, 1978; Young, Cohen, Caparulo, Brown, & Maas, 1979). The endogenous opioids of the brain regulate various functions and behaviors and also influence the neurotransmitters, such as serotonin, dopamine, and norepinephrine; these in turn regulate hormones and endocrine systems (for review, see Verebey, Volavka, & Clouet, 1978). For example, they are involved with the regulation of pain perception, as are the exogenous opiates. Therefore, it was hypothesized that the endogenous opioid systems (endorphins and enkephalins) also play a role in the development of self-mutilation (Coid, Allolio, & Rees, 1983; Davidson, Kleene, Carroll, & Rockowitz, 1983; Sandman *et al.*, 1983). Administration of naloxone, also an opiate antagonist, to a few retarded individuals with severe self-mutilation resulted in decreases of this symptom (Bernstein, Hughes, & Thompson, 1984; Davidson et al., 1983; Sandman et al., 1983). In recent years it has been hypothesized that abnormalities of brain-endogenous opioid systems represent the biochemical basis of certain behavioral symptoms and other abnormalities found in autistic children (Kalat, 1978; Panksepp, 1979). If this proves to be true, then treatment with an opiate antagonist—for example, naltrexone—may result in decreases of these symptoms.

To the present time, only one child with extremely severe behavioral symptoms, including aggressiveness, hyperactivity, withdrawal, stereotypies, and inability to focus, completed our open acute dose trial of naltrexone (Campbell, 1985). In this 5-year-old intellectually subnormal boy, who had no language skills, lower doses of naltrexone (0.5 and 1.0 mg/kg/day) had tranquilizing effects (decreases in hyperactivity, impulsivity, aggressiveness, and stereotypies), while at higher doses (2.0 and 3.0 mg/kg/day) the effects were rated as mainly stimulating and involved language and social behaviors. The child, for the first time, said words, babbled and vocalized, showed a marked decrease in withdrawal, and made social overtures (Campbell, 1985). These are preliminary results, based on one subject, whose behavior was quite variable even on baseline. However, he subsequently failed to respond to maintenance doses of haloperidol.

CONCLUSION

There is a need to develop more effective and safe treatments in infantile autism. Future research should put more emphasis on studying the interaction of safe and effective pharmacotherapy and psychosocial treatments (Campbell, Anderson, et al., 1978). We view an effective psychoactive drug as a treatment modality that, when given over a not excessive length of time, can render some autistic children more responsive or more amenable to special education and to behavior modification.

ACKNOWLEDGMENTS

This work was supported in part by NIMH grants MH-32212 and MH-40177, and by a grant from The Stallone Fund for Autism Research, and was aided by Social and Behavioral Sciences Research Grant No. 12-108 from March of Dimes Birth Defects Foundation (Dr. Campbell).

REFERENCES

Abbassi, V., Linscheid, T., & Coleman, M. (1978). Triiodothyronine (T3) concentration and therapy in autistic children. Journal of Autism and Childhood Schizophrenia, 8, 383–387.

Anderson, L. T., Campbell, M., Grega, D. M., Perry, R., Small, A. M., & Green, W. H. (1984). Haloperidol in infantile autism: Effects on learning and behavioral symptoms. American Journal of Psychiatry, 141, 1195–1202.

August, G. J., Raz, N., & Baird, T. D. (1985). Brief report: Effects of fenfluramine on behavioral, cognitive, and affective disturbances in autistic children. Journal of Autism and Developmental Disorders, 15, 97–107.

Bernstein, G. A., Hughes, J. R., & Thompson, T. (1984, October 13). *Naloxone reduces the self-injurious behavior of a mentally retarded adolescent.* Paper presented at the Annual Meeting of the American Academy of Child Psychiatry, Toronto.

Campbell, M. (1985, July). *Naltrexone in autistic children.* Paper presented at the Autism Research Symposium, Seventh Annual Meeting and Conference of the National Society for Children and Adults with Autism, Los Angeles.

Campbell, M., Anderson, L. T., Cohen, I. L., Perry, R., Small, A. M., Green, W. H., Anderson, L. & McCandless, W. (1982). Haloperidol in autistic children: Effects on learning, behavior, and abnormal involuntary movements. *Psychopharmacology Bulletin, 18*(1), 110–112.

Campbell, M., Anderson, L. T., Meier, M., Cohen, I. L., Small, A. M., Samit, C., & Sachar, E. J. (1978). A comparison of haloperidol, behavior therapy and their interaction in autistic children. *Journal of the American Academy of Child Psychiatry, 17,* 640–655.

Campbell, M., Anderson, L. T., Small, A. M., Perry, R., Green, W. H., & Caplan, R. (1982). The effects of haloperidol on learning and behavior in autistic children. *Journal of Autism and Developmental Disorders, 12,* 167–175.

Campbell, M., Cohen, I. L., & Anderson, L. T. (1981). Pharmacotherapy for autistic children. A summary of research. *Canadian Journal of Psychiatry, 26,* 265–273.

Campbell, M., Deutsch, S. I., Perry, R., Wolsky, B. B., & Palij, M. (1986). Short-term efficacy and safety of fenfluramine in hospitalized preschool-age autistic children: An open study. *Psychopharmacology Bulletin, 22*(1), 141–147.

Campbell, M., Fish, B., David, R., Shapiro, T., Collins, P., & Koh, C. (1972). Response to triiodothyronine and dextroamphetamine: A study of preschool schizophrenic children. *Journal of Autism and Childhood Schizophrenia, 2,* 343–358.

Campbell, M., Fish, B., David, R., Shapiro, T., Collins, P., & Koh, C. (1973). Liothyronine treatment in psychotic and non-psychotic children under 6 years. *Archives of General Psychiatry, 29,* 602–608.

Campbell, M., Fish, B., Korein, J., Shapiro, T., Collins, P., & Koh, C. (1972). Lithium and chlorpromazine: A controlled crossover study of hyperactive severely disturbed young children. *Journal of Autism and Childhood Schizophrenia, 2,* 234–263.

Campbell, M., Fish, B., Shapiro, T., & Floyd, A., Jr. (1970). Thiothixene in young disturbed children: A pilot study. *Archives of General Psychiatry, 23,* 70–72.

Campbell, M., Fish, B., Shapiro, T., & Floyd, A., Jr. (1971a). Study of molindone in disturbed preschool children. *Current Therapeutic Research, 13,* 28–33.

Campbell, M., Fish, B., Shapiro, T., & Floyd, A., Jr. (1971b). Imipramine in preschool autistic and schizophrenic children. *Journal of Autism and Childhood Schizophrenia, 1,* 267–282.

Campbell, M., Fish, B., Shapiro, T., & Floyd, A., Jr. (1972). Acute responses of schizophrenic children to a sedative and a "stimulating" neuroleptic: A pharmacologic yardstick. *Current Therapeutic Research, 14,* 759–766.

Campbell, M., Friedman, E., Green, W. H., Collins, P. J., Small, A. M., & Breuer, H. (1975). Blood serotonin in schizophrenic children. A preliminary study. *International Pharmacopsychiatry, 10,* 213–221.

Campbell, M., & Green, W. H. (1985). Pervasive developmental disorders of childhood. In H. I. Kaplan & B. J. Sadock (Eds.), *Comprehensive textbook of psychiatry* (4th ed., Vol. 2, pp. 1672–1683). Baltimore: Williams & Wilkins.

Campbell, M., Green, W., Caplan, R., & David, R. (1982). Psychiatry and endocrinology in children: Early infantile autism and psychosocial dwarfism. In P. J. V. Beumont & G. D. Burrows (Eds.), *Handbook of psychiatry and endocrinology* (pp. 50–62). Amsterdam: Elsevier Biomedical Press.

Campbell, M., Green, W. H., & Deutsch, S. I. (1985). *Childhood Pharmacology.* Beverly Hills: Sage Publications, 1985.

Campbell, M., Grega, D. M., Green, W. H., & Bennett, W. G. (1983). Neuroleptic-induced dyskinesias in children. *Clinical Neuropharmacology, 6,* 207–222.

Campbell, M., Hollander, C. S., Ferris, S., & Greene, L. W. (1978). Response to thyrotropin releasing hormone stimulation in young psychotic children: A pilot study. *Psychoneuroendocrinology, 3,* 195–201.

Campbell, M., & Palij, M. (1985a). Behavioral and cognitive measures used in psychopharmalogical studies of infantile autism. *Psychopharmacology Bulletin, 21*(4), 1047–1052.

Campbell, M., & Palij, M. (1985b). Measurement of untoward effects including tardive dyskinesia. *Psychopharmacology Bulletin, 21*(4), 1063–1066.

Campbell, M., Perry, R., Bennett, W. G., Small, A. M., Green, W. H., Grega, D., Schwartz, V., & Anderson, L. (1983). Long-term therapeutic efficacy and drug-related abnormal movements: A prospective study of haloperidol in autistic children. *Psychopharmacology Bulletin, 19*(1), 80–83.

Campbell, M., Perry, R., & Green, W. H. (1984). The use of lithium in children and adolescents. *Psychosomatics, 25,* 95–106.

Campbell, M., Petti, T. A., Green, W. H., Cohen, I. L., Genieser, N. B., & David, R. (1980). Some physical parameters of young autistic children. *Journal of the American Academy of Child Psychiatry, 19,* 193–212.

Campbell, M., Small, A. M., Collins, P. J., Friedman, E., David, R., & Genieser, N. (1976). Levodopa and levoamphetamine: A crossover study in young schizophrenic children. *Current Therapeutic Research, 19,* 70–86.

Campbell, M., Small, A. M., Hollander, C. S., Korein, J., Cohen, I. L., Kalmijn, M., & Ferris, S. (1978). A controlled crossover study of triiodothyronine in autistic children. *Journal of Autism and Childhood Schizophrenia, 8,* 371–381.

Campbell, M., Small, A. M., Palij, M., Perry, R., Polonsky, B. B., Lukashok, D., & Anderson, L. T. (in press). The efficacy and safety of fenfluramine in autistic children: Preliminary analysis of a double-blind study. *Psychopharmacology Bulletin, 23.*

Cohen, D. J., Caparulo, B. K., Shaywitz, B. A., & Bowers, M. B. (1977). Dopamine and serotonin metabolism in neuropsychiatrically disturbed children. *Archives of General Psychiatry, 34,* 545–550.

Cohen, D. J., Shaywitz, B. A., Johnson, W. T., & Bowers, M. (1974). Biogenic amines in autistic and atypical children. *Archives of General Psychiatry, 31,* 845–853.

Cohen, D. J., & Young, J. G. (1977). Neurochemistry and child psychiatry. *Journal of the American Academy of Child Psychiatry, 16,* 353–411.

Cohen, D. J., Young, J. G., Lowe, T. L., & Harcherik, D. (1980). Thyroid hormone in autistic children. *Journal of Autism and Developmental Disorders, 10,* 445–450.

Coid, J., Allolio, B., & Rees, L. H. Raised plasma metenkephalin in patients who habitually mutilate themselves. *Lancet II,* 1983 (September 3), 545–546.

Davidson, P. W., Kleene, B. M., Carroll, M., & Rockowitz, R. J. (1983). Effects of naloxone on self-injurious behavior: A case study. *Applied Research in Mental Retardation, 4,* 1–4.

DeMyer, M. K., Hintgen, J. N., & Jackson, R. K. (1981). Infantile autism reviewed: A decade of research. *Schizophrenia Bulletin, 7,* 388–451.

Denckla, M. B., Bemporad, J. R., & Mackay, M. C. (1976). Tics following methylphenidate administration. *Journal of the American Medical Association, 235,* 1349–1351.

Deutsch, S. I., Campbell, M., Perry, R., Green, W. H., Poland, R. E., & Rubin, R. T. (1986). Plasma growth hormone response to insulin-induced hypoglycemia in infantile autism: A pilot study. *Journal of Autism and Developmental Disorders, 16,* 59–68.

Deutsch, S. I., Campbell, M., Sachar, E. J., Green, W. H., & David, R. (1985). Plasma growth hormone response to oral L-dopa in infantile autism. *Journal of Autism and Developmental Disorders, 15,* 205–212.

Die Trill, M. L., Wolsky, B. B., Shell, J., Green, W. H., Perry, R., & Campbell, M. (1984, October). *Effects of long-term haloperidol treatment in intellectual functioning in autistic children: A pilot study.* Paper presented at the Thirty-First Annual Meeting of the American and Canadian Academy of Child Psychiatry, Toronto.

Engelhardt, D. M., & Polizos, P. (1978). Adverse effects of pharmacotherapy in childhood psychosis. In M. A. Lipton, A. DiMascio, & K. F. Killam (Eds.), *Psychopharmacology: A generation of progress.* New York: Raven Press.

Engelhardt, D. M., Polizos, P., Waizer, J., & Hoffman, S. P. (1973). A double-blind comparison of fluphenazine and haloperidol. *Journal of Autism and Childhood Schizophrenia, 3,* 128–137.

Faretra, G., Dooher, L., & Dowling, J. (1970). Comparison of haloperidol and fluphenazine in disturbed children. *American Journal of Psychiatry, 126,* 1670–1673.

Fish, B. (1970). Psychopharmacologic response of chronic schizophrenic adults as predictors of responses in young schizophrenic children. *Psychopharmacology Bulletin, 6,* 12–15.

Fish, B., Campbell, M., Shapiro, T., & Floyd, A., Jr. (1969a). Schizophrenic children treated with methysergide (Sansert). *Diseases of the Nervous System, 30,* 534–540.

Fish, B., Campbell, M., Shapiro, T., & Floyd, A., Jr. (1969b). Comparison of trifluperidol, trifluoperazine, and chlorpromazine in preschool schizophrenic children: The value of less sedative antipsychotic agents. *Current Therapeutic Research, 11,* 589–595.

Fish, B., & Ritvo, E. R. (1979). Psychoses of Childhood. In J. D. Noshpitz (Ed.), *Basic handbook of childhood psychiatry* (Vol. 2, pp. 249–304). New York: Basic Books.

Fish, B., Shapiro, T., Campbell, M. (1966). Long-term prognosis and the response of schizophrenic children to drug therapy: A controlled study of trifluoperazine. *American Journal of Psychiatry, 123,* 32–39.

Geller, E., Ritvo, E. R., Freeman, B. J., & Yuwiler, A. (1982). Preliminary observations on the effect of fenfluramine on blood serotonin and symptoms in three autistic boys. *New England Journal of Medicine, 307,* 165–169.

Gillberg, C., Terenius, C., & Lönnerholm, G. (1985). Endorphin activity in childhood psychosis: Spinal fluid levels in 24 cases. *Archives of General Psychiatry, 42,* 780–783.

Green, W. H., Campbell, M., Wolsky, B. B., Deutsch, S. I., Golden, R. R., & Cicero, S. D. (1984, October). *Effects of short- and long-term haloperidol administration on growth in young autistic children.* Paper presented at the Thirty-First Annual Meeting of the American and Canadian Academy of Child Psychiatry, Toronto.

Gualtieri, C. T., Quade, D., Hicks, R. E., Mayo, J. P., & Schroeder, S. R. (1984). Tardive dyskinesia and other clinical consequences of neuroleptic treatment in children and adolescents. *American Journal of Psychiatry, 141,* 20–23.

Kalat, J. W. (1978). Letter to the editor: Speculations on similarities between autism and opiate addiction. *Journal of Autism and Childhood Schizophrenia, 8,* 477–479.

Leventhal, B. L. (1985, May). *Fenfluramine administration to autistic children: Effects on behavior and biogenic amines.* Paper presented at the Annual Early Clinical Drug Evaluation Unit (ECDEU) (Anniversary) Meeting, Key Biscayne, Florida.

Panksepp, J. (1979). A neurochemical theory of autism. *Trends in Neuroscience, 2,* 174–177.

Perez-Cruet, J., Tagliamonte, A., Tagliamonte, P., & Gessa, G. L. (1971). Stimulation of serotonin synthesis by lithium. *Journal of Pharmacology and Experimental Therapeutics, 178,* 325–330.

Perry, R., Campbell, M., Green, W. H., Small, A. M., Die Trill, M. L., Meiselas, K., Golden, R. R., & Deutsch, S. I. (1985). Neuroleptic-related dyskinesias in autistic children: A prospective study. *Psychopharmacology Bulletin, 21*(1), 140–143.

Platt, J. E., Campbell, M., Green, W. H., & Grega, D. M. (1984). Cognitive effects of lithium carbonate and haloperidol in treatment-resistant aggressive children. *Archives of General Psychiatry, 41,* 657–662.

Ritvo, E. R., Freeman, B. J., Geller, E., & Yuwiler, A. (1983). Effects of fenfluramine on 14 outpatients with the syndrome of autism. *Journal of the American Academy of Child Psychiatry, 22,* 549–558.

Ritvo, E. R., Freeman, B. J., Yuwiler, A., Geller, E., Yokota, A., Schroth, P., & Novak, P. (1984). Study of fenfluramine in outpatients with the syndrome of autism. *Journal of Pediatrics, 105,* 823–828.

Ritvo, E. R., Yuwiler, A., Geller, E., Ornitz, E. M., Saeger, K., & Plotkin, S. (1970). Increased blood serotonin and platelets in early infantile autism. *Archives of General Psychiatry, 23,* 566–572.

Rutter, M., Bartak, M., & Newman, S. (1971). Autism—A central disorder of cognition and language? In M. Rutter (Ed.), *Infantile autism: Concepts, characteristics, and treatment* (pp. 148–171). Edinburgh: Churchill Livingstone.

Sandman, C. A., Dotta, P. C., Barron, J., Hochler, F. K., Williams, C., & Swanson, J. M. (1983). Naloxone attenuates self-abusive behavior in developmentally disabled clients. *Applied Research in Mental Retardation, 4,* 5–11.

Sherwin, A. C., Flach, F. F., & Stokes, P. E. (1958). Treatment of psychoses in early childhood with triiodothyronine. *American Journal of Psychiatry, 115,* 166–167.

Simeon, J., Saletu, B., Saletu, M., Itil, T. M., & DaSilva, J. (1973). *Thiothixene in childhood psychoses.* Paper presented at the Third International Symposium on Phenothiazines, Rockville, Maryland.

Verebey, K., Volavka, J., & Clouet, D. (1978). Endorphins in psychiatry. *Archives of General Psychiatry, 35,* 877–888.

Waizer, J., Polizos, P., Hoffman, S. P., Engelhardt, D. M., & Margolis, R. A. (1972). A single-blind evaluation of thiothixene with outpatient schizophrenic children. *Journal of Autism and Childhood Schizophrenia, 2,* 378–386.

Weizman, R., Weizman, A., Tyano, S., Szekely, G., Weissman, B. A., & Sarne, Y. (1984). Humoral-endorphin blood levels in autistic, schizophrenic and healthy subjects. *Psychopharmacology, 82,* 368–370.

Wing, L. (1972). *Autistic children.* New York: Brunner/Mazel.

Young, J. G., Cohen, D. J., Brown, S.-L., & Caparulo, B. K. (1978). Decreased urinary free catecholamines in childhood autism. *Journal of the American Academy of Child Psychiatry, 17,* 671–678.

Young, J. G., Cohen, D. J., Caparulo, B. K., Brown, S.-L., & Maas, J. W. (1979). Decreased 24-hour urinary MHPG in childhood autism. *American Journal of Psychiatry, 136,* 1055–1057.

Young, J. G., Kavanagh, M. E., Anderson, G. M., Shaywitz, B. A., & Cohen, D. J. (1982). Clinical neurochemistry of autism and associated disorders. *Journal of Autism and Developmental Disorders, 12,* 147–165.

Possible Brain Opioid Involvement in Disrupted Social Intent and Language Development of Autism

JAAK PANKSEPP and TONY L. SAHLEY

BACKGROUND INFORMATION

The underlying premise of this chapter is that a major dysfunction of the autistic brain resides in neural mechanisms that elaborate social motivation and thereby social intent. Although substantive understanding of brain mechanisms that mediate social emotions remains meager, animal brain research on fundamental processes such as separation distress and rough-and-tumble play has now yielded enough knowledge that some provisional hypotheses concerning the etiology and treatment of autism can be generated. Basically, our psychopharmacological work has affirmed the special importance of brain opioid activity in the elaboration of various social behaviors and social emotions, and convergent lines of reasoning suggest that opioid receptor blockade should be effective in alleviating and/or reversing the progress of certain autistic symptoms. In addition to summarizing evidence pertinent to the opioid-excess hypothesis, we discuss the possibility that certain cognitive symptoms of autism, such as problems in language development, may secondarily reflect disruption of underlying social emotions that dictate the intensity of social intent in the developing organism.

A Biological Overview

Accumulating evidence suggests that early childhood autism has a biological etiology. The disturbances appear to originate during gestation, are present at birth, and become manifest when they interfere with the normal course of development (Ciaranello, Vandenberg & Anders, 1982; Piggot, 1979). No single anatomical or biochemical lesion has yet been demonstrated to account for autistic behavior, although modest success in symptom reduction

JAAK PANKSEPP • Department of Psychology, Bowling Green State University, Bowling Green, Ohio 43403.   TONY L. SAHLEY • Coleman Memorial Laboratory, Department of Otolaryngology, University of California, San Francisco, California 94143.

has been achieved following the administration of antipsychotic drugs (e.g., Campbell, Cohen, & Anderson, 1981; Cohen, Campbell, & Posner, 1980), the anorexigenic drug fenfluramine, which releases and subsequently depletes brain serotonin (August, Raz, & Baird, 1985; Geller, Ritvo, Freeman, & Yuwiler, 1982; Ritvo, Freeman, Geller, & Yuwiler, 1983), and the B vitamin pyridoxine, which is a cofactor in the synthesis of many neurotransmitters (Lelord et al., 1981; Rimland, Callaway, & Dreyfus, 1978). Thus, the general consensus is that progress in treating autism will depend largely upon clarification of the neurochemical basis of this perplexing developmental disorder.

The specific hypothesis that excess brain opioid activity may contribute to the development of autistic symptoms was put forward several years ago (Kalat, 1978; Panksepp, 1979; Panksepp, Herman & Vilberg, 1978). Since that time, the hypothesis has continued to be supported by a growing body of evidence suggesting that autisticlike symptoms can be induced in animals (1) by the administration of exogenous opioids (Panksepp, 1981a), (2) by the apparent relationship between symptoms of opiate addiction and autistic symptoms (Kalat, 1978), and (3) by the fact that autisticlike symptoms in the severely mentally retarded can be attenuated by opioid blockade (Sandman et al., 1983). To clarify the conceptual basis of this neurochemical hypothesis, we would first address what is known at present regarding autism and delayed development of social signaling systems such as language.

Language Deficits in Autism

Even in the highest-functioning autistic individuals, problems in social interaction remain as the major obstacle to communicative competence (Akerly, 1974; Schopler & Mesibov, 1985). With respect to language development, autistic children exhibit a limited repertoire of communicative abilities (Wetherby & Prutting, 1984), although they may possess adequate linguistic ability (Wollner, 1983). The desire or intent to communicate in young children is displayed largely through preverbal gestures (Bates, Camaioni, & Volterra, 1975), and autistic children generally fail to use such gestures for communicative purposes (Kanner, 1943; Rutter, 1978). Instead, the communication of the autistic child appears to serve primarily instrumental or regulatory functions, related to their immediate biological needs (Schuler, 1980). They may engage other people as "object tools" in order to obtain environmental ends, and they may seem to exhibit a pervading developmental delay in their communicative ability to achieve social ends, and hence, to share feelings and knowledge. Thus, they fail to learn much from others (Wetherby & Prutting, 1984). One reasonable explanation for these observed behaviors is that the desire or need to communicate socially is disrupted or lacking in autistic children.

Herein we further discuss the possibility that the major disturbance in early childhood autism involves a blockade and/or a developmental disruption in primary, opioid-modulated social/emotional brain systems that mediate infant attachment behaviors and hence what Bates (1979a) refers to as social communicative intent. Such a deficit may prevent the secondary development of higher cortical regions that might otherwise serve language functions in these children (Damasio & Maurer, 1978; Wetherby, 1984).

The Neurochemistry of Social Attachment

Existing evidence suggests that the brain contains emotional/motivational systems specifically designed to mediate social cohesion (for summary, see Panksepp, Siviy, &

Normansell, 1985). Activation of these systems, triggered by a perceived loss of physical or emotional support from the environment, biases the organism toward behavior patterns that include social signaling (e.g., crying and smiling), orienting toward, and following the primary caregiver. Such behaviors serve to maintain the proximity of the parent–infant dyad and to promote caregiving behaviors, all of which help decrease the threat of species destruction.

Given the extended period of time that children remain dependent upon the primary caregiver, as compared to other mammals, many higher cortical human functions that subserve higher symbolic capacities may well have been naturally selected for via refinements in the developmental timing and growth of preexisting evolutionary capacities (Bates, 1979a)—a process labeled "heterochrony." According to Bates, the symbolic capacity, which evolved phylogenetically, may well be recapitulated ontogenetically as a "new evolutionary product" built from the interaction of available "old parts," of which communicative intent is a member. Normal development of speech and language in children probably proceeds from the infant's repeated attempts (which are initially reflexive, and later more purposive) to procure attention and caregiving from the adult. These goal-directed behaviors, which index social communicative intent, are presumably the impetus for the emergence of normal language (e.g., see Vygotsky, 1962).

In normal children, communicative intent is initially displayed through gestures and nonverbal, vocal utterances, and ultimately through referential (symbolic) language. The present argument is that if the underlying social/emotional intent is diminished or nonexistent at the beginning of life, any language that does emerge will lack a social or emotional referent (Bates, 1979b; Bates, Benigni, Bretherton, Camaioni, & Volterra, 1979; Bates et al., 1975). In other words, if the ability to fully appreciate the social/emotional relevance of other people is disrupted, as may occur in autistic children, the social pragmatics of an emergent language would be severely reduced. As a consequence, autistic children would be impaired in their ability to learn from other people (Schuler, 1980). They would also appear to be selectively impaired in certain aspects of the social domain that require the common sharing of a referent, and they would display a more limited repertoire of communicative functions than normal (Wetherby & Prutting, 1984), which could be attributed to a depressed or nonexistent desire or need to communicate on a social basis. If such a disruption places little ontogenetic demand on the functional development of higher brain regions, then we believe, as do others (Tanguay, Edwards, Buchwald, Schwafel, & Allen, 1982; Wetherby, 1984; Wetherby, Koegel, & Mendel, 1981), that the brain will fail to develop as it should in the service of socially relevant aspects of cognition and communication.

The disruption of subcortical functions could easily account for *many* of the symptoms of autistic children, including the failure of development in secondary cerebral cortical systems, subserving language. According to Rutter and Schopler (1978) and Werry (1972), autistic children appear apathetic and disinterested in their social surroundings and they derive little pleasure from social interaction. Indeed, they seem to lack the initiative to communicate (Maurer & Damasio, 1982). For example, they fail to smile or point as if to show (Bartak, Rutter, & Cox, 1975; Curcio, 1978), they fail to maintain eye contact, and they fail to orient toward others. During infancy, they fail to show appropriate anticipatory behaviors when picked up (Rimland, 1964). Consistent also with such disruptions are the observed disturbances in motility, such as the absence or poverty of movement (akinesia); slow initiation, termination, and alteration of motor patterns (bradykinesia); abnormalities of posture; intermittent dystonia of the extremities; hyper- and hypontia of the trunk and limbs; toe walking; and "emotional" facial paralysis, all of which have been observed in autistic children (Maurer & Damasio, 1982). Similarly, they appear unable to make sense of the world and cannot organize stimuli (Hermelin, 1976), they appear unable to give meaning (thematization) to their experiences (Prizant, 1982), and they fail to habituate (e.g., they perseverate) in speech (echolalia), in their motor behavior (motor flurries) (Ornitz, Guthrie, & Farley, 1978), and in their topics of conversation (Prizant, 1982). In the final analysis, autistic children fail to develop language for its intended purpose (Halliday, 1975).

Possible Neurologic Deficits in Autism

A variety of underlying derangements have been suggested as primary causes of autistic symptomology, and in general, they can be categorized into two camps: one that posits the primary difficulty to be within the realm of faulty information processing (Ornitz & Ritvo, 1968; Rimland, 1964; Rutter, 1968), and one that interprets the difficulty as arising from a constitutional emotional imbalance (Des Lauriers & Carlson, 1969; Kanner, 1943). It is noteworthy that the cognitive emphasis has come largely from experimentally oriented workers, while the emotional interpretation has come more from psychodynamically oriented therapists.

Rimland (1964) pioneered the idea that autism was primarily a cognitive disorder. Ornitz and Ritvo (1968) theorized that the defect in autism was due to a dysfunction of a homeostatic regulatory mechanism, which governs the constancy of perception. They claimed that autistic children suffer "perceptual inconstancy" in which sensations are dampened and amplified to abnormal degrees, resulting in an under- and overloading of neural activity. They believe also that this vascillation accounts for the autistic insistence upon sameness, as well as the apparent heightened sensitivity in one or more of their sensory modalities, that they seem to experience on certain occasions. Although these authors never specified which homeostatic mechanism was disrupted, their model can be well explained by a theory that posits a disruption in a primary emotional/motivational system as originally posited by Kanner (1943).

Little empirical evidence exists to draw any definitive statements regarding the nature or focus of a neurophysiological dysfunction in autism. Several investigators have attempted to account for the behavioral hyperactivity in autistic children by postulating maturational immaturity in primary and/or secondary sensory systems (Hermelin & O'Connor, 1968; Hutt, Hutt, Lee, & Ounsted, 1964). For example, it seems quite likely that a developmental delay, manifested as prolonged auditory transmission time (Fein, Skoff, & Mirsky, 1981; Rosenblum et al., 1980; Sohmer & Student, 1978; Student & Sohmer, 1978; Tanguay et al., 1982), or smaller event-related wave amplitudes (Courchesne, Lincoln, Kilman, & Galambos, 1985), as well as suppressed vestibular functioning (Freeman, Frankel, & Ritvo, 1976; Ornitz, 1974; Ritvo et al., 1969), may well contribute to deficits in forebrain sensory and cross-modality integration (DeMyer, Hingtgen, & Jackson, 1981). Such deficits could then conceivably result in disrupted language and cognition (Tanguay et al., 1982), an impaired ability to perceive environmental relationships, a failure to habituate, and the disruption and/or exaggeration of gross motor display (DeMyer et al., 1981).

Additional brain areas implicated in the etiology of autism include the brainstem reticular formation (Hutt et al., 1964; Rimland, 1964), the nucleus of the tractus solitarius of the dorsal brainstem (MacCulloch & Williams, 1971), the inferior colliculi (Simon, 1975), the mesial frontal and temporal lobes, including the amygdala (Hetzler & Griffin, 1981), and the thalamus and basal ganglia (Damasio & Maurer, 1978; Maurer & Damasio, 1982). The cerebral cortex itself has also been implicated (Wetherby et al., 1981), especially the left hemisphere (Blackstock, 1978), but such higher deficits may also be explicated by lower dysfunctions (Fein, Humes, Kaplan, Lucci, & Waterhouse, 1984).

The only established anatomical brain abnormality that could characterize some autistic children is provided by evidence of temporal horn enlargement in a region where the hippocampus typically bulges into the inferior horn of the lateral ventricle (Hauser, DeLong, & Rosman, 1975). Although such a disorder may exist in only 20% of children diagnosed as autistic, these authors reported that the abnormality was bilateral in most cases, but always present in the left hemisphere. The important point to be made here is that the disruption appears in an area of the brain associated with the higher organization of emotional processes (Gray, 1982). A disturbance of the hippocampus could easily explain the unusual persistence of behavior and apparent lack of satiation exhibited by autistic children. Just as in the hippocampal preparation, autistic children seem to have difficulty shifting from one idea to the next (Duchan & Palermo, 1982).

Such anatomical considerations are scientifically provocative, yet from a therapeutic perspective it may be more appropriate to (1) search for neurochemical disturbances that could explain most, if not all, of the major symptoms of autism and (2) search for a developmental disruption in a neurochemical system that may be common to many, if not all, of the subcortical anatomical structures previously implicated by others as possible sites of neural imbalance in this population.

POSSIBLE NEUROCHEMICAL DYSFUNCTIONS IN AUTISM

Serotonin and Autism

The major current neurochemical theory of autism is premised on the observation, in a subgroup of autistic children (approximately 40%), of abnormally elevated blood levels of serotonin (Ritvo, Rabin, Yuwiler, Freeman, & Geller, 1978; Ritvo et al., 1970). Ritvo, and Geller and associates (Geller et al., 1982; Ritvo et al., 1983) demonstrated that lowered blood concentrations of serotonin, which were induced by the administration of the anorexigenic drug fenfluramine, known to produce long-lasting but reversible decreases in brain serotonin in animals (Clineschmidt et al., 1978), was accompanied by significant improvements (from predrug baseline performance) in aberrant motor, social, affective, sensory, object use, and speech/language behavior, in three 3-year-old autistic children. It is noteworthy that the greatest improvements were made in the areas of social and visual curiosity (measured by eye contact and response to affection) while the smallest improvements were made in the area of speech and language. Fenfluramine has been shown to be therapeutic in about 25% of the autistic children tested to date.

The findings of serotonin receptor antibodies in some autistic children is another provocative line of evidence supporting an indoleamine hypothesis of autism (Todd & Ciaranello, 1985). Unfortunately, the serotonin hypothesis of autism remains without a coherent psychological foundation. Furthermore, while fenfluramine reduces autistic hyperactivity, its therapeutic benefit may be the result of an indirect reduction in arousal in those autistic children who are overactive, thus rendering them more accessible to behavioral intervention strategies (August et al., 1985). Accordingly, we herein discuss an alternative neuromodulatory system (brain opioids), the disruption of which could produce maturational immaturity and conceivably render a young organism emotionally indifferent to social stimuli.

Brain Opioid Systems and the Development of Social Behavior

Although there is now little doubt that endogenous opioid systems (see Table 1) control responsivity to pain (see Jessell, 1983), it has become increasingly clear that many other psychobehavioral processes are also under the control of opioid systems (for a review see Goodman, Fricker, & Snyder, 1983; Malick & Bell, 1982). Opioid systems (comprising at least three distinct families—see Table 1 and Dores *et al.*, 1984) exhibit a widespread distribution throughout the brain. Psychological effects produced by opioids strongly implicate them as modulators of emotional/motivational states (Barchas, Akil, Elliott, Holman, & Watson, 1978; Panksepp, Herman, & Vilberg, 1978; Panksepp, Vilberg, Bean, Coy, & Kastin, 1978), and they appear to be located in several strategic areas of the brain that are believed to integrate sensation with affect (Watson, Akil, Sullivan, & Barchas, 1977). Further, considerable evidence indicates the existence of a close functional relationship between endogenous opioid and serotonergic systems in the brain (e.g., Akil & Mayer, 1972; Samanin, Ghezzi, Mauron, & Valzelli, 1973). It is well known, for instance, that serotonin pathways in the brain modulate both morphine and enkephalin analgesia (e.g., Lee, Sewell, & Spencer, 1979; Samanin *et al.*, 1973).

From an evolutionary perspective, higher-order behavioral processes, such as the capacity for social attachment, may have arisen from existing neural systems that mediate pain, thus helping decrease the incidence of destruction to members of a species. In other words, primitive brain systems devoted to *individual* survival may be phylogenetic precursors to higher systems mediating *species* survival. To the extent that language development serves the same survival function, the location of opioid systems in the brain can provide a substrate by which emotions, as well as cognitions, may be directly influenced. Indeed, all brain areas that have been suggested to be incompletely developed or dysfunctioning in the autistic child have high concentrations of opioids (for a recent summary of opioid anatomy, see Khachaturian, Lewis, Schafer, & Watson, 1985).

Brain Opioids and Autism

As discussed below, symptoms of early childhood autism may result from excessive brain opioid activity, and this possibility is distinguished by a practical medical test of adequacy—i.e., opiate antagonist therapy with the opiate receptor blocker naloxone (Narcan) or the longer-acting orally effective antagonist naltrexone (Trexan). At least some of the physiologic deviations that characterize autism may be initiated during gestation (Ciaranello *et al.*, 1982; Piggott, 1979). From the present perspective, autism could reflect the failure of certain cleavage enzymes to appear, oversaturating the neonatal brain with powerful opioids, such as B-endorphin, leaving the brain and other organs of the developing child at earlier stages of development. For example, autistic children have often been reported to be cuter (Koegel, Egel, & Dunlap, 1980) and shorter (Campbell *et al.*, 1980) than normal, and have a variety of physical abnormalities suggestive of neoteny (Coleman, 1976).

Recent evidence indicates that endogenous opioids control developmental processes (Zagon & McLaughlin, 1978; Zagon, McLaughlin, Weaver, & Zagon, 1982), and chronic treatment with opiate antagonists promotes physical and social development (Najam, 1980; Najam & Panksepp, in press; Zagon & McLaughlin, 1984). Also, early exposure of young organisms to hypothalamic-pituitary-tropic hormones, which are cleaved from the same prohormone precursor (proopiomelanocortin) has a permanent effect on later development

Table 1. Summary of Brain Opioid Systems[a]

Opioid family	Precursor molecule	Endogenous ligands	Receptor type	Exogenous antagonist	Endogenous antagonist (putative)[b]
Endorphins	Pro-opiomelanocortin	B-Endorphin	mu	naloxone (Narcan) naltrexone (Trexan)	α-MSH MIF-1 FMRFamide
Enkephalins	Pro-enkephalin A	met-enkephalin leu-enkephalin	mu and delta	diprenorphine ICI 174864	?
Dynorphins	Pro-enkephalin B	dynorphin-A	kappa	Mr 2266 Mr 1452	?

[a]At present, only the mu receptor system is implicated in autism.

[b]α-MSH = α-melanocyte stimulating hormone, MIF-1 = melanocyte stimulating hormone inhibitory factor, FMRF amide = Phe-Met-Arg-Phe-NH$_2$.

and behavior. For instance, neonatal administration of α-MSH/ACTH 4-9 peptide fragments can produce lifelong enhancement of learning and memory (Champney, Sahley, & Sandman, 1976). On the other hand, prenatal exposure of rats to high levels of B-endorphin leads to profound physical and cognitive impairment, as well as delayed development (see Sandman & Kastin, 1981). Also, early neonatal exposure to B-endorphin permanently alters receptor binding affinity, leading to marked elevations in pain thresholds (Sandman et al., 1979), a characteristic of some autistic children. Interestingly enough, centrally administered B-endorphin produces a marked attenuation of the P1 component of the auditory evoked potential, while MSH/ACTH 4-10 not only reverses, but may enhance, the P1 component (Sandman & Kastin, 1981).

In addition to constitutional anomalies that could alter endorphin synthesis, receptor activity, and degradation, excess endorphin levels may also arise from conditions such as hypoxia and acidosis (Wardlaw, Stark, Daniel, & Frantz, 1981) and fetal distress (Gautray, Joliet, Viehl, & Guillemin, 1977). A large number of pre- and perinatal complications, including fetal hypoxia and bleeding, have been associated with childhood autism (see DeMyer et al., 1981, for a review). Interestingly, pretreatment of pregnant rats with naloxone protects fetuses from the retarding effects of experimentally induced hypoxia (Chernick & Craig, 1982).

One direct test of an endorphin hypothesis of autism was recently conducted by Weizman and colleagues (1984), and their measures of blood B-endorphin suggests that autistic children have reduced, rather than elevated, levels of circulating opioids. Unfortunately, this work cannot be clearly interpreted with regard to central levels of opioid tone. Considering that peripheral opioid levels may be reciprocally related to central opioid activity (e.g., the calming and stress-reducing effects of central opioid release would lead to a peripheral reduction of endorphins), Weizman's data may actually suggest high central opioid tone in autistic children. Indeed, reducing brain opioid tone with central injections of naloxone can markedly increase circulating levels of B-endorphin (Levin, Sharp, & Carlson, 1984). Indeed, more recent work measuring CSF opioid levels in autistic children suggests that a certain kind of enkephalin activity is elevated in such children (Gillberg, Terenius, & Lönnerholm, 1985).

Support for an endorphin theory of autism comes from (1) the symptom similarities between autistic children, and young animals treated with very low doses of opioids, and (2) clinical evidence in the mentally retarded suggesting that one of the defining characteristics of childhood autism, stereotypic behavior (Rimland, 1964), as well as self-abusive behavior, may be mediated and maintained by abnormally high levels of B-endorphin (Barron & Sandman, 1983, 1985; Sandman et al., 1983). For instance, autistic children appear insensitive to pain, as evidenced by their self-abusive behavior; they appear less emotional and cry less, except of course when their environment is disrupted; they seem to have a low desire for social companionship and fail to express physical affection; and they evidence an extreme resistance to extinction (Kanner, 1943; Koegel et al., 1980; Rutter, 1978; Werry, 1972).

Similarly, autisticlike symptoms can be produced by pharmacological alteration of opioid tone in experimental animals. Such treatment can (1) reduce pain sensitivity, (2) reduce crying (e.g., Herman & Panksepp, 1978; Newby-Schmidt & Norton, 1981; Panksepp, Bean, Bishop, Vilberg, & Sahley, 1980; Panksepp, Meeker, & Bean, 1980; Panksepp, Vilberg, et al., 1978), (3) reduce the desire for social companionship and diminish clinging behavior (Herman & Panksepp, 1978; Panksepp, Herman, & Vilberg, 1978a; Panksepp, Najam, & Soares, 1979; Plonsky & Freeman, 1982), (4) and evoke a variety of learning abnormalities characterized by extreme resistance to extinction (Panksepp & DeEskinazi, 1980). In animals, these opioid-induced effects are reversed by naloxone administration.

A growing body of clinical evidence indicates that naloxone is effective in alleviating self-injurious and autisticlike stereotypy (Barron & Sandman, 1983, 1985; Herman *et al.*, 1985; Richardson & Zaleski, 1983) as well as promoting interpersonal behaviors (Sandman *et al.*, 1983) in abnormal clinical populations. It has been suggested that stereotypy may prevent the symptoms of narcotic withdrawal in endorphin-addicted organisms, by stimulating the production and release of endogenous opioids. Certain kinds of stereotypy may therefore supply the "fix" for endogenous opioid addiction (Barron & Sandman, 1983).

Although there is no direct evidence for *tolerance* or *dependence* on high levels of endogenously released opioids, prolonged exogenous administration of B-endorphin does produce these two components of drug addiction (Wei & Loh, 1976). Also, it is noteworthy that self-injurious and stereotypic behaviors can occur when exogenous narcotics are withdrawn from addicted animals (Picker, Poling, & Parker, 1979). Additionally, vigorous exercise, which results in increased levels of plasma B-endorphin (Bortz *et al.*, 1981) has been shown to reduce stereotypy in autistic children (Kern, Koegel, & Dunlap, 1984; Kern, Koegel, Dyer, Blew, & Fenton, 1982), suggesting that vigorous exercise may act as an endorphin-releasing substitute for autistic stereotypy.

Of course, the above analysis only points toward one of many possible neurochemical abnormalities that may participate in the syndrome. Indeed, as in the control of pain (Sahley & Berntson, 1979; Samanin *et al.*, 1973), systems subserving social attachment are neither simply nor narrowly represented in the brain (Bishop, Panksepp, & Sahley, 1980; Panksepp, Meeker, & Bean, 1980; Rossi, Sahley, & Panksepp, 1983; Sahley, Panksepp, & Zolovick, 1981; Vilberg, Panksepp, Kastin, & Coy, 1984), and surely other brain systems should be considered as well. (For a more extensive review see Panksepp, 1986; Panksepp *et al.*, 1985).

In summary, high levels of opioid activity have been found in those brain areas that organize both sensory and social experience. An opioid theory of autism has the structural and functional breadth to handle most, if not all, of the symptoms of childhood autism, and it is compatible with the other existing neurochemical hypothesis (i.e., overactive serotonin). Thus, concurrent and/or linked dysfunctions in these systems could precipitate the many physiological and behavioral deficits associated with childhood autism.

Opioid Antagonist Pharmacotherapy of Autism

The opiate receptor antagonists, naloxone (Narcan) and naltrexone (Trexan) are generally safe drugs having no major contraindications. In the absence of narcotics, naloxone exhibits few physiological or psychological effects in adults and does not produce tolerance or cause physical or psychological dependence. Perhaps the major therapeutic shortcomings of Narcan are that it is ineffective when administered orally, and it has a relatively brief time course of biological activity (which apparently does not exceed a few hours in humans). The best available alternative is the long-lasting opiate receptor blocking agent naltrexone (Trexan). This drug is effective orally, it can yield opiate blockade for up to several days with a single administration, and it has just recently been approved for medical use by the FDA (for the purpose of narcotic detoxification).

It has recently come to our attention that Campbell, Small, Perry, Palij, Nobler, Polonsky, and Shore (1985) have conducted naltrexone trials on a 5-year-old autistic boy who exhibited the full syndrome by DSM-III criteria. The child had previously exhibited poor responses to Ritalin, Thorazine, and Mellaril, and had failed to respond to special educational programs. To quote Dr. Magda Campbell's unpublished observation:

> This patient showed a marked decrease of symptoms on naltrexone. . . . The lower doses (0.5 and 1.0 mg/kg per day) had tranquilizing effects and were characterized by decreases in aggressiveness, impulsivity, hyperactivity, and stereotypies. On higher dose (2.0 and 3.0 mg/kg per day) the effects observed were mainly stimulating and involved language and social behaviors: the patient, for the first time, said words (e.g., "mama," "juice," "bye"), vocalized a great deal, and babbled. He also was less withdrawn, made social overtures, and kissed this examiner, several times, upon request.

Opioid-antagonist therapy may be effective only for a subpopulation of autistic children having elevated brain opioid activity, just as it has been shown to be effective in the alleviation of psychotic symptoms such as auditory hallucinations in subpopulations of schizophrenics (Watson, Berger, Akil, Mills, & Barchas, 1978), some of which have been found to have elevated CSF levels of endorphinlike activity (for reviews, see Koob, LeMoal, & Bloom, 1984; Vereby, 1982; Watson, Albala, Berger, & Akil, 1983), although the drug is ineffective in most schizophrenics (see Mueser & Dysken, 1983, for review). If properly combined with clinical intervention in autistic patients, this pharmacotherapeutic approach may reduce or eliminate abnormal stereotypic behaviors, speed physiological development, and stimulate more normal ontogenetic organization of social behavior, as well as subsequent cortical functions subserving language, in autistic children.

CONCLUDING REMARKS

It seems likely that one neurophysiological deficit of autism is the reduced ability of brain emotional systems to mediate social affect and the consequent inability of related cognitive systems to mediate social intent. There is now abundant evidence that brain opioids modulate the activity of such poorly understood circuits (Panksepp, 1981a, 1986; Panksepp *et al.*, 1985). However, identification of new brain circuits, together with their diverse chemistries, is currently proceeding at a remarkable pace. Several new putative neurotransmitter systems are being revealed each year. Hence, there must be a continual winnowing of options to ensure the distillation of credible neurochemical hypotheses of autism.

In the absence of conclusive biological evidence from autistic children, autisticlike symptoms produced and alleviated by brain neurochemical manipulations in experimental animals remains the most reasonable alternative criterion for the credibility of any suggested neurochemical hypothesis. The behavioral symptoms of autism and those that can be produced by opioid administration in animals are remarkably similar (Panksepp, 1979). More importantly, opioid receptor blockade with drugs such as Narcan produces behavioral effects in animals similar to those that would most desirably be released in autistic children—increased vocalizations and increased solicitation of social companionship (Panksepp, 1981a). Although our initial attempt to treat poorly socialized, albeit neurologically sound, kennel dogs with naloxone therapy has yielded no evidence for a long-term therapeutic effect, the social "intent" of these animals increased in the short term (Panksepp, Conner, Forster, Bishop, & Scott, 1983). Whether this "therapeutic" trend can be magnified by more intensive treatment remains to be evaluated. In any event, the parallels between the symptoms of autism and the symptoms exhibited by normal animals treated with opioids, as well as the preliminary clinical evidence summarized herein, are sufficiently compelling to warrant thorough, long-term clinical trials with opiate antagonists, with the aim of halting, reversing, or preventing the further progression of this perplexing developmental brain disorder.

ACKNOWLEDGMENTS

Comments on earlier drafts of this manuscript by Roger J. Ingham, Robert L. Koegel, Maurice I. Mendel, Carol A. Prutting, and Michael P. Rastatter are greatly appreciated.

REFERENCES

Akerly, M. S. (1974). The near-normal autistic adolescent. *Journal of Autism and Childhood Schizophrenia, 4*, 347–356.

Akil, H., & Mayer, D. J. (1972). Antagonism of stimulation-produced analygesia by p-CPA, a serotonin synthesis inhibitor. *Brain Research, 44*, 692–697.

August, G. J., Raz, N., & Baird, T. D. (1985). Brief report: Effects of fenfluramine on behavioral, cognitive, and affective disturbances in autistic children. *Journal of Autism and Developmental Disorders, 15*, 97–107.

Barchas, J. D., Akil, H., Elliott, G., Holman, B., & Watson, S. J. (1978). Behavioral neurochemistry: Neuroregulators and behavioral states. *Science, 200*, 964–973.

Barron, J., & Sandman, C. A. (1983). Relationship of sedative-hypnotic response to self-injurious behavior and stereotypy by mentally retarded clients. *American Journal of Mental Deficiency, 88*, 177–186.

Barron, J., & Sandman, C. A. (1985). Paradoxical excitment to sedative-hypnotics in mentally regarded clients. *American Journal of Mental Deficiency, 90*, 124–129.

Bartak, L., Rutter, M., & Cox, A. (1975). A comparative study of infantile autism and specific developmental receptive language disorder: I. The children. *British Journal of Psychiatry, 126*, 127–145.

Bates, E. (1979a). On the evolution and development of symbols. In E. Bates, T. Benigni, I. Bretherton, L. Camaioni, & V. Volterra (Eds.), *The emergency of symbols: Cognition and communication in infancy.* New York: Academic Press.

Bates, E. (1979b). The biology of symbols: Some concluding thoughts. In E. Bates, T. Benigni, I. Brtherton, L. Camaioni, & V. Volterra (Eds.), *The emergence of symbols: Cognition and communication in infancy.* New York: Academic Press.

Bates, E., Benigni, T., Bretherton, I., Camaioni, L., & Volterra, V. (1979). *The emergence of symbols: Cognition and communication in infancy.* New York: Academic Press.

Bates, E., Camaioni, L., & Volterra, V. (1975). The acquisition of performatives prior to speech. *Merrill-Palmer Quarterly, 21*, 205–226.

Bishop, P., Panksepp, J., & Sahley, T. L. (1980). Opiate effects on social comfort and imprinting. *Society for Neuroscience Abstract, 6*, 105.

Blackstock, E. (1978). Cerebral asymmetry and the development of early infantile autism. *Journal of Autism and Childhood Schizophrenia, 8*, 339–353.

Bortz, W. M., Angivin, P., Mefford, I. N., Boarder, M. R., Noyce, N., & Barchas, J. D. (1981). Catecholamines, dopamine, and endorphin levels during extreme exercise. *New England Journal of Medicine, 305*, 466–467.

Campbell, M., Cohen, I. L., & Anderson, L. T. (1981). Pharmacotherapy for autistic children: A summary of research. *Canadian Journal of Psychiatry, 26*, 265–273.

Campbell, M., Petti, T. A., Green, W. H., Cohen, I. L., Genieser, N. B., & David, R. (1980). Some physical parameters of young autistic children. *Journal of the American Academy of Childhood Psychiatry, 19,* 193–212.

Campbell, M., Small, A. M., Perry, R., Palij, M., Nobler, M., Polonsky, B., & Shore, H. (1985, July). *Naltrexone in autistic children.* Paper presented at the 17th Annual Meeting and Conference of the National Society of Children and Adults with Autism, Autism Research Symposium, Los Angeles, CA.

Champney, T. F., Sahley, T. L., & Sandman, C. A. (1976). Effects of neonatal cerebral ventricular injection of ACTH 4-9 and subsequent adult injections on learning in male and female albino rats. *Pharmacology Biochemistry and Behavior, 5* (Suppl. 1, *The Neuropeptides*), 3–9.

Chernick, V., & Craig, R. J. (1982). Naloxone reverses neonatal depression caused by fetal asphyxia. *Science, 216,* 1252–1253.

Ciaranello, R. D., Vandenberg, S. R., & Anders, T. F. (1982). Intrinsic and extrinsic determinants of neuronal development: Relations to infantile autism. *Journal of Autism and Developmental Disorders, 12,* 115–145.

Clineschmidt, B. V., Zacchei, A. G., Totaro, J. A., Pflueger, A. B., McGuffin, J. C., & Wishonski, T. I. (1978). Fenfluramine and brain serotonin. *Annuals of the New York Academy of Sciences, 305,* 221–241.

Cohen, I. L., Campbell, M., & Posner, D. (1980). A study of haloperidol in young autistic children: A within subjects design using objective rating scales. *Psychopharmacological Bulletin, 16*(3), 63–65.

Coleman, M. (1976). *The autistic syndromes.* New York: Elsevier.

Courchesne, E., Lincoln, A. J., Kilman, B. A., & Galambos, R. (1985). Event-related brain potential correlates of the processing of novel visual and auditory information. *Journal of Autism and Developmental Disorders, 15,* 55–76.

Curcio, F. (1978). Sensorimotor functioning and communication in mute autistic children. *Journal of Autism and Childhood Schizophrenia, 8,* 281–292.

Damasio, A., & Maurer, R. (1978). A neurological model for childhood autism. *Archives of Neurology, 35,* 777–786.

DeMyer, M. K., Hingtgen, J. N., & Jackson, R. K. (1981). Infantile autism reviewed: A decade of research. *Schizophrenia Bulletin, 7,* 388–451.

Des Lauriers, A. M., & Carlson, C. F. (1969). *Your child is asleep: Early infantile autism.* Homewood, IL: Dorsey Press.

Dores, R. B., Akil, H., & Watson, S. J. (1984). Strategies for studying opioid peptide regulation at the gene, measure and protein levels. *Peptides 5* (Suppl. 1), 9–17.

Duchan, J. F., & Palermo, J. (1982). How autistic children view the world. *Topics in language disorders: Communication problems of autistic children: The role of context, 3*(1), 10–15.

Fein, D., Humes, M., Kaplan, E., Lucci, D., & Waterhouse, L. (1984). The question of left hemisphere dysfunction in infantile autism. *Psychological Bulletin, 95,* 258–281.

Fein, D., Skoff, B., & Mirsky, A. F. (1981). Clinical correlates of brainstem dysfunction in autistic children. *Journal of Autism and Developmental Disorders, 11,* 303–315.

Freeman, B. J., Frankel, F., & Ritvo, E. R. (1976). The effects of response-contingent vestibular stimulation on the behavior of autistic and related children. *Journal of Autism and Childhood Schizophrenia, 6,* 353.

Gautray, J. P., Joliet, A., Viehl, J. P., & Guillemin, R. (1977). Presence of immunoassayable B-endorphin on human amniotic fluid: Elevation in cases of fetal distress. *American Journal of Obstetrics and Gynecology, 129,* 211–212.

Geller, E., Ritvo, E., Freeman, B. J., & Yuwiler, A. (1982). Preliminary observations on the effect of fenfluramine on blood serotonin and symptoms in three autistic boys. *New England Journal of Medicine, 307,* 165–169.

Gillberg, C., Terenius, L., & Lönnerholm, G. (1985). Endorphin activity in childhood psychosis. *Archives of General Psychiatry, 42,* 780–783.

Goodman, R. R., Fricker, L. D., & Snyder, S. H. (1983). Enkephalins. In D. T. Krieger, M. J., Brownstein & J. B. Martin (Eds.), *Brain peptides* (pp. 827–849). New York: Wiley-Interscience.

Gray, J. A. (1982). *The neuropsychology of anxiety: An enquiry into the functions of the septo-hippocampal system.* Oxford: Oxford University Press.

Halliday, M. (1975). Learning how to mean. In E. Lenneberg & E. Lenneberg (Eds.), *Foundations of language development: A multidisciplinary approach.* New York: Academic Press.

Hauser, S., DeLong, G., & Rosman, N. (1975). Pneumographic findings in the infantile autism syndrome: A correlation with temporal lobe disease. *Brain, 98,* 667–688.

Herman, B. H., Hammock, M. K., Egan, J., Feinstein, C., Chatoor, I., Boeckx, R., Zelnick, N., Jack, R., & Rosenquist, J. (1985). Naltrexone induces dose-dependent decreases in self-injurious behavior. *Neuroscience Abstracts, 11,* 468.

Herman, B. H., & Panksepp, J. (1978). Effects of morphine and naloxone on separation distress and approach attachment: Evidence for opiate medication of social affect. *Pharmacology Biochemistry and Behavior, 9,* 213–220.

Hermelin, B. (1976). Coding and the sense modality. In L. Wing (Ed.), *Early childhood autism: Clinical educational, and social aspects* (pp. 135–168). New York: Pergamon Press.

Hermelin, B., & O'Connor, N. (1968). Measures of the occipital alpha rhythm in normal, subnormal, and autistic children. *British Journal of Psychiatry, 114,* 603–610.

Hetzler, B. E., & Griffin, J. L. (1981). Infantile autism and the temporal lobe of the brain. *Journal of Autism and Developmental Disorders, 11,* 317–330.

Hutt, C., Hutt, S., Lee, D., & Ounsted, C. (1964). Arousal and childhood autism. *Nature, 204,* 908.

Jessell, T. M. (1983). Nociception. In D. T. Krieger, M. J. Brownstein, & J. B. Martin (Eds.), *Brain peptides* (pp. 315–332). New York: Wiley-Interscience.

Kalat, J. W. (1978). Letter to the editor: Speculations on similarities between autism and opiate addiction. *Journal of Autism and Childhood Schizophrenia, 8,* 477–479.

Kanner, L. (1943). Autistic disturbances of affective content. *Nervous Child, 2,* 217–250.

Kern, L., Koegel, R. L., & Dunlap, G. (1984). The influence of vigorous versus mild exercise on autistic stereotyped behaviors. *Journal of Autism and Developmental Disorders, 14,* 57–67.

Kern, L., Koegel, R. L., Dyer, K., Blew, P. A., & Fenton, L. R. (1982). The effects of physical exercise on self-stimulation and appropriate responding in autistic children. *Journal of Autism and Developmental Disorders, 12,* 399–419.

Khachaturian, H., Lewis, M. E., Schafer, M. K. M., & Watson, S. J. (1985). Anatomy of the CNS opioid systems. *Trends in Neurosciences, 8,* 111–119.

Koegel, R. L., Egel, A. L., & Dunlap, G. (1980). Learning characteristics of autistic children. In W. Sailor, B. Wilcox, & L. Brown (Eds.), *Methods of instruction with severely handicapped students.* Baltimore: Brookes.

Koob, G., LeMoal, M., & Bloom, F. E. (1984). The role of endorphins in neurobiology, behavior and psychiatric disorders. In C. B. Nemeroff & A. J. Dunn (Eds.), *Peptides, hormones and behavior.* Jamaica: NY: Spectrum.

Kuhar, M. J., Pert, C. B., & Snyder, S. H. (1973). Regional distribution of opiate receptor binding in monkey and human brain. *Nature, 245,* 447–450.

Lee, R. L., Sewell, R. D., & Spencer, P. S. (1979). Antinociceptive activity of D-ala2-D-leu5-enkephalin (BW180C) in the rat after modification to central 5-hydroxytryptamine function. *Neuropharmacology, 18,* 711–717.

Lelord, G., Muh, J. P., Barthelemy, C., Martineau, Garreau, B., & Callaway, E. (1981). Effects of pyridoxine and magnesium on autistic symptoms—Initial observations. *Journal of Autism and Developmental Disorders, 11,* 219–230.

Levin, E. R., Sharp, B., & Carlson, H. E. (1984). Studies of naloxone-induced secretion of B-endorphin immunoactivity in dogs. *Life Sciences, 35,* 1535–1545.

Links, P. S., Stockwell, M., Abichandani, F., & Simeon, J. (1980). Minor physical anomalies in childhood autism. Part I. Their relationship to pre- and perinatal complications. *Journal of Autism and Developmental Disorders, 10,* 273–286.

MacCulloch, M., & Williams, C. (1971). On the nature of infantile autism. *Acta Psychiatrica Scandinavica, 47,* 295–314.

Malick, J. B., & Bell, R. M. S. (1982). *Endorphins: Chemistry, physiology, pharmacology and clinical relevance.* New York: Marcel Dekker.

Maurer, R. G., & Damasio, A. R. (1982). Childhood autism from the point of behavioral neurology. *Journal of Autism and Developmental Disorders, 12,* 195–205.

Mueser, K. T., & Dysken, M. W. (1983). Narcotic antagonists in schizophrenia. *Schizophrenia Bulletin, 9,* 213–225.

Najam, N. (1980). *A study of the effects of early postnatal exposure to opiate agonists and antagonists on motor and social behaviors of the young rat.* Unpublished doctoral dissertation, Bowling Green State University.

Najam, N., & Panksepp, J. (in press). Effect of chronic neonatal morphine and naloxone on sensorimotor and social development in young rats. *Pharmacology, Biochemistry and Behavior.*

Newby-Schmidt, M. D., & Norton, S. (1981). Development of opiate tolerance in the chick embryo. *Pharmacology, Biochemistry and Behavior, 15,* 773–778.

Ornitz, E. (1974). The modulation of sensory input and motor output in autistic children. *Journal of Autism and Childhood Schizophrenia, 4,* 197–215.

Ornitz, E., Guthrie, D., & Farley, A. (1978). The early symptoms of childhood autism. In G. Serban (Ed.), *Cognitive defects in the development of mental illness.* New York: Brunner/Mazel.

Ornitz, E., & Ritvo, E. (1968). Perceptual inconstancy in the syndrome of early infantile autism and its variants. *Archives of General Psychiatry, 18,* 76–98.

Panksepp, J. (1979). A neurochemical theory of autism. *Trends in Neuroscience, 2,* 174–177.

Panksepp, J. (1981a). Brain opioids—A neurochemical substrate for narcotic and social dependence. In S. J. Cooper (Ed.), *Theory in psychopharmacology* (Vol. 1). London: Academic Press.

Panksepp, J. (1981b). Hypothalamic integration of behavior. In *Handbook of the hypothalamus, Vol. III-Part B, Behavioral studies of the hypothalamus.* New York: Marcel Dekker.

Panksepp, J. (1982). Toward a general psychobiological theory of emotions. *Behavioral and Brain Sciences, 5*(3). New York: Cambridge University Press.

Panksepp, J. (1986). The psychobiology of prosocial behaviors: Separation distress, play and altruism. In C. Zahn-Waxler (Ed.), *Social and biological origins of altruism and aggression.* New York: Cambridge University Press.

Panksepp, J., Bean, J. J., Bishop, P., Vilberg, T., & Sahley, T. L. (1980). Opioid blockade and social comfort in chicks. *Pharmacology, Biochemistry and Behavior, 13,* 673–683.

Panksepp, J., Conner, R., Forster, P. K., Bishop, P., & Scott, J. P. (1983). Opioid effects on social behavior of kennel dogs. *Applied Animal Ethology, 10,* 63–74.

Panksepp, J., & DeEskinazi, F. G. (1980). Opiates and homing. *Journal of Comparative and Physiological Psychology, 94,* 650–663.

Panksepp, J., Herman, B., & Vilberg, T. (1978). An opiate excess model of autism. *Neuroscience Abstract, 4,* 500.

Panksepp, J., Herman, B., Vilberg, T., Bishop, P., & DeEskinazi, F. G. (1980). Endogenous opioids and social behavior. *Neuroscience and Biobehavioral Reviews, 4,* 473–487.

Panksepp, J., Meeker, R., & Bean, N. J. (1980). The neurochemical control of crying. *Pharmacology, Biochemistry and Behavior, 12,* 437–443.

Panksepp, J., Najam, N., & Soares, F. (1979). Morphine reduces social cohesion in rats. *Pharmacology, Biochemistry and Behavior, 11,* 131–134.

Panksepp, J., Siviy, S. M., & Normansell, L. A. (1985). Brain opioids and social emotions. In M. Reite & T. Fields (Eds.), *The psychobiology of attachment.* New York: Academic Press.

Panksepp, J., Vilberg, T., Bean, N. J., Coy, D. H., & Kastin, A. J. (1978). Reductions of distress vocalizations in chicks by opiate-like peptides. *Brain Research Bulletin, 3,* 663–667.

Picker, M., Poling, A., & Parker, A. (1979). A review of children's self-injurious behavior. *Psychological Record, 29,* 435–452.

Piggott, L. R. (1979). Overview of selected basic research in autism. *Journal of Autism and Developmental Disorders, 9,* 199–218.

Plonsky, M., & Freeman, P. R. (1982). The effects of methadone on the social behavior and activity of the rat. *Pharmacology, Biochemistry and Behavior, 16,* 569–571.

Prizant, B. M. (1982). Gestalt language and gestalt processing in autism. *Topics in Language Disorders, 3,* 16–23.

Richardson, J. S., & Zaleski, W. A. (1983). Naloxone and self-mutilation. *Biological Psychiatry, 18,* 99–101.

Rimland, B. (1964). *Infantile autism.* New York: Appleton-Century-Crofts.

Rimland, B. (1978). Inside the mind of an autistic savant. *Psychology Today, 12,* 68–80.

Rimland, B., Callaway, E., & Dreyfus, P. (1978). The effects of high doses of vitamin B6 of autistic children: A double-blind crossover study. *American Journal of Psychiatry, 135,* 472–475.

Ritvo, E. O., Freeman, B. J., Geller, E., & Yuwiler, A. (1983). Effects of fenfluramine on 14 autistic outpatients. *Journal of the American Academy of Child Psychiatry, 17,* 565–576.

Ritvo, E. R., Ornitz, E. M., Eviatar, A., Markham, C. H., Crown, M. B., & Mason, A. (1969). Decreased postrotary nystagmus in early infantile autism. *Neurology, 19,* 653.

Ritvo, E. R., Rabin, K., Yuwiler, A., Freeman, B. J., & Geller, E. (1978). Biochemical and hematologic studies: A critical review. In M. Rutter & E. Schopler (Eds.), *Autism: A reappraisal of concepts and treatment* (pp. 163–183). New York: Plenum Press.

Ritvo, E. R., Yuwiler, A., Geller, E., Ornitz, E. M., Saeger, K., & Plotkin, S. (1970). Increased blood serotonin and platelets in early infantile autism. *Archives of General Psychiatry, 23,* 566–572.

Rosenblum, S. M., Arick, J. R., Krug, D. A., Stubbs, E. G., Young, N. B., & Pelson, R. O. (1980). Auditory brainstem evoked responses in autistic children. *Journal of Autism and Developmental Disorders, 10,* 215–225.

Rossi, J., Sahley, T. L., & Panksepp, J. (1983). The role of brain norepinephrine in clonidine suppression of isolation-induced distress in the domestic chick. *Psychopharmacology, 79,* 338–342.

Rutter, M. (1968). Concepts of autism: A review of research. *Journal of Child Psychology and Psychiatry, 9,* 1–25.

Rutter, M. (1978). Diagnosis and definition of childhood autism. *Journal of Autism and Childhood Schizophrenia, 8,* 139–161.

Rutter, M., & Schopler, E. (Eds.). (1978). *Autism: A reappraisal of concepts and treatment,* New York: Plenum Press.

Sahley, T. L., & Berntson, G. G. (1979). Antinociceptive effects of central and systemic administrations of nicotine in the rat. *Psychopharmacology, 65,* 279–283.

Sahley, T. L., Panksepp, J., & Zolovick, A. J. (1981). Cholinergic modulation of separation distress in the domestic chick. *European Journal of Pharmacology, 72,* 261–264.

Samanin, R., Ghezzi, D., Mauron, C., & Valzelli, L. (1973). Effect of midbrain raphe lesion on the antinociceptive action of morphine and other analgesics in rats. *Psychopharmacologia (Berlin), 33,* 365–368.

Sandman, C. A., Data, P. C., Barron, J., Hoehler, F. K., Williams, C., & Swanson, J. M. (1983). Naloxone attenuates self-abusive behavior in developmentally disabled clients. *Applied Research in Mental Retardation, 4,* 5–11.

Sandman, C. A., & Kastin, A. J. (1981). The influence of fragments of the LPH chains on learning, memory, and attention in animals and man. *Pharmacological Therapy, 13,* 39–60.

Sandman, C. A., McGivern, R. F., Berka, C., Walker, J. M., Coy, D. H., & Kastin, A. J. (1979). Neonatal administration of B-endorphine produces "chronic" insensitivity to thermal stimuli. *Life Sciences, 25,* 1755–1760.

Schopler, E., & Mesibov, G. B. (Eds.). (1985). *Communication problems in autism.* New York: Plenum Press.

Schuler, A. L. (1980). Aspects of communication. In W. Fay & A. Schuler, *Emerging language in autistic children* (pp. 87–113). Baltimore: University Park Press.

Scott, J. P. (1974). Effects of psychotropic drugs on separation distress in dogs. *Neuropsychopharmacology, Proceedings of the IX Congress of the CINP*. Paris: Excerpta Medica Amsterdam.

Simon, N. (1975). Echolalic speech in childhood autism: Considerations of possible underlying loci of brain damage. *Archives of General Psychiatry, 32*, 1439–1446.

Sohmer, H., & Student, M. (1978). Auditory nerve and brain-stem evoked responses in normal, autistic, minimal brain dysfunction and psycho-motor retarded children. *Electroencephalography and Clinical Neurophysiology, 44*, 380–388.

Student, M., & Sohmer, H. (1978). Evidence from auditory nerve and brainstem evoked responses for an organic brain lesion in childhood with autistic traits. *Journal of Autism and Childhood Schizophrenia, 8*, 13–20.

Tanguay, P. E., Edwards, R. M., Buchwald, J., Schwafel, J., & Allen, V. (1982). Auditory brainstem evoked responses in autistic children. *Archives of General Psychiatry, 39*, 174–180.

Todd, R. D., & Ciaranello, R. D. (1985). Demonstration of inter- and intra species differences in serotonin binding sites by antibodies from autistic children. *Proceedings of the National Academy of Sciences, U.S.A., 82*, 612–616.

Verebey, K. (Ed.). (1982). Opioids in mental illness: Theories, clinical observations, and treatment possibilities. *Annals of the New York Academy of Sciences, 398*.

Vilberg, T. R., Panksepp, J., Kastin, A. J., & Coy, D. C. (1984). The pharmacology of endorphin modulation of chick distress vocalization. *Peptides, 5*, 823–827.

Vygotsky, T. (1962). *Thought and language*, Cambridge, MA: MIT Press.

Wardlaw, S. L., Stark, R. I., Daniel, S., & Frantz, A. F. (1981). Effects of hypoxia on B-lipotropin release in fetal, newborn and maternal sheep. *Endocrinology, 108*, 1710–1715.

Watson, S. J., Akil, H., Sullivan, S. O., & Barchas, J. D. (1977). Immunocytochemical localization of methionine enkephalin: Preliminary observations. *Life Sciences, 21*, 733–738.

Watson, S. J., Albala, A. A., Berger, P., & Akil, H. (1983). Peptides and psychiatry. In D. T. Krieger, M. J. Brownstein, & J. B. Martin (Eds.), *Brain peptides*. New York: Wiley-Interscience

Watson, S. J., Berger, P. A., Akil, H., Mills, M. J., & Barchas, J. P. (1978). Effect of naloxone on schizophrenia: Reduction in hallucinations in a subpopulation of subjects. *Science, 201*, 73–75.

Wei, E., & Loh, H. (1976). Physical dependence of opiate-like peptides. *Science, 193*, 1242–1263.

Weizman, R., Weizman, A., Tyano, S., Szekely, G., Weissman, B. A., & Sarne, Y. (1984). Humoral-endorphin blood levels in autistic schizophrenic and healthy subjects. *Psychopharmacology, 82*, 368–370.

Werry, J. S. (1972). Childhood psychosis. In H. Quay & J. Werry (Eds.), *Psychopathological disorders of childhood*. New York: Wiley.

Wetherby, A. M. (1984). Possible neurological breakdown in autistic children. *Topics in Language Disorders, 4* (Suppl. 32), 19–33.

Wetherby, A. M., Koegel, R. L., & Mendel, M. (1981). Central auditory nervous system dysfunction in echolalic autistic individuals. *Journal of Speech and Hearing Research, 24*, 420–429.

Wetherby, A. M., & Prutting, C. A. (1984). Communicative, cognitive and social development in autistic children. *Journal of Speech and Hearing Research, 27*, 364–377.

Wollner, S. G. (1983). Communicating intentions: How well do language-impaired children do? *Topics in Language Disorders: Pragmatics in Language Disordered Children, 4*(1), 1–14.

Zagon, I. S., & McLaughlin, P. J. (1978). Perinatal methadone exposure and its influence on the behavioral ontogeny of rats. *Pharmacology, Biochemistry and Behavior, 9*, 665.

Zagon, I. S., & McLaughlin, P. J. (1984). Naltrexone modulates body and brain development in rats: A role for endogenous opioid systems in growth. *Life Sciences, 35*, 2057–2064.

Zagon, I. S., McLaughlin, P. J., Weaver, D. J., & Zagon, E. (1982). Opiate endorphins and the developing organism: A comprehensive bibliography. *Neuroscience and Biobehavioral Reviews, 6*.

The Medical Treatment of Autistic People

Problems and Side Effects

THOMAS GUALTIERI, RANDALL W. EVANS, and DEBRA R. PATTERSON

The proper study of risks attendant on a particular medical treatment, or on a class of treatments, can only be made if proper deference is paid to the potential benefits that may reasonably be expected to accrue. In considering the risks and side effects of medical treatments that are brought to bear in the management of autistic persons, therefore, there is a fatal irony since little direct benefit is known to derive from *any* somatic treatment. There is no rational chemotherapy for autism. There is no medical intervention that can reverse or undo the physiological basis of the disorder. Indeed, the disorder is not known to be characterized by any specific pathophysiologic defect. From the biologist's perspective, autism is an impossible concept, one that embraces a wide range of individual deficits and individual patients who differ widely in clinical presentation (Wing, 1969), developmental level, etiology, associated disorders, and prognosis. A generation of research has failed to uncover any single biological mechanism by dint of which such diversity might be reconciled. In the face of such ambiguity, the hope for a specific biological "treatment" is vain.

In fact, autistic people are treated with medication not by virtue of their autistic diagnosis but rather for the associated problems that may develop during the course of their lives. Treatment is never "specific," in an etiopathogenic sense, but symptomatic. There is no medical treatment for autism; there are treatments for the seizure disorders that afflict a substantial number of autistic people, and there are also medical treatments that can mitigate, at least for a while, many of the destructive behaviors that they develop. When these treatments are properly used there is, in all probability, no greater toxicity for autistic persons than for other patients who are treated for seizures or behavior disorders.

THOMAS GUALTIERI • Department of Psychiatry, and RANDALL W. EVANS and DEBRA R. PATTERSON • Biological Sciences Research Center, University of North Carolina, Chapel Hill, North Carolina 27514.

The first principle of medical treatment for autistic persons is taken from the biologist's perspective: the biological heterogeneity of the disorder, and the absence of any current treatment that is rationally derived from an established biological deficit. A corollary to this principle is taken from the physician's perspective: All medical treatments for autistic persons are symptomatic and are aimed at reducing seizures or undesirable behaviors or attributes. (Proponents of "megavitamin" treatment or of fenfluramine might take exception to this corollary since they have asserted that these treatments may actually confer a surge of developmental acceleration in some patients, but their claims are probably extravagant and they have not been substantiated.)

An additional observation on the state of current neuropsychiatric care for autistic people in particular and for developmentally handicapped people in general is the relative unavailability of experienced and sensitive physicians. The neuropsychiatric problems of these patients occupy a very low status in the training priorities of pediatricians, neurologists, and psychiatrists, at least in the United States. As a result, anticonvulsant and psychophar- macologic regimes are often dealt with clumsily, to the dismay of families and physicians alike. The careful integration of a medical treatment regime into a comprehensive habilitative program, with good communication between physician and other caregivers, is the rare exception and not the rule. This deficit is a national phenomenon. Advances in modern neuropsychiatry have been dramatic over the last 25 years, but the fruits of this advance have hardly been tasted by the vast population of developmentally handicapped people.

This relative lack of experienced neuropsychiatic care has as a necessary consequence not only dismay among caregivers but also some serious medical problems for patients. Anticonvulsant and psychopharmacologic drugs and even vitamin combinations are not inherently dangerous, if they are managed correctly. But serious problems may arise with unnecessary polypharmacy, excessive doses, failure to monitor treatment, and failure to integrate medical treatment into the patient's overall treatment program.

Parental dismay over the marginal quality of traditional medical services and treatments has led to an understandable receptiveness to new and unorthodox treatments, such as "megavitamins" and fenfluramine. The unique clinical picture of the autistic child has always fed vain hopes of a single, dramatic "cure." One's willingness to entertain fantasies of "doubling the IQ" of mentally retarded (Harrell, Capp, Davis, Peerless, & Ravitz, 1981) and autistic persons (Ritvo, 1985), and the disappointment that attends such fantasies, is an ironic consequence, a side effect if you will, of the failure of conventional medical treatments for autistic people.

With respect to specific side effects of medical treatments—conventional and experimental—the ensuing discussion will cover four topics: neuroleptic or antipsychotic drugs, fenfluramine, "megavitamins," and anticonvulsant drugs.

NEUROLEPTIC DRUGS

Neuroleptics are the most commonly prescribed psychotropics to autistic children (Rimland, 1977). Although autism is a relatively uncommon disorder, the existence of specialized referral centers for autistic children—for example, at New York University— has permitted the development of a solid body of psychopharmacologic research on this kind of treatment. Neuroleptics (especially haloperidol in low doses) have been shown to reduce symptoms of stereotypy, withdrawal, hyperactivity, abnormal relatedness, and fidgetiness in young (age 2 to 8) autistic children (Campbell et al., 1982). Clinical improvement in such areas would naturally be expected to render children more tractable in the classroom and presumably more amenable to a learning environment. There is at least tentative evidence that discrimination learning in a laboratory task may also be improved in autistic children on haloperidol (Campbell *et al.*, 1982), although it is an open question whether this putative learning effect is a direct consequence of improved cognitive function or an indirect effect— for example, the result of diminished stereotyped responding.

Haloperidol may be superior to certain types of behavior therapy in reducing specific symptoms in autistic children, while the combination of haloperidol and behavioral treatments has been found to be superior in facilitating the acquisition of adaptive functions (Campbell *et al.*, 1978).

There is a common belief that less "sedating," high-potency neuroleptics may be superior to the more sedating, low-potency neuroleptics like chlorpromazine and thioridazine (Fish, Campbell, Shapiro, & Floyd, 1969). On the other hand, Rimland (1977) reported that chlorpromazine and thioridazine are the most commonly used neuroleptics for autistic children.

Although autism has, in the past, been described as an infantile variant of schizophrenia, there is, in fact, little support for a common basis to the two disorders. Therefore, the antipsychotic effects of neuroleptics, which are best appreciated in acutely schizophrenic patients, are not necessarily germane to the case of autism. What is common to both disorders is a pattern of disorganization and unusual behavior that is described as "psychotic," and antipsychotic drugs are the psychotropes most frequently administered to autistic and schizophrenic patients.

It is not known whether neuroleptics exercise the positive benefit they have for some autistic children as a consequence of a specific antipsychotic effect, or whether they simply exercise a nonspecific sedating or tranquilizing effect (Winsberg & Yepes, 1978). Neuroleptics exert a specific effect on the stereotypies that arise in autistic children, but this effect is probably analogous to their specific effect on tics in patients with Tourette syndrome, which is not related to a specific antipsychotic action.

The occasional utility of neuroleptic drugs in low doses for some autistic patients with severe behavior problems, at least over the short and intermediate terms, cannot be gainsaid. Since it is not possible to predict which patients will respond favorably, a brief therapeutic trial is hardly ever contraindicated. However, the long-term efficacy of neuroleptics in autistic children has not been established, and there is no reason to resort to high doses in patients who fail to respond to low doses of medication. Autistic children are known to develop transient neuroleptic-induced withdrawal dyskinesias (Campbell *et al.*, 1984) and persistent tardive dyskinesia (Gualtieri, Quade, Hicks, Mayo, & Schroeder, 1984).

What guarantees the continued prescription of neuroleptic drugs for autistic children and for other children with developmental handicaps is the dearth of suitable pharmacologic alternatives. The risk of tardive dyskinesia has certainly impelled pediatric psychiatrists to seek alternative pharmacologic treatments—unfortunately, however, with only limited success (Gualtieri, Golden, & Fahs, 1983).

Neuroleptic Side Effects

There is little difference between children and adults in the occurrence of most of the untoward effects of neuroleptic drugs. Hypotension, cholestatic jaundice, leukopenia, weight gain, seizures, constipation, and dysphoria have all been noted in greater or lesser degree in children. Particularly troublesome side effects for children are coryza, which may be attributed to allergy or infection; photosensitivity, since children spend so much time outdoors; and urinary incontinence (especially with thioridazine). Sedation and cognitive impairment may interfere with classroom performance. Many Tourette syndrome patients on neuroleptics experience "cognitive blunting" and diminished energy.

The occurrence of *acute extrapyramidal symptoms* in children has been reviewed by Winsberg and Yepes (1978) and by Gualtieri, Barnhill, McGimsey, and Schell (1980); their data base comprised case studies or reports of side effects in clinical drug trials. The full range of extrapyramidal side effects may occur, especially dystonia, and children are sensitive even to low doses of high-potency neuroleptics in this regard (Gualtieri *et al.*, 1980). In contrast, Parkinsonian symptoms may be less frequent. Whether this pattern does indeed characterize the response of children to neuroleptics is an open question; it may simply be the consequence of patterns of reporting, the sensitivity of examiners, or the idiosyncrasies of a few clinical studies. The comparative sensitivity of adults and children has not been the topic of systematic study. It is tempting to predict that were such work done, it would show an increased vulnerability to dystonia and diminished sensitivity to tremor, rigidity, and bradykinesia in children (Gualtieri *et al.*, 1980). The point is not a trivial one, because extrapyramidal symptoms may be related to the early development of tardive dyskinesia (Kane, Woerner, Weinhold, Wegner, & Kinon, 1984).

The treatment of extrapyramidal symptoms with anticholinergic drugs is not dissimilar to that for adults, although children appear to be particularly sensitive to some anticholinergic side effects like dry mouth, blurred vision, and urinary retention.

Tardive Dyskinesia

Severe, persistent tardive dyskinesia does occur in autistic people, sometimes after relatively short treatment periods. The reader is referred to two recent reviews of the subject (Campbell, Grega, Green, & Bennett, 1983; Gualtieri *et al.*, 1980). Studies of tardive dyskinesia refer to three additional neuroleptic withdrawal syndromes or "withdrawal emergent symptoms": (1) transient withdrawal dyskinesia, (2) withdrawal symptoms like nausea, vomiting, anorexia, diaphoresis, and seizures, and (3) a behavioral analogue of tardive dyskinesia (Davis & Rosenberg, 1979), "tardive dysbehavior" (Gualtieri & Guimond, 1981), or "supersensitivity psychosis" (Chouinard & Jones, 1980; Gualtieri *et al.*, 1984).

The early work of Polizos and Engelhardt was quite influential; they coined the term *withdrawal emergent symptoms* in psychotic children, many of whom were autistic (Polizos & Engelhardt, 1978; Engelhardt, Polizos, & Waizer, 1975). Such symptoms occurred in 51% of a group of autistic and schizophrenic children within 2 weeks of neuroleptic withdrawal. However, the authors' belief that dyskinetic movements in children were topographically different from those that arise in adults has not been affirmed in other research (Gualtieri *et al.*, 1984; Paulson, Rizvi, & Crane, 1975). Buccal-lingual-masticatory and facial movements predominate in cases of tardive dyskinesia and withdrawal dyskinesia in chidren (Gualtieri *et al.*, 1984) and in developmentally handicapped young adults (Gualtieri, Quade, Schroeder, & Hicks, 1986). Recent research indicates that while withdrawal dyskinesia (duration 4 months or less) is the more common form of neuroleptic-induced dyskinesia in children (Campbell *et al.*, 1984; Gualtieri *et al.*, 1984), persistent tardive dyskinesia, sometimes of alarming intensity, may also occur (Gualtieri *et al.*, 1984; Polizos & Engelhardt, 1980). Female sex and cumulative neuroleptic dose appear to be relevant factors in the development of same (Gualtieri *et al.*, 1984, 1986).

The occurrence of a transient period of behavioral instability in patients who are withdrawn from neuroleptic drugs has fed speculation concerning the existence of a "behavioral equivalent" of tardive or at least of withdrawal dyskinesia (Gualtieri & Guimond, 1981).

It is not possible to estimate the prevalence or the incidence of tardive dyskinesia or of related disorders in autistic children and adults with any degree of assurance. Sufficient to emphasize that tardive dyskinesia, even severe and persistent forms, may occur in children treated with long-term neuroleptic drugs.

Recommendations for Neuroleptic Treatment

1. There are no absolute indications for neuroleptic treatment in developmentally handicapped people, with the exceptions of acute psychosis, agitation, and severe Tourette syndrome.

2. There is, however, a broad range of relative indications for neuroleptic treatment, and autism may be one such indication, especially when the following problem behaviors are apparent: hyperactivity, aggression, severe disorganization, agitation, or insomnia.

3. Neuroleptic treatment must be guided by the exigencies of the individual clinical situation, by the severity of the problem, and by the failure of reasonable alternative treatments.

4. Short-term success with neuroleptics does not spell a requirement for continued treatment over the long term. Careful reevaluation of therapeutic benefit and periodic monitoring for side effects are essential.

5. Clinicians are well advised to use only the lowest effective doses, to eschew unnecessary polypharmacy, and to taper maintenance doses on regular basis, if possible.

6. The informed consent of responsible adult(s) (i.e., parents, guardians) should be obtained if long-term treatment is necessary. Ideally, the patient should assent to treatment.

7. Neuroleptic treatment in autistic people is by no means an ordinary kind of treatment. It should be undertaken and supervised by physicians who have special skills in psychopharmacology, who can properly evaluate the potential benefits of alternative treatments and the risk of withholding neuroleptics, and who are capable of monitoring the occurrence of side effects.

FENFLURAMINE

A preliminary report of the clinical efficacy of the atypical stimulant fenfluramine (Geller, Ritvo, Freeman, & Yuwiler, 1982) was greeted with extraordinary enthusiasm by the medical (Ciaranello, 1982) and lay press. The preliminary report was based on an uncontrolled study of two children, one of whom "almost doubling his IQ during the course of the experiment" (Geller et al., 1982, pp. 166–167). The attention that greeted this report, which appeared in a prestigious medical journal, seemed appropriate by virtue of a proposed rational basis for fenfluramine treatment in autism. The drug lowers serotonin levels in the brain, and serotoninemia is not an infrequent concomitant of the disorder.

A multicenter trial of fenfluramine was soon assembled, but the initial results of this trial, reported at scientific meetings, have not supported the initial impressions of Geller et al. (1982). For example, the beneficial effects of fenfluramine in allaying problem behaviors, when they occur, do not correlate with pretreatment hyperserotoninemia or posttreatment reduction in blood serotonin levels (Gualtieri, 1986). The clinical impressions of participants in the multicenter study are by no means unanimous in support of the efficacy of the drug (Leventhal, 1985). It is not yet known which autistic patients will respond favorably to fenfluramine, in which problem areas improvement may be expected to occur, or to what degree, or how the drug compares in efficacy to neuroleptics like haloperidol, for example.

The safety of fenfluramine is an open question, and a serious one. Since the only previous indication for the drug was short-term appetite suppression in obese people, the question of long-term safety in human populations, and especially in children, has never been addressed. Fenfluramine is, however, known to be *neurotoxic* in contained animal studies. Even short-term treatment courses have been associated with long-lasting changes in the neurochemical constituents of brain—for example, depletion of serotonin in hippocampus, caudate, and cerebral cortex (Schuster & Seiden, 1985). It is conceivable that fenfluramine lowers serotonin by exercising a neurotoxic effect on serotoninergic neurons (Harvey & McMaster, 1977). Long-term alterations in certain neurotransmitter metabolites have been noted in autistic children treated with short courses of fenfluramine (Leventhal, 1985). This suggests that the animal data, though based on high-dose studies, may not be entirely irrelevant to the clinical situation. If fenfluramine were neurotoxic to children, the effect might not be clinically apparent as an overt, toxic occurrence. There is at least one neuropathic model, that of Parkinson disease, where traumatic or toxic injury to nervous tissue has no immediately apparent effects but does have devastating consequences after a latent period of several years. The issue of fenfluramine neurotoxicity, therefore, may not be resolved in humans until the drug has been used for many years and conceivably not until after thousands of patients have been treated.

Other toxic effects of fenfluramine include pulmonary hypertension (Douglas, Munro, Kitchin, Muir, & Proudfoot, 1981), hyperactivity, irritability, insomnia (Volkmar, Paul, Cohen, & Shaywitz, 1983), and hyperprolactinemia (Slater, de la Vega, Skyler, & Murphy, 1976). Fenfluramine may cause "hallucinatory states" in human subjects (Griffith, 1977), and overdosage may lead to convulsions, coma, and death (Von Muhlendahl & Krienke, 1979).

It is impossible to know how the publicity over fenfluramine in autism may have influenced physicians around the world to treat children with this untested drug. Nor is it possible to recommend treatment guildelines for a drug that has no respectable literature based on carefully controlled studies. In light of concerns over the potential neurotoxicity of the drug, it is the authors' opinion that further human trials of fenfluramine be delayed until the question of long-term toxicity can be tested in laboratory animals. There is, at this time, no clinical justification for the prescription of fenfluramine to any autistic child. One is not at all certain whether human research studies with fenfluramine should be continued until the safety of the drug is established.

"MEGAVITAMIN" THERAPY

The "therapeutic" or "prophylactic" use of high doses of water-soluble vitamins has grown immeasurably, largely at the urging of food faddists, the "holistic health" movement, and "orthomolecular" physicians. It has been claimed that "mega" doses of certain vitamins will ameliorate or prevent or cure cancer, schizophrenia, mental retardation, and the common cold, as well as autism. Conventional wisdom holds that because excess amounts of water-soluble vitamins are excreted in urine, they are therefore nontoxic. In fact, the water-soluble vitamins (C, B1, B2, B3, B6, B12, folate, biotin, pantothenic acid, and para-aminobenzoic acid) are much less toxic than the lipid-soluble vitamins (A, D, K, and E) that accumulate in body fat. However, it is not known that high doses of water-soluble vitamins may indeed have toxic effects (Alhadeff, Gualtieri, & Lipton, 1984).

There are five discrete mechanisms by which high doses of water-soluble vitamins can cause toxic effects in humans:

1. High doses of water-soluble vitamins may lead to dependency states and withdrawal symptoms may develop if they are abruptly discontinued.
-2. Vitamins or their metabolites may have direct toxic effects.
3. Vitamins may mask the symptoms or signs of a concurrent disease.
4. Vitamins may interact with drugs or with other vitamins.
5. The use of "mega" doses of water-soluble vitamins may be associated with concurrent use of fat-soluble vitamins.

High Doses of Water-Soluble Vitamins May Induce a Dependency State and Withdrawal Symptoms May Arise When They Are Discontinued

Water-soluble vitamins taken in high doses over long periods of time may induce dependency states, and users may show signs of deficiency or withdrawal symptoms when the dose is lowered or the substance is discontinued (American Pharmaceutical Association, 1979; APA Task Force on Vitamin Therapy, 1973; Coronary Drug Project Research Group, 1975; Gilman, Goodman, & Gilman, 1980; Richens, 1971). Although the mechanism for this is not well understood, it may be related to the fact that most of the water-soluble vitamins induce the enzymes of their own metabolism. It is also possible that target tissues grow "accustomed" to operating in the presence of high concentrations of a particular vitamin, and physiologic mechanisms for "sparing" the vitamin are inactivated (Wentzler, 1979). Most of the water-soluble vitamins are converted in the body to coenzymes. High levels of coenzymes may induce the formation of new protein enzymes (apoenzymes). When the coenzyme level falls rapidly after discontinuation of high-dose vitamin intake, excessive quantities of apoenzyme may remain unsaturated and this may cause withdrawal symptoms. Two vitamins associated with such problems are pyridoxine (B6) and ascorbic acid (C).

Dependency and withdrawal reactions have been described in people who grew accustomed to daily doses of vitamin C as low as 200 mgm. "Rebound scurvy" has been reported after withdrawal from chronic ascorbic acid administration (Gilman et al., 1980; Schrauzer & Rhead, 1971). There was an increased incidence of scurvy among individuals who received extra dietary ascorbic acid during the siege of Leningrad when the siege was lifted and they returned to their normal diets. There are also reports of scurvy in infants of mothers who took high doses of vitamin C during pregnancy (DiPalma & Ritchie, 1977; Gilman et al., 1980; Schrauzer & Rhead, 1971).

There are three case reports of babies with infantile seizures whose mothers took pyridoxine (5-300/day) during pregnancy (Williams & Kalita, 1977). These infantile seizures respond to pyridoxine treatment.

The occurrence of withdrawal symptoms after megavitamin treatment certainly diminishes the credibility of one controlled study of pyridoxine in autistic children (Ref). In this study, the efficacy of pyridoxine was based on the emergence of behavior problems after withdrawal from high doses of the substance. A more cogent interpretation of these data is that the children experienced a withdrawal syndrome.

Direct Toxic Effects and Toxic Effects Mediated by a Metabolite or an Intermediate Substance

High doses of vitamin B3 (nicotinic acid, niacin, nicotinamide, niaciamide) have been recommended for the treatment of hypercholesterolemia (Coronory Drug Project Research Group, 1975) and schizophrenia (APA Task Force on Vitamin Therapy, 1973; Williams & Kalita, 1977) in doses up to 3 gm/day (the recommended daily allowance RDA is 20 mgm/ day; Committee on Dietary Allowances, 1980). Nicotinic acid (but not niacinamide) causes the release of the vasodilator histamine from mast cells, and as a consequence, flushing is a common side effect (DiPalma & Ritchie, 1977). Flushing within 15 minutes after an oral dose may occur at doses as low as 100 mgm/day (Lesser, 1980); flushing may occur in 92% of patients taking niacin (3 grams/day) (APA Task Force, 1973). Because niacin may release histamine, it has been suggested that caution should be exercised by asthmatics and patients with peptic ulcer disease. Other toxic niacin effects on the GI tract include stomach pain (13.9%), nausea (8.5%), and diarrhea (4.6%) (Coronary Drug Project Research Group, 1975). Niacin has also been associated with toxic effects on the liver (DiPalma & Ritchie, 1977). Large doses of niacin have been reported to cause cholestatic jaundice; this usually disappears after the vitamin is discontinued (Finstein, Balsen, Galper, & Wolfe, 1975). Niacin may also increase serum uric acid levels, and the vitamin has been associated with certain cardiac arrhythmias, and dermatologic problems including pruritus, rash, and hyper-keratosis (American Pharmaceutical Association, 1979); APA Task Force, 1973; Coronary Drug Project Research Group, 1975). Acanthosis nigricans is a rare but serious skin condition that has been reported to occur in about 5% of patients taking niacin (Mosher, 1970). Plasma glucose levels in the fasting state and 1 hour after glucose challenge can be elevated by niacin (American Pharmaceutical Association, 1979; APA Task Force, 1973; Coronary Drug Project, 1975).

Vitamin C (ascorbic acid) in high doses has been recommended for the treatment of the common cold, anxiety, cancer, hypercholesterolemia, schizophrenia, heavy metal intoxication, shock, urethritis, arthritis, and heroin addition (Williams & Kalita, 1977). Vitamin C has been shown to be uricosuric (Stein, Hasan, & Fox, 1976). Significant uricosuria (about 200% of control values) has been reported with single doses of 4 grams of vitamin C, but not with doses of 0.5 to 2 grams (Stein et al., 1976). Excessive intake of vitamin C may also be associated with the formation of oxalate stones (Stein et al., 1976).

Chronic high doses of vitamin C may affect the function and viability of various constituents of blood. Increased lytic sensitivity of red blood cells was noted in 14 healthy volunteers taking 5 grams of vitamin C per day for only 2 days (Fersdyke, 1975). It has been suggested that high doses of vitamin C may lead to hemolysis in patients with glucose-6 phosphate dehydrogenase (G6PD) deficiency, and reports of vitamin C-induced hemolysis exist. It has also been reported that high doses of vitamin C may impair the bactericidal activity of white blood cells. Although doses around 200 mgm per day will not exert such an effect, a dose of 2 grams per day over 15 days has done so (Campbell, Steinberg, & Beven, 1975). This reaction is readily reversible.

It is well known that vitamin C at high doses may cause diarreha (Williams & Kalita, 1977). In fact, it is suggested by some faddists that the proper dose of vitamin C is one that is slightly below the diarrhea threshold.

Three other water-soluble vitamins may also show direct toxicity:

Vitamin B1 is currently used in treatment of alcoholics to prevent or reverse Wernicke encephalopathy. Though this indication makes thiamine a relatively popular vitamin, it is rarely used by itself by faddists. The only side effect mentioned in the more recent literature is anaphylaxis (Sebrell & Harris, 1968) secondary to parenteral use.

In the 1940s and 1950s there were frequent episodes of thiamine toxicity. According to Mills (1941), thiamine toxicity could occur in doses as low as 5 mgm for 4½ weeks (thiamine's RDA is 0.5 mg/100 kcal in nonpregnant adults). The side effects were said to resemble an overdose of thyroid extract: headache, irritability, insomnia, rapid pulse, and weakness. The decrease of thiamine use in recent times is probably responsible for the decreased incidence of toxicity.

Vitamin B6 is a collective term for three naturally occurring pyridines: pyridoxine, pyridoxal, and pyridoxamine. Large doses of B6 are advocated to treat depression, muscle fatigue, parasthesias, and autism. Unlike B3 and C, vitamin B6 has almost no direct toxicity. In one report B6 is associated with peptic ulcer disease (Williams & Kalita, 1977). In another, it is suggested that high doses may cause seizures (DiPalma & Ritchie, 1977), but this effect might have been a withdrawal reaction second to B6 dependency and withdrawal (see below). Sensory neuropathy has been reported as a consequence of very high-dose pyridoxine treatment (Schaumberg, et al., 1983).

Vitamins May Mask the Symptoms or Signs of a Preexisting Disease Process

The Food and Drug Administration restricts vitamin manufacturers from including more than 0.4 mg of folate/dose in over-the-counter vitamin preparations because high doses of folic acid may mask the hematological signs of mebaloblastic anemia secondary to vitamin B12 (cyanocobalamin) deficiency. This is a serious problem because the neurological deterioration attendant on persistent B12 deficiency may progress in spite of a normal hemogram, and the damage may be irreversible. In the presence of a normal hemogram, the neurologic and psychiatric manifestations of B12 deficiency may be nonspecific and proper diagnosis may be delayed (Pfeiffer, 1975).

High doses of vitamin C can complicate the treatment of diabetic patients, because the vitamin may cause clinisticks to read false negatives or Clinitest tablets/Benedict's solution to read false positives (American Pharmaceutical Association, 1979).

Because of the uricosuric effects of vitamin C in very high doses, serum uric acid levels may decrease and the diagnosis of gout may be missed (Stein et al., 1976).

Vitamins Interact with Drugs and Other Vitamins

Vitamins, like drugs, may interact with other drugs or vitamins. Several mechanisms may be operative here; they include interference with absorption, metabolism, effectiveness at the target site, and excretion.

Vitamin C may decrease the absorption of vitamin B12 (Hines, 1975). Interference with the absorption of vitamin B12 is dose-related. In sample meals containing moderate amounts of vitamin B12 (0.1 grams, 0.25 grams, and 0.5 grams), vitamin C destroyed 43%, 81%, and 91% of the B12 (Herbert & Jacob, 1974). It has been estimated that 3% of subjects on doses of vitamin C ranging from 0.5 to 1 gram per day are at risk of developing B12 deficiency (Hines, 1975).

Several studies designed to confirm this interaction did not find a clinically significant interaction on doses from 1 gram/day to 10 grams/day of ascorbic acid. However, one study found a 17.9% mean decrease in total plasma Warfarin concentration (Feetam, Leach, & Meynell, 1975). It was claimed, however, that this drop in plasma Wafarin levels was not clinically significant. Decrease in Warfarin levels seemed to be a dose-dependent phenomenon, so it seems fair to say there may be vitamin C effect at higher doses, although its clinical significance is an open question.

Vitamin C is known to increase iron absorption. The effect can lead to hemochromatosis. For example, the Bantu people of South Africa brew a drink that is strong in vitamin C and drink it from iron vessels to contract the disease. It is possible that some preparations of multivitamins plus iron can result in the absorption of too much iron (Gilman et al., 1980). The ratio of iron absorption with vitamin C (100 mg) to iron absorption without vitamin C is 4.5 to 1. Normal individuals can probably regulate their iron intake effectively, whatever the concomitant dose of vitamin C. However, in people with idiopathic hemochromatosis, thalassemia major, and sideroblastic anemia, vitamin C might compound the problem of iron overload (Cook & Monsen, 1977).

Because vitamin C acidifies the urine, it may influence the excretion of other drugs. In general, acidic drugs such as aspirin tend to be resorbed to a greater extent in patients on high doses of vitamin C, and basic drugs such as the tricyclic antidepressants or amphetamines are excreted at a higher rate (American Pharmaceutical Association, 1979). Vitamin C may also decrease the antibacterial effect of aminoglycoside antibiotics in the urinary tract, although a dose–response relationship is not available (Rubenstein & Federman, 1981).

Vitamin C has been reported to lower blood levels of the neuroleptic fluphenazine (Stockley, 1981). A patient who was taking 15 mg of fluphenazine was given 1 gram of ascorbic acid daily. In 2 weeks, his phenothiazine level dropped by 90%.

Pyridoxine in doses as small as 10 to 25 mg can increase the peripheral metabolism of L-dopa to dopamine; dopamine cannot cross the blood brain barrier (Leue & Bachy, 1976). (The RDA for vitamin B6 is 0.02 mg/day per 1 gram of protein consumed per day in nonpregnant, nonlactating individuals.) This premature conversion of L-dopa to dopamine may diminish the effectivenesses of L-dopa in the treatment of Parkinsonism. Because of this interaction, a multivitamin formulation that does not contain pyridoxine has been created for Parkinsonian patients on L-dopa. Pyridoxine may also antagonize penicillamine in the treatment of Wilson disease (DiPalma & Ritchie, 1977).

Both folic acid and vitamin B6 reduce serum levels of phenytoin. Folate is often used in patients who are on anticonvulsant medications because anticonvulsants depress serum folate levels. However, folate (5–15 mg/day) may in turn reduce serum phenytoin levels by 16 to 50%. Phenytoin metabolism (hydroxylation) is dependent on folate as a cofactor (Stockley, 1981).

Pyridoxine (200 mgm/day) has also been shown to reduce phenytoin blood levels up to 50%; the mechanism is not certain. It is possible that pyridoxine induces enzymes that metabolize the anticonvulsant (Stockley, 1981).

Vitamin H (pantothenic acid) has been reported to prolong neuromuscular blockade. A patient who had been given 500 mg of vitamin H intramuscularly while recovering from anesthesia with suxamethonium (a neuromuscular blocker), cyclopropane, and nitrous oxide suffered severe respiratory embarrassment. However, a subsequent study of six patients given the same dose of vitamin H after neuromuscular blockade were unaffected (Stockley, 1981).

Vitamin B2 (riboflavin) also deserves mention here. The RDA for this vitamin has been set at 0.6 mg/1000 kcal for adults and children. Riboflavin in large doses may cause a yellow discoloration of the urine, which can be misleading or alarming (Leue & Bachy, 1976). Riboflavin has also been shown to inhibit the uptake of methotrexate by neoplastic cells (DiPalma & Ritchie, 1977).

It is not known whether PABA (paraaminobenzoic acid) is a vitamin or not, so there is no RDA for it. But even if humans do not really need PABA, bacteria do. Sulpha drugs resemble PABA so closely that bacteria absorb the drugs and die of relative PABA deficiency. Vitamin preparations that include PABA should not be taken concurrently with sulpha drugs (Stockley, 1981).

The Use of "Mega" Doses of Water-Soluble Vitamins May Be Accompanied by Concurrent Use of Other, More Toxic Vitamins

Some multivitamin preparations contain both water- and fat-soluble vitamins. The ingestion of high doses of water-soluble vitamins in such preparations may be accompanied by the concurrent ingestion of the more toxic fat-soluble vitamins (Willett et al., 1981). Patients on high doses of water-soluble vitamins should be carefully questioned about concurrent ingestion of other vitamin supplements.

It is probably true that megavitamin or, more specifically, pyridoxine treatment for autistic people is less troublesome, from a medical point of view, than treatment with neuroleptics, for example. The relatively low toxicity profile of the water-soluble vitamins is a truism. That is why they are freely available at grocery stores and pharmacies without a physician's prescription. However, the administration of megavitamin preparations is not entirely free of toxic effects, and the ready availability of these chemicals through commercial outlets may, in some cases, spell danger to individuals whose "treatment" is not supervised by a competent physician.

There is no way of knowing how frequently toxic effects to megavitamin therapy occur in autistic individuals, or how severe occasional megavitamin side effects may be, and this is regrettable. Professionals who work with autistic people should try to guarantee that megavitamin treatments are medically supervised, and they ought to try to educate physicians to regard megavitamin trials with less than unbridled hostility. After all, it is not outlandish to suggest that some vitamin preparations *might* have psychoactive or behavioral effects. The brain is the most metabolically active organ in the human body. It is conceivable that subtle alterations in brain metabolism could influence behavior and developmental performance in some autistic people. One is left to wish for more in the way of research on the topic.

Since autistic people are most likely to be treated with pyridoxine (B6) in combination with other B vitamins and nutritional supplements, the side effects that are most salient are these: (1) withdrawal reactions after the vitamin regime is abruptly discontinued, seizures, or behavioral deterioration; (2) sensory neuropathy; (3) interactions with phenytoin and possibly with other drugs; (4) gastric distress, nausea, diarrhea; (5) excitability, irritability, sound sensitivity; (6) enuresis and daytime incontinence; (7) increased autistic symptoms or hyperactivity; (8) insomnia.

Megavitamin treatment of autistic people may be relatively safe, but it is not completely free of untoward effects, and some effects may be quite serious. Megavitamin treatment should be undertaken—or discontinued—only under the supervision of a knowledgeable physician.

ANTICONVULSANT DRUGS

Autistic children are particularly vulnerable to the development of seizure disorders; seizures may begin in infancy or early childhood, or in early adolescence. The most common seizure disorder in autistic people is the complex-partial type. The seizures derive, in all probability, from the same encephalopathic processes that are responsible for autistic symptoms and developmental retardation. Epilepsy is probably no more common in autistic people than in matched groups of retarded people who are not autistic. In both groups, however, the seizure disorder is likely to carry a poor prognosis: Evidence of focal brain damage, low IQ, and seizures of the complex partial type are poor prognosis mediators in epilepsy. Thus, autistic people who develop seizures are likely to require long-term anticonvulsant polypharmacy.

It is not feasible to review the wide range of anticonvulsant side effects, but it is important to reiterate and to emphasize the cognitive and behavioral toxicity of anticonvulsants. Developmentally handicapped people are not more likely to incur medical side effects of anticonvulsants than epileptic patients of normal capacity, but they are, by virtue of their limited cognitive "reserve," and their proclivity to behavior problems, especially vulnerable to the negative cognitive and behavioral effects of anticonvulsants. The facts that anticonvulsant therapy may be lifelong and that multiples of drugs may be required amplify the potential dangers of anticonvulsant therapy.

The anticonvulsants of particular relevance are phenytoin, phenobarbital and related barbituates, clonazepam, carbamazepine, and valproic acid. The first three drugs are widely known to exercise negative cognitive effects, although it is also appreciated that appropriate seizure management may be of benefit both to learning and to behavioral stability. Phenobarbital and other barbiturate anticonvulsants may cause hyperactivity or sedation in vulnerable patients (Stores, Hart, & Piran, 1978). Dilantin may be a sedative, it may impair motor coordination and performance, and it has well-established negative effects on memory and learning (Smith & Lowery, 1972). Clonazepam, like other benzodiazepines, may cause sedation and memory impairment, depression, motor deficits, and paradoxical excitement on disinhibition (Rivinius, 1982).

Carbamazepine and valproic acid are generally conceded to exercise fewer sedative effects than other anticonvulsants that are administered to patients with complex partial epilepsy (Evans & Gualtieri, 1985). However, they are not without serious toxicity, and the prevailing belief, for example, that carbamazepine does not cause such problems is almost certainly an overstatement of the case. Memory impairment can occur with carbamazepine, although probably not to the same degree as with phenytoin (Evans & Gualtieri, 1985). Both carbamazepine and valproate may cause hyperactivity, irritability, and insomnia (Evans & Gualtieri, 1985; Rivinius, 1982). Carbamazepine may also lead to assaultive behavior, agitation, and motor and phonic tics (Evans & Gualtieri, 1985). Although such effects are, in the main, dose-related, they may occur at low doses, and a low blood level does not exclude the possibility of anticonsulvant toxicity.

The major problem of anticonvulsant treatment in autistic people is the availability of competent and sensitive medical management. Physicians who prescribe anticonvulsants are not necessarily well versed in the proper treatment of developmentally handicapped patients, and they may not appreciate the importance of integrating a medical treatment regime into a total care program. The negative cognitive and behavioral effects of anticonvulsants may be devastating to such a program, and many physicians are insufficiently attentive to this aspect of anticonvulsant pharmacotherapy. It is not uncommon for a physician to prescribe a psychotropic to control behavioral reactions to anticonvulsant drugs, when a change in the anticonvulsant regime would be a more appropriate decision. Nor is it uncommon for a retarded person to continue on multiple anticonvulsants for prolonged periods when single-drug therapy would be entirely sufficient. Although the consequences of uncontrolled epilepsy may be catastrophic, the occurrence of an occasional seizure may be an acceptable price to pay to maintain the quality of an individual's day-to-day life. Perfect seizure control is not necessarily worth the price of severe cognitive blunting, especially in a person who is not very smart to begin with.

The availability of competent modern epileptology is as important to autistic and retarded people as the availability of competent, modern psychopharmacology. There is no point to railing against the evils of drug treatment in autism; there is, however, every reason to decry the generally poor level of medical care these people receive, the low status their proper care has in medical schools and training programs, and the relative unavailability of psychosocial programs that may reduce the necessity of pharmacologic solutions to behavioral difficulties. The toxic consequences of medical treatments administered to autistic people would be reduced considerably if the quality of medical care were improved. The influence of mountebanks and ideologues would be reduced were there more in the way of competent professionalism in the field.

REFERENCES

Alhadeff, L., Gualtieri, C. T., & Lipton, M. (1984). Toxic effects of water-soluble vitamins. *Nutrition Reviews, 42*(2), 33–40.

American Pharmaceutical Association. (1979). *Handbook of non prescription drugs* (6th ed.). Washington, DC: Author.

APA Task Force on Vitamin Therapy in Psychiatry. (1973). *Megavitamin and orthomolecular therapy in psychiatry.* Washington, DC: American Psychiatric Association.

Campbell, G. D., Steinberg, M. H., & Beven, J. D. (1975). Ascorbic acid induced hemolysis in G6PD deficiency. *Annual of Internal Medicine, 82*, 810.

Campbell, M., Anderson, L. T., Cohen, I. L., Perry, R., Small, A. M., Green, W.H., Anderson, L. & McCandless, W. H. (1982). Haloperidol in autistic children: Effects on learning, behavior, and abnormal involuntary movements. *Psychopharmacology Bulletin, 18*, 110–112.

Campbell, M., Anderson, L., Meier, M., Cohen, I., Small, A., Samit, C., & Sachan, E. (1978). A comparison of haloperidol and behavior therapy and their interaction in autistic children. *Journal of the American Academy of Child Psychiatry, 12*, 55–67.

Campbell, M., Grega, D. M., Green, W. H., & Bennett, W. G. (1983). Neuroleptic-induced dyskinesias in children. *Clinical Neuropharmacology, 6*, 207–222.

Campbell, M., Perry, R., Bennett, W. G., Small, A. M., Green, W. H., Grega, D., Schwartz, V., & Anderson, L. (1984). Long-term therapeutic efficacy and drug-related abnormal movements: A prospective study of haloperidol in autistic children. *Psychopharmacology Bulletin, 19*, 80–83.

Chouinard, G., & Jones, B. D. (1980). Neuroleptic-induced supersensitivity psychosis: Clinical and pharmacologic characteristics. *American Journal of Psychiatry, 137*, 16–21.

Ciaranello, R. D. (1982). Hyperserotoninemia and early infantile autism. *New England Journal of Medicine, 307*, 181–183.

Committee on Dietary Allowances. (1980). *Food and Nutrition Board: Recommended dietary allowance* (9th ed.). Washington, DC: National Academy of Science.

Cook, J., & Monsen, E. (1977). Vitamin C, the common cold and iron absorption. *American Journal of Clinical Nutrition, 30*, 235–241.

Coronary Drug Project Research Group, The. (1975). Clofibrate and niacin in coronary heart disease. *Journal of the American Medical Association, 231*, 360–381.

Davis, K. L., & Rosenberg, G. S. (1979). Is there a limbic system equivalent of tardive dyskinesia? *Biological Psychiatry, 14*, 699–703.

DiPalma, J. R., & Ritchie, D. M. (1977). Vitamin toxicity. *Annual Review of Pharmacological Toxicity, 17*, 133.

Douglas, J. G., Munro, J. F., Kitchin, A. H., Muir, A. L., & Proudfoot, A. T. (1981). Pulmonary hypertension and fenfluramine. *British Medical Journal, 283*, 881–883.

Engelhardt, D. M., Polizos, P., & Waizer, J. (1975). CNS consequences of psychotropic drug withdrawal in autistic children: A follow-up report. *Psychopharmacology Bulletin, 11*(1), 6–7.

Evans, R. W., & Gualtieri, C. T. (1985). Carbamazepine: A neuropsychological and psychiatric profile. *Clinical Neuropharmacology, 83*, 221–241.

Feetam, C., Leach, R., & Meynell, M. (1975). Lack of clinically important interactions between Warfarin and ascorbic acid. *Toxicology and Applied Pharmacology, 31*, 522–527.

Fersdyke, D. R. (1976). Ascorbic acid effects on erythrolytes. *Annual of Internal Medicine, 84*, 490.

Finstein, N., Balsen, A., Galper, J., & Wolfe, H. (1975). Jaundice due to nicotinic acid therapy. *American Journal of Digestive Disease, 20*, 282–286.

Fish, B., Campbell, M., Shapiro, T., & Floyd, A. (1969). Comparison of trifluperidol, trifluoperazine, and chlorpromazine in preschool schizophrenic children. *Current Therapeutic Research, 11*, 589–595.

Geller, E., Ritvo, E. R., Freeman, B. J., & Yuwiler, A. (1982). Preliminary observations on the effect of fenfluramine on blood serotonin and symptoms in three autistic children. *New England Journal of Medicine, 307*, 165–169.

Gilman, A. G., Goodman, L. S., & Gilman, A. (1980). *The pharmacologic basis of therapeutics*: Toronto: MacMillan.

Griffith, J. D. (1977). Structure–activity relationships of several amphetamine drugs in man. In E. H. Ellinwood & M. M. Kilbey (Eds.), *Cocaine and other stimulants*: New York: Plenum Press.

Gualtieri, C. T. (1986). Fenfluramine and autism: A careful reappraisal is in order. *Journal of Pediatrics, 108*, 417–419.

Gualtieri, C. T., Barnhill, J., McGimsey, J., & Schell, D. (1980). Tardive dyskinesia and other movement disorders in children treated with psychotropic drugs. *Journal of the American Academy of Child Psychiatry, 19*, 491–510.

Gualtieri, C. T., & Evans, R. W. (1984). Carbamazepine-induced tics. *Developmental Medicine and Child Neurology, 26*, 546–548.

Gualtieri, C. T., Golden, R. N., & Fahs, J. J. (1983). New developments in pediatric psychopharmacology. *Developmental and Behavioral Pediatrics, 4*, 202–209.

Gualtieri, C. T., & Guimond, M. (1981). Tardive dyskinesia and the behavioral consequences of chronic neuroleptic treatment. *Developmental Medicine and Child Neurology, 23*, 255–259.

Gualtieri, C. T., Quade, D., Hicks, R. E., Mayo, J. P., & Schroeder, S. R. (1984). Tardive dyskinesia and other clinical consequences of neuroleptic tratment in children and adolescents. *American Journal of Psychiatry, 141*, 20–23.

Gualtieri, C. T., Quade, D., Schroeder, S. R., & Hicks, R. E. (1986). Tardive dyskinesia in mentally retarded young adults. *Archives of General Psychiatry, 43*, 335–340.

Harrell, R. F., Capp, R. H., Davis, D. R., Peerless, J., & Ravitz, L. R. (1981). Can nutritional supplements help mentally retarded children? An exploratory study. *Proceedings of the National Academy of Sciences, USA, 78*, 574–578.

Harvey, J. A., & McMaster, S. E. (1977). Fenfluramine: Cumulative neurotoxicity after chronic treatment with low dosages in the rat. *Communications in Psychopharmacology, 1*, 3–17.

Herbert, V., & Jacob, E. (1974). Destruction of vitamin B_{12} by ascorbic acid. *Journal of the American Medical Association, 230*, 41–241.

Hines, S. (1975). Ascorbic acid and vitamin B_{12} deficiency. *Journal of the American Medical Association, 234*, 24.

Ho, H. H., Lockitch, G., Eaves, L., & Jacobson, B. (1986). Blood serotonin concentrations and fenfluramine therapy in autistic children. *Journal of Pediatrics, 108*, 465–469.

Kane, J. M., Woerner, M., Weinhold, P., Wegner, J., & Kinon, B. (1984). Incidence of tardive dyskinesia: Five year data from a prospective study. *Psychopharmacology Bulletin, 20*(1), 39–40.

Lesser, M. (1980). *Nutrition and vitamin therapy.* New York: Grove Press.

Leue, J., & Bachy, R. (1976). *Vitamins, their use and abuse.* New York: Liveright.

Leventhal, B. L. (1985, May 2). *Fenfluamine administration to autistic children: Effects on behavior and biogenic amines.* Paper presented at the NCDEU Annual Meeting, Key Biscayne.

Mosher, L. (1970). Nicotinic acid side effects and toxicity; a review. *American Journal of Psychiatry, 126*, 1290–1296.

Mills, C. (1941). Thiamine overdose and toxicity. *Journal of the American Medical Association, 116*, 2101.

Paulson, G. W., Rizvi, C. A., & Crane, G. E. (1975). Tardive dyskinesia as a possible sequel of long-term therapy with phenothiazines. *Clinical Pediatrics, 14*, 953–955.

Pfeiffer, C. (1975). *Mental and elemental nutrients.* New Canaan, CT: Keats.

Polizos, P., & Engelhardt, D. (1978). Dyskinetic phenomena in children treated with psychotropic medications. *Psychopharmacology Bulletin, 14*(4), 65–68.

Polizos, P., & Engelhardt, D. M. (1980). Dyskinetic and neurological complications in children treated with psychotropic medication. In W. E. Fann, R. E. Smith, J. M. Davis, & E. F. Domino (Eds.), *Tardive dyskinesia. Research and treatment* (pp. 193–199). Jamaica, NY: Spectrum.

Richens, A. (1971). Toxicology of folic acid. *Lancet, 1*, 912.

Rimland, B. (1977). *Comparative effects of treatment on child's behavior* (Vol. 34). San Diego: Institute for Child Behavior Research.

Ritvo, E. R. (1985, May). *The efficacy and safety of fenfluramine in autism: A multicenter trial.* Paper presented at the NCDEU Annual Meeting, Key Biscayne.

Ritvo, E. R., Freeman, B. J., Yuwiler, A., Geller, E., Yokota, A., Schroth, P., & Novak, P. (1984). Study of fenfluramine in outpatients with the syndrome of autism. *Journal of Pediatrics, 105*, 823–828.

Rivinius, T. M. (1982). Psychiatric effects of the anticonvulsant regimens. *Journal of Clinical Psychopharmacology, 2*, 165–192.

Rubenstein, E., & Federman, D. D. (1981). *Scientific American Medicine.* New York: Scientific American.

Schaumberg, H., Kaplan, J., Windebank, A., Vick, N., Rasmus, S., Pleasure, D., & Brown, M. (1983). Sensory neuropathy from pyridoxine abuse: A new megavitamin syndrome. *New England Journal of Medicine, 309*, 445–454.

Schrauzer, G. N., & Rhead, W. J. (1971). Risks of long term ascorbic acid overdosage. *Nutrition Review, 29*, 262–263.

Schuster, C. R., & Seiden, L. S. (1985, May 2). *Assessment of neurotoxicity of fenfluramine.* Paper presented at the NCDEU Annual Meeting, Key Biscayne.

Sebrell, W. J., Jr., & Harris, R. S. (1968). *The vitamins* (2nd ed., Vol. 2). London/New York: Academic Press.

Slater, S., de la Vega, C. E., Skyler, J., & Murphy, D. L. (1976). Plasma prolactin stimulation by fenfluramine and amphetamine. *Psychopharmacology Bulletin, 12*(4), 26.

Smith, W. L., & Lowery, J. B. (1972). The effects of diphenylhydantoin on cognitive functions in man. In W. L. Smith (Ed.), *Drugs, development and cerebral function* (pp. 344–351). Springfield, IL: Charles C Thomas.

Stein, H., Hasan, A., & Fox, L. (1976). Ascorbic acid induced uricosuria. *Annual of Internal Medicine, 84*, 385–388.

Stockley, I. (1981). *Drug interactions*. London: Blackwell Scientific.

Stores, G., Hart, J., & Piran, N. (1978). Inattentiveness in school children with epilepsy. *Epilepsia, 19* 169–175.

Volkmar, F. R., Paul, R., Cohen, D. J., & Shaywitz, B. A. (1983). Irritability in autistic children treated with fenfluramine. *New England Journal of Medicine, 309*, 187.

Von Muhlendahl, K. E., & Krienke, E. G. (1979). Fenfluramine poisoning. *Clinical Toxicology, 14*, 96–106.

Wentzler, R. (1979). *The vitamin book*: New York: Doubleday.

Willett, W., Sampson, C., Bain, B., Rosner, C. H., Hennekins, J., Witschie, J., & Speizer, F. E. (1981). Vitamin supplement use among registered nurses. *Annual Journal of Clinical Nutrition, 34*, 1121–1125.

Williams, R. J., & Kalita, D. K. (1977). *A physicians handbook of orthomolecular medicine*. New Canaan, CT: Keats.

Winsberg, B., & Yepes, L. E. (1978). Antipsychotics. In J. S. Werry (Ed.), *Pediatric psychopharmacology* (pp. 234–273). New York: Brunner/Mazel.

Wing, L. (1969). The handicaps of autistic children: A comparative study. *Journal of Child Psychology and Psychiatry, 10*, 1–40.

Megavitamin B6 and Magnesium in the Treatment of Autistic Children and Adults

BERNARD RIMLAND

The idea that a commonplace, nontoxic vitamin can often ameliorate so profound, baffling, and severely disabling a condition as autism is incredible to many people. Yet despite its initial implausibility, the evidence is clear and compelling: Vitamin B6, when given in large amounts, especially when given with moderate amounts of magnesium and the other B vitamins, can safely bring about substantial improvement in a significant proportion of children and adults diagnosed as autistic. The improvement is seen not only in behavior but also in laboratory measurements of brain waves and urinary constituents. In this chapter I will review the available evidence bearing on the use of megadose vitamin B6 in the treatment of autistic children and adults.

My first exposure to the idea that massive supplements of the B vitamins might be helpful in improving the learning and behavior of autistic children came about in 1964, soon after my book *Infantile Autism* was published. I had begun to receive hundreds of letters from parents and professionals throughout the United States, as well as overseas. Among these letters were several from mothers of autistic children who had read popular books on nutrition by such authors as Adelle Davis, Roger Williams, and Carlton Fredericks. My reaction to the first few letters that described significant improvement in autistic children given vitamins in large amounts was skepticism. However, as more letters arrived in the ensuing months, my skepticism mellowed, my curiosity was aroused, and I became convinced that further study of the matter was required.

Within a few years I had a list of names and addresses of over 1000 parents, primarily from throughout the United States, Canada, and England. Thinking that perhaps a considerable number of parents had tried megavitamin therapy on their children with negative results but had not bothered to tell me about their informal experiments, I decided to collect information on megavitamin therapy in a systematic manner. Accordingly, I sent a questionnaire to over 1000 parents on my mailing list, asking for detailed information on any

---

BERNARD RIMLAND • Institute for Child Behavior Research, San Diego, California 92116.

vitamins they might have tried on their children. (I knew too little, then, to ask about minerals.) I asked which vitamins, if any, had been tried, what the dosage levels were, for how long the vitamins had been administered, what benefits, if any, had been observed, and what adverse effects, if any, had been noted. The survey brought in detailed case studies on the use of high-dosage vitamins from the parents of 57 children, as well as from the seven physicians I had learned of who had used vitamins in high dosage in treating children with severe behavior disorders. Some of the parents had experimented with as many as nine individual vitamins. I was struck by the extent to which the trial-and-error efforts had so often converged to the same four vitamins: ascorbic acid, niacin (or niacinamide), pyridoxine, and, to a lesser extent, pantothenic acid. Over half of the children for whom we received reports had shown significant improvement, and in some cases the improvement was quite remarkable.

The reports showed enormous diversity in the combinations and in the range of dosages used by the parents and physicians who had experimented with the vitamins. In most cases in which the vitamins appeared beneficial, increasing the dosage beyond a certain level did not bring about commensurate improvement, although the dosage levels that appeared best were markedly above the usual levels. In the case of vitamin B6, for example, the amounts exceeded 200 times the recommended dietary allowance (RDA). It was also quite clear from our reports that no significant ill effects had occurred in any of the children, despite the use, in many cases, of very high dosage levels of these vitamins. There were a number of individual case reports that showed striking examples of behavioral improvement associated with the use of the vitamins, and equally striking examples of behavioral deterioration that were clearly associated with the cessation of the use of the vitamins.

At about this time a study was published in England by Heeley and Roberts (1966) in which 11 of 19 autistic children were found to exhibit an abnormality of their tryptophan metabolism. When each of the 11 children was given 30 mg of vitamin B6, the tryptophan load test produced normal results. Despite the favorable results of the one-time administration of vitamin B6 to these children, no attempt was made by the researchers to continue the administration of B6 or to determine the possible beneficial effects of the B6 on the children's behavior. However, 1 of the 11 children who had shown benefits from the administration of vitamin B6 was the son of professor Jeremy Noakes, who reasoned that if his son's urine showed benefits from the administration of vitamin B6 supplements, perhaps his son's behavior might also show some benefits. Accordingly, he continued to give his son 30 mg a day of vitamin B6. His son's behavior showed such remarkable improvement that Professor Noakes wrote a long letter to the London *Observer* describing the changes in behavior and sudden onset of speech. The text of Noakes's letter appears in Rimland (1973).

The result of my survey of parents and physicians, together with the findings of Heeley and Roberts, convinced me that it was necessary to do systematic research on the effects of megavitamin therapy on autistic children.

THE FIRST INSTITUTE FOR CHILD BEHAVIOR RESEARCH VITAMIN STUDY

Since our first study has been reported in detail elsewhere (Rimland, 1973, 1974), only the broad outline will be provided here.

The subjects in our study were several hundred children in the United States and

Canada who were considered autistic by their parents and by their physicians (usually a pediatrician or a psychiatrist). The parents were recruited from our mailing list and were required to obtain cooperation from their physicians. The study took 4½ months. The parents agreed to submit a detailed behavioral checklist every 2 weeks. The physicians agreed to submit the checklist every month.

Each child was given the same vitamin regimen, the dosage varying with the weight of the child. The children were started on a multiple B vitamin tablet plus several grams per day of vitamin C. The multiple B tablet was given prior to the child's being given megadoses of the B vitamins because we felt that it was reasonably well established that megadoses of any of the B vitamins could induce deficiencies of the other B vitamins, unless the other B vitamins were supplemented in at least moderate amounts.

After 2 weeks, niacinamide and pyridoxine were added, each in quantities several hundred times the usual dosage. Finally, after 2 more weeks, several hundred milligrams of pantothenic acid were added. We thought that by staggering the onset of each vitamin, we would be in a better position to determine the differential effects of the vitamins, as well as to observe their effects in combination.

After 3 months on the vitamins, a "no-treatment" period was instituted, so that any changes that resulted from the discontinuance of the vitamins could be observed. The vitamins were then reinstated briefly as the final stage of the design.

In addition to the one-page questionnaire/checklist completed by the parents every 2 weeks and by the physicians every month, the parents completed a more intensive questionnaire at the conclusion of their child's participation in the study.

Although an intensive review of the literature had convinced me that all of the vitamins used were nontoxic, even in large quantities, we required the parents to obtain the participation of a physician of their choice, both as protection against the possibility of adverse reaction and to provide an independent opinion on the child's response to the vitamins.

Complete data were available for 191 children. The major criterion of the effectiveness of the treatment was a two-digit score, assigned systematically by two independent judges, which ranged from 10 to 99, with 99 meaning maximum possible improvement. These overall improvement scores were assigned and independently checked by the two judges, after intensive study of all parent and doctor reports for each child. Discrepant or ambiguous ratings were resolved by discussion or excluded from the analysis.

The design of the study is quite unusual. Critics with a limited understanding of statistics and experimental design have incorrectly categorized our study as "open" and "uncontrolled." In fact, the study used a highly sophisticated computer-clustering principle that precluded the possibility of finding significant results as a consequence of placebo effects or parental hopes or expectations (see Rimland, 1973, for details).

The customary double-blind control group and placebo crossover design has many limitations. Some of the many shortcomings of the traditional experimental designs are discussed in my chapter in *Orthomolecular Psychiatry* (Rimland, 1973). One important reason for our not using a double-blind crossover design is that most conventional double-blind designs presuppose that the subjects constitute a homogeneous group that will respond (or fail to respond) uniformly to the treatment. Such an assumption is obviously false.

Our computer-clustering design used detailed case history information about each child, collected before the treatment was initiated, to group the children into a number of homogeneous clusters. At the completion of the study, it was found that the various computer-created subgroups had responded differentially to the vitamins, to a statistically significant extent. That is, as predicted, some subgroups showed large treatment effects, while others showed little or none. The analyses were repeated at three different computer centers, using different clustering programs, with highly significant results reported from each computer center (Rimland, 1973).

Table 1 presents a summary of the overall results. As may be seen from the table, 41 (21.5%) of the children were reported to have shown some improvement, while 86 (45.3%) were reported to have shown definite improvement. Thus, approximately two-thirds (66.5%) of the children showed at least some improvement.

Some critics of our study have suggested that our findings may reflect only wishful thinking, and have suggested that our positive results might stem from the fact that many parents would be inclined to overrate the vitamins because they want so badly to see their child improve. This criticism is not valid, since parent expectation could not influence the computer grouping. The children were grouped by the computer from data collected prior to the initiation of the vitamins, and the improvement ratings were not used in the analysis until after the subgroups had been formed.

A quite unexpected side effect of the vitamins was, in many cases, an improvement in the child's physical well-being. Many parents reported improved skin condition or hair texture, better muscle tone, and the cessation of teeth grinding. But, of course, of most interest was the sought-for behavioral improvement that constituted the basic reason for doing this study. In many children the improvement was striking. It shows up most clearly in contrasting the behavior of the child during the several months he or she was on the vitamins— during which time there was often a gradual improvement—with his or her behavior during the no-treatment period when the vitamins were suddenly stopped.

I am frequently asked what kinds of changes the vitamins bring about in the children. It is hard to characterize such changes in any simple way, except to say that the children who are helped are moved in the direction of being more *normal*. There is more social interaction with parents and siblings, more general awareness, fewer tantrums and disruptive acts, greater interest in speech and other means of communication, better sleeping and eating

Table 1. Distribution of "Overall Improvement" Ratings in First Megavitamin Study (Magnesium Not Used)

	Scores	Description	No. of cases
Definite improvement 45.3%	90–99	Maximum improvement in all areas	3
	80–89	Very good improvement	38
	70–79	Significant (definite) improvement	45
Some improvement 21.6%	60–69	Some improvement	41
Possible improvement 19.5%	50–59	Possible improvement	37
No improvement 10.5%	40–59	No change	20
Adverse effects 3.2%	30–39	Some behavior deterioration	4
	20–29	Much deterioration	2
	10–19	Great deterioration	1
Totals 100%			191

habits, and other improvements. The entire spectrum of the child's behavior moves toward that seen in nonautistic children—sometimes strikingly so. Examples are given in Rimland (1973, 1974).

Also impressive, beyond the statistical data, are the reports we received from teachers who in their records documented improvements when the children were on the vitamins and deterioration when the children were taken off the vitamins—even though these teachers had been unaware that the children were in our study or that the children were on or off treatment at any time. We had asked the parents to keep secret from the school the child's being in the study until it was over.

Soon after the study started, we began receiving parental reports of some side effects: bed-wetting in previously dry children, sound sensitivity, and irritability. These side effects were not severe enough to warrant curtailing the study or removing the children showing the side effects from the study, but they were somewhat worrisome. Puzzled by these unexpected adverse findings, we consulted professors of neurology at the nearby medical school, but they were unable to shed light on the problem.

Then, toward the end of the study, I received a telephone inquiry on the progress of the research from nutritionist Adelle Davis, who had served as a consultant to us in the design of the study. I told her that we had over 200 children enrolled and that the study was about three-quarters completed.

She asked what supplements the children were getting, and I told her that we were giving them the multiple B tablet that she had designed for us, plus several grams a day of vitamin C and niacinamide and several hundred milligrams a day of vitamin B6 and pantothenic acid. She expressed surprise on learning we were not using the several hundred milligrams of magnesium per day that she had recommended. When I explained that none of our seven consultant physicians had supported her recommendation to use magnesium, she asserted that we were "going to have problems." Some of the children would show enuresis, sound sensitivity, and irritability, she predicted.

Startled by her prescience, I explained that we had indeed been seeing these problems and were puzzled by them. After chiding me for failing to take her advice, she called my attention to a section in one of her books in which she pointed out that individuals taking large amounts of vitamin B6 ran the risk of an induced magnesium deficiency unless magnesium supplements were also used. Enuresis, sound sensitivity, and irritability were signs of magnesium deficiency.

When we added the magnesium, the effects of the magnesium deficiency disappeared, literally overnight. Further, in many cases children who had improved on the vitamin regimen showed still greater improvement when the magnesium was added.

In furtherance of her concept that nutrients work in synergistic combinations, Adelle Davis had also emphasized in her books and in her lectures that one could easily induce a B-vitamin deficiency by giving large amounts of any one of the B vitamins without also administering the entire B complex in small or moderate amounts. I will return to this point later, in my discussion of the safety of vitamin B6.

Our reason for having staggered the onset of the different vitamins was to help us and the parents determine which of the vitamins was most effective. At the conclusion of the study, many of the parents whose children had showed marked improvement asked us which vitamins they should continue, and at what dosage levels. We suggested to them that they experiment with the different vitamins that had seemed to them to be most effective by doubling the dosage level, and by halving the dosage levels of the vitamins that did not appear to them to be especially helpful.

The results of these trial-and-error experiments by the parents, as well as of our own observations during the study, implicated vitamin B6 as having the most profound effects on the largest number of children. Very often the effects were seen most clearly after the parent had doubled the 150 mg per 50-pound body weight initial dosage of B6. In particular, remarkable improvement in the child's speech was commented upon as a frequent consequence of doubling the B6 dosage.

At about the same time our study of vitamin therapy in autistic children was being conducted, a German investigator, Bonisch (1968), reported his experience with B6 treatment of 16 children diagnosed as autistic, out of a larger group of 200 "brain-damaged" children. Twelve of the 16 were reported as becoming more interested and accessible. Like our cases, the German children showed dramatic improvement in speech. Three children spoke for the first time while on the B6 treatment, and language development reportedly improved for two others. Nine children grew restless and showed disturbances of sleep until the B6 dosage was reduced. Bonisch used 100 mg to 600 mg of B6 per day, with most of the dosages at the 300- to 400-mg level.

THE INSTITUTE FOR CHILD BEHAVIOR RESEARCH/UNIVERSITY OF CALIFORNIA MEDICAL SCHOOL VITAMIN B6 STUDY

As noted earlier, our first large-scale study used a computer-clustering technique, rather than a double-blind placebo crossover design, largely because we could not be assured of the homogeneity of the sample. Once the study was complete, it became possible to identify a relatively homogeneous group that had responded to the vitamin B6 and could therefore be utilized in a double-blind crossover study. Such a study was undertaken with Enoch Callaway, of the Department of Psychiatry at the University of California Medical School in San Francisco, and Pierre Dreyfus, of the Department of Neurology, University of California Medical School in Sacramento.

I selected 16 responders from the children in the first study and matched them as closely as possible on age and sex, so as to make up eight matched pairs of subjects. The children were located throughout the United States. Contact with the families and physicians was primarily by mail or phone, although a research assistant traveled to many of the families' homes to help in constructing the "target symptom checklist" that provided an individualized means of evaluating each child's behavioral change.

The 16 names and addresses (8 pairs) were submitted to Dreyfus, who randomly assigned one member of each pair to group A and the other to group B. Only Dreyfus knew whether a given child was in the A or B group. Each family was sent two bottles by Dreyfus, one marked A and one marked B. The children in the A group received in bottle A a vitamin supplement identical to the one they were already taking, including the same amount of vitamin B6 their parents had decided was best for them, as well as the other B vitamins and magnesium. In the B bottle for this group was tablets that resembled the A bottle tablets in all respects, except that they did not contain vitamin B6. For the children in the B group, the tablets in the bottle marked A were the placebos and contained all the vitamins and minerals that the child was ordinarily getting, except for the B6. The B bottle for this group contained the full range of supplements the child was taking, including the B6. In summary, group A received the vitamin B6 in bottle A, which was taken during period A, while group B received the vitamin B6 from bottle B, during period B.

A target symptom checklist was individually prepared for each child in the study. The checklist provided a means of recording the frequency of occurrence of each of a number of specific symptoms for each child that were considered particularly troublesome by that child's parents and teacher. The completed checklists were submitted periodically to the Institute for Child Behavior Research, in San Diego, which accumulated them for study. When all of the target symptom checklists had been collected for all 16 children, for both periods A and B, and for the 3-week-long (average) "washout" period between periods A and B, the data were ready for analysis.

After the data were collected, Callaway joined Rimland in San Diego to evaluate each child's differential response during periods A and B. Only after all of the behavioral ratings had been made by Callaway and Rimland was Dreyfus telephoned so he could compare the Callaway/Rimland behavioral ratings with his own records of vitamin/placebo status of each child during periods A and B.

On the basis of the target symptom checklist data, Callaway and Rimland classified each of the 16 children into predicted groups A or B, except for case No. 16. For case No. 16, they could find no difference between the behavior under condition A and that under condition B.

The Callaway/Rimland ratings of the children were found to be correct in 11 of the 15 comparisons. In the case of the 16th child, where they could not differentiate his behavior during phase A from phase B, it turned out that both of the bottles contained B6! Additionally, in case No. 14, the urine showed three times as much pyridoxic acid during period B, when the child was supposedly on placebo. Nevertheless, we counted case No. 14 as a "miss," (against our hypothesis) in the statistical analysis.

Statistical analysis of the behavioral data demonstrated significance at the .05 level, despite the problem with case No. 14. The second study, like the first, had produced positive results.

ADDITIONAL STUDIES IN THE UNITED STATES OF VITAMIN B6 WITH AUTISTIC INDIVIDUALS

Two additional studies of the use of vitamin B6 in autistic individuals have since been done in the United States. One of these, an open clinical pilot study (Gualtieri, van Bourgondien, Martz, Schopler, & Marcus, 1981), included 15 autistic children, ages 6 to 16, widely dispersed throughout the state of North Carolina. The B6 was given in a powdered supplement that also contained magnesium and other background nutrients. Only the B6 was given in "mega" quantities ranging from 300 to 900 mg per day, depending on body weight. The main effects were seen during a 12-week full-treatment period, followed by a variable-length no-treatment period.

Six of the children were described as responders: "parents were all quite convinced that substantial changes . . . had occurred in the children, and that continued treatment with pyridoxine and Nuthera was important and desirable. Further, in all of the responders, there was consensus among parents, teachers, and therapists that a favorable response had occurred. . . . The improvements were noted in the following areas: less moodiness, decreased hyperactivity, fewer tantrums, more attentiveness, more play, increased appetite, decreased self stimulation, increase in spontaneous speech, more cooperation and improved general health."

In this study, despite the fact that the parents of the responders reported improved general health as a "side effect," four families reported negative side effects during the treatment phase; two children had diarrhea and two experienced increased urinary incontenence. "In all these cases, the symptoms disappeared when the dose was decreased or the vitamins were discontinued."

Gualtieri *et al.* reported two additional interesting findings. The first was that, despite the marked improvement reported for the responders, the improvement in no case was reported as global, and many of the more severe autistic symptoms and mannerisms remained: "Relative to normal children, they were still gravely handicapped. However, relative to their condition prior to initiating treatment, they had improved markedly."

The second finding was that basal serum prolactin (PRL) levels were lower in the responders than in the nonresponders. The difference was significant at the .05 level, despite the small number of cases. This finding warrants further investigation.

Ellman (1981) reported a double-blind crossover study of vitamin B6 among adult and adolescent patients at a California State Hospital. Eight of these subjects were given 1 gram per day of vitamin B6 and ½ gram per day of magnesium lactate for 30 days, then switched to a placebo. The other 8 subjects received the placebo first and the B6 and magnesium during the second 30-day period. Four of the 16 subjects were reported to show significant improvement when on the B6–magnesium combination. Five additional subjects showed improvement on some of the evaluation scales, but the improvement was less significant and not as marked as in the clear responders. Analysis of the urine of the responders as compared to the nonresponders did not suggest a pyridoxine deficiency in the responders.

THE FRENCH STUDIES OF VITAMIN B6 AND MAGNESIUM

Soon after completing the study with Rimland and Dreyfus, Callaway spent a sabbatical at the Bretonneau Psychiatric Hospital in Tours, France, where he undertook a series of collaborative studies of vitamin B6 with Gilbert Lelord and colleagues. Callaway reported that there was an initial reluctance—in fact, resistance—on the part of many of the staff to the idea of administering vitamins to the children at the institution. Many staff members felt that they were dealing with very severe disorders, and substances as innocuous as vitamins could obviously have no worthwhile beneficial effects on children so profoundly impaired as those at Bretonneau. Nevertheless, an open clinical trial of vitamin B6 was tried on 44 institutionalized children "with autistic symptoms" at the hospital (Lelord *et al.*, 1981).

Fifteen of the group were rated as improved, showing better social behavior, increased alertness, reduced negativism, less self-injurious behavior, and fewer tantrums. The improvement disappeared within 10 days after the treatment was terminated in 10 of the children, and in 3 weeks in 14 of the 15. In several cases, according to Callaway (personal communcation) the improvement in the behavior of the children was so striking that some of the staff members, who had originally resisted initiating the study, insisted that the children be kept on the vitamin B6 because they were so much more alert and easier to manage.

Urinary homovanillic acid levels were measured before and during treatment for 37 of the autistic patients and 11 normal control children. The autistic children showed elevated HVAs initially, dropping to near-normal levels during B6 administration. In contrast, the HVA mean for the normal children *rose* slightly, largely as a result of an increase in the children with initially low levels. Thus, the B6 seems to *normalize* the HVA level, in both autistic and control children, by moving the means in opposite directions.

Of the 13 children who had responded to B6 in the open trial, 10 responded again during the double-blind placebo crossover study, while only 2 of the 8 nonresponders showed a positive response to B6 in the double-blind study ($p < .01$).

Preliminary auditory evoked potential (AEP) studies on 12 of the autistic patients, compared to 11 normal controls, suggested tendencies toward normalization (lowering) of the AEP amplitudes in the autistic children.

The Bretonneau group, intrigued by these findings, began an important series of follow-up studies designed to elucidate the effects of vitamin B6 and magnesium, used separately and jointly, on the behavior, HVA levels, and AEPs of both autistic children and autistic adults.

Barthelemy et al. (1981) followed up the original study by conducting three therapeutic crossed-sequential double-blind trials on 52 autistic children. In trial A, B6 and magnesium were compared with placebo, in trial B, magnesium alone was compared with placebo, and in trial C, B6 alone was compared with placebo. Behavioral rating scales showed marked improvement in the B6–magnesium combination, but not on B6 or magnesium alone. Responsiveness increased and bizarre behavior decreased significantly, while verbal behavior increased and sleeping, eating, and incontinence improved, at the .01 level. HVA excretion normalized (lowered), at the .02 level.

A similar but larger study was reported by Martineau, Barthelemy, Garreau, and Lelord (1985), who performed four therapeutic crossed-sequential double-blind trials on 60 autistic children, again to compare the effectiveness of B6 and magnesium with various combinations of B6 and magnesium alone or with placebos. Again the combination of B6 and magnesium was found to be better than any of the alternatives. Significant improvements were seen in behavior ($p < .02$) and in evoked potentials ($p < .05$).

The electrophysiological effects of B6 and magnesium were investigated by Martineau, Garreau, Barthelemy, and Lelord (1982) in a study involving conditioned evoked potentials. During trial A, 12 autistic children received either 30 mg/kg of B6 and 15 mg/kg of magnesium or placebo. During trial B another group of 12 received either 15 mg/kg of magnesium alone or placebo. Each trial lasted 30 days, with a crossover of 15 days. EPs were recorded on the 11th and 26th days. B6 and magnesium together lengthened (normalized) the N_1 and P_2 latency ($p < .05$); little effect was seen from magnesium alone.

Jonas, Etienne, Barthelemy, Jouve, and Mariotte (1984) performed a 22-week therapeutic trial of B6 and magnesium on eight autistic adults. Communication and affective reaction showed significant improvement ($p < .05$ and $p < .01$, respectively). A nonsignificant trend toward improvement of the urinary metabolites of dopamine, especially HVA, was observed.

The first systematic long-term follow-up of an autistic child on B6 and magnesium was reported by Martineau, Barthelemy, and Lelord (1986), who studied a 4-year-old boy over a period of 8 months. The child had proven to be responsive to B6 and magnesium in the earlier group experiments. His behavior was rated twice a week by two raters, and seven periodic HVA and EP measurements were made (including one each before and after treatment). Improvement ranging from 85 to 50% in symptom reduction was observed in various sections of the rating scales. The urinary HVA level increased during the B6–magnesium treatment, owing to a strong augmentation of the conjugated fraction. AEP findings were inconsistent.

Six weeks after the end of the B6–magnesium treatment, the child's autistic symptoms returned to such a degree that it was decided to place him back on the treatment. At the time of the report, "He is a more socially adapted 6-year-old boy. His intellectual evolution

Table 2. Studies of High-Dosage Vitamin B6 and Magnesium in Autistic Children and Adults

Author/year	Subjects/dosage	Design/outcome
Heeley & Roberts 1966	16 autistic children; 30 mg B6 one time (1 child continued)	Tryptophan load test, 11 of 16 children normalized urine (child who continued showed "remarkable" progress)
Bonisch 1968	16 autistic children; 100 mg– 600 mg B6 (mostly 300– 400 mg)	Open trial; 12 of 16 improved, 3 spoke for the time
Rimland 1973	191 autistic children; 4 megavitamins, 150 mg– 450 mg B6	Computer cluster subgroups; 45% "definite improvement" ($p < 02$).
Rimland, Callway, & Dreyfus 1978	16 autistic children; 75 mg– 3000 mg B6 (mostly 300– 500 mg)	Double-blind placebo crossover; 11 of 15 better on B6 ($p < .05$)
Gualtieri et al. 1981	15 autistic children; 300 mg– 900 mg B6, 80 mg–400 mg magnesium, plus other vitamins and minerals	Open trial 12 weeks, then no-treatment period; 6 children showed "substantial" improvement, basal serum prolactin levels (PRL) were lower in responders ($p < .05$)
Ellman 1981	16 autistic adults and adolescents; 1 gram/day B6, 500 mg/day magnesium	Double-blind placebo crossover, 4 showed global improvement, 5 showed partial improvement
Barthelemy et al. 1981	52 autistic children, 11 normal controls; 30 mg/kg/day B6 (up to 1 gram), 10–15 mg/ kg/day magnesium	Three double-blind crossovers, comparing B6 alone, magnesium alone, and B6 + magnesium with placebo, B6 + magnesium was best, highly significant ($p < .01$– $p < .001$) decreases in autistic behaviors, significant ($p < .02$) decreases in urinary HVA
Lelord et al. 1981	Study 1: 44 children with autistic symptoms; Study 2: 21 children selected from above 44; 600 mg– 1125 mg/day B6, 400 mg– 500 mg/day magnesium	Study 1: open trial to identify responders; Study 2: double-blind placebo crossover comparing responders and nonresponders; 15 of 44 improved, in 14 of 15, improvement disappeared 3 weeks after cessation of treatment; double-blind study confirmed behavior improvement ($p < .01$), HVA levels ($N = 37$) also improved ($p < .01$)

(continued)

Table 2. (Continued)

Author/year	Subjects/dosage	Design/outcome
Martineau et al. 1982	24 autistic children; 30 mg/kg/ day B6, 15 mg/kg/day magnesium	Compared electrophysiological effects of magnesium given alone or with B6, in conditioning experiment, B6 + magnesium significantly improved brain response latencies and amplitudes ($p < .05$)
Jonas et al. 1984	8 autistic adults; 1 gram/day B6, 380 mg/day magnesium	Double-blind crossover; behavior improved significantly, nonsignificant improvement in HVA excretion.
Martineau et al. 1985	60 autistic children; 30 mg/kg/ day B6 (up to 1 gram/day), 10 mg–15 mg/kg/day magnesium	4 crossed sequential double-blind trials, comparing B6 alone, magnesium alone, and B6 + magnesium with placebo; B6 + magnesium was best, significant improvement in behavior, HVA excretion, and evoked potentials
Martineau et al. 1986	1 4-year-old autistic child; 30 mg/kg/day B6, 15 mg/ kg/day magnesium	Long-term (8 months) study; clear improvement in behavior, HVA levels, evoked potentials over the 8 months; deterioration 6 weeks after cessation resulted in reinstating B6 + magnesium treatment.

is appropriate for his age (verbal 4 years, nonverbal 4.6 years, symbolic expression 5 years) with language appearing with well-constructed sentences."

The reports of vitamin B6 use in autism are summarized in Table 2.

CRITICISMS OF VITAMIN B6 THERAPY WITH AUTISM

All 12 of the published reports cited in Table 2 provided positive results; no studies have failed to report benefits from the use of vitamin B6 and magnesium in cases of autism. Why is this treatment not in wide use? The reason is, unfortunately, that most medically trained people are committed to the idea that vitamins are to be used only in cases of overt vitamin deficiency, and then only in small amounts. Discussion with hundreds of parents of autistic children and scores of physicians over a period of years discloses the following four reasons to be commonly given to parents by physicians who wish to discourage the therapeutic trial of vitamin B6 and magnesium on autistic patients: (1) not scientifically proven, (2) helpful to only a very small fraction of autistic children, (3) improvement not clinically significant, and (4) megadose vitamin B6 said to be unsafe. In the following sections we will address each of these criticisms.

1. *Criticism: Not scientifically proven.* Physicians or other professionals who say this are admitting that they have not done their homework. It is quite obvious from the

evidence provided in this chapter that there is indeed a considerable body of unrefuted scientific evidence favoring the use of vitamin B6.

2. *Criticism: Helps only a few children.*   Since the diagnosis of autism covers a variety of different metabolic disorders, only some of which can be expected to respond to a specific treatment, such as vitamin B6 and magnesium, it is true that only a fraction of the population of children diagnosed as autistic will be helped by the vitamin approach. In our first study (Rimland, 1973) two-thirds of the nearly 200 children in the study were reported to have shown *some* benefit, although in some cases the benefit was not great. A more conservative estimate, using a criterion of "definite improvement," resulted in 45.3% being classified as improved. It must be remembered that in this study a multiple vitamin tablet containing all of the B vitamins and several minerals was employed along with the B6, although magnesium was not used. The multiple B tablet was expected to potentiate the B6, as well as to protect the child from any B-vitamin deficiency that might be induced by the large amount of B6. None of the subsequent studies by other researchers, except Gualtieri *et al.*, have used multiple vitamins to supplement the B6, so these studies may underestimate the effectiveness of B6 and magnesium.

Judging from the available data in both the published studies and from the author's contacts with literally hundreds of parents and physicians who have tried the vitamin approach on autistic children, it is estimated that between 40 and 50% of any substantial size sample of autistic children would be helped by the vitamin B6–magnesium combination, particularly if a comprehensive vitamin and mineral supplement were also provided.

3. *Criticism: Improvement not clinically significant.*   Among the autistic children and adults who show improvement on vitamin B6, the degree of improvement ranges from small to highly significant. While no patient has been cured (apparently vitamin B6 and magnesium are only part of the solution), there have been many instances where enormous benefits have been achieved. In one such instance, the vitamin treatment was tried in desperation by a psychiatrist whose 18-year-old autistic patient was so violent that he was about to be evicted from the third—and last—institution in his city. While even massive drug dosages had not calmed down the patient, the B6 and magnesium helped so dramatically that he was able to return to a quiet and pleasant life at his parents' home. In another case, a 29-year-old autistic adult who was about to be expelled from a sheltered workshop responded so well to B6 and magnesium that he began receiving pay raises and "worker of the week" awards.

4. *Criticism: Vitamin B6 is unsafe.*   When I reviewed the literature on the safety of the water-soluble vitamins prior to my first study in the late 1960s, it was obvious that vitamin B6 (as well as the other water-soluble vitamins I investigated) was quite safe. Correspondence with Paul Gyorgy, the discoverer of B6, and our own intensive search of the literature showed no adverse effects of vitamin B6 in humans, even at high levels. A 1966 review published by the American Academy of Pediatrics came to the same conclusion: "To date there has been no report of deleterious effects associated with daily oral ingestion of large doses of vitamin B6 (0.2 to 1.0 g per day)." In dealing with literally hundreds of parents and physicians who were using vitamin B6 on autistic children, in a few cases in amounts exceeding a gram a day, we encountered very few reports of significant adverse effects, other than the enuresis, sound sensitivity, and irritability mentioned earlier in conjunction with our failure to use magnesium supplements along with the vitamin B6. An upset stomach has occasionally been reported, and there were 3 cases, out of perhaps 600 at that time, of children who became whiny and began crying unexplainably soon after the B6 was

initiated. We advised those parents to discontinue the B6 and start over later at a lower dosage level. It is possible that those 3 instances were children who were catching a cold or were upset for some other reason, but since the onset coincided with the onset of the B6, it is at least possible that the B6 did cause the symptoms in those children. It is also possible that the children were reacting to fillers, binders, or other substances in the tablets.

In 1983 Schaumburg *et al.* published a brief article on "vitamin B6 abuse" in the *New England Journal of Medicine* that attracted an enormous amount of attention and media coverage. Even the *Readers' Digest* carried an article on how vitamin B6 had been found to be "toxic." Schaumburg, from the Albert Einstein Medical College, had joined with six other neurologists from such geographically diverse medical centers as the Mayo Clinic, Northwestern University, and the University of Pennsylvania in presenting the findings on seven patients who had been taking from 2 to 6 grams of vitamin B6 per day for extended periods. The patients had complained of numbness and tingling in their hands and feet, which bothered some of them to the point of interfering with their walking. Interestingly, the muscular strength of their hands and feet was not impaired —only the sensory abilities suffered.

When it was learned that these patients had been taking large amounts of vitamin B6, their doctors requested them to discontinue the B6, and slowly, over a period of many months, the symptoms subsided. It is of particular interest that the patients' symptoms were treated by their neurologists by discontinuing the B6. If the neurologists had been nutritionally sophisticated, they would have given the patients, at minimum, a vitamin B complex supplement, along with supplements of magnesium. As early as 1959, in her book *Let's Have Healthy Children*, Adelle Davis had written, "When an excess of any one B vitamin is taken for a prolonged period . . . it increases the need for the other B vitamins and can produce deficiencies of them." In *Let's Get Well* (1965) she was more specific: "If large amounts of vitamin B6 alone are given, the need for the other B vitamins, particularly B2 and pantothenic acid, is so increased that harm can be done unless they, too, are supplied."

Schaumburg *et al.* made an alarming, but unjustified, recommendation in their paper when they said, "Megavitamin therapy with vitamin B6 for behavioral disorders should be strongly discouraged . . . until the value of such treatment has been clearly determined through controlled studies. . . ." Schaumburg *et al.* apparently were not aware of the fact that they were in all likelihood looking at an induced deficiency of the other B vitamins brought on by megadose vitamin B6, rather than vitamin B6 toxicity. They apparently were also unaware of the controlled studies by me, by Lelord, and by others cited earlier in this chapter, nor were they aware, apparently, of the double-blind controlled study comparing vitamin B6 and methylphenidate on hyperactive children, in which vitamin B6 was found to be safer than, at least as effective as, and longer-lasting than, the methylphenidate (Coleman *et al.*, 1979).

During the period when Schaumburg and his coauthors were collecting their data, writing their article about their seven patients, and waiting for it to be published, literally thousands of patients died as a result of the use of prescription psychoactive drugs. In addition, many more thousands suffered permanent damage, including impaired vision, impaired liver function, and tardive dyskinesia. Tardive dyskinesia is of particular concern in the drug treatment of autistic children, some 26% of the treated children manifesting the movement disorder (Gualtieri, Quade, Hicks, Mayo, & Schroeder, 1984; Ornitz, 1985; Perry *et al*, 1985). Only about 50% of patients with TD recover (Hawkins, 1986).

Several researchers (e.g., Devaugh-Geiss & Manion, 1978) have reported that high-dose vitamin B6 may be an effective means to reduce the frequency and severity of involuntary movements in tardive dyskinesia. Tkacz and Hawkins (1981) reported no cases of tardive dyskinesia in over 10,000 adult schizophrenics given high doses of vitamin C, B3, E, and B6, even though many also had been given neuroleptic drugs, and Hawkins (1986) reported only 26 possible cases of tardive dyskinesia in 58,000 patients treated by physicians who use high-dosage vitamins along with neuroleptic drugs.

Wilcken and Turner (1973) reported a decrease in the level of blood folate in homocystinuric children receiving megadoses of B6 for an extended time, but they reported no anemia, morphological changes in blood cells, or other problems. They recommended accompanying the B6 with a small supplement of folate in order to avoid any problems that might be associated with a folate deficiency. Numbness and tingling in the extremities, such as Schaumburg et al. noted, may be a sign of folate deficiency.

Similarly, Coleman et al. (1985) have reported an apparent lowering of niacin levels in patients given high-dose vitamin B6. It seems evident, or at least likely, from these studies, that Adelle Davis was correct in insisting that large amounts of vitamin B6, or any other B vitamin, should not be taken unless one also takes moderate-size supplements of the other B vitamins.

As noted earlier, in our experience it has almost never been necessary for an autistic patient to take more than 1 gram a day of vitamin B6 (most seem to need between 250 and 750 mg per day, depending largely on body weight), while the patients reported by Schaumburg et al. consumed 2 to 6 grams a day, over an extended period of time, without additional vitamin/mineral supplementation. (Berger & Schaumburg later, 1984, reported similar numbness and tingling complaints in a woman who had taken over 500 mg of B6 daily for some time. This is the only report known to me of adverse effects of any consequence at less than 2 grams daily intake. The woman may have had a severe preexisting B-vitamin deficiency, or it might simply be a rare case of a hypersensitive individual.)

It seems that the Schaumburg et al. report could arguably be said to demonstrate the safety, not the toxicity, of megadose B6. Despite massive doses (2–6 grams, for most of the patients), despite the failure to take other vitamins and minerals, no life-threatening symptoms were seen, and even the symptoms observed started to reverse when the massive intake of B6 was stopped. A far cry from the often lethal toxicity of drugs! Deaths from the use of prescription drugs rank with breast cancer as a major cause of mortality in the United States (Silverman & Lee, 1974). Vitamin B6 has in fact been used to save patients from what would otherwise be lethal overdoses of various drugs. Single doses of 50 grams of B6 have been used in such cases (Sievers & Herrier, 1984).

DISCUSSION

It is important to understand that if extra B6 helps an autistic child, it helps only because that child *requires* more B6 than does a normal child. Of the various genetic neurological conditions that require large amounts of vitamins, B6 is the vitamin most often required in massive amounts (Rosenberg, 1970). There is a crucial distinction between therapy with vitamins and therapy with drugs. Vitamins are substances that are essential to the body's function. They are enabling or facilitating agents that permit metabolism to take place. In contrast, most drugs are foreign to the body and thus can serve only to block or interfere with ongoing natural processes. This vital difference in function between vitamins and drugs helps explain the enormous difference between them in toxicity, and the virtual absence of significant side effects of vitamins (especially water-soluble vitamins) as compared to drugs. Even the non-water-soluble vitamins are considerably safer than generally believed. Davis (1978), after an intensive search of the medical literature, reports fewer than five cases of hypervitaminosis A in the United States each year, and the only death he could discover was that of a "suicidal" Ph.D. chemist in England.

That vitamin B6 helps to normalize the metabolism in many autistic children is evident from the fact that the studies cited earlier show not only behavioral improvement, but also partial normalization of evoked potentials and of metabolic byproducts in the urine.

Another important—but often overlooked—difference between vitamins and drugs is that drugs, as blocking agents designed to interfere with some metabolic step, can be administered alone, although other drugs are often jointly administered to help offset the side effects of the first drug. (I am aware of some autistic children who have been given eight drugs concurrently!) When a vitamin or other nutrient is given, it rarely acts as a single agent within the body. It must join with other molecules—become part of a metabolic team—to do its job properly. Since one can never be sure that a patient's diet contains an abundance of magnesium, zinc, the B vitamins, and so forth, knowledgeable practioners of nutrient therapy almost never give a single nutrient by itself. To practitioners of traditional medical treatment ("one disease, one drug"), the idea of routinely giving a combination of nutrients seems like a shotgun approach and is easily dismissed as quackery.

I am often asked what mechanisms account for the usefulness of vitamin B6 in those autistic children who are helped. At present, no one knows the answer to that question. There are at least five hypothesized mechanisms, but which, if any, of these is the appropriate explanation is not known (Barthelemy et al., 1983). Unraveling the biochemistry of B6 as it applies to autistic children should, in my opinion, be given highest priority on the agenda of researchers in the field of autism. (For an excellent current review of B6 metabolism as it applies to autism, see Coleman & Gillberg, 1985. For a recent review of HVA in autism, see Garnier et al., 1986.)

Another question I am frequently asked is whether there are laboratory tests that will indicate which children will be most likely to respond to the B6–magnesium treatment. Opinions differ on this matter, but my own feeling is that a simple 20-dollar, 2-month trial of the treatment is far more informative, safer, less painful, and less expensive than a laboratory workup that may or may not lead to an appropriate answer to the question. If the child is helped, the dosage level should be adjusted to the smallest amount that maintains the gains in learning and behavior. If the child is not helped, the trial can be discontinued, and little has been lost.

Although the present state of the art in laboratory testing makes such testing a questionable investment, I hope that in a few years diagnostic tests will be routinely available that will tell us not only if a child requires more B6 but also if the child may be helped by modifying the intake of other vitamins, minerals, amino acids, fatty acids, or other substances. Such research is long overdue.

Parents and professionals interested in receiving current information on the use of vitamin B6 in the treatment of autism and related conditions are invited to write to the Institute for Child Behavior Research, 4182 Adams Avenue, San Diego, California 92116, and ask for our publication No. 39, which is updated from time to time as new information becomes available. The Institute also maintains a list of nutritionally oriented physicians who have experience in working with autistic patients.

REFERENCES

Barthelemy, C., Garreau, B., Leddet, I., Ernouf, D., Muh, J. P., & Lelord, G. (1981). Behavioral and biological effects of oral magnesium, vitamin B6, a combined magnesium - B6 administration in autistic children. *Magnesium Bulletin, 3*, 150–153.

Barthelemy, C., Garreau, B., Leddet, I., Sauvage, D., Muh, J. P., Lelord, G., & Callaway, E. (1983). Intérèt des echelles de comportement et des dosages de l'acide homovanillique urinaire pour le contrôle des effets d'un traitement associant vitamine B6 et magnesium chez des enfants ayant un comportement autistique. *Neuropsychiatrie de l'Enfance, 31*, 289–301.

Berger, A., & Schaumburg, H. H. (1984). More on neuropathy from pyridoxine abuse. *New England Journal of Medicine, 311*, 986–987.

Bonisch, V. E. (1968). Erfahrungen met pyrithioxin bei hirngeschadigten kindern mit autistischem syndrom. *Praxis der Kinderpsychologie, 8*, 308–310.

Coleman, M., & Gillberg, C. (1985). *The biology of the autistic syndromes.* New York: Praeger.

Coleman, M., Sobel, S., Bhagavan, H., Coursin, D., Marquardt, M., Guay, M., & Hunt, C. (1985). A double-blind study of vitamin B6 in Down's syndrome infants. Part 1—Clinical and biochemical results. *Journal of Mental Deficiency Research, 29*, 233–240.

Coleman, M., Steinberg, G., Tippett, J., Bhagavan, H. N., Coursin, D. B., Gross, M., Lewis, C., & DeVeau, L. (1979). A preliminary study of the effect of pyridoxine administration in a subgroup of hyperkinetic children: A double-blind crossover comparison with methylphenidate. *Biological Psychiatry, 141*, 741–751.

Davis, A. (1959). *Let's have healthy children.* New York: Harcourt Brace Jovanovich.

Davis, A. (1965). *Let's get well.* New York: Harcourt, Brace, and World.

Davis, D. (1978). Using vitamin A safely. *Osteopathic Medicine, 3*, 31–43.

DeVeaugh-Geiss, J., & Manion, L. (1978). High-dose pyridoxine in tardive dyskinesia. *Journal of Clinical Psychiatry, 39*, 573–575.

Ellman, G. (1981, November). *Pyridoxine effectiveness on autistic patients at Sonoma State Hospital.* Paper presented at the Research Conference on Autism, San Diego.

Garnier, C., Comoy, E., Barthelemy, C., Leddet, I., Garreau, B., Muh, J. P., & Lelord, G. (1986). Dopamine-beta-hydroxylase (DBH) and homovanillic acid (HVA) in autistic children. *Journal of Autism and Developmental Disorders, 16*, 23–29.

Gualtieri, C. T., Quade, D., Hicks, R. E., Mayo, J. P., & Schroeder, S. R. (1984). Tardive dyskinesia and other clinical consequences of neuroleptic treatment in children and adolescents. *American Journal of Psychiatry, 141*, 20–23.

Gualtieri, C. T., van Bourgondien, M. E., Hartz, C., Schopler, E., & Marcus, L. (1981, May). *A pilot study of pyridoxine treatment in autistic children.* Paper presented at the American Psychiatric Association meeting, New Orleans.

Hawkins, D. R. (1986). The prevention of tardive dyskinesia with high dosage vitamins: A study of 58,000 patients. *Journal of Orthomolecular Medicine, 1*, 24–26.

Heeley, A. F., & Roberts, G. E. (1966). A study of tryptophan metabolism in psychotic children. *Developmental Medicine and Child Neurology, 3*, 708–718.

Jonas, C., Etienne, T., Barthelemy, C., Jouve, J., & Mariotte, N. (1984). Intérèt clinique et biochimique de l'association vitamine B6 + magnesium dans le traitement de l'autisme résiduel è l'âge adults. *Therapie, 39*, 661–669.

Lelord, G., Muh, J. P., Barthelemy, C., Martineau, J. Garreau, B., & Callaway, E. (1981). Effects of pyridoxine and magnesium on autistic symptoms—Initial observations. *Journal of Autism and Developmental Disorders, 11*, 219–230.

Martineau, J., Barthelemy, C., Garreau, B., & Lelord, G. (1985). Vitamin B6, magnesium and combined B6-Mg: Therapeutic effects in childhood autism. *Biological Psychiatry, 20*, 467–468.

Martineau, J., Barthelemy, C., & Lelord, G. (1986). Long-term effects of combined vitamin B6-magnesium administration in an autistic child. *Biological Psychiatry, 21*, 511–518.

Martineau, J., Garreau, B., Barthelemy, C., & Lelord, G. (1982). Comparative effects of oral B6, B6-Mg, and Mg administration on evoked potentials conditioning in autistic children. In A. Rothenberger (Ed.) *Proceedings: Symposium and event-related potentials in children*, Essen, F.R.G. June 11–13, 1982, (pp. 411–416). Amsterdam: Elsevier Biomedical Press.

Ornitz, E. (1985). Should autistic children be treated with haloperidol? *American Journal of Psychiatry, 142*, 883.

Perry, R., Campbell, M., Green, W. H., Small, A. M., Die Trill, M. L., Meiselas, K., Golden, R., & Deutsch, S. I. (1985). Neuroleptic-related dyskinesias in autistic children: A prospective study. *Psychopharmacology Bulletin, 21*, 140–143.

Rimland, B. (1973). High dosage levels of certain vitamins in the treatment of children with severe mental disorders. In D. R. Hawkins & L. Pauling (Eds.), *Orthomolecular psychiatry* (pp. 513–539). New York: W. H. Freeman.

Rimland, B. (1974). An orthomolecular study of psychotic children. *Orthomolecular Psychiatry, 3*, 371–377.

Rimland, B., Callaway, E., & Dreyfus, P. (1978). The effects of high doses of vitamin B6 on autistic children: A double-blind crossover study. *American Journal of Psychiatry, 135*, 472–475.

Rosenberg, L. (1970). Vitamin-dependent genetic disease. *Hospital Practice, July*, 59–66.

Schaumburg, H., Kaplan, J., Windebank, A., Vick, N., Rasmus, S., Pleasure, D., & Brown, M. J. (1983). Sensory neuropathy from pyridoxine abuse. *New England Journal of Medicine, 309*, 445–448.

Sievers, M. L., & Herrier, R. N. (1984). Sensory neuropathy from pyrodoxine abuse. *New England Journal of Medicine, 310*, 198.

Silverman, M., & Lee, P. R. (1974). *Pills, profits and politics*. Berkeley: University of California Press.

Tkacz, C., & Hawkins, D. R. (1981). A preventive measure for tardive dyskinesia. *Orthomolecular Psychiatry, 10*, 119–123.

Wilcken, B., & Turner, B. (1973). Homocystinuria: Reduced folate levels during pyridoxine treatment. *Archives of Diseases of Children, 48*, 58–62.

Index

Accident, maternal, as autism risk factor, 181, 184
Achondroplasia, 171
Acidosis, lactic, 53, 170
Acoustic spectral analysis, 48, 54
Activity level, sex differences in, 193
Adenylosuccinase lyase, 169, 170
Affectionate bonding deficits, 24, 25, 26, 27
Affective development, hemispheric specialization basis, 221–223
Aggressiveness, lithium control, 343, 348
Allergic reactions, food-related, 329
Ambidexterity, 112, 113
Amniotic fluid, meconium in, 181, 185
Amphetamines
    adverse effects, 275, 344, 348
    clinical response, 344
    stereotypic behavior and, 108–109
Amygdala
    in autism, 360
        functional deficits, 27
        structure, 20
Anesthesia, use during childbirth, 181, 185
Animal models
    of autism, 49–50
        behavioral, 45
        neurochemical, 250
        social impairment, 50
    of Lesch–Nyhan syndrome, 149–152
Antibody screening, see Serotonin antibody receptor, screening
Anticonvulsant therapy, see also Epilepsy; Seizures, in autism
    adverse effects, 332, 384–385
Antidepressants
    adverse effects, 334
    efficacy, 275
Antipsychotic drugs, efficacy, 252
Antisocial behavior, sex ratio, 193
Apgar score, 181,1 86
Aphasia, 48
Applied research, 3–5
Arousal, see Overarousal
Asperger syndrome, 87

Attentional deficits, neurophysiological factors, 285–286, 312–318
    event-related potential recording, 306–310
Autism
    animal models, 49–50
        behavioral, 45
        neurochemical, 250
        social impairment, 50
    autopsy studies, 84, 248
    basic versus applied research in, 3–5
    behavioral pathology
        characterization, 44–47
        classification, 44–47
        neural development dysfunction and, 35–36
        nutritional factors, 327–330
        in overarousal, 107–109
        sex differences in, 193, 204–205
    biological mechanisms, 16
    brain lesions in, 229–242
        aphasia and, 48
        clinical studies, 230–231
        computerized tomographic scan, 234–235, 236, 237–238
        congenital rubella and, 231
        encephalopathy and, 230–235
        of frontal lobes, 135
        localization, 170–171
        of medial temporal lobes, 21–22, 235–237, 238–240
        neuroanatomical studies, 237–238
        pneumoencephalography, 232, 233–234
        significance, 229–230
    characterization, 84–86
    classification, 44–47
    cognitive dysfunction in
        familial factors, 193
        perceptual inconstancy, 360
        sex differences, 205
        siblings, 89–90
        social impairment and, 46, 128–130
    diagnosis, 44, 83
        Diagnostic and Statistical Manual III criteria, 15
        differential, 163–164

Autism *(cont.)*
  diagnosis *(cont.)*
    sex differences in, 206–207
  drug therapy, 341–356, 374–378, 384–385
    adverse effects, 342–345
    anticonvulsants, 332, 384–385
    dosage, 346
    fenfluramine, 250, 251, 271–272, 342,
      346, 348–349, 350–351, 361, 377–378
    historical background, 346–348
    neurochemical effects, 52
    neuroleptics, 331, 334–334, 346–347, 374–
      377
    nutrition and, 330–334
    opiate antagonists, 345, 351–352, 362,
      364–367
    recent studies, 348–352
    serotonergic transmission effects, 270–272
  encephalopathy and, 166–167, 230–235
  ethology, 45
  etiology, 83–84
    multiple, 163, 264
  familial factors, 86–87, 89–90, 165, 193
  genetic counseling, 53, 99
  genetic evaluation, 96–99
  genetic factors, 84
    autosomal, 165, 198–199
    dominant, 198
    epistasis, 197
    family studies, 86–87
    fragile X chromosome disorder, 89, 90, 91,
      93–95, 98–99, 165–166, 196, 247
    histocompatibility antigen, 32–33
    linkage analysis, 90–91
    lyonization, 197
    multifactorial polygenic threshold, 199–201
    penetrance, 197
    recessive, 86, 90, 97, 98, 165, 197–199
    segregation analysis, 90
    sex ratios and, 196–201
    single gene disorders, 91–96
    twin studies, 32, 86–89, 164–165, 198,
      247
    X-linked, 86, 90, 96, 97, 165, 196–198
    XYY syndrome, 171
  hemispheric specialization, 213–227
    research evidence, 213–227
    theories, 215–221
  homeostatic mechanism, 360
  idiopathic, 86, 91
  immunological factors, 174, *see also* Sero-
    tonin antibody receptor
  infantile
    brain lesions, 229–242
    cerebral–brainstem relations, 107–125
    peripheral laterality, 113–114
  intelligence quotient, 83, 85, 90, 194–195,
    200, 350–351
  megavitamin therapy, 326, 378–384
    vitamin B1, 381

Autism *(cont.)*
  megavitamin therapy *(cont.)*
    vitamin B2, 383
    vitamin B3, 380
    vitamin B6, 381, 383–384, 389–405
    vitamin C, 379, 380–381
  mental retardation and, 83, 84–85, 86
    fragile X chromosome disorder and, 93–94
    intelligence quotient and, 194–195, 200
    sex differences in, 193–195
    in siblings of autistic children, 90
  models, 13–42
    biological mechanisms, 16
    critique of, 33–34
    developmental, 5, 34–36
    etiological specificity, 15–16
    genetic, 32–33
    neuroanatomical, 16–29
    neurochemical, 29, 31–32
    specificity, 14–15
  neonatal factors, 181, 186–187, 231
  neuroanatomy of, 16–29, 170–171, 360–361
    autistic symptoms, 21–29
    computerized tomographic evaluation, 22,
      48–49, 137, 234–235, 236, 237–238,
      248
    functional deficits, 24–29, 30
    localization research, 47–52
    magnetic resonance imaging, 49, 255
    research, 47–52
  neurobiological research priorities, 43–61
    behavioral pathology, 44–47
    localization research, 47–52
    neurochemistry, 52–53
  neurochemistry of, 29, 31–32, 95–96, 174,
    245–261, 361–367
    animal models, 250
    brain opioids, 357–372
    definition, 29
    Huntington chorea and, 145, 146, 148–149
    Lesch–Nyhan syndrome and, 145–160
    Parkinsonism and, 145, 146–147, 148–149
    research, 52–53
    research techniques, 254–256
    risk factors, 247–248
    social attachment, 358–360
  neurofibromatosis and, 93, 171
  neurological dysfunction, 179, 202–204, 229–
    230, 360–361
    cerebral cortex-related, 111–112
    sex differences in, 202–204
    social impairment and, 127–144
  neurological subgroups, 163–178
    birth injury, 167
    blindness, 173
    brain structural changes, 170–171
    congenital syndromes, 171–173
    deafness, 173
    genetic disorders, 164–166
    infectious disorders, 166–167

Autism (*cont.*)
  neurological subgroups (*cont.*)
    metabolic disorders, 167–170
  neuropathology of, 248
    research, 51–52
    techniques, 21
  neurophysiology of, 285–324
    attentional deficits, 312–318
    event-related potential recording, 287–311, 314
    positron emission tomography, 31–32, 50–51, 254–255
  techniques, 249
  nonneurological factors, 229–230
  onset age, 84
  organic brain disease and, 179, 230, 231
  perinatal factors, 181, 184–186, 230–231
    sex differences in, 203–204
  phenylketonuria and, 91, 92, 167, 168–169, 247–248, 326
  prenatal factors, 180–184, 231
    birth order, 182–183
    bleeding during pregnancy, 181, 183
    maternal accident/injury, 181, 184
    maternal age, 180, 182
    maternal drug use, 181, 184
    maternal infectious disease, 181, 183
    preeclampsia, 181, 183–184
    toxemia, 181, 184
  prevalence, 246–247
  risk factors, 247–248
  rubella and, 84, 91, 166, 173, 231, 247
  sex differences, 191–211
    genetic factors and, 196–201
    incidence, 192
    incidence of related disorders, 192–194
    intelligence quotient, 194–195, 200
    mental retardation, 194–195
    normal development, 202–206
    referral rates, 206
    skills, 204–205
  symptoms, 14–15
    neuroanatomy and, 21–29
  tuberous sclerosis and, 92–93, 171
  twin studies, 32, 86–89, 164–165, 198, 247
Autistic syndromes, 15
Autoimmunity, 270
Autopsy studies, 84, 248
Autosomal genetic transmission, of autism
  dominant, 198
  recessive, 165
  sex ratios and, 198–199
Axon
  development dysfunction, 34–35
  structure, 17, 19

Baby Doe case, 64
Barbiturates, for seizure control, 384

Basal ganglia
  dysfunction
    in autism, 23, 133, 360
    in Lesch–Nyhan syndrome, 146–147
    in Parkinson disease, 133
  structure, 17, 18, 20
Basic research, 3–5
Behavior, brain control of, 21
Behavioral pathology, in autism
  characterization, 44–47
  classification, 44–47
  compulsive behavior, 23
  imitative behavior, 215, 217, 222–223
  neural development dysfunction and, 35–36
  nutritional factors, 327–330
  in overarousal, 107–109
  repetitive behavior, 25, 44, 163, 164
  ritualistic, 23
  self-injurious, 146, 148, 149–151, 152, 153, 154, 365
  sex differences in, 193, 204–205
  stereotyped, 25, 26, 27, 28–29, 108–110, 365
Biedl-Bardet syndrome, 171
Bilaterality, 116
Biochemical factors, in autism, *see* Neurochemistry, of autism
Biological mechanisms, of autism, 16
Birth injury, 167
Birth order, 182–183
Blindness, 173
Blood
  dopamine content, 31
  B-endorphin content, 364
  norepinephrine content, 31
  serotonin content, 31, 250–251, 265–269
Brain, *see also* Neuroanatomy; Neurochemistry; Neurologic dysfunction; Neurologic subgroups; Neuropathology; Neurophysiology; *specific areas of the brain*
  behavioral control by, 21
  development, sex differences in, 202–204
  glucose utilization, 31–32, 254–255
  hemispheric specialization, *see* Hemispheric specialization
  metabolic process mapping, 31–32, 254–255
  "new," 20–21
  "old," 20, 21
  opioids, *see* Opioids, brain content
  serotonergic systems, 251–252, *see also* Serotonin
  structure, 17–21
Brain lesions, in autism, 229–242
  aphasia and, 48
  clinical studies, 230–231
  computerized tomographic evaluation, 234–235, 236, 237–238
  congenital rubella and, 231
  encephalopathy and, 230–235
  of frontal lobes, 135
  localization, 170–171

Brain lesions (*cont.*)
  of medial temporal lobes, 21–22, 235–237,
      238–240
    bilateral anterior, 235–236
    neuroanatomic studies, 237–238
    pneumoencephalography, 232, 233–234
    significance, 229–230
Brainstem, in autism, 360
  auditory deficits and, 293–295
  cerebrum relations, 107–125
    activational pathology, 111
    hemispheric specialization, 114–117, 119–
        120
    neurologic deficits, 111–112
    overarousal, 107–110, 117–119
    peripheral laterality, 112–114
  diencephalon interaction, 22–23
  event-related potential recording, 293–295
  hemispheric specialization and, 119–120,
      218–219
  vestibular system interaction, 22–23

Carbamazepine, 384–385
Carbohydrate metabolism disorders, 53, 170
Caregiving, communication and, 359
Catecholamines, *see also names of specific*
      catecholamines
  synthesis, 272–273, 328
Catechol-O-methyl transferase, 253
Central gray lesions, 29
Central nervous system
  in autism, 246–249
    developmental dysfunctions, 34–36
  functional components, 17, 18
  neurotransmitter activity, 29, 31
  structure, 17, 18
Cerebellum, in autism, 237–238
  atrophy, 49
  neuropathology, 51–52, 317–318
Cerebral cortex
  in autism, 360–361
  structure, 17, 18
Cerebrospinal fluid
  homovanillic acid content, 31, 252–253, 273–
      274
  5-hydroxyindoleacetic acid content, 251–252,
      269
  neurotransmitter content, 29
Cerebrum
  brainstem relations, 107–125
    activational pathology, 111
    hemispheric specialization, 114–117, 119–
        120
    neurologic deficits, 111–112
    overarousal, 107–110, 117–119
    peripheral laterality, 112–114
  hemispheric specialization, *see* Hemispheric
      specialization
Cesarean section, 181, 185

Child Behavior Research Vitamin Study, 390–
    395
Childhood Autism Rating Scale, 14–15
Chlorpromazine, 334, 346, 375
Cholecystokinin, 265
Choroid plexus, papilloma, 170
Clonazepam, 384
Coffin Siris syndrome, 171
Cognitive dysfunction, in autism
  familial factors, 193
  perceptual inconstancy, 360
  sex differences, 205
  of siblings of autistic children, 89–90
  social impairment and, 46, 128–130
Communication, *see also* Language disorders;
      Speech
  caregiving and, 359
  nonverbal, 47
    limbic system in, 134
    preverbal gestures, 358, 359
  physician–patient, 66–68
  social attachment and, 359–360
Communicative intent, 25, 26, 27, 28, 134, 359
Communities, health care-related value conflicts
      in, 74–75
Compulsive behavior, 23
Computerized tomographic evaluation
  of autism, 22, 137, 234–235, 236, 237–238,
      248
    quantitative studies, 48–49
  of development disorders, 22
  of Tourette syndrome, 22
Conceptual orientation deficits, 286
  event-related potential recording, 302–305
Conflict values, 66–68, 69–70, 71
Cord complications, as autism risk factor, 181,
    185
Corpus striatum, functional deficits, 28
Coryza, neuroleptic-related, 375–376
Criminality, sex ratio, 193
CT, *see* Computerized tomographic evaluation
Cultural factors, in development disorder-related
      health care, 68–70
Cytomegalovirus infection, 166

Dandy Walker syndrome, 170
Deafness, 173
deLange syndrome, 171
Delivery complications, as autism risk factors,
    167, 181, 184–185
Dendrite
  development dysfunction, 34–35
  structure, 19
Dependency
  in development disorder-related health care,
      70–72
  megavitamin-related, 379
Developmental disorders
  autistic symptomatology, 14

Developmental disorders (cont.)
  computerized tomographic evaluation, 22
  health care-related ethical issues, 63-79
    case approach, 66-79
    conflict values, 66-68, 69-70
    cultural factors, 68-70
    dependency, 70-72
    informed consent, 72-74
    moral conflicts, 71
    moral principles, 63, 71-72, 73
    sexual abuse, 75-78
    values conflicts in communities, 74-75
  hemispheric specialization and, 220-221
  immunological factors, 203
  Lesch-Nyhan syndrome and, 155
  nutritional factors, 325-338
Developmental factors, in autism, 5, 34-36
Diagnostic and Statistical Manual-III, autism
    criteria, 15
Diencephalon, brainstem interaction, 22-23
Displacement behavior, 108-109
Dominant genetic transmission, of autism, 198
Dopa, serotonergic transmission effects, 271
L-Dopa
  adverse effects, 342, 348
  clinical response, 342, 344
Dopamine
  in autism, 52, 118
    blood content, 31
    cholecystokinin coexistence, 265
    in neurotransmitter abnormality research,
      264-265
    pharmacological basis, 274
    pyridoxine interaction, 382
    synthesis, 272
    tissue content, 273-274
  in Lesch-Nyhan syndrome, 147, 148, 149-
    150
  receptors, 150-152, 154, 155
  in schizophrenia, 252
Dopamine agonists, 344
Dopamine antagonists, 343
Dopamine-beta-hydroxylase, 31, 253, 272, 274
Drug therapy, 341-356, 374-378, 384-385, see
    also Megavitamin therapy
  adverse effects, 342-345
  anticonvulsants, 332, 284-285
  dosage, 346
  fenfluramine, 250, 251, 271-272, 342, 346,
    348-349, 350-351, 361, 377-378
  historical background, 346-348
  neurochemical effects, 52
  neuroleptics
    adverse effects, 333-334, 375-376
    efficacy, 374-375
    historical background, 346-347
    metabolism, 331
    withdrawal, 376-377
  nutrition and, 330-334

Drug therapy (cont.)
  opiate antagonists, 345, 362, 365-367
    naloxone, 154, 345, 362, 364
    naltrexone, 345, 351-352, 362, 365-366
  recent studies, 348-352
  serotonergic transmission effects, 270-272
Drug-nutrient interaction, 332-334
Drug-vitamin interaction, 381-383
Drugs, use during pregnancy, 181, 184
Dynorphin, 363
Dyskinesia, drug-related, 349-350

Ear preference, 116
Echolalia, 14, 25, 233
Electroencephalogram (EEG) abnormality, in
    autism, 138, 249
  arousal mechanisms, 109
  event-related potential recording, 287
  hemispheric specialization measurement, 214-
    215
Emotional expression, hemispheric involvement,
    217-218, 221-222
Emotional facial paralysis, 23
Encephalitis, of medial temporal lobe, 236-237
Encephalopathy, congenital, autism and, 230-
    235
  epidemiological factors, 231
  herpes simplex infection and, 166-167
  neuroradiological studies, 231-235
Endorphin(s), 174
  characteristics, 363
  deficiency, 53
Endorphin H, 276
Endorphin system, hyperactivity, 276
B-Endorphin
  blood content, 364
  neonatal exposure effects, 364
  self-injurious behavior and, 365
Enkephalin(s)
  characteristics, 363
  neurotransmitter coexistence, 265
Enkephalin system, hyperactivity, 276
Environmental stimuli
  modulatory response, 24, 25, 26, 27
  response deficits
    attentional, 285-286
    conceptual, 286
    event-related potential recording, 287-311,
      314
    neuroanatomical factors, 24, 25, 26, 27, 28
    neurophysiological factors, 285-286
    novel stimuli and, 299-302
Epilepsy, autism and, 384
  abnormal neural activity, 312, 313-314, 316
Epinephrine, 31
Epistasis, 197
Ethical issues, in developmental disorder-related
    health care, 63-79
  case approach, 65-79

Ethical issues (*cont.*)
  case approach (*cont.*).
    conflict values, 66–68, 69–70
    cultural values, 68–70
    dependency, 70–72
    informed consent, 72–74
    moral conflicts, 71
    moral principles, 63, 71–72, 73
    sexual abuse, 75–78
    value conflicts in communities, 74–75
  terminology, 63–64
Ethology, of autism, 45
Event-related potential recording (ERP), 287–
    311, 314
  advantages, 290–291
  description, 287–288
  interpretation, 291–292
  long-latency components, 296–310
    attentional deficits, 306–310
    auditory stimuli, 293–299, 300–301, 303–
      305, 306, 307–310, 311
    concept modification, 302–305
    event importance, attention to, 302–305
    novel stimuli orientation, 299–302
    visual, 296, 299, 300–301, 303–305, 306,
      307–310
  records
    description, 288
    illustration, 288–290
    types, 290, 292
  research requirements, 292–293
  short-latency components, 293–295
  somatosensory components, 296
  terminology, 287–288
Experimentation, informed consent for, 72–74
Extrapyramidal symptoms, neuroleptic-related,
    376

Face, emotional paralysis of, 23
Faces, recognition of, 128, 129, 130, 313, 132
Familial factors, in autism, 86–87, 89–90, 165,
    193, *see also* Siblings
Family history, 96–97, 98
Family studies, of autism, 86–87
Feingold diet, 329
Fenfluramine, 248–249, 377–378
  adverse effects, 342, 351, 378
  clinical response, 342
  dosage, 346
  efficacy, 361
  hyperserotonemia control, 250, 251
  intelligence quotient effects, 350–351
  serotonergic transmission effects, 271–272
Fetal alcohol syndrome, 171
Fetus, *see also* Prenatal factors
  malposition, 181, 184
Fluphenazine, 343, 346
Folic acid, megadose, 381
  phenytoin interaction, 382

Folic acid deficiency, 332
Food additives, 329
Food allergy, 329
Food cravings, 327–328, 329–330
Forcep delivery, as autism risk factor, 181, 185
Forebrain, structure, 17, 18
Fornix, 20
Fragile X chromosome disorder, 89, 90, 91, 93–
    95, 196
  chromosome culture test, 165–166
  incidence, 247
  mental retardation and, 93–94
  physical examination for, 98–99
Frontal lobes
  dysfunction, 24, 25, 26
    social impairment and, 135
  function, 17
  structure, 17, 18

Gamma-aminobutyric acid (GABA), 254, 255
Gaze aversion, 14, 127, 128
Genetic counseling, 99
  antibody screening, 53, *see also* Serotonin
      antibody receptor
Genetic evaluation, 96–99
  early injury/illness history, 97–98
  family history, 96–97, 98
  neurological examination, 98–99
  physical examination, 98–99
Genetic factors, in autism, 84
  autosomal transmission, 165, 198–199
  dominant transmission, 198
  epistasis, 197
  family studies, 86–87
  histocompatibility antigens, 32–33
  linkage analysis, 90–91
  lyonization, 197
  multifactorial polygenic threshold, 199–201
  penetrance, 197
  recessive transmission, 86, 90, 97, 98, 165,
      197–199
  segregation analysis, 90
  sex ratios and, 196–201
  single gene disorders, 91–96
  twin studies, 32, 86–89, 164–165, 198, 247
  X-linked transmission, 86, 90, 96, 97, 165,
      196–198
    fragile X chromosome disorder, 89, 90, 91,
      93–95, 98–99, 165–166, 196, 247
  XYY syndrome, 171
Gestures, preverbal, 358, 359
Glossary, 54–57
Glucose utilization, by brain, 31–32, 254–255

Haloperidol, 348
  adverse effects, 343, 349
  clinical response, 349–350, 374, 375
  dosage, 346, 374
Hand preference, 112–114, 116

Health care, of developmental disorders, ethical
issues in, 63–79
case approach, 66–79
conflict values, 66–68, 69–70
cultural factors, 68–70
dependency, 70–72
informed consent, 72–74
moral conflicts, 71
moral principles, 63, 71–72, 73
sexual abuse, 75–78
value conflicts in communities, 74–75
Hearing disorders, event-related potential recording, 293–295, 296–299
Hemispheric specialization, 213–227
approach versus withdrawal, 119–120
cerebral–brainstem relations, 114–117, 119–
120
emotional expression control, 217–218, 221–
222
language disorders and, 114–116, 118, 214,
216, 217, 219–220, 221
laterality and
ascending activation, 117–118
bilaterality, 116
central, 115–117
peripheral, 112–114
testing, 116
of medial temporal lobe, 240
neurologic deficits and, 111–112
research evidence, 213–215
in social impairment, 131–133, 221–223
theories, 215–221
developmental, 220–221
left hemisphere hypothesis, 215–216
reduced hemispheric specialization, 216–
218
subcortical dysfunction relationship, 218–
219
testing, 219–220
types of abnormalities, 110–111
Herpes simplex virus infection, 166–167
Heterochrony, 359
Hindbrain, structure, 17, 18
Hippocampus
in autism, 361
functional deficits, 27–28
neuropathology, 316–317
structure, 20
Histocompatibility antigen, 32–33
Homeostatic mechanisms, of autism, 360
Homovanillic acid, 52
cerebrospinal fluid content, 31, 252–253,
273–274
vitamin B6 megadose therapy effects, 396,
398, 398, 399
Huntington chorea
Lesch–Nyhan syndrome and, 148–149
neurochemical factors, 145, 146, 148–149
onset age, 149, 155

Hydrocephalus, 170
5-Hydroxyindoleacetic acid, 31, 265, 267, 268
cerebrospinal fluid content, 251–252, 269
5-Hydroxytryptamine, see Serotonin
5-Hydroxytryptophan, 265, 270
5-Hydroxytryptophol, 265
Hyperactivity, see also Overarousal
Feingold diet for, 329
fenfluramine therapy, 361
stimuli response in, 22
Hyperbilirubinemia, 181, 186
Hyperlactatemia, 170
Hyperlalia, 233
Hyperserotonemia, 250, 267–269, see also
Serotonin
autoimmunity and, 270
Hypocalcinuria, 174
Hypothalamic-pituitary-tropic hormones, 362,
364
Hypothalamus
function, 17
structure, 17, 18, 20
Hypoxanthine-guanine-phosphoribosyltransferase
deficiency, 145, 146, 147–148, 153

Imipramine
adverse effects, 342, 347
clinical response, 342
serotonergic neurotransmission effects, 270–
271
Imitative behavior, hemispheric basis, 215, 217,
222–223
Immunochemistry, 52–53
Immunological factors
in autism, 174, see also Serotonin antibody
receptor
in developmental disorders, 203
Infection, as autism risk factor
maternal, 166, 181, 183
postnatal, 166–167
prenatal, 166, 181, 183
Informed consent, 72–74
Injury, maternal, as autism risk factor, 181, 184
Inosinate dehydrogenase, 169
Intelligence quotient, in autism, 83, 85
behavioral pathology and, 44–45
fenfluramine effects, 350–351
mental retardation and, 194–195, 200
sex differences in, 194–195, 200
of siblings of autistic children, 90

Kanner syndrome, 318
Karyotyping, 99
Kluver–Bucy syndrome, 21, 23, 134
Korsakoff psychosis, 21

Labor, prolonged, as autism risk factor, 181,
185

Language disorders, in autism
  brain opioids and, 358–360
  characteristics, 46–47
  developmental, 22, 46
  hemispheric specialization and, 114–116, 118,
      214, 216, 217, 219–220, 221
  neuroanatomical factors, 21–22, 25, 26, 27,
      28
  pneumoencephalographic findings in, 232–233
  primary, 21
  sex differences in, 193, 194
  social attachment and, 359–360
Laterality
  ascending activation, 117–118
  bilaterality, 116
  central, 115–117
  peripheral, 112–114
  testing, 116
Lead poisoning, 329–330
Learning disabilities, 89
Lesch–Nyhan syndrome, 145–160
  definition, 145
  developmental disorders and, 155
  dopamine deficiency and, 147, 148, 149–150
  dopamine receptors and, 150–152, 154, 155
    supersensitivity, 152
  Huntington chorea and, 148–149
  hypoxanthine-guanine-phosphoribosyltransfer-
      ase deficiency and, 145, 146, 147–148,
      153
  mental retardation and, 145, 148
  neurochemical assessment of, 146–148
  neurochemical deficit modeling of, 149–152
    age-dependent responses, 150–152
  neurological symptoms, 146
  onset age, 146, 149
  Parkinsonism and, 148–149
  self-biting behavior in, 146, 148, 149–151,
      152
    purinergic mechanisms, 147, 153
  treatment, 153–155
Limbic system
  nonverbal communication and, 134
  septum, 20, 28, 33
  social impairment and, 131, 133–135
  speech and, 133
  structure, 17, 20
Linkage analysis, 90–91
Lithium, clinical response, 343, 348
Localization, neuroanatomical, 47–52
Low birth weight, as autism risk factor, 181,
      186
Lyonization, 197

Magnesium, in vitamin B6 megavitamin ther-
      apy, 389, 393, 396, 397–403
Magnesium deficiency, 174
Magnetic resonance imaging, 49, 255
Malnutrition, causes, 326

Mammillary body, 20
Maternal factors, in autism, 181, 183–184
  age, 180, 182
  infection, 166, 181, 183
Meconium, in amniotic fluid, 181, 185
Medulla, structure, 17, 18
Megavitamin therapy, 378–384
  dependency and, 379
  direct toxic effects, 380–381
  increased nutritional requirements and, 326
  mediated toxic effects, 381–384
  vitamin B1, 381
  vitamin B2, 383
  vitamin B3, 380
  vitamin B6, 389–405
    adverse effects, 381, 383–384, 392, 393,
        396, 400–402
    Child Behavior Research Vitamin Study,
        390–395
    criticisms of, 399–402
    drug interaction, 382
    efficacy, 390, 392–393, 394, 395–397,
        398–399
    magnesium combined with, 389, 393, 396,
        397–403
  vitamin C, 391–394
    adverse effects, 380–381
    dependency on, 379
    disease masking by, 381
    drug interaction, 382
    "rebound" scurvy and, 379
  vitamin H, 383
  withdrawal, 379–380
Meningitis, 167
Mental retardation
  autism-associated, 83, 84–85, 86
    fragile X chromosome disorder and, 93–94
    intelligence quotient and, 194–195, 200
    sex differences in, 193–195
  of siblings of autistic children, 90
  Lesch–Nyhan syndrome-associated, 145, 148
  reproductive rights and, 75–78
Mesocortex, dysfunction, 23
Metabolic disorders, 95–96, 167–170
  carbohydrates, 53, 170
  increased nutritional requirements and, 326
  phenylketonuria, 91, 92, 167, 168–169, 247–
      248, 326
  positron emission tomographic evaluation, 31–
      32, 254–255
  purine, 53, 147, 153, 169–170
3-Methoxy-4-hydroxyphenylethylene glycol,
      253, 275
Methylphenidate, 275
Methysergide
  adverse effects, 347
  clinical response, 342
  serotonergic transmission effects, 271
Midbrain, structure, 17, 18

Moebius syndrome, 171
Molindone, 346
Monoamine oxidase, 31, 253, 265, 273, 275
Moral conflicts/principles, in developmental
    disorder-related health care, 63, 66–68,
    69–70, 71–72, 73
Motivational dysfunction, 24, 25, 26, 27
Motor activity disorders
    motor studies of, 48
    neuroanatomical factors, 23, 25, 26, 27, 28
Multifactorial threshold model, of autism genetic
    transmission, 199–201
Mutism, 23
Myelin basic protein, 270

Naloxone
    brain opioid activity test, 362
    clinical response, 345
    prenatal administration, 364
    self-mutilation inhibition by, 154
Naltrexone, 351–352, 362
    clinical response, 345, 352
    efficacy, 365–366
Narcan, see Naloxone
Neocortex, development, 34
Neonatal factors, in autism, 181, 186–187, 231
Neostriatum, dysfunction, 23
Neuroanatomy, of autism, 16–29, 170–171,
    360–361
    autistic symptoms and, 21–29
    computerized tomographic evaluation, 22, 48–
        49, 137, 234–235, 236, 237–238, 248
    functional deficits, 24–29, 30
        amygdala, 27
        frontal lobes, 24, 26
        hippocampus, 27–28
        temporal lobes, 26–27
    localization research, 47–52
    magnetic resonance imaging, 48, 255
Neurobiology, of autism, research priorities, 43–
    61
    behavioral pathology, 44–47
    localization research, 47–52
    neurochemistry, 52–53
Neurochemistry, of autism, 29, 31–32, 95–96,
    174, 245–261, 361–367, see also names
    of specific chemicals
    animal model, 250
    definition, 29
    Huntington chorea and, 145, 146, 148–149
    Lesch–Nyhan syndrome and, 145–160
    Parkinsonism and, 145, 146–147, 148–149
    research, 52–53
        techniques, 254–256
    risk factors, 247–248
    serotonin hypothesis, see Serotonin, in autism
    of social attachment, 358–360
Neurofibromatosis, see von Recklinghausen
    disease

Neuroleptics
    adverse effects, 333–334, 375–377
    efficacy, 374–375
    historical background, 346–347
    metabolism, 331
    withdrawal, 376–377
Neurologic dysfunction, in autism, 179, 202–
    204, 229–230, 360–361
    cerebral cortex-related, 111–112
    sex differences in, 202–204
    social impairment and, 127–144
        basal ganglia involvement, 133
        cognitive impairment versus, 128–130
        frontal lobe lesions and, 135
        limbic system involvement, 131, 133–135
        prosopagnosia, 132
        right hemisphere involvement, 131–133
Neurologic examination, 98–99
Neurologic subgroups, in autism, 163–178
    birth injury, 167
    blindness, 173
    brain structural changes, 170–171
    congenital syndromes, 171–173
    deafness, 173
    genetic disorders, 164–166
    infectious disorders, 166–167
    metabolic disorders, 167–170
Neuron
    developmental dysfunction, 35
    structure, 17, 18, 19
Neuropathology, of autism, 248
    research, 51–52
    techniques, 21
Neuropeptides, 253, 275–276
Neurophysiology, of autism, 285–324
    of attentional deficits, 312–318
    techniques, 249
        event-related potential recording, 287–311,
            314
        positron emission tomographic evaluation,
            31–32, 50–51, 254–255
Neuropsychology, clinical, 45–46
Neurotransmitters, see also names of specific
        neurotransmitters
    activity measurement, 29
    assay, 263–264
    interconnections, 265
    synthesis, 327–328
Niacin, see Vitamin B3
Noonan syndrome, 171
Norepinephrine
    blood content, 31
    in neurotransmitter abnormality research,
        264–265
    synthesis, 253, 272
    tissue content, 274–275
Nosology, clinical, 44–45
Nuclei, of central nervous system, 17
    dentate, 317–318

Nutrition, 325–338
  behavior and, 327–330
  definition, 325–326
  dietary adequacy, 327
  drug therapy and, 330–334
    drug–nutrient interaction, 332–334
    nutrient–drug interaction, 330–331
  food preferences/idiosyncracies, 327–328,
      329–330
  food reactions, 329–330
Nystagmus
  postrotary, 118
  vestibular, 249

Obesity, 326, 328, 333
Opiate antagonists, 362, 365–367
  clinical response, 345
  naloxone, 154, 345, 362, 364
  naltrexone, 345, 351–352, 365–366
Opioids, brain content, 347–372
  language deficits and, 358–360
  play behavior and, 254
  social dysfunction and, 357–360, 362–365
  stereotypy and, 365
  systems, 363
Organic brain disease, see also Brain lesions
  autism and, 230, 231
  incidence, 179
Orienting response deficits
  attentional, 285–286
  conceptual, 286
  event-related potential recording, 287–311,
      314
  neuroanatomical factors, 24, 25, 26, 27, 28
  neurophysiological factors, 285–286
  to novel stimuli, 299–302
Overarousal, 107–110
  activational pathology, 111
  autistic symptomatology and, 117–119
  behavioral factors, 107–109
  psychopathological factors, 109–110
Overnutrition, causes, 326

Pantothenic acid, see Vitamin H
Papilloma, of choroid plexus, 170
Paraaminobenzoic acid, 383
Parents' rights, 64
Parkinsonism
  basal ganglia dysfunction in, 133
  Lesch–Nyhan syndrome and, 148–149
  neurochemical factors, 145, 146–147, 148–
      149
PEG, see Pneumoencephalography
PET, see Positron emission tomography
Penetrance, genetic, 197
Perception
  hemispheric involvement, 217–218
  inconstancy of, 360
  neuroanatomical factors, 23, 24, 25, 26, 27

Perinatal factors, in autism, 181, 184–186, 230–
      231
  birth injury, 167
  sex differences in, 203–204
Peripheral laterality, 112–114
Personal values, 64
Pharmacology, see Drug therapy
Phenobarbital, for seizure control, 384
Phenylketonuria, autism and, 91, 92, 167, 168,
      247–248, 326
  screening, 168
  treatment, 168–169
Phenylpyruvic acid, 168
Phenytoin, 384
Phosphoribosylpyrophosphate synthetase, 169
Photosensitivity, neuroleptic-related, 376
Physical examination, of autistic children, 98–99
Pica, 329–330
Pituitary gland, structure, 18
Play, brain opioids and, 254
Pneumoencephalography, 232, 233–234
  psychotic symptoms and, 138
  of temporal lobe lesions, 21–22
Polygenic model, of autism genetic transmis-
      sion, 199–204
Porencephaly, 170
Positron emission tomography, 31–32, 50–51,
      254–255
Posturing, neuroanatomical basis, 25, 26, 27, 28
Preeclampsia, as autism risk factor, 181, 183–
      184
Prenatal factors, in autism, 180–184, 231
  birth order, 182–183
  bleeding during pregnancy, 181, 183
  maternal accident/injury, 181, 184
  maternal age, 180, 182
  maternal drug use, 181, 184
  maternal infections, 166, 181, 183
  preeclampsia, 181, 183–184
  toxemia, 181, 184
Probenecid, 251–252
Proenkephalin A, 275–276
Proenkephalin B, 276
Proopiomelanocortin, 276
Prosody, 48
Prosopagnosia, 132
Psychopathological factors, in overarousal, 109–
      110
Purine metabolism disorder, 53, 147, 153, 169–
      170
Pyridine, see Vitamin B6
Pyridoxine, see Vitamin B6

Reading disabilities, 89
Recessive genetic transmission, of autism, 86,
      90, 97, 98, 165, 197–199
Recognition disorders
  facial recognition, 128, 129, 130, 131, 132
  neuroanatomical factors, 24, 25, 26, 27

Referral, 206
Repetitive behavior, 163, 164
  as diagnostic criteria, 44
  neuroanatomical factors, 25
Reproductive rights, 75–78
Respiratory distress, neonatal, 181, 186
Rett syndrome, 171–172
Riboflavin, *see* Vitamin B2
Right hemisphere, *see also* Hemispheric
    specialization
  social impairment and, 131–133
Right to life movement, 64
Rights
  of parents, 64
  of patients, 63–64
  reproductive,75–78
Ritualistic behavior, 23, *see also* Repetitive
    behavior
Rubella, congenital, autism and, 84, 91, 166,
    247
  brain lesions and, 231
  deafness and, 173
  prevalence, 231
Rules, ethical, 63

Schizophrenia
  dopamine and, 252, 253
  onset age, 84
  sex differences, 192
Sclerosis, tuberous, 92–93, 171
Scurvy, "rebound," 379
Segregation analysis, of autism genetic factors,
    90
Seizures, in autism, 384
  onset age, 84
Self-injurious behavior
  in autism
    B-endorphin and, 365
    naloxone inhibition, 154
  in Lesch–Nyhan syndrome, 146, 148, 149–
    151, 152
  purinergic mechanisms, 153
Sensory disorders
  event-related potential recording, 296
  vestibular system and, 22–23
Septum, of limbic system, 20
  functional deficits, 28
  lesions, 33
Serotonin
  in autism, 250–252, 265, 361
    blood content, 31, 250–251, 265–269
    brain content, 269
    in neurotransmitter abnormality research,
      264–265
    pharmacological studies, 270–272
    substance P coexistence, 265
    synthesis, 265, 328
  in Lesch–Nyhan syndrome, 147, 148
Serotonin agonist, 342

Serotonin antagonist, 342
Serotonin antibody receptor, 52–53, 174, 252,
    269–270, 361
  screening, 53
Sex differences/ratios
  in autism, 191–211
    activity level, 193
    antisocial behavior, 193
    behavior problems, 193
    diagnosis, 206–207
    genetic factors and, 196–201
    incidence, 192
    incidence of related disorders, 192–194
    intelligence quotient, 194–195
    language disorders, 193, 194
    mental retardation, 194–195
    normal development and, 202–206
    sex hormones and, 202
  in criminality, 193
  in schizophrenia, 192
Sex hormones, sex differences and, 202
Sexual abuse,75–78
Sexual behavior, in autism, 202
Siblings, of autistic children
  autism prevalence among, 246–247
  autism risk among, 165
  cognitive abnormalities among, 89–90
  intelligence quotients of, 90
  mental retardation among, 90
Single gene disorders, 91–96
  biochemical abnormalities, 95–96
  fragile X chromosome disorder, *see* Fragile X
    chromosome disorder
  neurofibromatosis and, 93
  phenylketonuria, 91, 92
  tuberous sclerosis, 92–93
Sleep cycles, in autism, 249
Smiling, 128
Social attachment
  language development and, 359–360
  neurochemistry of, 358–360
Social behavior development, brain opioids and,
    362
Social impairment
  animal model, 50
  brain opioid involvement, 357–350, 362–
    365
  cognitive deficits and, 46, 128–130
  as diagnostic criteria, 44
  hemispheric specialization and, 221–223
  neurological dysfunction and, 127–144
    basal ganglia involvement, 133
    cognitive impairment versus, 128–130
    frontal lobe lesions, 135
    limbic system involvement, 131, 133–135
    prosopagnosia, 132
    right hemisphere involvement, 131–133
  types, 127
Social interaction, social approach and, 45

Speech, autistic
  acoustic spectral analysis, 48
  -characteristics, 132
  hemispheric specialization and, 219–220, 221
  limbic system and, 133
Spinal cord, structure, 17
Stereotypy
  amphetamine-related, 108–109
  dearousal function, 108–110
  neuroanatomical factors, 25, 26, 27, 28–29
  opioids and, 365
Stimulation, avoidance of, 107–108, 110
Stimuli, see Environmental stimuli
Subcortical dysfunction, 218–219
Substance P, 265
Syphilis, as autism risk factor, 166, 247

Tardive dyskinesia, 375, 376–377
Temporal horn, enlargement, 361
Temporal lobe
  function, 17
  functional deficits, 26–27
  lesions, 21–22, 235–237, 238–240
    autistic symptoms and, 21–22
    bilateral anterior, 235–236
  structure, 17, 18
Thalamus
  in autism, 360
    functional deficits, 28
  structure, 20
Thiamin, see Vitamin B1
Thioridazine, 375, 376
Thiothixene, 346
Thyrotropin-releasing hormone, 347–348
Tourette syndrome
  computerized tomographic evaluation, 22
  neuroleptics and, 349, 376
Toxemia, as autism risk factor, 181, 184
Toxoplasmosis, as autism risk factor, 247
Trexan, see Naltrexone
Trifluoperazine, 346–347
Triiodothyronine, 344, 347
Trisomy 21, 171
Trisomy 22, 171
Tryptophan
  blood content, 267–268
  conversion to serotonin, 265, 328
Twin studies, of autism, 32, 86–89, 164–165,
    247
  sex ratio, 198

Umbilical cord complications, as autism risk
    factor, 181, 185
Undernutrition, causes, 326
Unresponsiveness, 128

Valproic acid, 384
Vanillymandelic acid, 275
Verbal skills, in autism, 204, 205, see also Lan-
    guage disorders; Speech
Vestibular system
  functional deficits, 28–29
  nystagmus suppression by, 249
  sensory disturbances and, 22–23
Vision, event-related potential recording, 296,
    299, 300–301, 303–305, 306, 307–310
Visuospatial skills
  right hemisphere function and, 132
  sex differences in, 204–205
Vitamin(s), neurochemical functions, 328
Vitamin B deficiency, lead poisoning and, 330
Vitamin B1, megadose, 381
Vitamin B2
  deficiency, 334
  megadose, 383
Vitamin B3, megadose, 380
Vitamin B6, megadose, 389–405
  adverse effects, 381, 383–384, 392, 393, 396,
    400–402
  Child Behavior Research Vitamin Study, 390–
    395
  criticisms of, 399–402
  drug interaction, 382
  efficacy, 390, 392–393, 394, 395–397, 398–
    399
  magnesium combined with, 389, 393, 396,
    397–403
Vitamin B12 deficiency, 381
Vitamin C, megadose, 390–394
  adverse effects, 380–381
  dependency, 379
  disease masking by, 381
  drug interaction, 382
  "rebound" scurvy and, 379
Vitamin D deficiency, 332
Vitamin H, megadose, 383
Vitamin–drug interaction, 381–383
von Recklinghausen disease, 93, 171

Williams syndrome, 171
Withdrawal
  from megavitamins, 379–380
  from neuroleptics, 376–377

X-linked genetic transmission, of autism, 86,
    90, 96, 97
  dominant, 197
  fragile X chromosome disorder, see Fragile X
    chromosome disorder
  recessive, 196–198
  sex ratio, 196–198
XYY syndrome, 171